I0044650

A Practical Approach to Intensive Care

Editor: Damien Newman

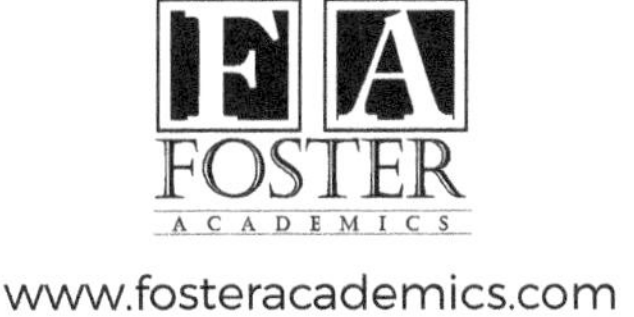

www.fosteracademics.com

www.fosteracademics.com

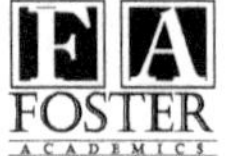

Cataloging-in-Publication Data

A practical approach to intensive care / edited by Damien Newman.
p. cm.
Includes bibliographical references and index.
ISBN 978-1-63242-635-2
1. Critical care medicine. 2. Emergency medicine. 3. Intensive care units.
I. Newman, Damien.
RC86.7 .P73 2019
616.025--dc23

Foster Academics,
118-35 Queens Blvd., Suite 400,
Forest Hills, NY 11375, USA

ISBN 978-1-63242-635-2 (Hardback)

Contents

Preface.......IX

Chapter 1 **Overview of point-of-care abdominal ultrasound in emergency and critical care**.......1
Toru Kameda and Nobuyuki Taniguchi

Chapter 2 **Diaphragm thickening fraction to predict weaning—a prospective exploratory study**.......10
Sujay Samanta, Ratender Kumar Singh, Arvind K. Baronia, Banani Poddar, Afzal Azim and Mohan Gurjar

Chapter 3 **Acute traumatic coagulopathy and traumainduced coagulopathy**.......19
Shigeki Kushimoto, Daisuke Kudo and Yu Kawazoe

Chapter 4 **The impact of changes in intensive care organization on patient outcome and costeffectiveness**.......26
Alexander F. van der Sluijs, Eline R. van Slobbe-Bijlsma, Stephen E. Chick, Margreeth B. Vroom, Dave A. Dongelmans and Alexander P. J. Vlaar

Chapter 5 **Usefulness of plasminogen activator inhibitor-1 as a predictive marker of mortality in sepsis**.......34
Kota Hoshino, Taisuke Kitamura, Yoshihiko Nakamura, Yuhei Irie, Norihiko Matsumoto, Yasumasa Kawano and Hiroyasu Ishikura

Chapter 6 **Early mobilization of mechanically ventilated patients in the intensive care unit**.......42
Shunsuke Taito, Nobuaki Shime, Kohei Ota and Hideto Yasuda

Chapter 7 **Early versus late tracheostomy after decompressive craniectomy for stroke**.......49
Michael P. Catalino, Feng-Chang Lin, Nathan Davis, Keith Anderson, Casey Olm-Shipman and J. Dedrick Jordan

Chapter 8 **C-terminal proendothelin-1 (CT-proET-1) is associated with organ failure and predicts mortality in critically ill patients**.......58
Lukas Buendgens, Eray Yagmur, Jan Bruensing, Ulf Herbers, Christer Baeck, Christian Trautwein, Alexander Koch and Frank Tacke

Chapter 9 **Evolved role of the cardiovascular intensive care unit (CICU)**.......67
Shunji Kasaoka

Chapter 10 **Damage control resuscitation: a practical approach for severely hemorrhagic patients and its effects on trauma surgery**.......72
Yasumitsu Mizobata

Chapter 11 **Make it SIMPLE: enhanced shock management by focused cardiac ultrasound**.......81
Ka Leung Mok

Chapter 12 **Predicting contrast-induced nephropathy after CT pulmonary angiography in the critically ill** 98
Kwok M. Ho and Yusrah Harahsheh

Chapter 13 **Monitoring the coagulation status of trauma patients with viscoelastic devices** 106
Yuichiro Sakamoto, Hiroyuki Koami and Toru Miike

Chapter 14 **Lung ultrasound—a primary survey of the acutely dyspneic patient** 117
Francis Chun Yue Lee

Chapter 15 **Procalcitonin: a promising diagnostic marker for sepsis and antibiotic therapy** 130
Ashitha L. Vijayan, Vanimaya, Shilpa Ravindran, R. Saikant, S. Lakshmi, R. Kartik and Manoj. G

Chapter 16 **Fluid responsiveness prediction using Vigileo FloTrac measured cardiac output changes during passive leg raise test** 137
Anton Krige, Martin Bland and Thomas Fanshawe

Chapter 17 **Achieving the earliest possible reperfusion in patients with acute coronary syndrome** 146
Takahiro Nakashima and Yoshio Tahara

Chapter 18 **Evaluating the discriminating capacity of cell death (apoptotic) biomarkers in sepsis** 156
Christopher Duplessis, Michael Gregory, Kenneth Frey, Matthew Bell, Luu Truong, Kevin Schully, James Lawler, Raymond J. Langley, Stephen F. Kingsmore, Christopher W. Woods, Emanuel P. Rivers, Anja K. Jaehne, Eugenia B. Quackenbush, Vance G. Fowler, Ephraim L. Tsalik and Danielle Clark

Chapter 19 **Daily use of extracorporeal CO_2 removal in a critical care unit: indications and results** 167
Hadrien Winiszewski, François Aptel, François Belon, Nicolas Belin, Claire Chaignat, Cyrille Patry, Cecilia Clermont, Elise David, Jean-Christophe Navellou, Guylaine Labro, Gaël Piton and Gilles Capellier

Chapter 20 **Treatment of patients with sepsis in a closed intensive care unit is associated with improved survival** 175
Takayuki Ogura, Yoshihiko Nakamura, Kunihiko Takahashi, Kazuki Nishida, Daisuke Kobashi and Shigeyuki Matsui

Chapter 21 **Cefepime dosing regimens in critically ill patients receiving continuous renal replacement therapy: a Monte Carlo simulation study** 185
Weerachai Chaijamorn, Taniya Charoensareerat, Nattachai Srisawat, Sutthiporn Pattharachayakul and Apinya Boonpeng

Chapter 22 **Accuracy of the first interpretation of early brain CT images for predicting the prognosis of post-cardiac arrest syndrome patients at the emergency department** 196
Mitsuaki Nishikimi, Takayuki Ogura, Kota Matsui, Kunihiko Takahashi, Kenji Fukaya, Keibun Liu, Hideo Morita, Mitsunobu Nakamura, Shigeyuki Matsui and Naoyuki Matsuda

Chapter 23 **Epidemiology, clinical characteristics, resistance and treatment of infections by *Candida auris*** 202
Andrea Cortegiani, Giovanni Misseri, Teresa Fasciana, Anna Giammanco, Antonino Giarratano and Anuradha Chowdhary

Chapter 24 **Transient hyperlactatemia during intravenous administration of glycerol** 215
Shinshu Katayama, Ken Tonai, Yuya Goto, Kansuke Koyama, Toshitaka Koinuma, Jun Shima, Masahiko Wada and Shin Nunomiya

Chapter 25 **High red blood cell distribution width as a marker of hospital mortality after ICU discharge** 222
Rafael Fernandez, Silvia Cano, Ignacio Catalan, Olga Rubio, Carles Subira, Jaume Masclans, Gina Rognoni, Lara Ventura, Caroline Macharete, Len Winfield and Josep M[a]. Alcoverro

Chapter 26 **Studying the effect of abdominal massage on the gastric residual volume in patients hospitalized in intensive care units** 228
Farzad Momenfar, Alireza Abdi, Nader Salari, Ali Soroush and Behzad Hemmatpour

Permissions

List of Contributors

Index

Preface

Care meant for patients suffering from severe and life-threatening illnesses is known as intensive care. The departments in hospitals specifically designed for the care and treatment of patients requiring intensive care are known as intensive care units (ICUs). Intensive care units are usually equipped with advanced medical resources and equipments. The common equipments in an intensive care unit include mechanical ventilators, cardiac monitors, feeding tubes, intravenous lines, nasogastric tubes, catheters, drains and suction pumps. Intensive care is generally offered only in the cases where there is a strong possibility of survival and improvement under the support of intensive care. This book brings forth some of the most innovative concepts and elucidates the unexplored aspects of intensive care. The topics included herein on intensive care are of utmost significance and bound to provide incredible insights to readers. This book will prove to be immensely beneficial to students, doctors and researchers in this field.

The researches compiled throughout the book are authentic and of high quality, combining several disciplines and from very diverse regions from around the world. Drawing on the contributions of many researchers from diverse countries, the book's objective is to provide the readers with the latest achievements in the area of research. This book will surely be a source of knowledge to all interested and researching the field.

In the end, I would like to express my deep sense of gratitude to all the authors for meeting the set deadlines in completing and submitting their research chapters. I would also like to thank the publisher for the support offered to us throughout the course of the book. Finally, I extend my sincere thanks to my family for being a constant source of inspiration and encouragement.

Editor

1

Overview of point-of-care abdominal ultrasound in emergency and critical care

Toru Kameda[1*] and Nobuyuki Taniguchi[2]

Abstract

Point-of-care abdominal ultrasound (US), which is performed by clinicians at bedside, is increasingly being used to evaluate clinical manifestations, to facilitate accurate diagnoses, and to assist procedures in emergency and critical care. Methods for the assessment of acute abdominal pain with point-of-care US must be developed according to accumulated evidence in each abdominal region. To detect hemoperitoneum, the methodology of a focused assessment with sonography for a trauma examination may also be an option in non-trauma patients. For the assessment of systemic hypoperfusion and renal dysfunction, point-of-care renal Doppler US may be an option. Utilization of point-of-care US is also considered in order to detect abdominal and pelvic lesions. It is particularly useful for the detection of gallstones and the diagnosis of acute cholecystitis. Point-of-case US is justified as the initial imaging modality for the diagnosis of ureterolithiasis and the assessment of pyelonephritis. It can be used with great accuracy to detect the presence of abdominal aortic aneurysm in symptomatic patients. It may also be useful for the diagnoses of digestive tract diseases such as appendicitis, small bowel obstruction, and gastrointestinal perforation. Additionally, point-of-care US can be a modality for assisting procedures. Paracentesis under US guidance has been shown to improve patient care. US appears to be a potential modality to verify the placement of the gastric tube. The estimation of the amount of urine with bladder US can lead to an increased success rate in small children. US-guided catheterization with transrectal pressure appears to be useful in some male patients in whom standard urethral catheterization is difficult. Although a greater accumulation of evidences is needed in some fields, point-of-care abdominal US is a promising modality to improve patient care in emergency and critical care settings.

Keywords: Point-of-care ultrasound, Abdominal ultrasound, Emergency, Critical care, Review

Background

Due to the portability and accessibility of ultrasound (US), point-of-care US, which is performed by clinicians at the bedside, is increasingly being used to facilitate accurate diagnoses, to monitor the fluid status, and to guide procedures in emergency and critical care [1]. The main applications in abdominal regions include trauma, biliary, urinary tract, intrauterine pregnancy, and abdominal aortic aneurysm (AAA), which can be evaluated by a transabdominal approach [2, 3]. Additionally, new applications with point-of-care abdominal US have also been assessed and recently proposed. This article provides an up-to-date overview of point-of-care abdominal US performed by clinicians in emergency and critical care settings.

* Correspondence: kamekame@pb3.so-net.ne.jp
[1]Department of Emergency Medicine, Red Cross Society Azumino Hospital, 5685 Toyoshina, Azumino, Nagano 399-8292, Japan
Full list of author information is available at the end of the article

Review

Clinical manifestations and point-of-care US

Acute abdominal pain

As a single imaging strategy, computed tomography (CT) is overall superior to US in patients with acute abdominal pain [4]. Laméris et al. reported that conditional strategy with CT after negative or inconclusive radiology US resulted in the highest overall sensitivity, with only 6 % missed urgent conditions, and the lowest overall exposure to radiation by performing CT in only half of adult patients with acute abdominal pain [4]. In this regard, imaging strategies including point-of-care abdominal US must also be evaluated.

A pilot observational study showed that emergency physician (EP)-performed US appears to positively impact decision-making and the diagnostic workup of patients with nonspecific abdominal pain as determined by the nursing triage. In 128 patients, 58 (45 %; 95 % confidence interval (CI), 36–54 %) had an improvement in diagnostic accuracy and planned diagnostic workup using US [5]. In a randomized study including 800 adult patients with acute abdominal pain, Lindelius et al. reported the utility of US performed by surgeons who underwent a 4-week US training program. The proportion of correct primary diagnoses was 7.9 % higher in the group undergoing surgeon-performed US than in the control group (64.7 vs 56.8 %; $p = 0.027$) [6]. The number of US performed in the radiology department was significantly lower in the group receiving surgeon-performed US, while there was no difference between the groups regarding the number of ordered CT scans or other examinations [7].

Evidence on detection of each lesion causing acute abdominal pain with point-of-care abdominal US is reviewed in the "Detection of abdominal and pelvic lesions" section. Methods for the assessment of acute abdominal pain with point-of-care US must be developed according to the accumulated evidence in each abdominal region.

Hemoperitoneum

Abdominal US in trauma patients is typically performed with the methodology of a focused assessment with sonography for trauma (FAST) examination. FAST provides a quick overview of the peritoneal cavity to detect free fluid, which is a direct sign of hemoperitoneum and an indirect sign of organ injuries. The sensitivity and specificity of FAST for the detection of free intraperitoneal fluid were 64–98 and 86–100 %, respectively. These ranging results may be explained by differences in the levels of clinical experience and in the reference standards [8]. The sensitivity may be higher, and time needed to perform may be shorter in patients with hemodynamic collapse. Wherrett et al. demonstrated that an abdominal assessment with FAST required 19 ± 5 s in the positive group and 154 ± 13 s in the negative group ($p < 0.001$) with high accuracy in 69 hypotensive blunt trauma patients [9].

It is also reasonable to consider the usage of a complete or partial FAST examination in evaluating spontaneous hemoperitoneum in non-trauma patients. The etiology of spontaneous hemoperitoneum can vary, and the causes may be classified as gynecologic, hepatic, splenic, vascular, or coagulopathic conditions [10]. Spontaneous hemoperitoneum frequently presents with acute abdominal pain with or without hemodynamic collapse. In some patients, the collapse becomes obvious after the initial evaluation; therefore, spontaneous hemoperitoneum should be detected rapidly during the evaluation. Case reports comment on the use of bedside US to detect intra-abdominal free fluid to aid in the diagnosis of the causes; however, few original studies have explored its use [11].

Hemoperitoneum caused by gynecologic conditions, such as rupture of the gestational sac in ectopic pregnancy and hemorrhage or rupture of an ovarian cyst, is common in women of childbearing age, in whom US is selected as the primary imaging modality [10]. In a retrospective study, Rodgerson et al. demonstrated that identifying patients with a suspected ectopic pregnancy and fluid in Morison's pouch by EP-performed abdominal US decreased the time to diagnosis and treatment [12]. In a prospective observational study, Moore et al. reported that ten of 242 patients with suspected ectopic pregnancy were found to have fluid in Morison's pouch with EP-performed abdominal US, and nine of the ten patients underwent immediate operative intervention for ruptured ectopic pregnancy. They concluded that free intraperitoneal fluid in Morison's pouch in patients with suspected ectopic pregnancy may be rapidly identified by US and predicts the need for intervention [13].

However, US is not sensitive at identifying a focus of extravasation from a vessel or organ [8]. Therefore, FAST may be an option for the initial evaluation to detect hemoperitoneum in non-trauma patients (Fig. 1).

Hypoperfusion and renal dysfunction

Doppler US is indicated as a tool to assess renal perfusion. The Doppler-based resistive index (RI) is calculated using the following formula: (peak systolic velocity − end-diastolic velocity)/peak systolic velocity in an interlobar or arcuate artery, with a normal value of 0.58 ± 0.10. It is broadly accepted that values >0.70 are considered to be abnormal [14]. Corradi et al. reported that in normotensive polytrauma patients without biochemical signs of hypoperfusion, a renal Doppler RI greater than 0.7 at admittance into the emergency department was predictive of hemorrhagic shock within the first 24 h (odds ratio, 57.8; 95 % CI, 10.5–317.0; $p < 0.001$). However, the inferior vena cava (IVC) diameter and caval index were not predictive in these patients. They hypothesized that most of the patients were normovolemic at arrival [15]. Although larger comparative studies are needed, a high renal Doppler RI may be more predictive of hemorrhagic shock than the IVC diameter and caval index [15].

A renal Doppler RI may also help in detecting early renal dysfunction or predicting short-term reversibility of acute kidney injury (AKI) in critically ill patients [16–18]. A preliminary study showed that a semi-quantitative assessment of renal perfusion using color Doppler was

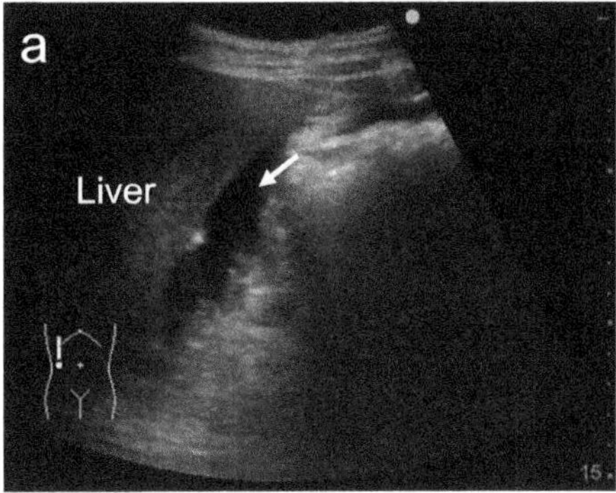

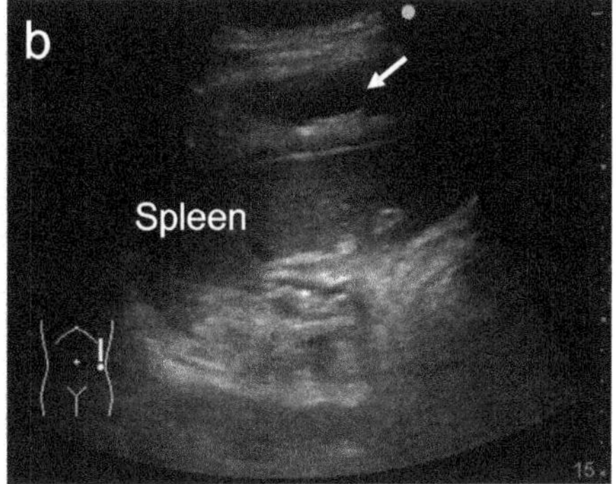

Fig. 1 Ultrasound images in a 47-year-old man who presented with left upper continuous abdominal pain. The patient began to feel pain after heavy physical labor without awareness of a traumatic event. Bedside ultrasound after history taking and a physical examination revealed free fluid in Morison's pouch (**a**, *arrow*), perisplenic space (**b**, *arrow*), and rectovesical pouch. Contrast-enhanced computed tomography showed hemoperitoneum and splenomegaly with a low-density, striped area in the lower pole. He was diagnosed as having splenic rupture and treated conservatively

easier to perform than the RI and may provide similar information [16]. That study also found that both the semi-quantitative assessment using color Doppler and the RI could be performed with good feasibility and reliability by inexperienced operators, such as intensive care residents following a half-day training session [16]. Doppler US may be useful in assessing renal perfusion; however, larger studies with standardized methods are needed to confirm these results and reveal its roles in the management of patients with AKI [19].

Detection of abdominal and pelvic lesions

Gallstone and acute cholecystitis

It is well known that radiology US is very useful for the detection of gallstones and the diagnosis of acute cholecystitis [20]. A systematic review and meta-analysis was conducted to compare surgeon-performed US for suspected gallstone disease to radiology US or a pathological examination as the gold standard investigation. The search criteria resulted in eight studies with 1019 patients. The pooled sensitivity was 96 % (95 % CI, 93.4–97.9 %), and the specificity was 99 % (95 % CI, 98.3–99.8 %) [21]. On the other hand, EP interpretation for the identification of gallstones is reported to have a sensitivity of 86–96 % and specificity of 78–98 % [22].

Gallstones are found in approximately 95 % of patients with acute cholecystitis; however, the detection of gallstones is not specific for the diagnosis of acute cholecystitis. When performing US, secondary findings such as gallbladder wall thickening, pericholecystic fluid, and sonographic Murphy sign provide more specific information [20]. Summers et al. reported in a prospective observational study with 164 enrolled patients that the test characteristics of EP-performed US for the detection of acute cholecystitis had a sensitivity of 87 % (95 % CI, 66–97 %), specificity of 82 % (95 % CI, 74–88 %), positive predictive value of 44 % (95 % CI, 29–59 %), and negative predictive value of 97 % (95 % CI, 93–99 %). Additionally, the test characteristics of EP-performed US were similar to those of radiology US. According to the high negative predictive value, the study indicated that patients with a negative result are unlikely to require cholecystectomy or admission within 2 weeks of their initial presentation [23].

Appendicitis

CT was found to have a superior test performance to US in the diagnosis of acute appendicitis; however, US is recommended as the first-line imaging modality in young, female, and slender patients in view of the radiation exposure [24]. Recent studies from the field of emergency medicine addressed the diagnostic performance of point-of-care US performed by EPs or pediatric EPs in the evaluation of suspected appendicitis [25–30] (Table 1). In these studies, no visualization of the appendix with US was coded as a negative result, and the final diagnosis of appendicitis was made with operative or pathology findings. Chen et al. demonstrated a high sensitivity in their study, where more extensive US training was provided and the prevalence of appendicitis was higher [25]. Several studies demonstrated the feasibility of reducing the length of stay in the emergency department [28] and avoiding CT according to the result of a high positive predictive value in some patients [30] when using point-of-care US as the first-line imaging modality. To date, the diagnosis of appendicitis with point-of-care US by clinicians has not been fully accepted. A large prospective study is necessary to investigate methods to increase the accuracy of point-of-care US through more effective educational techniques and safety of the addition to sequential radiology imaging [28, 30].

Table 1 Diagnostic performance of ultrasound performed by emergency physicians in the evaluation of suspected acute appendicitis

Author	Sample size	Prevalence (%)	Sensitivity (%)	Specificity (%)	PPV (%)	NPV (%)
Chen et al. [25]	147	75	96	68	90	86
Fox et al. [26]	155	45	39	90	75	65
Fox et al. [27]	126	45	65	90	84	76
Elikashvili et al. [28]	150	33	60	94	86	82
Sivitz et al. [29]	264	32	85	93	85	93
Mallin et al. [30]	97	35	68	98	96	85

Four studies [25, 27–30] were performed prospectively. The final diagnosis of appendicitis was made according to operative or pathology findings
PPV positive predictive value, *NPV* negative predictive value

Small bowel obstruction

The utility of surgeon-performed US for the diagnosis of bowel obstruction and early recognition of strangulation was evaluated in the 1990s [31]. In recent years, some studies showed the accuracy of EP-performed US for the diagnosis of small bowel obstruction. Unlüer et al. demonstrated in a prospective study with 168 patients that the sensitivity and specificity were 97.7 % (95 % CI, 94.5–100 %) and 92.7 % (95 % CI, 87.0–98.3 %), respectively. Additionally, the diagnostic accuracy of EP-performed and radiology-performed US were not statistically different from one another [32]. Jang et al. demonstrated in a prospective study with 76 patients that the sensitivity and specificity were 90.9 % (95 % CI, 74.5–97.6 %) and 83.7 % (95 % CI, 68.7–92.7 %), respectively [33]. These studies also showed that EP-performed US had a superior test performance compared with an X-ray in the diagnosis of small bowel obstruction [32, 33]. However, large prospective studies are needed to alter the management of small bowel obstruction with its use.

Gastrointestinal perforation

The diagnosis of gastrointestinal perforation is based on the evidence of pneumoperitoneum, which is usually detected with an X-ray or CT. A US sign of pneumoperitoneum (Fig. 2) has also been recognized following a comprehensive study on visualizing pneumoperitoneum with US reported from Germany over 30 years ago [34]. In the 21st century, the utility of clinician-performed US for the detection of pneumoperitoneum was reported from Asian countries. Prospective studies have demonstrated the sensitivity and specificity to be 85–93 % and 53–100 %, respectively [35–37]. Moreover, Chan et al. also reported that US was more sensitive than an X-ray for the detection [36]. However, large prospective trials are needed to validate the accuracy of this modality and whether the concept can be generalized among clinician sonographers.

Ureterolithiasis and pyelonephritis

Pain due to ureterolithiasis is a common problem in the emergency room. CT has become the most common initial imaging modality for suspected ureterolithiasis because of its high accuracy [38]. However, CT exposes patients to ionizing radiation, which is especially concerning for patients with ureterolithiasis as they are prone to recurrence and repeated imaging. Moreover, no evidence has shown that increased CT use is associated with an improved patient outcome [38]. The diagnostic performance of bedside US performed by EPs or medical staff members in the diagnosis of ureterolithiasis has been prospectively studied, as shown in Table 2 [39–42]. These studies, which used CT as the reference standard, showed that the diagnostic performance using US finding of hydronephrosis was generally modest. In one of the articles, Herbst et al. also demonstrated that attending physicians with fellowship training had significantly

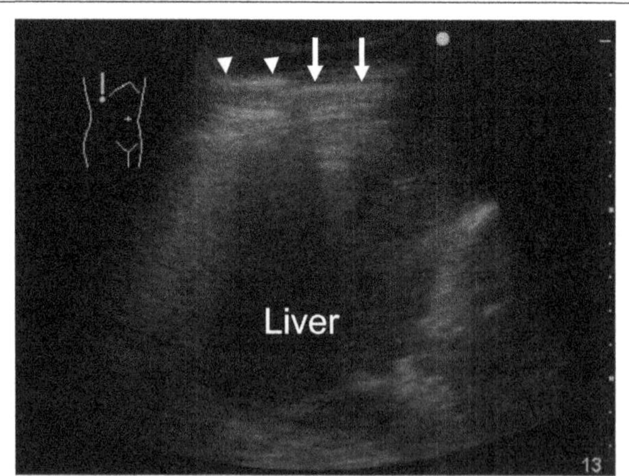

Fig. 2 An ultrasound image in a 43-year-old man who presented with sudden onset of abdominal pain. The patient had a history of a duodenal ulcer and was aware of black stool prior to the presentation. On physical examination, he had diffuse abdominal tenderness with guarding. Bedside ultrasound was performed with the patient in the left lateral decubitus position. Reverberation artifacts on the ventral surface of the liver (*arrows*) indicated intraperitoneal free air. The artifacts were distinguished from other artifacts with respiratory movement (*arrowheads*), which originated at the lung surface

Table 2 Diagnostic performance of ultrasound performed by emergency clinicians in the evaluation of suspected ureterolithiasis

Author	Sample size	Prevalence (%)	Sensitivity (%)	Specificity (%)	PPV (%)	NPV (%)
Gaspari et al. [39]	104	51	87	82	84	86
Watkins et al. [40]	57	68	80	83	91	65
Moak et al. [41]	107	36	76	78	66	86
Herbst et al. [42]	670	47	73	73	71	75

PPV positive predictive value, *NPV* negative predictive value

better sensitivity than all other users (93 vs 68 %) [42]. A large, multicenter, randomized trial conducted in the USA showed that initial US performed by EPs was associated with lower cumulative radiation exposure than initial CT, without significant differences in high-risk diagnoses with complications, serious adverse events, pain scores, return emergency department visits, or hospitalizations [38]. Although US was less sensitive than CT for the diagnosis of ureterolithiasis, bedside US in emergency departments is justified as the initial imaging modality. Moreover, whether the detection of the stone itself in addition to hydronephrosis with point-of-care US actually improves the accuracy of the diagnosis requires further investigation [43].

Acute pyelonephritis is also a common disease encountered in emergency departments. For complicated acute pyelonephritis, such as obstructive uropathy due to ureterolithiasis, delayed management can lead to high morbidity and mortality. Chen et al. showed that EP-performed US was able to detect significant abnormalities such as hydronephrosis, polycystic kidney disease, renal abscess, and emphysematous pyelonephritis in 40 % of patients finally diagnosed with acute pyelonephritis. The early utilization of US in emergency departments may impact on the management of these patients or initial assessment of septic patients [44] (Fig. 3).

Adnexa and uterus

It has been generally accepted that transvaginal US is superior to transabdominal US for evaluating adnexa and uterus, and transvaginal US is generally selected as the initial technique among gynecological imaging modalities [45]. In some institutions and countries, EPs perform transvaginal US in daily practice; however, EP-performed transvaginal US is not common globally. They may have the opportunity to perform transabdominal US in women who may have genital problems [45].

A systematic review and meta-analysis showed that the use of bedside transabdominal US and/or transvaginal US performed by EPs consistently exhibits excellent test characteristics for ruling out ectopic pregnancy. In this investigation, the positive and negative results were defined as the absence of a definite intrauterine pregnancy and a visible intrauterine pregnancy, respectively. Ten studies were included with a total of 2057 patients, of whom 152 (7.5 %) had an ectopic pregnancy. The pooled sensitivity and negative predictive value were reported to be 99.3 % (95 % CI, 96.6 to 100 %) and 99.96 % (95 % CI, 99.6 to 100 %), respectively [46].

As mentioned previously, point-of-care transabdominal US is useful to detect hemoperitoneum due to gynecologic diseases. Moreover, it is reasonable to investigate its efficacy to detect genital lesions themselves, because the use of point-of-care transabdominal US as an

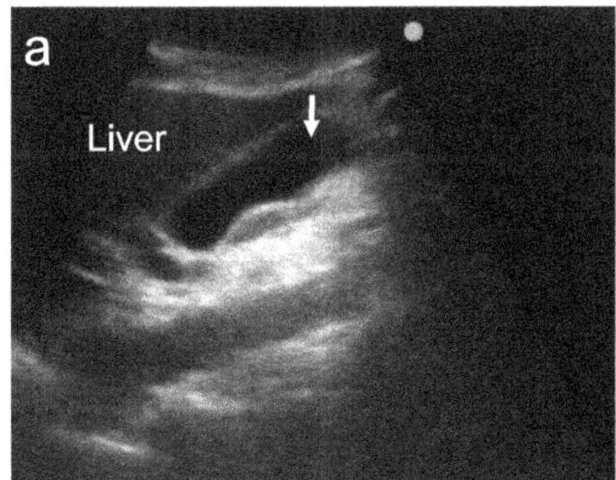

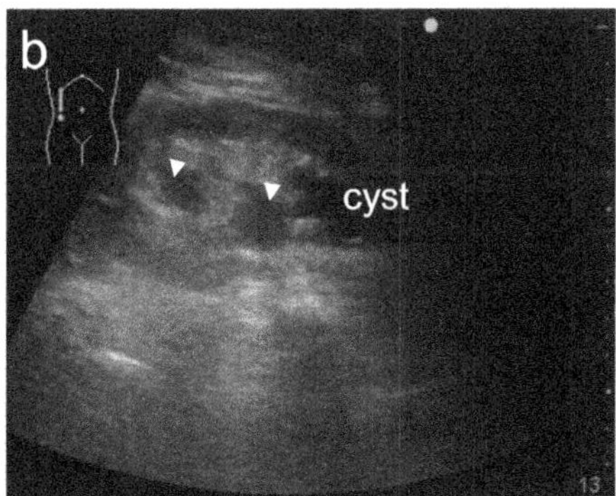

Fig. 3 Ultrasound images in an 88-year-old man who presented with shaking chills. The patient had a history of acute cholecystitis with percutaneous transhepatic gallbladder drainage. On physical examination, he had no abdominal or costovertebral angel tenderness. Bedside ultrasound showed a normal gallbladder (**a**, *arrow*) and pelvic dilatation in the right kidney (**b**, *arrowheads*). A subsequent computed tomography scan revealed the stone at the right ureterovesical junction. A complicated urinary tract infection was strongly suspected, and emergent urological consultation was ordered. He fell into shock soon after the initial evaluation

extension of the physical examination is rapidly growing with widespread application [45].

AAA

The use of US performed by EPs to diagnose AAA has been well studied prospectively since the 2000s. A systematic review and meta-analysis published in 2013 showed that the search criteria resulted in seven studies with 655 patients, and the pooled operating characteristics of EP-performed US for the detection of AAA had a sensitivity of 99 % (95 % CI, 96–100 %) and specificity of 98 % (95 % CI, 97–99 %) [47]. Bedside US can be used with great accuracy to detect AAA in symptomatic patients; therefore, it is justified as the initial imaging modality to rapidly detect AAA in emergency departments.

Usages assisting procedures

Paracentesis

US guidance enables visualization of the needle insertion site to perform paracentesis safely. An observational cohort study using a nationally representative database was conducted to examine the effect of US guidance on the risk of bleeding complications after paracentesis. Of 69,859 patients undergoing paracentesis, 0.8 % ($n = 565$) experienced bleeding complications. After adjusting for the inpatient or outpatient procedures, the duration of hospitalization before the paracentesis, and the admission diagnoses, US guidance reduced the risk of bleeding complications by 68 % (odds ratio, 0.32; 95 % CI, 0.25–0.41). The data indicated that US guidance is associated with a decreased risk of complications after paracentesis [48]. A randomized study with 100 enrolled patients demonstrated that the success rate of US-assisted paracentesis performed by EPs with varying levels of experience and the traditional technique were 95 and 65 %, respectively ($p = 0.0003$) [49]. Case series indicated that emergent US-guided paracentesis may lead to a significant management change in selected unstable patients with a positive FAST examination [50]. As mentioned above, paracentesis under US guidance is shown to improve patient care. Furthermore, localization of the inferior epigastric artery before paracentesis may provide a more reliable means to avoid complications [51].

Conformation of gastric tube placement

Gastric tube insertion is commonly performed in emergency and critical care settings. Immediately after the procedure, the placement of the tube is typically evaluated using a visual inspection of aspirate contents and auscultation with instillation of air in the tube. Additionally, a chest X-ray is recommended in most cases to confirm correct placement. However, a chest X-ray has issues, including radiation exposure, delayed confirmation, and cost. Several recent studies showed that US is a potential modality to verify the placement of the gastric tube. The methods include confirmation of the tube in the stomach [52], the stomach or duodenum with or without instillation of normal saline mixed with air [53], and the cervical esophagus and stomach with or without instillation of air [54] or normal saline with air [55]. The visualization can be affected by the size of the tube [52] and volume of gas in the gastrointestinal tract [55]. If the presence of the tip of the tube in the stomach is verified with direct visualization or an indirect finding of dynamic fogging made by the instillation, US in addition to physical examinations appears to be a substitute imaging modality for a chest X-ray in some patients.

Urethral catheterization

Urethral catheterization is frequently performed for a urinalysis and culture, management of acute urinary retention, and monitoring of the urine output in emergency and critical care settings.

If there is little certainty of the presence or amount of urine in the bladder before urethral catheterization, then this procedure to obtain urine for an analysis and culture often needs to be repeated. The estimation of the amount of urine using bedside bladder US has been reported to lead to an increased success rate during the first attempt in children younger than 2 years of age [56, 57].

In adult male patients, difficulty with standard catheterization is occasionally encountered. In such cases, repeated and unsuccessful blind attempts can cause patient distress and damage to the urethra, usually requiring a urological consultation. Kameda et al. mentioned in their pilot study that transabdominal US performed by emergency medical personnel can reveal the tip of the catheter in a part of the posterior and bulbar urethra, and US-guided catheterization with transrectal pressure appears to be safe and useful in some male patients in whom standard urethral catheterization is difficult [58] (Fig. 4).

Conclusions

Methods for the assessment of acute abdominal pain with point-of-care abdominal US must be developed according to the accumulated evidence in each abdominal region. To detect hemoperitoneum, a FAST examination may be a helpful option in non-trauma patients. For the assessment of systemic hypoperfusion and renal dysfunction, point-of-care renal Doppler US may be an option. The utilization of point-of-care US is also considered in order to detect abdominal and pelvic lesions. It is useful for the detection of gallstones and the diagnosis of acute cholecystitis. It is justified as the initial imaging modality for the diagnosis of ureterolithiasis and the assessment of pyelonephritis. It can be used with great accuracy to

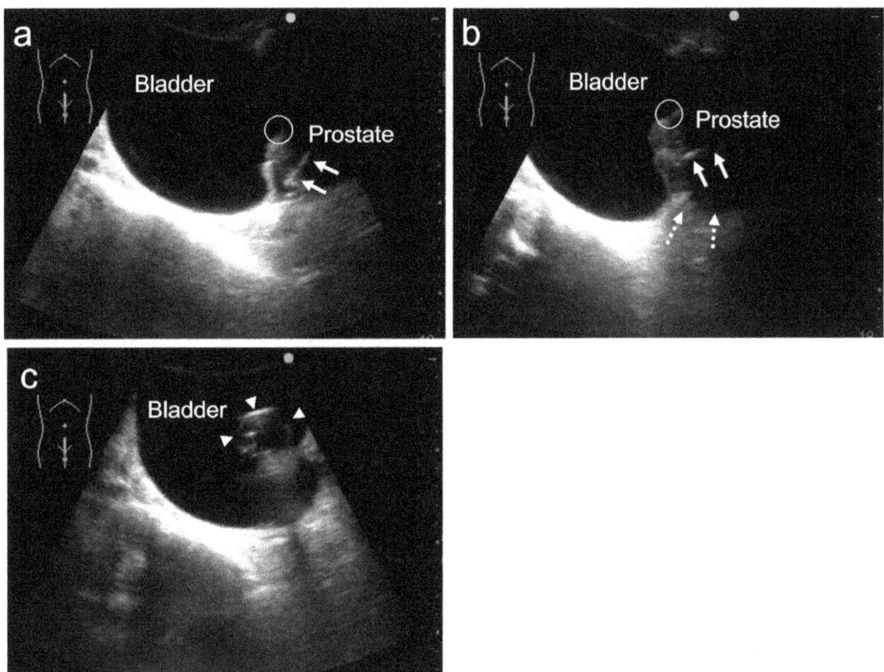

Fig. 4 Ultrasound images in a 78-year-old man who presented with difficult urination. The patient had a history of benign prostatic hypertrophy. Standard urethral catheterization attempted by an experienced emergency nurse and an experienced emergency physician failed due to complicated urethral bleeding. **a** Bedside ultrasound revealed the tip of the catheter in a part of the posterior and bulbar urethra (*arrows*) while the progress was obstructed. Judging from the location of the internal urethral orifice, a part of the urethra was thus determined to be bent. The *circle* denotes the location of the internal urethral orifice. **b** The bent part of the urethra had become blunt with transrectal pressure using an inserted index finger (*broken arrows*). The *arrows* denote the tip of the catheter, and the *circle* denotes the location of the internal urethral orifice. **c** Ultrasound-guided catheterization with transrectal pressure without forceful manipulation was successful on the first attempt. *Arrowheads* denote the inflated balloon

detect the presence of AAA in symptomatic patients. It may also be useful for the diagnoses of digestive tract diseases. Additionally, point-of-care US can be a modality for assisting procedures. Paracentesis under US guidance is shown to improve patient care. US appears to be a potential modality to verify the placement of a gastric tube. Moreover, the estimation of the amount of urine with bladder US can lead to an increased success rate in small children. US-guided catheterization with transrectal pressure appears to be useful in some male patients in whom standard urethral catheterization is difficult. Although a greater accumulation of evidence is needed in some fields, point-of-care abdominal US is a promising modality to improve patient care in emergency and critical care settings.

Abbreviations
AAA, abdominal aortic aneurysm; AKI, acute kidney injury; CI, confidence interval; CT, computed tomography; EP, emergency physician; FAST, focused assessment with sonography for trauma; IVC, inferior vena cava; RI, resistive index; US, ultrasound

Funding
No funding.

Authors' contributions
TK wrote the manuscript and revised the manuscript. NT revised the manuscript. All authors read and approved the final manuscript.

Competing interests
The authors declare that they have no competing interests.

Author details
[1]Department of Emergency Medicine, Red Cross Society Azumino Hospital, 5685 Toyoshina, Azumino, Nagano 399-8292, Japan. [2]Department of Clinical Laboratory Medicine, Jichi Medical University, 3311-1, Yakushiji, Shimotsuke, Tochigi 329-0498, Japan.

References
1. Moore CL, Copel JA. Point-of-care ultrasonography. N Engl J Med. 2011;364:749–57.
2. American College of Emergency Physicians. Emergency ultrasound guidelines. Ann Emerg Med. 2009;53:550–70.
3. Boniface KS, Calabrese KY. Intensive care ultrasound: IV. Abdominal ultrasound in critical care. Ann Am Thorac Soc. 2013;10:713–24.

4. Laméris W, van Randen A, van Es HW, van Heesewijk JP, van Ramshorst B, Bouma WH, et al. Imaging strategies for detection of urgent conditions in patients with acute abdominal pain: diagnostic accuracy study. BMJ. 2009; 338:b2431.
5. Jang T, Chauhan V, Cundiff C, Kaji AH. Assessment of emergency physician-performed ultrasound in evaluating nonspecific abdominal pain. Am J Emerg Med. 2014;32:457–60.
6. Lindelius A, Törngren S, Sondén A, Pettersson H, Adami J. Impact of surgeon-performed ultrasound on diagnosis of abdominal pain. Emerg Med J. 2008;25:486–91.
7. Lindelius A, Törngren S, Pettersson H, Adami J. Role of surgeon-performed ultrasound on further management of patients with acute abdominal pain: a randomised controlled clinical trial. Emerg Med J. 2009;26:561–6.
8. Körner M, Krötz MM, Degenhart C, Pfeifer KJ, Reiser MF, Linsenmaier U. Current role of emergency US in patients with major trauma. Radiographics. 2008;28:225–42.
9. Wherrett LJ, Boulanger BR, McLellan BA, Brenneman FD, Rizoli SB, Culhane J, et al. Hypotension after blunt abdominal trauma: the role of emergent abdominal sonography in surgical triage. J Trauma. 1996;41:815–20.
10. Lucey BC, Varghese JC, Anderson SW, Soto JA. Spontaneous hemoperitoneum: a bloody mess. Emerg Radiol. 2007;14:65–75.
11. Jackson HT, Diaconu SC, Maluso PJ, Abell B, Lee J. Ruptured splenic artery aneurysms and the use of an adapted fast protocol in reproductive age women with hemodynamic collapse: case series. Case Rep Emerg Med. 2014. doi:10.1155/2014/454923.
12. Rodgerson JD, Heegaard WG, Plummer D, Hicks J, Clinton J, Sterner S. Emergency department right upper quadrant ultrasound is associated with a reduced time to diagnosis and treatment of ruptured ectopic pregnancies. Acad Emerg Med. 2001;8:331–6.
13. Moore C, Todd WM, O'Brien E, Lin H. Free fluid in Morison's pouch on bedside ultrasound predicts need for operative intervention in suspected ectopic pregnancy. Acad Emerg Med. 2007;14:755–8.
14. Barozzi L, Valentino M, Santoro A, Mancini E, Pavlica P. Renal ultrasonography in critically ill patients. Crit Care Med. 2007;35(Suppl):S198–205.
15. Corradi F, Brusasco C, Vezzani A, Palermo S, Altomonte F, Moscatelli P, et al. Hemorrhagic shock in polytrauma patients: early detection with renal Doppler resistive index measurements. Radiology. 2011;260:112–8.
16. Schnell D, Reynaud M, Venot M, Le Maho AL, Dinic M, Baulieu M, et al. Resistive index or color-Doppler semi-quantitative evaluation of renal perfusion by inexperienced physicians: results of a pilot study. Minerva Anestesiol. 2014;80:1273–81.
17. Lerolle N, Guérot E, Faisy C, Bornstain C, Diehl JL, Fagon JY. Renal failure in septic shock: predictive value of Doppler-based renal arterial resistive index. Intensive Care Med. 2006;32:1553–9.
18. Darmon M, Schortgen F, Vargas F, Liazydi A, Schlemmer B, Brun-Buisson C, et al. Diagnostic accuracy of Doppler renal resistive index for reversibility of acute kidney injury in critically ill patients. Intensive Care Med. 2011;37:68–76.
19. Schnell D, Darmon M. Bedside Doppler ultrasound for the assessment of renal perfusion in the ICU: advantages and limitations of the available techniques. Crit Ultrasound J. 2015;7:24. doi:10.1186/s13089-015-0024-6.
20. Bortoff GA, Chen MY, Ott DJ, Wolfman NT, Routh WD. Gallbladder stones: imaging and intervention. Radiographics. 2000;20:751–66.
21. Carroll PJ, Gibson D, El-Faedy O, Dunne C, Coffey C, Hannigan A, et al. Surgeon-performed ultrasound at the bedside for the detection of appendicitis and gallstones: systematic review and meta-analysis. Am J Surg. 2013;205:102–8.
22. Scruggs W, Fox JC, Potts B, Zlidenny A, McDonough J, Anderson CL, et al. Accuracy of ED bedside ultrasound for identification of gallstones: retrospective analysis of 575 studies. West J Emerg Med. 2008;9:1–5.
23. Summers SM, Scruggs W, Menchine MD, Lahham S, Anderson C, Amr O, et al. A prospective evaluation of emergency department bedside ultrasonography for the detection of acute cholecystitis. Ann Emerg Med. 2010;56:114–22.
24. van Randen A, Bipat S, Zwinderman AH, Ubbink DT, Stoker J, Boermeester MA. Acute appendicitis: meta-analysis of diagnostic performance of CT and graded compression US related to prevalence of disease. Radiology. 2008; 249:97–106.
25. Chen SC, Wang HP, Hsu HY, Huang PM, Lin FY. Accuracy of ED sonography in the diagnosis of acute appendicitis. Am J Emerg Med. 2000;18:449–52.
26. Fox JC, Hunt MJ, Zlidenny AM, Oshita MH, Barajas G, Langdorf MI. Retrospective analysis of emergency department ultrasound for acute appendicitis. Cal J Emerg Med. 2007;8:41–5.
27. Fox JC, Solley M, Anderson CL, Zlidenny A, Lahham S, Maasumi K. Prospective evaluation of emergency physician performed bedside ultrasound to detect acute appendicitis. Eur J Emerg Med. 2008;15:80–5.
28. Elikashvili I, Tay ET, Tsung JW. The effect of point-of-care ultrasonography on emergency department length of stay and computed tomography utilization in children with suspected appendicitis. Acad Emerg Med. 2014; 21:163–70.
29. Sivitz AB, Cohen SG, Tejani C. Evaluation of acute appendicitis by pediatric emergency physician sonography. Ann Emerg Med. 2014;64:358–64.
30. Mallin M, Craven P, Ockerse P, Steenblik J, Forbes B, Boehm K, et al. Diagnosis of appendicitis by bedside ultrasound in the ED. Am J Emerg Med. 2015;33:430–2.
31. Ogata M, Mateer JR, Condon RE. Prospective evaluation of abdominal sonography for the diagnosis of bowel obstruction. Ann Surg. 1996;223: 237–41.
32. Unlüer EE, Yavaşi O, Eroğlu O, Yilmaz C, Akarca FK. Ultrasonography by emergency medicine and radiology residents for the diagnosis of small bowel obstruction. Eur J Emerg Med. 2010;17:260–4.
33. Jang TB, Schindler D, Kaji AH. Bedside ultrasonography for the detection of small bowel obstruction in the emergency department. Emerg Med J. 2011;28:676–8.
34. Seitz K, Reising KD. Ultrasound detection of free air in the abdominal cavity. Ultraschall Med. 1982;3:4–6.
35. Chen SC, Wang HP, Chen WJ, Lin FY, Hsu CY, Chang KJ, et al. Selective use of ultrasonography for the detection of pneumoperitoneum. Acad Emerg Med. 2002;9:643–5.
36. Chen SC, Yen ZS, Wang HP, Lin FY, Hsu CY, Chen WJ. Ultrasonography is superior to plain radiography in the diagnosis of pneumoperitoneum. Br J Surg. 2002;89:351–4.
37. Moriwaki Y, Sugiyama M, Toyoda H, Kosuge T, Arata S, Iwashita M, et al. Ultrasonography for the diagnosis of intraperitoneal free air in chest-abdominal-pelvic blunt trauma and critical acute abdominal pain. Arch Surg. 2009;144:137–41.
38. Smith-Bindman R, Aubin C, Bailitz J, Bengiamin RN, Camargo Jr CA, Corbo J, et al. Ultrasonography versus computed tomography for suspected nephrolithiasis. N Engl J Med. 2014;371:1100–10.
39. Gaspari RJ, Horst K. Emergency ultrasound and urinalysis in the evaluation of flank pain. Acad Emerg Med. 2005;12:1180–4.
40. Watkins S, Bowra J, Sharma P, Holdgate A, Giles A, Campbell L. Validation of emergency physician ultrasound in diagnosing hydronephrosis in ureteric colic. Emerg Med Australas. 2007;19:188–95.
41. Moak JH, Lyons MS, Lindsell CJ. Bedside renal ultrasound in the evaluation of suspected ureterolithiasis. Am J Emerg Med. 2012;30:218–21.
42. Herbst MK, Rosenberg G, Daniels B, Gross CP, Singh D, Molinaro AM, et al. Effect of provider experience on clinician-performed ultrasonography for hydronephrosis in patients with suspected renal colic. Ann Emerg Med. 2014;64:269–76.
43. Kameda T, Kawai F, Taniguchi N, Mori I, Ono M, Tsukahara N, et al. Ultrasonography for ureteral stone detection in patients with or without caliceal dilatation. J Med Ultrason. 2010;37:9–14.
44. Chen KC, Hung SW, Seow VK, Chong CF, Wang TL, Li YC, et al. The role of emergency ultrasound for evaluating acute pyelonephritis in the ED. Am J Emerg Med. 2011;29:721–4.
45. Kameda T, Kawai F, Taniguchi N, Kobori Y. Usefulness of transabdominal ultrasonography in excluding adnexal disease. J Med Ultrason. 2016;43:63–70.
46. Stein JC, Wang R, Adler N, Boscardin J, Jacoby VL, Won G, et al. Emergency physician ultrasonography for evaluating patients at risk for ectopic pregnancy: a meta-analysis. Ann Emerg Med. 2010;56:674–83.
47. Rubano E, Mehta N, Caputo W, Paladino L, Sinert R. Systematic review: emergency department bedside ultrasonography for diagnosing suspected abdominal aortic aneurysm. Acad Emerg Med. 2013;20:128–38.
48. Mercaldi CJ, Lanes SF. Ultrasound guidance decreases complications and improves the cost of care among patients undergoing thoracentesis and paracentesis. Chest. 2013;143:532–8.
49. Nazeer SR, Dewbre H, Miller AH. Ultrasound-assisted paracentesis performed by emergency physicians vs the traditional technique: a prospective, randomized study. Am J Emerg Med. 2005;23:363–7.

50. Blaivas M. Emergency diagnostic paracentesis to determine intraperitoneal fluid identity discovered on bedside ultrasound of unstable patients. J Emerg Med. 2005;29:461–5.
51. Stone JC, Moak JH. Feasibility of sonographic localization of the inferior epigastric artery before ultrasound-guided paracentesis. Am J Emerg Med. 2015;33:1795–8.
52. Chenaitia H, Brun PM, Querellou E, Leyral J, Bessereau J, Aimé C, et al. Ultrasound to confirm gastric tube placement in prehospital management. Resuscitation. 2012;83:447–51.
53. Vigneau C, Baudel JL, Guidet B, Offenstadt G, Maury E. Sonography as an alternative to radiography for nasogastric feeding tube location. Intensive Care Med. 2005;31:1570–2.
54. Brun PM, Chenaitia H, Lablanche C, Pradel AL, Deniel C, Bessereau J, et al. 2-point ultrasonography to confirm correct position of the gastric tube in prehospital setting. Mil Med. 2014;179:959–63.
55. Kim HM, So BH, Jeong WJ, Choi SM, Park KN. The effectiveness of ultrasonography in verifying the placement of a nasogastric tube in patients with low consciousness at an emergency center. Scand J Trauma Resusc Emerg Med. 2012;20:38. doi:10.1186/1757-7241-20-38.
56. Chen L, Hsiao AL, Moore CL, Dziura JD, Santucci KA. Utility of bedside bladder ultrasound before urethral catheterization in young children. Pediatrics. 2005;115:108–11.
57. Milling Jr TJ, Van Amerongen R, Melville L, Santiago L, Gaeta T, Birkhahn R, et al. Use of ultrasonography to identify infants for whom urinary catheterization will be unsuccessful because of insufficient urine volume: validation of the urinary bladder index. Ann Emerg Med. 2005;45:510–3.
58. Kameda T, Murata Y, Fujita M, Isaka A. Transabdominal ultrasound-guided urethral catheterization with transrectal pressure. J Emerg Med. 2014;46:215–9.

2

Diaphragm thickening fraction to predict weaning—a prospective exploratory study

Sujay Samanta, Ratender Kumar Singh*, Arvind K. Baronia, Banani Poddar, Afzal Azim and Mohan Gurjar

Abstract

Background: Diaphragm ultrasound (DUS) is a well-established point of care modality for assessment of dimensional and functional aspects of the diaphragm. Amongst various measures, diaphragmatic thickening fraction (DT*f*) is more comprehensive. However, there is still uncertainty about its capability to predict weaning from mechanical ventilation (MV). The present prospective observational exploratory study assessed the diaphragm at variable negative pressure triggers (NPTs) with US to predict weaning in ICU patients.

Methods: Adult ICU patients about to receive their first T-piece were included in the study. Linear and curvilinear US probes were used to measure right side diaphragm characteristics first at pressure support ventilation (PSV) of 8 cmH2O with positive end expiratory pressure (PEEP) of 5 cmH2O against NPTs of 2, 4, and 6 cmH2O and then later during their first T-piece. The measured variables were then categorized into simple weaning (SW) and complicated weaning (CW) groups and their outcomes analyzed.

Results: Sixty-four (M:F, 40:24) medical (55/64, 86%) patients were included in the study. Sepsis of lung origin (65.5%) was the dominant reason for MV. There were 33 and 31 patients in the SW and CW groups, respectively. DT*f* predicts SW with a cutoff ≥ 25.5, 26.5, 25.5, and 24.5 for 2, 4, and 6 NPTs and T-piece, respectively, with ≥ 0.90 ROC AUC. At NPT of 2, DT*f* had the highest sensitivity of 97% and specificity of 81% [ROC AUC (CI), 0.91 (0.84–0.99); $p < 0.001$].

Conclusions: DT*f* may successfully predict SW and also help identify patients ready to wean prior to a T-piece trial.

Keywords: Weaning, Diaphragm ultrasound, Diaphragm thickening fraction

Background

Weaning from mechanical ventilation (MV) is one of the major challenges faced by intensivists. Premature [1, 2] and delayed [3, 4] weaning are both detrimental in patients admitted in the intensive care unit (ICU). Weaning consumes approximately 40% time of ventilation [5]. While majority weaning is simple, difficult weaning is encountered in 20–25% of patients [6]. The diaphragm, the main inspiratory muscle, is affected by multiple factors in critical illness [7, 8], including disuse atrophy as a result of MV itself [9–12]. Diaphragm dysfunction also results in prolonged MV, weaning failure [13, 14], and increased mortality [15].

In 2007, the International Task Force of Respiratory and Critical Care Societies categorized weaning into simple, difficult, and prolonged [16]. Later in 2010, the incidence and outcomes of these new weaning categories were further studied [17]. In spite of subjective and objective extubation and weaning criteria, predicting a successful outcome is still difficult. Although several traditional tools to predict successful outcomes exist, their precision and accuracy are variable [18–20]. Diaphragm ultrasound (DUS) is a well-established point of care modality for assessment of dimensional and functional aspects of the diaphragm [14, 21]. Diaphragmatic thickening fraction (DT*f* (%)) reflects the magnitude of diaphragmatic effort and may predict successful weaning [22, 23].

We proposed to confirm the utility of DUS to assess muscle function in response to a maximal volitional inspiratory effort. In order to test the hypothesis that DUS-based measurements can successfully predict weaning, we conducted the present prospective exploratory study in adult critically ill ICU patients at variable negative pressure triggers (NPTs) both prior and during a T-piece trial. We in our present study also attempted

* Correspondence: ratender@sgpgi.ac.in; ratenderrks70@gmail.com
Department of Critical Care Medicine, Sanjay Gandhi Post Graduate Institute of Medical Sciences (SGPGIMS), Raebareli Road, Lucknow, Uttar Pradesh 226014, India

to explore DUS-based parameters in the above-mentioned weaning categories.

Methods

Ethics and consent

After prior approval from the ethics committee (Sanjay Gandhi Post Graduate Institute of Medical Sciences, Lucknow, UP, India) and obtaining patient's written informed consent, we conducted the present prospective exploratory study. The study period was from January 2015 to June 2016. A 12-bed closed, medical, surgical, adult, and pediatric ICU of a tertiary care referral hospital and academic institute in north of India was used for this purpose. The clinical management of patients was at the discretion of the ICU treating team in accordance with the contemporary best ICU practices. No interventions or therapy was modified based on the study findings.

Inclusion criteria

Patients aged ≥ 18 years, admitted to ICU and receiving MV longer than 24 h and about to be subjected to their first T-piece after satisfying conventional criteria for ready to wean from ventilator, were enrolled in the study. DUS examinations were performed initially at pressure support ventilation (PSV) with variable NPTs, and then 6–12 h later during the first T-piece trial.

Exclusion criteria

Patients aged < 18 years, ventilated for less than 24 h, with preexisting diaphragm disease, increased intra-abdominal pressure, any breach in skin preventing DUS examinations in subcostal area, phrenic nerve palsy, and refusal of consent were excluded from study. Patients who deteriorated with application of PSV at NPTs or during the T-piece were also excluded.

Study protocol

Patients on MV received their first T-piece when they were afebrile, alert, cooperative, and hemodynamically stable without vasopressor support and PaO_2/FiO_2 ratio > 200 was achievable at $FiO_2 < 0.5$ with positive end expiratory pressure (PEEP) ≤ 5 cmH2O and respiratory rate of < 30 breaths per minute. The patients who were considered ready to wean from MV as per the above indices were included in the assessment of increasing ventilatory burden by subjecting them to non-randomized NPTs of 2, 4, and 6 during PSV of 8 cmH2O with PEEP 5 cmH2O. A period of 30 min of PSV without NPT was mandated to prevent exhaustion from burden of the test. Patients who successfully tolerated the variable NPT trial subsequently received their first T-piece trial after 6–12 h to prevent influence of any burden of test on the outcome of T-piece. Both PSV at NPTs and the T-piece trials were performed in semi-recumbent position. Decisions about tolerability of NPTs, T-piece, extubation, repeat T-piece, and or tracheostomy were as per the clinical judgment of the physician in-charge of the patient and were not in any way based on DUS measurements.

Diaphragm ultrasound

DUS measurements were performed on the right subcostal side using both brightness (B) and motion (M) mode.

Ultrasound machine and probe

High-resolution linear and curvilinear US probes of 10 and 3.5–5 MHz (FUJIFILM SonoSite, Inc.) were used to measure the diaphragm thickness (DT) and diaphragmatic excursion [amplitude (AMP)] respectively using both B and M modes.

Probe placement

Both the amplitude and speed of contraction were assessed by placing the curvilinear probe on the right subcostal margin between the mid-clavicular and anterior axillary line allowing placement of the M mode line parallel to the excursion of the diaphragm. DT was measured in the zone of apposition of the diaphragm and rib cage in the mid-axillary line between the eighth and tenth intercostal space. The right-sided DUS measurements were used because of their reproducibility and feasibility in MV patients [21].

Measurements

DT [at end of inspiration (*i*) and expiration (*e*)], AMP [centimeters (cm)], and speed of contraction [SP*cont* (cm/s)] were measured. The DT*f* (%) was calculated as the difference between DT*i* and DT*e* divided by DT*e* × 100. These measurements were performed by a single intensivist experienced in performing DUS. In order to minimize intra-observer variability to less than 10% and establish reproducibility, an average of three readings measured in at least three sessions each lasting 10–15 min was ensured.

Inspiratory effort capacity

Within 6–12 h preceding the first T-piece, each patient was subjected to NPTs of 2, 4, and 6 cmH_2O at PSV of 8 and 5 cmH2O PEEP for a minimum period of 20 min each to achieve a steady state. The measurements were recorded at the end of the 20th minute. Cooperative patient was instructed to perform breathing to total lung capacity (TLC) and then to exhale to residual volume (RV). DUS measurements at TLC and RV were then recorded. These points were considered as surrogates of end-inspiration and end-expiration respectively [22]. Several images of the diaphragm were captured and stored, including at least three at the point of maximum thickening at TLC and at least three at minimum thickening at RV. Diaphragm measurements were taken at PSV at three different NPTs and during the period of the first T-piece and at TLC and RV. Between each change over to a higher NPT, a rest period of 30 min on previous ventilatory support was mandatory to prevent exhaustion. The protocol was also interrupted for 30 min with increased pressure support after each trigger if signs of respiratory distress like respiratory rate > 35 breaths/min, SpO2 < 90%, heart rate > 140 beats/min, variation of > 30% from baseline, systolic blood pressure > 180 or < 90 mmHg, diaphoresis, or anxiety occurred. The time gap of 6–12 h between NPT trials and T-piece was incorporated to provide enough rest between the two procedures. SERVO-i-Maquet ventilator was used for mechanical ventilation of all patients included in the study.

Definitions

Patients were categorized based on the following weaning classification [16].

Simple weaning

Patients who proceeded from initiation of weaning to successful extubation on their first SBT without any difficulty were categorized as simple weaning (SW).

Difficult weaning

Patients who failed initial weaning and required up to three SBTs or as long as 7 days from the first SBT to achieve successful weaning were categorized as having difficult weaning.

Prolonged weaning

Patients who failed at least three weaning attempts or required 7 days of weaning after the first SBT were said to have prolonged weaning.

Weaning failure

It was defined as resumption of ventilatory support within 48 h of liberation from MV.

Complicated weaning

We grouped all patients with difficult, prolonged, and failed weaning together as complicated weaning (CW).

Data collection

Demographic (age, gender, category of patient, care received prior to present admission, source of admission, type of illness, coexisting illness, and source of sepsis), severity [Acute Physiologic and Chronic Health Evaluation (APACHE-II) and Sequential Organ Dysfunction Assessment (SOFA)] scores, organ failure at admission, indication for intubation, ventilation-related characteristics like tracheostomy, spontaneous breathing trials (SBTs), time before initiation of T-piece, length of MV, and ICU stay, along with DUS-based parameters of thickness, amplitude, thickening fraction, and outcomes relating to SW and CW and 28-day survival, were all recorded.

Sample size and statistical analysis

Sample size

Sample size was calculated assuming simple weaning proportion of 0.5 and 25% relative error of the proportion at two-sided 95% confidence interval (CI). Finally, a minimum sample size of 62 was calculated for the study. Sample size was calculated using software power analysis and sample size (PASS version 8).

Statistical analysis

Normality of continuous data was tested using Shapiro-Wilk test. Non-normal, continuous data was expressed as median (interquartile range), while categorical data was expressed as frequency and percentage. Mann-Whitney *U* test was used to compare the medians between SW and CW. Kruskal-Wallis test was used for comparison of continuous variables between more than two groups. Chi-square test was used to compare the proportions/test the association between groups. For repeated observations over variable NPTs, Friedman analysis of variance (ANOVA) was used to estimate the significance. If in Friedman ANOVA the p value was observed to be significant, then the difference in medians between individual groups was further assessed using the Wilcoxon signed rank test. A two-tailed p value of < 0.05 was considered statistically significant. IBM, SPSS version 23 (SPSS Inc., Chicago, IL, USA), was used for statistical analysis.

Results

Sixty-four patients, 40 (62.5%) males, were included in the study. Baseline characteristics of the studied population were as depicted in Table 1. Approximately, 86% of patients were with medical illness. Prior to present ICU admission, nearly 73 and 48% received ICU and MV support, respectively. Nearly 45% of the studied patients had been transferred from ICUs of other hospitals. Sepsis was the predominant (17/64, ~ 27%) reason for admission, with nearly 66% of respiratory origin. Nearly 58% of patients had no coexisting illness. There were 33 and 31 patients in SW and CW group, respectively. The groups were not significantly different, except for the type of illness (p, 0.01) (Table 1). Amongst the CW group, there were 16, 10, and 5 patients with difficult, prolonged, and failed weaning, respectively. Their baseline characteristics were also comparable with SW (Table not shown).

The attributes of severity, MV, and outcomes were as depicted in Table 2. APACHE-II and SOFA scores were

Table 1 Baseline characteristics of patients with different weaning outcomes

Variables	All weaning ($N = 64$)	Simple weaning ($n = 33$)	Complicated weaning ($n = 31$)	*p* value
Age, years	37 (22–56)	39 (21–54)	37 (22–58)	0.37
Gender, male, *n* (%)	40 (62.5)	22 (66.7)	18 (58.1)	0.60
Category of patients, *n* (%)				0.29
Medical	55 (85.9)	30 (90.9)	25 (80.6)	
Surgical	9 (14.1)	3 (9.1)	6 (19.3)	
Care received prior to admission, *n* (%)				
Intensive care	47 (73.4)	24 (72.7)	23 (74.2)	1
Mechanical ventilation	31 (48.4)	13 (39.4)	18 (58.1)	0.21
Source of admission, *n* (%)				0.05
Emergency	12 (18.8)	5 (15.1)	7 (22.6)	
Intra-hospital ICU	14 (21.9)	11 (33.3)	3 (9.7)	
Inter-hospital ICU	29 (45.3)	11 (33.3)	18 (58.1)	
Intra-hospital ward	9 (14.1)	6 (18.2)	3 (9.7)	
Type of illness, *n* (%)				
Sepsis	17 (26.6)	11 (33.3)	6 (19.3)	0.01
Neurological	16 (25)	3 (9.1)	13 (41.9)	
Cardiovascular	3 (4.7)	3 (9.1)	0	
Gastrointestinal	3 (4.7)	0	3 (9.7)	
Hepatic	4 (6.3)	2 (6.1)	2 (6.4)	
Respiratory	3 (4.7)	2 (6.1)	1 (3.2)	
SAP	4 (6.3)	1 (3.0)	3 (9.7)	
Tropical	7 (10.9)	5 (15.1)	2 (6.4)	
Others	7 (10.9)	6 (9.1)	1 (3.2)	
Coexisting illness, *n* (%)				0.66
CKD	3 (4.7)	3 (9.1)	0	
COPD	3 (4.7)	1 (3.0)	2 (6.4)	
Hypertension	6 (9.4)	2 (6.1)	4 (12.9)	
Hypertension, diabetes mellitus	7 (10.9)	3 (9.1)	4 (12.9)	
Hypothyroidism	1 (1.6)	0	1 (3.2)	
Multiple (≥ 3)	3 (4.7)	2 (6.1)	1 (3.2)	
None	37 (57.8)	20 (60.6)	17 (54.8)	
Other	4 (6.3)	2 (6.1)	2 (6.4)	
Source of sepsis, *n* (%)				0.60
Intra-abdominal	8 (12.5)	3 (9.1)	5 (16.1)	
Central nervous system	8 (12.5)	5 (15.1)	3 (9.7)	
Hepatic	1 (1.6)	1 (3.0)	0	
Respiratory	42 (65.6)	20 (60.6)	22 (71.0)	
None	1 (1.6)	1 (3.0)	0	
Unknown	4 (6.3)	3 (9.1)	1 (3.2)	

Data is expressed in median (interquartile range), unless specified. Test for statistical significance (*p* value) used is Pearson chi-square for categorical data and Mann-Whitney *U* test for continuous measurements
Abbreviations: *IQR* interquartile range, *ICU* intensive care unit

Table 2 Severity, ventilation, and outcome-related characteristics in weaning groups

Variables	All weaning ($N = 64$)	Simple weaning ($n = 33$)	Complicated weaning ($n = 31$)	*p* value
Severity scores at admission				
APACHE-II	12 (10–16)	12 (10–15)	14 (10–16)	0.47
SOFA	8 (6–10)	8 (6–10)	8 (6–10)	0.74
No of organ failure at admission, *n* (%)				0.04
1	3 (4.7)	0	3 (9.7)	
2	29 (45.3)	18 (54.5)	11 (35.5)	
3	23 (35.9)	13 (39.4)	10 (32.2)	
4	9 (14.1)	2 (6.1)	7 (22.6)	
Indication for intubation, *n* (%)				0.44
Central nervous system	20 (31.3)	9 (27.3)	11 (35.5)	
Respiratory	35 (54.7)	20 (60.6)	15 (48.4)	
Combination	2 (3.1)	0	2 (6.4)	
Others	7 (10.9)	4 (12.1)	3 (9.7)	
Onset of illness requiring ICU admission, days	7 (5–11.7)	7 (5–12)	7 (6–10)	0.79
Tracheostomy, *n* (%)	24 (37.5)	1 (3.0)	23 (74.2)	< 0.001
1st T-piece failure, *n* (%)	20 (31.3)	0	20 (64.5)	< 0.001
Time to T-piece, days	8 (5–14)	6 (4–8.5)	13 (8–22)	< 0.001
MLV, days	12.5 (6–21.7)	6 (5–9)	22 (14–28)	< 0.001
LOS-ICU, days	14.5 (8–28)	8 (7–14.5)	28 (15–35)	< 0.001
Survival at 28 days, *n* (%)	60 (93.8)	33 (100)	27 (87.1)	0.05
Final outcome, *n* (%)				0.07
Death	4 (6.3)	0	4 (12.9)	
Discharged to home	39 (60.9)	20 (60.6)	19 (61.3)	
Transferred to ward	21 (32.8)	13 (39.4)	8 (25.8)	

Data is expressed in median (interquartile range), unless specified. Test for statistical significance (*p* value) used is Pearson chi-square for categorical data and Mann-Whitney *U* test for continuous measurements

Abbreviations: *APACHE* Acute Physiological and Chronic Health Evaluation, *SOFA* Sequential Organ Failure Assessment, *ICU* intensive care unit, *MLV* mechanical lung ventilation, *LOS* length of stay

comparable. Nearly 95% (61/64) of patients had two or more organ failures at admission, and they differed significantly between SW and CW (*p*, 0.04). Nearly 37% (24/64) required tracheostomy (SW, 1 vs. CW, 23; $p < 0.001$) during ICU stay. Significantly delayed [CW, 13 (8–22) day vs. 6 (4–8.5) day in SW; $p < 0.001$)] and failed first T-piece [CW, 20 (64.5%) vs. Nil in SW; $p < 0.001$] along with prolonged MV [CW, 22 (14–28) vs. 6 (5–9) in SW; $p < 0.001$] and ICU stay [CW, 28 (15–35) days vs. 8 (7–14.5) days in SW; $p < 0.001$] were observed in CW relative to SW (Table 2). Similar significance ($p < 0.001$) for these characteristics were also observed when comparing SW with difficult, prolonged, and failed weaning (Table not shown). Only one patient in the SW group got re-intubated and was later tracheostomized during the follow-up period of 28 days. All patients in CW group (*n*, 31) failed the first T-piece trial, and 23 (23/31, 74%) were tracheostomized. The remaining eight patients were extubated following more than one T-piece trial in the follow-up period. Post extubation non-invasive ventilation was used in eight patients in the CW group.

While 100% of patients in SW, difficult and prolonged weaning, survived 28 days, one of five (20%) in the failed weaning died within this period ($p < 0.001$) (Table not shown). The 28-day survival and final outcomes were comparable (Table 2). However, the four patients with CW who finally died were also the ones who had failed weaning and three of them died beyond 28 days of ICU stay.

The measurements of diaphragm (DT*i*, DT*e*, DT*f*, AMP, and SP*cont*) at NPTs of 2, 4, and 6 and during first T-piece for SW and CW were as depicted in Table 3. Also depicted in the same table were inter- and intra-differences between groups. DT*i* exceeded DT*e* at all NPTs. The intergroup variability between SW and CW was statistically significant for DT*i*, DT*f*, AMP, and SP*cont*, at variable NPTs and T-piece (for each, $p < 0.001$). Similar comparison of SW with difficult, prolonged, and failed

Table 3 Differences between groups at variable negative pressure

Diaphragm parameters	Weaning groups ($N = 64$)	Negative pressure trigger ($N = 64$)							
Median (IQR)	Simple ($n = 33$) Complicated ($n = 31$)	2	4	6	T-piece	$p^{\#\#}$	$p^{\#\#\#}$		
							Δ2–4	Δ4–6	Δ2–6
DT*i*, mm	Simple	2.2 (2.1–2.3)	2.2 (2.2–2.3)	2.2 (2.2–2.3)	2.2 (2.2–2.2)	< 0.001*	< 0.001*	< 0.001*	<0.001*
	Complicated	2.0 (2.0–2.1)	2.1 (2–2.2)	2.0 (2.0–2.2)	2.0 (2.0–2.2)	< 0.001*	< 0.001*	< 0.001*	0.004
	$p^{\#}$	< 0.001	< 0.001	< 0.001	< 0.001				
DT*e*, mm	Simple	1.7 (1.6–1.7)	1.7 (1.7–1.8)	1.7 (1.7–1.8)	1.7 (1.6–1.8)	< 0.001*	< 0.001*	0.82	<0.001*
	Complicated	1.6 (1.5–1.7)	1.7 (1.6–1.8)	1.6 (1.6–1.8)	1.7 (1.6–1.8)	0.001	< 0.001*	0.03	0.006
	$p^{\#}$	0.22	0.31	0.10	0.16				
DT*f*, %	Simple	31 (28–32)	31 (28–35)	29 (26–32)	29 (26–33)	0.010	0.40	0.001	0.05
	Complicated	22 (17–24)	22 (18–27)	23 (18–25)	21 (17–25)	0.34	0.94	0.28	0.50
	$p^{\#}$	< 0.001	< 0.001	< 0.001	< 0.001				
AMP, cm	Simple	1.3 (1.3–1.5)	1.3 (1.3–1.5)	1.3 (1.2–1.4)	1.3 (1.2–1.4)	< 0.001*	< 0.001*	< 0.001*	0.49
	Complicated	1.2 (1.1–1.2)	1.2 (1.1–1.3)	1.2 (1.1–1.2)	1.2 (1.1–1.2)	< 0.001*	< 0.001*	0.01	<0.001*
	$p^{\#}$	< 0.001	< 0.001	< 0.001	< 0.001				
SP*cont*, cm/s	Simple	1.3 (1.3–1.3)	1.3 (1.3–1.4)	1.3 (1.3–1.4)	1.3 (1.2–1.3)	< 0.001*	0.001	< 0.001*	0.36
	Complicated	1.2 (1.1–1.2)	1.2 (1.1–1.3)	1.2 (1.1–1.3)	1.2 (1.1–1.3)	0.001	< 0.001*	0.97	<0.001*
	$p^{\#}$	< 0.001	< 0.001	< 0.001	< 0.001				

Note: Tests of statistical significance used for *p* values: $p^{\#}$, Mann-Whitney *U* test; $p^{\#\#}$, Friedman ANOVA test; $p^{\#\#\#}$, Wilcoxon signed rank test; p^{*}, < 0.001 highly significant
Abbreviations: *DTi* thickness of diaphragm during inspiration, *DTe* thickness of diaphragm during expiration, *TP* T-piece, *DTf* diaphragm thickening fraction, *AMP* amplitude of diaphragm, *SPcont* speed of contraction of diaphragm

weaning patients was also significant ($p < 0.001$) (Table not shown). The intra-group variability at different triggers and T-piece as assessed by Friedman ANOVA was statistically significant ($p \leq 0.001$) for all the measured diaphragm parameters except in the CW for DT*f* (*p*, 0.34). Similar results of significance were also observed when SW was compared with difficult and prolonged weaning ($p \leq 0.001$), except that patients with failed weaning had a somewhat lower significance ($p < 0.05$) (Table not shown). The Δ2–4, Δ4–6, and Δ2–6 variables for SW and CW were as depicted in Table 3. For most, the significance was ≤ 0.001, except for 2, 3, and 4 variables in Δ2–4, Δ4–6, and Δ2–6 respectively, wherein it was comparable. However, the Δ variability (Table 3) increased when patients in SW were compared with difficult, prolonged, and failed weaning (Table not shown).

The sensitivity and specificity of various diaphragm measurements to predict SW was analyzed using the receiver operative characteristics (Table 4). With a cutoff at or above 25.5, 26.5, 25.5, and 24.5 for 2, 4, and 6 NPTs and T-piece, respectively, the DT*f* had a ROC AUC of ≥ 0.90. At NPT of 2, DT*f* had the highest sensitivity of 97%, albeit 81% specificity [ROC AUC, 0.91 (0.84–0.99); $p < 0.001$] compared to AMP and SP*cont*.

Discussion

DUS is an acknowledged investigative tool for assessment of diaphragm in critically ill patients. The present prospective study utilized DUS measurements at variable inspiratory efforts to predict successful weaning. The main findings of our study were as follows: (1) DT*f* predicts simple weaning; (2) DUS parameters at variable NPTs can identify patients ready to wean; and (3) DUS can help analyze patients with complicated weaning.

DT*f* predicts simple weaning

In recent years, several DUS-based measurements and some derived parameters have been validated for predicting weaning in critically ill patients [13, 14, 21–23]. Similar to majority of previous studies [21, 24, 25], we too assessed the more feasible and highly reproducible right hemi-diaphragm via DUS. DT*i*, DT*f*, AMP, and SP*cont* were all significantly higher in SW compared to CW (Table 3) or difficult, prolonged, and failed weaning (Table not shown), both at variable NPTs and during T-piece ($p < 0.001$). These parameters were also relatively better at different NPTs than during T-piece for predicting SW. The DT*f* cutoff ≥ 25.5% with AUC of 0.91 had sensitivity and specificity of 97 and 81% respectively at NPT of 2 for predicting SW. This sensitivity was higher than the AMP (cutoff ≥ 1.21 cm) and SP*cont* (cutoff ≥ 1.24 cm/s) at same NPT, desirable to predict SW. Variable DT*f* cutoffs have been used previously. DiNino et al., in 2014, studied DUS in 63 patients before extubation, during SBT or pressure support trial [23]. They suggested that a threshold DT*f* of greater or equal to 30%, with a positive predictive value (PPV) and negative

Table 4 Prediction of simple weaning

Diaphragm parameter	Cutoff	ROC of AUC (95% CI)	Sensitivity (%)	Specificity (%)	*p* value
DT*f*, % NPT					
2	≥ 25.5	0.91 (0.84–0.99)	97	81	< 0.001
4	≥ 26.5	0.93 (0.87–0.99)	87	75	< 0.001
6	≥ 25.5	0.91 (0.84–0.99)	90	88	< 0.001
T-piece	≥ 24.5	0.90 (0.82–0.97)	87	75	< 0.001
AMP, inspiration, cm					
2	≥ 1.21	0.87 (0.78–0.96)	87	75	< 0.001
4	≥ 1.27	0.81 (0.71–0.92)	81	81	< 0.001
6	≥ 1.24	0.77 (0.66–0.88)	84	59	< 0.001
T-piece	≥ 1.20	0.76 (0.65–0.88)	72	55	< 0.001
SP*cont*, cm/s					
2	≥ 1.24	0.94 (0.88–0.99)	84	91	< 0.001
4	≥ 1.27	0.94 (0.89–0.99)	93	78	< 0.001
6	≥ 1.24	0.89 (0.81–0.96)	78	71	< 0.001
T-piece	≥ 1.23	0.86 (0.77–0.94)	87	68	< 0.001

Abbreviations: *ROC* receiver operative characteristics, *AUC* area under curve, *CI* confidence interval, DTf diaphragm thickening fraction, *AMP* amplitude of diaphragm, *SPcont* speed of contraction of diaphragm

predictive value (NPV) of 91 and 63%, respectively, for extubation success, performed similarly during SBT or pressure support ventilation. Similarly, Ferrari et al., in 46 patients of repeated weaning failure, suggested that a cutoff DT*f* greater or equal to 36%, during SBT in tracheostomized patients, was associated with a PPV and NPV of 92 and 75%, respectively, for successful or failed weaning at 48 h [22]. By comparison, rapid shallow breathing index (RSBI) < 105 had sensitivity, specificity, PPV, and NPV of 93, 88, 93, and 88%, respectively, for determining successful SBT. The plausible explanation of a lower DT*f* threshold in our study is due to differences in methodology, variable inspiratory efforts, patient population, and severity of illness at ICU admission, metabolic conditions, and duration of MV. Several studies report superiority of DT*f* over diaphragm excursions as a marker of diaphragm function [26, 27]. However, we studied predictability of weaning via DUS at variable inspiratory efforts and observed a higher sensitivity and comparable AUC for DT*f* to predict SW.

DUS parameters at variable NPTs can identify patients ready to wean

The ROC AUC, sensitivity, and specificity during T-piece for DT*f*, AMP, and SP*cont* were lower as compared to NPTs at comparable cutoffs (Table 4). DUS measurements at NPT of 2 were observed to be more favorable for predicting SW compared to T-piece. Both, DT*f* and AMP, showed higher or comparable sensitivity and specificity at NPT of 2 relative to NPT of 6. Hence, SW prediction can be performed prior to T-piece and at lower NPTs. No previous studies have reported this.

DUS can help analyze patients with complicated weaning

Diaphragm excursion [13], twitch tracheal pressure [15], and trans-diaphragmatic twitch pressure [26, 27] have all been used to quantify diaphragm dysfunction. These studies have reported increased mortality and morbidity associated with diaphragm dysfunction. However, we categorized our patients into SW and CW. All DUS parameters were significantly lower in the CW group, and these patients also had delayed and failed SBT and prolonged MV and length of ICU stay. Similar outcomes were observed in the difficult, prolonged, and failed weaning patients. These were similar to findings of earlier study [17]. Only patients with failed weaning died.

Limitations

Several limitations of our study were as follows: (1) single-center study with a small sample size; (2) DT*f* cutoff not validated; (3) illness- and severity-specific variability not ascertained due to a small sample size; (4) minimal differences between measurements altered the weaning categorization; (5) small number of patients in difficult, prolonged, and failed weaning may have overestimated the differences; (6) trigger sensitivity not randomized; (7) due to small sample size, independent trigger sensitivity for each patient group could not be individually tested; (8) workload increase contributed by the burden of test and its impact on T-piece outcome could not be clearly ascertained; ideally, these two observations should have been done separately to avoid influence; (9) rest period of 30 min between variable triggers may have been insufficient to relieve the fatigue imposed; (10) DUS-based measurements were not compared against traditional weaning indices; (11) trends of DUS measurements overtime in CW group may have better correlated with outcomes; (12) inter-observer variability not assessed; (13) due to non-availability of ventilator-coupled USG machine, only cooperative patients could be included in the study; (14) factors affecting the DT*f*, their impact on weaning, and how they could be modified to optimize weaning were not studied.

Despite the abovementioned shortcomings, our study is a humble exploratory attempt to use DUS measurements to identify patients with SW even before their first T-piece trial. DT*f*, AMP, and SP*cont* with cutoffs ≥ 25.5%, ≥ 1.2 cm, and ≥ 1.24 cm/s, respectively, at NPT of 2 may help to not only determine which patient will safely endure the T-piece but also predict a successful T-piece trial. These measures may also help to further analyze patients with CW. Furthermore, DT*f* values could also be of use to optimize CW patients for further extubation trials.

Conclusion

Ultrasound-based diaphragm measurements at variable inspiratory efforts can help identify patients safe and ready to wean even without enduring a T-piece. Amongst these parameters, DT*f*, apart from recognizing readiness to wean, can also predict simple weaning. However, a larger multicenter study is still required to validate the observed DT*f* cutoff in our study. Research on factors which affect the DT*f* and their modification to optimize weaning need to be further explored.

Abbreviations

AMP: Amplitude; APACHE: Acute Physiology and Chronic Health Evaluation; CW: Complicated weaning; DT: Diaphragm thickening; DT*e*: Diaphragm thickening during expiration; DT*f*: Diaphragm thickening fraction; DT*i*: Diaphragm thickening during inspiration; DUS: Diaphragm ultrasound; ICU: Intensive care unit; MV: Mechanical ventilation; NPTs: Negative pressure triggers; PSV: Pressure support ventilation; RV: Residual volume; SOFA: Sequential Organ Failure Assessment; SP*cont*: Speed of contraction; SW: Simple weaning; TLC: Total lung capacity

Acknowledgements

The authors wish to thank the Department of Biostatistics and Health Informatics, Sanjay Gandhi Post Graduate Institute of Medical Sciences (SGPGIMS), Lucknow, Uttar Pradesh, India, for the support provided in the statistical analysis of the results.

Funding

The author(s) received no financial support for this study.

Authors' contributions

RKS and SS contributed equally to the design, data acquisition, statistical calculations, and manuscript preparation. AKB, BP, AZ, and MG contributed equally to the manuscript preparation. All authors read and approved the final manuscript.

Competing interests

The authors declare that they have no competing interests.

References

1. Epstein SK, Ciubotaru RL, Wong JB. Effect of failed extubation on the outcome of mechanical ventilation. Chest. 1997;112:186–92.
2. Seymour CW, Martinez A, Christie JD, Fuchs BD. The outcome of extubation failure in a community hospital intensive care unit: a cohort study. Crit Care. 2004;8:R322–7.
3. Coplin WM, Pierson DJ, Cooley KD, Newell DW, Rubenfeld GD. Implications of extubation delay in brain-injured patients meeting standard weaning criteria. Am J Respir Crit Care Med. 2000;161:1530–6.
4. Esteban A, Alía I, Tobin MJ, Gil A, Gordo F, Vallverdú I, Blanch L, Bonet A, Vázquez A, de Pablo R, Torres A, de La Cal MA, Macías S. Effect of spontaneous breathing trial duration on outcome of attempts to discontinue mechanical ventilation. Spanish Lung Failure Collaborative Group. Am J Respir Crit Care Med. 1999;159:512–8.
5. Esteban A, Alía I, Ibañez J, Benito S, Tobin MJ. Modes of mechanical ventilation and weaning. A national survey of Spanish hospitals. The Spanish Lung Failure Collaborative Group. Chest. 1994;106:1188–93.
6. Esteban A, Frutos F, Tobin MJ, Alía I, Solsona JF, Valverdú I, Fernández R, de la Cal MA, Benito S, TomásR, et al. A comparison of four methods of weaning patients from mechanical ventilation. Spanish Lung Failure Collaborative Group. N Engl J Med. 1995;332:345–50.
7. Tobin MJ, Laghi F, Jubran A. Narrative review: ventilator-induced respiratory muscle weakness. Ann Intern Med. 2010;153:240–5.
8. Laghi F, Tobin MJ. Disorders of the respiratory muscles. Am J Respir Crit Care Med. 2003;168:10–48.
9. Powers SK, Shanely RA, Coombes JS, Koesterer TJ, McKenzie M, Van Gammeren D, Cicale M, Dodd SL. Mechanical ventilation results in progressive contractile dysfunction in the diaphragm. J Appl Physiol. 2002; 92:1851–8.
10. Sassoon CS, Caiozzo VJ, Manka A, Sieck GC. Altered diaphragm contractile properties with controlled mechanical ventilation. J Appl Physiol. 2002;92: 2585–95.
11. Levine S, Nguyen T, Taylor N, Friscia ME, Budak MT, Rothenberg P, Zhu J, Sachdeva R, Sonnad S, Kaiser LR, Rubinstein NA, Powers SK, Shrager JB. Rapid disuse atrophy of diaphragm fibers in mechanically ventilated humans. N Engl J Med. 2008;358:1327–35.
12. Jaber S, Petrof BJ, Jung B, Chanques G, Berthet JP, Rabuel C, Bouyabrine H, Courouble P, Koechlin-Ramonatxo C, Sebbane M, Similowski T, Scheuermann V, Mebazaa A, Capdevila X, Mornet D, Mercier J, Lacampagne A, Philips A, Matecki S. Rapidly progressive diaphragmatic weakness and injury during mechanical ventilation in humans. Am J Respir Crit Care Med. 2011;183:364–71.
13. Kim WY, Suh HJ, Hong SB, Koh Y, Lim CM. Diaphragm dysfunction assessed by ultrasonography: influence on weaning from mechanical ventilation. Crit Care Med. 2011;39:2627–30.
14. Matamis D, Soilemezi E, Tsagourias M, Akoumianaki E, Dimassi S, Boroli F, Richard JC, Brochard L. Sonographic evaluation of the diaphragm in critically ill patients. Technique and clinical applications. Intensive Care Med. 2013;39:801–10.
15. Demoule A, Jung B, Prodanovic H, Molinari N, Chanques G, Coirault C, Matecki S, Duguet A, Similowski T, Jaber S. Diaphragm dysfunction on admission to the intensive care unit. Prevalence, risk factors, and prognostic impact—a prospective study. Am J Respir Crit Care Med. 2013;188:213–9.
16. Boles JM, Bion J, Connors A, Herridge M, Marsh B, Melot C, Pearl R, Silverman H, Stanchina M, Vieillard-Baron A, Welte T. Weaning from mechanical ventilation. EurRespir J. 2007;29:1033–56.
17. Funk GC, Anders S, Breyer MK, Burghuber OC, Edelmann G, Heindl W, Hinterholzer G, Kohansal R, Schuster R, Schwarzmaier-D'Assie A, Valentin A. Incidence and outcome of weaning from mechanical ventilation according to new categories. Eur Respir J. 2010;35:88–94.
18. Conti G, Montini L, Pennisi MA, Cavaliere F, Arcangeli A, Bocci MG, Proietti R, Antonelli M. A prospective, blinded evaluation of indexes proposed to predict weaning from mechanical ventilation. Intensive Care Med. 2004;30:830–6.
19. Yang KL, Tobin MJ. A prospective study of indexes predicting the outcome of trials of weaning from mechanical ventilation. N Engl J Med. 1991;324:1445–50.
20. Lee KH, Hui KP, Chan TB, Tan WC, Lim TK. Rapid shallow breathing (frequency-tidal volume ratio) did not predict extubation outcome. Chest. 1994;105:540–3.

21. Goligher EC, Laghi F, Detsky ME, Farias P, Murray A, Brace D, Brochard LJ, Bolz SS, Rubenfeld GD, Kavanagh BP, Ferguson ND. Measuring diaphragm thickness with ultrasound in mechanically ventilated patients: feasibility, reproducibility and validity. Intensive Care Med. 2015;41:642–9.
22. Ferrari G, De Filippi G, Elia F, Panero F, Volpicelli G, Aprà F. Diaphragm ultrasound as a new index of discontinuation from mechanical ventilation. Crit Ultrasound J. 2014;6:8.
23. DiNino E, Gartman EJ, Sethi JM, McCool FD. Diaphragm ultrasound as a predictor of successful extubation from mechanical ventilation. Thorax. 2014;69:423–7.
24. Houston JG, Morris AD, Howie CA, Ried JLNM. Technical report: quantitative assessment of diaphragmatic movement—a reproducible method using ultrasound. Clin Radiol. 1992;46:405–7.
25. Gerscovich EO, Cronan M, McGahan JP, Jain K, Jones CD, McDonald C. Ultrasonographic evaluation of diaphragmatic motion. J Ultrasound Med. 2001;20:597–604.
26. Umbrello M, Formenti P, Longhi D, Galimberti A, Piva I, Pezzi A, Mistraletti G, Marini JJ, Iapichino G. Diaphragm ultrasound as indicator of respiratory effort in critically ill patients undergoing assisted mechanical ventilation: a pilot clinical study. Crit Care. 2015;19:161.
27. Vivier E, Mekontso Dessap A, Dimassi S, Vargas F, Lyazidi A, Thille AW, Brochard L. Diaphragm ultrasonography to estimate the work of breathing during non-invasive ventilation. Intensive Care Med. 2012;38:796–803.

3

Acute traumatic coagulopathy and trauma-induced coagulopathy

Shigeki Kushimoto[1,2*], Daisuke Kudo[1,2] and Yu Kawazoe[1,2]

Abstract

Hemorrhage is the most important contributing factor of acute-phase mortality in trauma patients. Previously, traumatologists and investigators identified iatrogenic and resuscitation-associated causes of coagulopathic bleeding after traumatic injury, including hypothermia, metabolic acidosis, and dilutional coagulopathy that were recognized as primary drivers of bleeding after trauma. However, the last 10 years has seen a widespread paradigm shift in the resuscitation of critically injured patients, and there has been a dramatic evolution in our understanding of trauma-induced coagulopathy. Although there is no consensus regarding a definition or an approach to the classification and naming of trauma-associated coagulation impairment, trauma itself and/or traumatic shock-induced endogenous coagulopathy are both referred to as acute traumatic coagulopathy (ATC), and multifactorial trauma-associated coagulation impairment, including ATC and resuscitation-associated coagulopathy is recognized as trauma-induced coagulopathy. Understanding the pathophysiology of trauma-induced coagulopathy is vitally important, especially with respect to the critical issue of establishing therapeutic strategies for the management of patients with severe trauma.

Keywords: Acute traumatic coagulopathy, Trauma-induced coagulopathy, Disseminated intravascular coagulation

Background

Trauma remains a leading cause of death and permanent disability in adults despite advances in systematic approaches including prevention, resuscitation, surgical management, and critical care [1]. Trauma-related death and disability have also been suggested to have a great impact on global productivity.

Bleeding accounts for 30–40% of all trauma-related deaths and typically occurs within hours after injury [2]. Although the mortality of trauma patients requiring massive transfusion exceeds 50% [3], at least 10% of deaths after traumatic injury are potentially preventable, and 15% of those are due to hemorrhage; many of these deaths occur within the first few hours of definitive care, with coagulopathy playing a crucial role [4–6].

Regarding the management of patients requiring massive transfusion, it has been repeatedly suggested that patients are more likely to die from intraoperative metabolic failure than from the failure to complete organ repairs [7, 8]. Coagulopathy is one of the most preventable causes of death in trauma and has been implicated as the cause of almost half of hemorrhagic deaths in trauma patients [8, 9].

Previous landmark studies identified iatrogenic and resuscitation-associated causes of coagulopathic bleeding after traumatic injury, of which hypothermia, metabolic acidosis, and dilutional coagulopathy were recognized as primary drivers of bleeding after trauma [9–11]. However, endogenous acute coagulopathy, which occurs within minutes following injury, before and independent of iatrogenic factors, is clearly recognized and accepted as the primary cause of perturbed coagulation after injury [12]. Coagulopathy is present at the time of admission to the emergency department in up to 25–35% of trauma patients [9, 10, 13]. Understanding the pathophysiology of trauma-induced coagulopathy is vitally important, especially with respect to the critical issue of establishing therapeutic strategies for the management of patients with severe trauma [14].

* Correspondence: kussie@emergency-medicine.med.tohoku.ac.jp
[1]Division of Emergency and Critical Care Medicine, Tohoku University Graduate School of Medicine, Seiryo-machi 2-1, Aoba-ku, Sendai, Miyagi 980-8574, Japan
[2]Department of Emergency and Critical Care Medicine, Tohoku University Hospital, Seiryo-machi 1-1, Aoba-ku, Sendai, Miyagi 980-8574, Japan

Coagulopathy in the acute phase of trauma: not a simple dilutional and resuscitation-related coagulopathy

Coagulopathy in the acute phase of trauma has long been known to coexist with severe hemorrhage and has been recognized as a co-phenomenon and unavoidable sequela of resuscitation for patients requiring massive transfusion, and accompanied by hypothermia, metabolic acidosis, and dilutional coagulopathy. However, our understanding of the mechanisms and clinical importance of coagulopathy changed significantly after the identification of an endogenous coagulation abnormality, i.e., acute traumatic coagulopathy (ATC), nearly a decade ago [9, 10]. The presence of this impairment early after trauma has been demonstrated to be an independent predictor for increased organ dysfunction, infection, and overall mortality [15]. Trauma itself and/or traumatic shock can directly induce endogenous ATC, in contrast with the indirect mechanisms such as hypothermia, metabolic acidosis, and dilutional coagulopathy [16–18]. These contributing factors of hemostatic impairment exacerbate ATC and may participate collectively to the clinical features of trauma-induced coagulopathy [16–18]. Acute coagulopathy has recently been identified at admission before trauma resuscitation in one in four trauma patients [10, 13, 19], and is associated with a fourfold increase in mortality [9, 10, 13, 19].

Coagulopathy in the acute phase of trauma patients consists of two core components: (1) trauma itself and/or traumatic shock-induced endogenous ATC and (2) resuscitation-associated coagulopathy [20] (Fig. 1).

Although no consensus has been reached regarding a definition and there are different approaches to the classification and naming of trauma-associated coagulation impairment, in this manuscript, we define ATC as trauma itself (directly trauma-induced) and/or traumatic shock-induced endogenous ATC and trauma-induced coagulopathy as multifactorial trauma-associated coagulation impairment, including ATC and resuscitation-associated coagulopathy associated with hypothermia, metabolic acidosis, and dilutional coagulopathy [11, 18]. Gando and Hayakawa summarized the important components of trauma-induced coagulopathy, consisting of endogenously (trauma- and traumatic shock-induced) primary pathologies and exogenous secondary pathologies (Table 1) [21].

Cap and Hunt classified trauma-associated coagulopathies into three phases [11]. The first phase is immediate activation of multiple hemostatic pathways, with increased fibrinolysis, in association with tissue injury and/or tissue hypoperfusion. The second phase involves therapy-related factors during resuscitation. The third, post-resuscitation, phase is an acute-phase response leading to a prothrombotic state predisposing to venous thromboembolism.

Of these three phases, the first phase corresponds to ATC, and the clinical features of the first phase along with the pathophysiologic factors of the second phase provide the characteristics of trauma-induced coagulopathy (Fig. 2) [22]. Recently, the clinical features and pathophysiology of trauma-induced coagulopathy have been recognized as the comprehensive condition of ATC involving resuscitation-associated coagulopathy, a systemic inflammatory response to tissue injury, and predisposing factors [23]. Currently recommended management lists for the first and second phases based on The European guideline on management of major bleeding and coagulopathy are summarized as Table 2 [24]. It is also recommended that early mechanical thromboprophylaxis

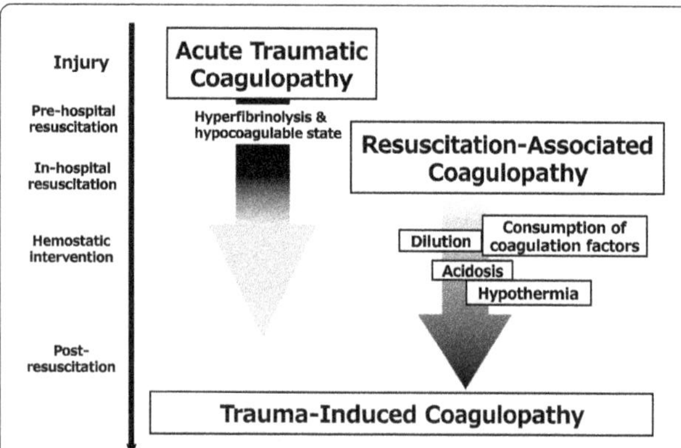

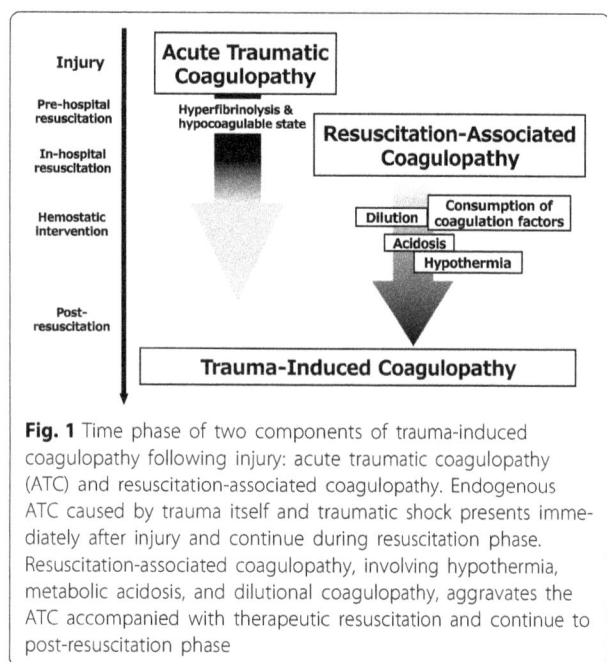

Fig. 1 Time phase of two components of trauma-induced coagulopathy following injury: acute traumatic coagulopathy (ATC) and resuscitation-associated coagulopathy. Endogenous ATC caused by trauma itself and traumatic shock presents immediately after injury and continue during resuscitation phase. Resuscitation-associated coagulopathy, involving hypothermia, metabolic acidosis, and dilutional coagulopathy, aggravates the ATC accompanied with therapeutic resuscitation and continue to post-resuscitation phase

Table 1 Summary of trauma-induced coagulopathy (cited from [21])

1 Physiological changes
- Hemostasis and wound healing

2 Pathological changes
- Endogenously induced primary pathologies
  - o Disseminated intravascular coagulation (DIC)
    - Activation of coagulation
    - Insufficient anticoagulation mechanisms
    - Increased fibrin(ogen)olysis (early phase)
    - Suppression of fibrinolysis (late phase)
    - Consumption coagulopathy
  - o Acute coagulopathy trauma-shock (ACOTS)
    - Activated protein C-mediated suppression of coagulation
    - Activated protein C-mediated increased fibrinolysis
- Exogenously induced secondary pathologies that modify DIC and ACOTS
  - o Anemia-induced coagulopathy
  - o Hypothermia-induced coagulopathy
  - o Acidosis-induced coagulopathy
  - o Dilutional coagulopathy
  - o Others

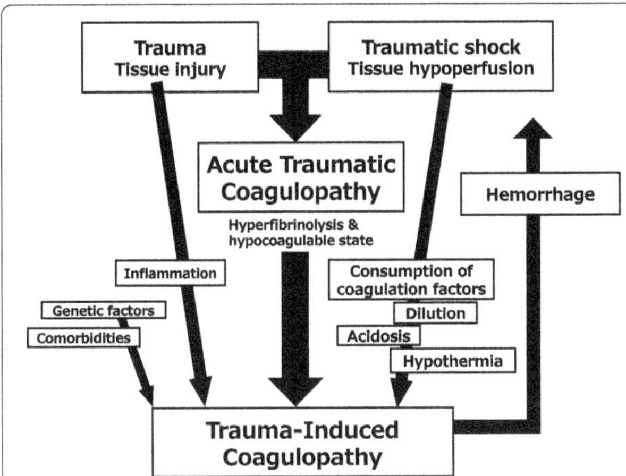

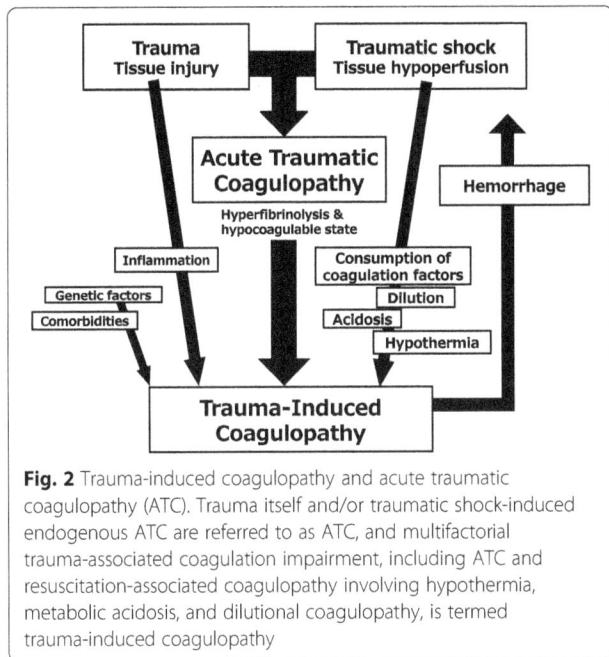

Fig. 2 Trauma-induced coagulopathy and acute traumatic coagulopathy (ATC). Trauma itself and/or traumatic shock-induced endogenous ATC are referred to as ATC, and multifactorial trauma-associated coagulation impairment, including ATC and resuscitation-associated coagulopathy involving hypothermia, metabolic acidosis, and dilutional coagulopathy, is termed trauma-induced coagulopathy

Table 2 Currently recommended management for trauma-induced coagulopathy (cited from [24] with modification)

Initial assessment and management
Extent of traumatic hemorrhage assessed
Patient in shock with identified source of bleeding treated immediately
Patient in shock with unidentified source of bleeding sent for further investigation
Coagulation, hematocrit, serum lactate, base deficit assessed
Antifibrinolytic therapy (tranexamic acid within 3 h after injury) initiated
Patient history of anticoagulant therapy assessed
Resuscitation
Systolic blood pressure of 80–90 mmHg achieved in absence of traumatic brain injury
Measures to achieve normothermia implemented
Target hemoglobin level 7–9 g/dl achieved
Surgical intervention
Damage control surgery performed in hemodynamically unstable patient
Coagulation management
Massive transfusion protocol with high plasma: red blood cell ratio employed
Target fibrinogen level 1.5–2 g/l achieved
Target platelet level achieved
Prothrombin complex concentrate administered if indicated due to vitamin K antagonist, oral anticoagulant or evidence from viscoelastic monitoring

with intermittent pneumatic compression or anti-embolic stockings followed by pharmacological thromboprophylaxis within 24 h after bleeding has been controlled [24].

Pathophysiology of ATC and its clinical impact on patients with severe trauma

Although the pathophysiology of coagulation impairment in the acute phase of trauma has not yet been elucidated, ATC plays a pivotal role. It has been repeatedly demonstrated that ATC is a frequent complication in patients with severe trauma [9, 10, 13, 25].

Clinical features of ATC

ATC that is caused by trauma-induced tissue injury and/or traumatic shock (generalized tissue hypoperfusion) presents as systemic activation of coagulation responses associated with increased fibrinolysis [19, 26, 27]. The clinical features of ATC can be summarized as follows [11, 18, 28–30]:

- Increased activation of coagulation (as a background pathophysiologic characteristic) leading to uncontrolled coagulation
- Coagulation impairment secondary to coagulation factor deficiency (consumption coagulopathy) leading to a hypocoagulable state
- Increased fibrin(ogen)olysis

The increased fibrin(ogen)olysis constitutes the most prominent feature of ATC.

Clinical impact of ATC

Coagulopathy in trauma patients is associated with higher transfusion requirements, longer intensive care unit and hospital stays, prolonged mechanical ventilation support, and a greater incidence of multiple organ dysfunction. Compared with patients without coagulopathy, those with coagulopathy have a three- to fourfold greater mortality and up to eight times higher mortality within the initial 24 h of injury [9, 10, 31, 32].

Mechanisms of ATC

It has been argued that activated protein C plays a central role in the mechanism of ATC. In initial observations in trauma patients with systemic hypoperfusion, defined by an elevated base deficit, a correlation was found between ATC and increased levels of activated protein C, reduced levels of protein C, and elevated soluble thrombomodulin [31]. The activation of the thrombomodulin-protein C system has been suggested as a principle pathway mediating ATC, characterized as hyperfibrinolysis and a hypocoagulable state, and this proposed mechanism is distinct from clotting factor consumption or dysfunction [31, 33].

However, authors only speculated increase in the levels of activated protein C based on the lower levels of protein C. The precise pathophysiologic mechanisms are still under investigation. Other mechanisms have been suggested and may contribute to this pathologic condition [34, 35].

ATC is mediated by dysregulated activation of the thrombomodulin-protein C system

Physiologic response to tissue injury by the thrombomodulin-protein C system

In physiologic conditions, tissue injury leads to thrombin generation and fibrin and clot formation through the extrinsic coagulation pathway. Although the clotting process is initially localized at the site of injury, systemic activation of coagulation secondary to the escape of thrombin from the injury site is inhibited by circulating antithrombin or by the binding of thrombin to constitutively expressed thrombomodulin on intact endothelial cells [36]. Protein C is converted from an inactive to an active form by the complex of thrombin with thrombomodulin on the endothelial cell surface. Activated protein C serves a protective function to maintain tissue perfusion by inhibiting thrombosis through inactivation of factors Va and VIIIa and inhibiting plasminogen activator inhibitor-1 (PAI-1) during periods of decreased flow [33, 37].

Tissue hypoperfusion due to traumatic shock and activation of protein C

Sustained tissue hypoperfusion is associated with elevated levels of soluble thrombomodulin secondary to endothelial damage, which can increase the availability of thrombomodulin to bound thrombin [31]. As a result of complex formation with thrombomodulin, the role of thrombin can be diverted from procoagulant to anticoagulant by excess activation of protein C [31, 38]. This hypothetical condition has been named acute coagulopathy of trauma-shock (ACOTS) [39, 40]. Although the precise pathophysiology remains to be elucidated, these mechanisms may lead to the hyperfibrinolytic state in patients with ATC, which is reflected in increased tissue plasminogen activator (t-PA), decreased PAI, and increased D-dimer levels [31, 33].

ATC as disseminated intravascular coagulation with a fibrinolytic phenotype

Disseminated intravascular coagulation (DIC) is characterized by activation of the tissue factor-dependent coagulation pathway and insufficient anticoagulant mechanisms, leading to consumption of platelets and coagulation factors and associated with coagulopathic clinical features [41–43]. The Scientific and Standardization Committee (SSC) on DIC of the International Society on Thrombosis and Haemostasis (ISTH) defined DIC as follows: DIC is an acquired syndrome characterized by the intravascular activation of coagulation with loss of localization arising from different causes. It can originate from and cause damage to the microvasculature, which, if sufficiently severe, can produce organ dysfunction. The most important points of the definition of DIC are "intravascular activation of coagulation with loss of localization" and "damage to the microvasculature", which means thrombin generation and its activation in the circulation and extensive damage to the microvascular endothelium give rise to insufficient coagulation control [18, 44].

Although there is no consensus regarding the classification of the pathophysiology and clinical features of DIC, it may be divided into fibrinolytic and antifibrinolytic phenotypes [41–43]. The characteristics of ATC are essentially the same as DIC with the fibrinolytic phenotype, which contributes to massive bleeding and patients' prognoses [45, 46]. DIC in the late phase of trauma is a thrombotic phenotype, which can be complicated with the development of multiple organ dysfunction syndrome [43, 47, 48].

The synergistic activation of primary and secondary fibrin(ogen)olysis causes DIC with the fibrinolytic phenotype [42, 46], whereas both depression of the inhibitory system of coagulation and PAI-1-mediated inhibition of fibrinolysis cause DIC with the thrombotic phenotype [41, 42].

The Scientific and Standardization Committee on DIC of ISTH commented on two concepts regarding the hemostatic changes occurring early after trauma: DIC with the fibrinolytic phenotype and coagulopathy of trauma (COT) and ACOTS. Although there are differences between these two conditions and more information is needed to elucidate the pathogenesis of these entities, it has been suggested that COT/ACOTS is not a new concept but a disease entity similar to or the same as DIC with the fibrinolytic phenotype [49].

Acute traumatic coagulopathy may not be a DIC

DIC is defined as a clinicopathologic syndrome characterized by widespread activation of coagulation resulting in intravascular formation of fibrin and thrombotic occlusion of vessels [50, 51]. Almost all severely traumatized patients, especially those with ATC, are diagnosed as having DIC according to the scoring systems of the ISTH and Japanese Association for Acute Medicine [48, 52, 53]. However, no anatomopathologic evidence, e.g., intravascular formation of fibrin and thrombotic occlusion of vessels, has been demonstrated, and consumption coagulopathy leading to platelet and coagulation factor deficiency is not a common finding in patients with ATC [27].

Rizoli and colleagues reported the relationship between a clinical diagnosis of DIC using the ISTH score and pathologic findings in a prospective observational cohort study of severely injured patients (injury severity score ≥16) [53]. All organs surgically removed within 24 h of trauma were reviewed by two independent pathologists. All autopsy reports were also reviewed. Because D-dimer levels have a disproportional influence in trauma DIC scores, most patients have DIC scores that indicate overt DIC or are suggestive of DIC within 24 h of trauma. However, decreased platelet counts, fibrinogen levels, clotting times, and factor VIII levels were not evident. In addition, no anatomopathologic evidence of DIC was identified in the first 24 h, even after additional histochemical staining, in 40 excised organs and 27 autopsy reports.

Although diffuse intravascular fibrin formation and deficiencies in coagulation factors are suggested to be specific findings for DIC, these clinical and pathologic features were not observed in patients with ATC. Therefore, the pathophysiologic mechanism of ATC has been emphasized as being different from that of DIC [13, 27, 41, 54]. However, thrombin generation with marked decrease in fibrinogen and D-dimer elevation was observed [13, 27, 41, 54], suggested to be consistent with the pathophysiology of DIC.

DIC with the fibrinolytic phenotype as a pathophysiologic mechanism for ATC has been definitively denied by researchers emphasizing activation of the thrombomodulin-protein C system as a principle pathway mediating ATC [43]. Some researchers suggested that ATC is not a DIC because there is no clear evidence of diffuse anatomopathologic intravascular fibrin deposition and also because the "DIC hypothesis with a fibrinolytic phenotype" is a confusion of terms and should be abandoned. They suggested that a state in which fibrinolytic activity exceeds the capacity of the hemostatic system to make stable clots, resulting in excess or uncontrolled hemorrhage, should be termed systemic activation of fibrinolysis with poor hemostasis [27]. However, they misunderstand the concept of DIC, leading to inappropriate conclusion. DIC is intravascular activation of coagulation with loss of localization and damage to the microvasculature, which means thrombin generation, not fibrin clot formation and its activation in the circulation and extensive damage to the microvascular endothelium that give rise to insufficient coagulation control [18, 44].

Trauma-induced coagulopathy, especially ATC, is a dynamic entity that evolves over time, and it has been suggested that no single hypothesis explains the different manifestations of coagulopathy [27]. Many problematic issues have been suggested regarding the activation of the thrombomodulin-protein C system mechanism, and a pathophysiologic overlap with DIC has also been proposed in recent reviews [18, 55].

Pathophysiologic mechanism of increased fibrinolysis in ATC

ATC presents as systemic activation of coagulation associated with increased fibrinolysis [19, 26, 27], and the increased fibrin(ogen)olysis is the most characteristic feature.

Thrombin is a central molecule in hemostasis. Thrombin generation converts fibrinogen to fibrin, resulting in fibrin strand formation, and activates platelets, leukocytes, and endothelium. However, thrombin also stimulates the production of t-PA from the endothelium, an effect previously known as secondary fibrinolysis. Stimulation of t-PA release from the endothelium by other factors such as hypoxia, adrenaline, and vasopressin is known as primary fibrinolysis [11]. Traumatic shock-induced tissue hypoperfusion has also been demonstrated to promote the production of t-PA from the endothelium, and increased t-PA levels have been reported in coagulopathic trauma patients [42, 56].

Additionally, it has been demonstrated that fibrin(ogen)olysis is accelerated by α2-plasmin inhibitor deficiency secondary to increased plasmin production [30]. These multiple factors are suggested to contribute to the fibrinolytic status in patients with severe trauma.

The critical point in the pathogenesis of fibrinolysis in patients with ATC is the difference in timing of onset between the immediate t-PA release from the endothelium and later expression of PAI-1 mRNA, which results in an extreme imbalance of these molecules [43, 57, 58]. The difference of several hours may play an important role in the fibrinolytic condition. This difference in timing is supported by the findings that the levels of PAI-1 are identical immediately after trauma in almost all severely traumatized patients regardless the diagnosis of DIC, whereas the levels of t-PA and plasmin generation were both significantly increased in patients diagnosed as having DIC [41, 59–61].

Conclusions

Exsanguinating hemorrhage is the most common preventable cause of death after trauma [7, 62, 63]. Many of these deaths occur within the first few hours of definitive care, with coagulopathy playing a major role. A widespread paradigm shift in the resuscitation of critically injured patients with hemorrhagic shock has changed the management of severe trauma from a definitive surgical approach to damage control surgery during the past two decades [7, 62, 63]. Rewarming efforts, early correction of acidosis, and aggressive crystalloid resuscitation in patients requiring damage control surgery have been the prime tenets of a trauma resuscitation strategy. This focus on early correction of physiologic abnormalities has prompted the era of damage control surgery [17, 20, 23, 64–68]. However, improvement of clinical outcomes in patients requiring damage control surgery, even accompanied by aggressive correction of physiologic derangements, is still insufficient.

Although trauma-induced coagulopathy, consisting of ATC and resuscitation-associated coagulopathy, is multifactorial, it is definitively the most important issue for the management of severe trauma patients. Damage control surgery accompanied by sophisticated damage control resuscitation [17, 69, 70], including hypotensive/hypovolemic resuscitation and hemostatic resuscitation based on an understanding of the pathophysiology of ATC and trauma-induced coagulopathy, must be the central theme of the management of severely traumatized patients with ATC.

Abbreviations

ACOTS: Acute coagulopathy of trauma-shock; ATC: Acute traumatic coagulopathy; COT: Coagulopathy of trauma; DIC: Disseminated intravascular coagulation; ISTH: International Society of Thrombosis and Haemostasis; PAI: Plasminogen activator inhibitor; t-PA: Tissue plasminogen activator

Acknowledgements

The authors are grateful to Satoshi Akaishi, Takashi Irinoda, Takeaki Sato, Ryosuke Nomura, and Noriko Miyagawa for their support in review and drafting the article for important intellectual content.

Funding

This study was supported by the fund of Tohoku Kyuikai and departmental fund of the Division of Emergency and Critical Care Medicine, Tohoku University Graduate School of Medicine.

Authors' contributions

SK conducted the article search and drafted the manuscript. All authors substantially contributed to the conception of the review and drafting or critically revising the article for important intellectual content. All authors finally approved the version to be published.

Competing interests

The authors declare that they have no competing interests.

References

1. Mathers CD, Loncar D. Projections of global mortality and burden of disease from 2002 to 2030. PLoS Med. 2006;3:e442.
2. Holcomb JB, Tilley BC, Baraniuk S, et al. Transfusion of plasma, platelets, and red blood cells in a 1:1:1 vs a 1:1:2 ratio and mortality in patients with severe trauma: the PROPPR randomized clinical trial. JAMA. 2015;313:471–82.
3. Sauaia A, Moore FA, Moore EE, Haenel JB, Read RA, Lezotte DC. Early predictors of postinjury multiple organ failure. Arch Surg. 1994;129:39–45.
4. Diaz Jr JJ, Dutton WD, Ott MM, et al. Eastern Association for the Surgery of Trauma: a review of the management of the open abdomen—part 2 "Management of the open abdomen". J Trauma. 2011;71:502–12.
5. Diaz Jr JJ, Cullinane DC, Dutton WD, et al. The management of the open abdomen in trauma and emergency general surgery: part 1—damage control. J Trauma. 2010;68:1425–38.
6. Gruen RL, Jurkovich GJ, McIntyre LK, Foy HM, Maier RV. Patterns of errors contributing to trauma mortality: lessons learned from 2,594 deaths. Ann Surg. 2006;244:371–80.
7. Wyrzykowski AD, Feliciano DV. Trauma damage control. In: Feliciano DVMK, Moore EE, editors. Trauma 7th edition. 7th ed. New York: McGraw-Hill; 2013. p. 725–46.
8. Duchesne JC, McSwain Jr NE, Cotton BA, et al. Damage control resuscitation: the new face of damage control. J Trauma. 2010;69:976–90.
9. MacLeod JB, Lynn M, McKenney MG, Cohn SM, Murtha M. Early coagulopathy predicts mortality in trauma. J Trauma. 2003;55:39–44.
10. Brohi K, Singh J, Heron M, Coats T. Acute traumatic coagulopathy. J Trauma. 2003;54:1127–30.
11. Cap A, Hunt B. Acute traumatic coagulopathy. Curr Opin Crit Care. 2014;20:638–45.
12. Floccard B, Rugeri L, Faure A, et al. Early coagulopathy in trauma patients: an on-scene and hospital admission study. Injury. 2012;43:26–32.
13. Maegele M, Lefering R, Yucel N, et al. Early coagulopathy in multiple injury: an analysis from the German Trauma Registry on 8724 patients. Injury. 2007; 38:298–304.
14. Brohi K. Diagnosis and management of coagulopathy after major trauma. Br J Surg. 2009;96:963–4.
15. Cohen MJ, Call M, Nelson M, et al. Critical role of activated protein C in early coagulopathy and later organ failure, infection and death in trauma patients. Ann Surg. 2012;255:379–85.
16. Geeraedts Jr LM, Demiral H, Schaap NP, Kamphuisen PW, Pompe JC, Frolke JP. 'Blind' transfusion of blood products in exsanguinating trauma patients. Resuscitation. 2007;73:382–8.
17. Holcomb JB, Jenkins D, Rhee P, et al. Damage control resuscitation: directly addressing the early coagulopathy of trauma. J Trauma. 2007;62:307–10.
18. Gando S, Otomo Y. Local hemostasis, immunothrombosis, and systemic disseminated intravascular coagulation in trauma and traumatic shock. Crit Care. 2015;19:72.
19. Frith D, Goslings JC, Gaarder C, et al. Definition and drivers of acute traumatic coagulopathy: clinical and experimental investigations. J Thromb Haemost. 2010;8:1919–25.
20. Kutcher ME, Kornblith LZ, Narayan R, et al. A paradigm shift in trauma resuscitation: evaluation of evolving massive transfusion practices. JAMA Surg. 2013;148:834–40.
21. Gando S, Hayakawa M. Pathophysiology of trauma-induced coagulopathy and management of critical bleeding requiring massive transfusion. Semin Thromb Hemost. 2016;42:155–65.
22. Davenport R, Khan S. Management of major trauma haemorrhage: treatment priorities and controversies. Br J Haematol. 2011;155:537–48.
23. Spahn DR, Bouillon B, Cerny V, et al. Management of bleeding and coagulopathy following major trauma: an updated European guideline. Crit Care. 2013;17:R76.
24. Rossaint R, Bouillon B, Cerny V, et al. The European guideline on management of major bleeding and coagulopathy following trauma: fourth edition. Crit Care. 2016;20:100.
25. Davenport RA, Brohi K. Cause of trauma-induced coagulopathy. Curr Opin Anaesthesiol. 2016;29:212–9.
26. Cohen MJ, Kutcher M, Redick B, et al. Clinical and mechanistic drivers of acute traumatic coagulopathy. J Trauma Acute Care Surg. 2013;75:S40–7.
27. Dobson GP, Letson HL, Sharma R, Sheppard FR, Cap AP. Mechanisms of early trauma-induced coagulopathy: the clot thickens or not? J Trauma Acute Care Surg. 2015;79:301–9.
28. Kashuk JL, Moore EE, Sawyer M, et al. Primary fibrinolysis is integral in the pathogenesis of the acute coagulopathy of trauma. Ann Surg. 2010;252: 434–42. discussion 43-4.
29. Kutcher ME, Ferguson AR, Cohen MJ. A principal component analysis of coagulation after trauma. J Trauma Acute Care Surg. 2013;74:1223–9. discussion 9-30.
30. Raza I, Davenport R, Rourke C, et al. The incidence and magnitude of fibrinolytic activation in trauma patients. J Thromb Haemost. 2013;11:307–14.
31. Brohi K, Cohen MJ, Ganter MT, Matthay MA, Mackersie RC, Pittet JF. Acute traumatic coagulopathy: initiated by hypoperfusion: modulated through the protein C pathway? Ann Surg. 2007;245:812–8.
32. Niles SE, McLaughlin DF, Perkins JG, et al. Increased mortality associated with the early coagulopathy of trauma in combat casualties. J Trauma. 2008; 64:1459–63. discussion 63-5.
33. Chesebro BB, Rahn P, Carles M, et al. Increase in activated protein C mediates acute traumatic coagulopathy in mice. Shock. 2009;32:659–65.
34. Campbell JE, Meledeo MA, Cap AP. Comparative response of platelet fV and plasma fV to activated protein C and relevance to a model of acute traumatic coagulopathy. PLoS One. 2014;9:e99181.
35. Jesmin S, Gando S, Wada T, Hayakawa M, Sawamura A. Activated protein C does not increase in the early phase of trauma with disseminated intravascular coagulation: comparison with acute coagulopathy of trauma-shock. J Intensive Care. 2016;4:1.

36. Cadroy Y, Diquelou A, Dupouy D, et al. The thrombomodulin/protein C/protein S anticoagulant pathway modulates the thrombogenic properties of the normal resting and stimulated endothelium. Arterioscler Thromb Vasc Biol. 1997;17:520–7.
37. Esmon CT. Protein C, pathway in sepsis. Ann Med. 2002;34:598–605.
38. Rezaie AR. Vitronectin functions as a cofactor for rapid inhibition of activated protein C by plasminogen activator inhibitor-1. Implications for the mechanism of profibrinolytic action of activated protein C. J Biol Chem. 2001;276:15567–70.
39. Bouillon B, Brohi K, Hess JR, Holcomb JB, Parr MJ, Hoyt DB. Educational initiative on critical bleeding in trauma: Chicago, July 11-13, 2008. J Trauma. 2010;68:225–30.
40. Hess JR, Brohi K, Dutton RP, et al. The coagulopathy of trauma: a review of mechanisms. J Trauma. 2008;65:748–54.
41. Maegele M, Schochl H, Cohen MJ. An update on the coagulopathy of trauma. Shock. 2014;41 Suppl 1:21–5.
42. Marder VJFD, Colman RW, Levi M. Consumptive thrombohemorrhagic disorders. In: Colman RWMV, Clowes AW, George JN, Goldhaber SZ, editors. Hemostasis and thrombosis basic principles and clinical practice. 5th ed. Philadelphia: Lippincott Williams & Wilkins; 2006. p. 1571–600.
43. Levi M, ten Cate H, van der Poll T, van Deventer SJ. Pathogenesis of disseminated intravascular coagulation in sepsis. JAMA. 1993;270:975–9.
44. Taylor Jr FB, Toh CH, Hoots WK, Wada H, Levi M. Towards definition, clinical and laboratory criteria, and a scoring system for disseminated intravascular coagulation. Thromb Haemost. 2001;86:1327–30.
45. Sawamura A, Hayakawa M, Gando S, et al. Disseminated intravascular coagulation with a fibrinolytic phenotype at an early phase of trauma predicts mortality. Thromb Res. 2009;124:608–13.
46. Gando S, Wada H, Kim HK, et al. Comparison of disseminated intravascular coagulation in trauma with coagulopathy of trauma/acute coagulopathy of trauma-shock. J Thromb Haemost. 2012;10:2593–5.
47. Gando S. Disseminated intravascular coagulation in trauma patients. Semin Thromb Hemost. 2001;27:585–92.
48. Gando S. Acute coagulopathy of trauma shock and coagulopathy of trauma: a rebuttal. You are now going down the wrong path. J Trauma. 2009;67:381–3.
49. Gando S, Wada H, Thachil J, Scientific, Standardization Committee on DICotISoT, Haemostasis. Differentiating disseminated intravascular coagulation (DIC) with the fibrinolytic phenotype from coagulopathy of trauma and acute coagulopathy of trauma-shock (COT/ACOTS). J Thromb Haemost. 2013;11:826–35.
50. Levi M. Disseminated intravascular coagulation. Crit Care Med. 2007;35:2191–5.
51. Levi M, Ten Cate H. Disseminated intravascular coagulation. N Engl J Med. 1999;341:586–92.
52. Hayakawa M, Sawamura A, Gando S, et al. Disseminated intravascular coagulation at an early phase of trauma is associated with consumption coagulopathy and excessive fibrinolysis both by plasmin and neutrophil elastase. Surgery. 2011;149:221–30.
53. Rizoli S, Nascimento Jr B, Key N, et al. Disseminated intravascular coagulopathy in the first 24 hours after trauma: the association between ISTH score and anatomopathologic evidence. J Trauma. 2011;71:S441–7.
54. Maegele M, Lefering R, Wafaisade A, et al. Revalidation and update of the TASH-Score: a scoring system to predict the probability for massive transfusion as a surrogate for life-threatening haemorrhage after severe injury. Vox Sang. 2011;100:231–8.
55. Coagulopathy associated with trauma. 2016. (at https://www.uptodate.com/contents/coagulopathy-associated-with-trauma?source=search_result&search=Coagulopathy%20associated%20with%20trauma&selectedTitle=1~150. Accessed 14 Mar 2016)
56. Lowenstein CJ, Morrell CN, Yamakuchi M. Regulation of Weibel-Palade body exocytosis. Trends Cardiovasc Med. 2005;15:302–8.
57. Gando S, Kameue T, Nanzaki S, Nakanishi Y. Massive fibrin formation with consecutive impairment of fibrinolysis in patients with out-of-hospital cardiac arrest. Thromb Haemost. 1997;77:278–82.
58. Stump DC, Taylor Jr FB, Nesheim ME, Giles AR, Dzik WH, Bovill EG. Pathologic fibrinolysis as a cause of clinical bleeding. Semin Thromb Hemost. 1990;16:260–73.
59. Gando S, Nakanishi Y, Tedo I. Cytokines and plasminogen activator inhibitor-1 in posttrauma disseminated intravascular coagulation: relationship to multiple organ dysfunction syndrome. Crit Care Med. 1995;23:1835–42.
60. Gando S, Tedo I, Kubota M. Posttrauma coagulation and fibrinolysis. Crit Care Med. 1992;20:594–600.
61. Yanagida Y, Gando S, Sawamura A, et al. Normal prothrombinase activity, increased systemic thrombin activity, and lower antithrombin levels in patients with disseminated intravascular coagulation at an early phase of trauma: comparison with acute coagulopathy of trauma-shock. Surgery. 2013;154:48–57.
62. Raeburn CD, Moore EE, Biffl WL, et al. The abdominal compartment syndrome is a morbid complication of postinjury damage control surgery. Am J Surg. 2001;182:542–6.
63. Nagy KK, Fildes JJ, Mahr C, et al. Experience with three prosthetic materials in temporary abdominal wall closure. Am Surg. 1996;62:331–5.
64. Borgman MA, Spinella PC, Perkins JG, et al. The ratio of blood products transfused affects mortality in patients receiving massive transfusions at a combat support hospital. J Trauma. 2007;63:805–13.
65. Murad MH, Stubbs JR, Gandhi MJ, et al. The effect of plasma transfusion on morbidity and mortality: a systematic review and meta-analysis. Transfusion. 2010;50:1370–83.
66. Cotton BA, Reddy N, Hatch QM, et al. Damage control resuscitation is associated with a reduction in resuscitation volumes and improvement in survival in 390 damage control laparotomy patients. Ann Surg. 2011;254:598–605.
67. Duchesne JC, Kimonis K, Marr AB, et al. Damage control resuscitation in combination with damage control laparotomy: a survival advantage. J Trauma. 2010;69:46–52.
68. Undurraga Perl VJ, Leroux B, Cook MR, et al. Damage control resuscitation and emergency laparotomy: findings from the PROPPR study. J Trauma Acute Care Surg. 2016;80:568–74.
69. Duchesne JC, Islam TM, Stuke L, et al. Hemostatic resuscitation during surgery improves survival in patients with traumatic-induced coagulopathy. J Trauma. 2009;67:33–7. discussion 7-9.
70. Holcomb JB, Wade CE, Michalek JE, et al. Increased plasma and platelet to red blood cell ratios improves outcome in 466 massively transfused civilian trauma patients. Ann Surg. 2008;248:447–58.

4

The impact of changes in intensive care organization on patient outcome and cost-effectiveness

Alexander F. van der Sluijs[1], Eline R. van Slobbe-Bijlsma[2], Stephen E. Chick[3], Margreeth B. Vroom[1], Dave A. Dongelmans[1] and Alexander P. J. Vlaar[1,3*]

Abstract

The mortality rate of critically ill patients is high and the cost of the intensive (ICU) department is among the highest within the health-care industry. The cost will continue to increase because of the aging population in the western world. In the present review, we will discuss the impact of changes in ICU department organization on patient outcome and cost-effectiveness. The general perception that drug and treatment discoveries are the main drivers behind improved patient outcome within the health-care industry is in general not true. This is especially the case for the ICU department, in which the past decades' organizational changes were the main drivers behind the reduction of ICU mortality. These interventions were at the same time able to reduce cost, something which is rare for drug and treatment discoveries. The organization of the intensive care department has been changed over the past decades, resulting in better patient outcome and reduction of cost. Major changes are the implementation of the "closed format" and electronic patient record. Furthermore, we will present possible future options to improve the organization of the ICU department to further reduce mortality and cost such as pooling of dedicated ICU into mixed ICU and embedding business strategies such as lean and total quality management. Challenges are ahead as the ICU is taking up the largest share of national health-care expenditure, and with the aging of the population, this will continue to increase. Besides future improvements of organizational structures within the ICU, the focus should also be on the implementation of and compliance with proven beneficial organizational structures.

Keywords: Intensive care department, Critically ill, Lean, Management, Organization, Total quality management, Six Sigma, Pooling, Closed and open format

Background

Intensive care units (ICUs) are among the most complex and expensive departments in a hospital. The innate complexity of the ICU makes organizational structuring of care an attractive target for performance improvement strategies. One improvement in the past is assigning "intensivists" (specialists in critical care medicine) in managing ICU patients instead of specialists from the referral medical departments, which is also called "closed format" ICU departments. This closed format transformation has shown a beneficial impact on patient outcomes in a number of studies [1–3]. However, due to an aging population and the increasing acuity of illness of hospitalized patients, both the total number of ICU patients and their proportional share of hospital admissions overall are expected to keep growing [4]. Furthermore, although mortality rates have significantly reduced after assigning intensivists to these patients, mortality rates are still relatively high, at up to 28% for a general ICU population [5]. This implies that additional improvements in survival of patients and cost-effectiveness of the ICU departments are necessary. In the present review, an overview will be given on changes in organizational models in the ICU departments in the past and their impact on quality of patient care and cost. Furthermore, possible future improvements will be discussed.

* Correspondence: a.p.vlaar@amc.uva.nl
[1]Department of Intensive Care Medicine, Academic Medical Center, Room C3-343, Meibergdreef 9, Amsterdam 1105 AZ, The Netherlands
[3]INSEAD Healthcare Management Initiative, INSEAD, Fontainebleau, France
Full list of author information is available at the end of the article

Methods—systematic search of the literature

The Medline database was used to identify Medical Subject Headings (MeSH) to select search terms. In addition to MeSH terms, we also used free-text words. Search terms referred to aspects of the ICU organization ("Intensive Care department", "organization", "management", "staffing") as well as related topics ("cost reduction", "patient outcome", "lean", "Toyota", "total quality management", "Toyota Production System", and "monitoring"). Relevance of each paper was assessed using the online abstracts. In addition, the reference lists of retrieved papers were screened for potentially important papers.

The cost of intensive care health-care services

The intensive care department is the most expensive hospital department. In the US alone, annual critical care medicine costs nearly doubled from 2000 to 2010 (from $56.6 to an estimated amount of $108 billion). Although the proportion of hospital cost allocated to critical care medicine (13.2%) decreased by 1.5% and the proportion of national health expenditures (4.14%) remained stable, the proportion of the gross domestic product used by critical care medicine increased from 0.66% in 2005 to 0.74% in 2010 [6, 7]. In highly developed European health-care systems, the average cost per ICU patient is around €1200 per day and €17,000 per admission [8, 9]. The main drivers of cost are personnel cost followed by infrastructure and pharmaceutical expenditure. This illustrates that reduction of cost should be aimed at the improvement of the utilization of personnel, processes, and infrastructure. We will now discuss the interventions in the past on organizational structures in the ICU department and the impact on patient outcome and cost.

The impact of the intensivist

Closed format vs. open format

In the early days of the ICU, patients admitted to the ICU were treated by the referring physicians. Although referring physicians had extensive knowledge on the specific disease the patient was suffering from, there was a lack of knowledge concerning the intensive care treatment these patients needed. Another issue was the lack of continuity of care for these critically ill patients, as the referring physicians were not providing 7-day-per-week coverage of care. This issue was recognized in the 1990s and resulted in the development of the "Leapfrog initiative" [10]. In short, the Leapfrog initiative proposed that the "intensivist" (specialists in critical care medicine) is present in the ICU during the daytime hours 7 days/week, with no other clinical duties during this time. Hence, the intensivist was assigned to manage ICU patients rather than specialists from the referral medical departments. This closed format transformation has shown a beneficial impact on patient outcomes in a number of studies (see Table 1). A systematic review on the effect of physician staffing on the ICU showed that the assignment of intensivist to the ICU led to an overall 0.61 relative risk (RR) (95%CI 0.50–0.75) reduction of ICU mortality [11]. Furthermore, the assignment of intensivists in some studies led to a reduction of intensive care stay and hospital stay, and, subsequently, a

Table 1 The impact of the intensivist on patient outcome and cost in the adult intensive care unit

Reference	Country	Design	Population	Year	Reduction in ICU LOS	Reduction in hospital LOS	Reduction in hospital mortality	Reduction in cost
Multz [1]	USA	Prospective	Medical	1998	Yes, <0.0001	Yes, <0.01	No	n/a
Dimick [2]	USA	Retrospective	Surgical	1994–1998	n/a	Yes, <0.05[a]	Yes, <0.001	Yes, 61%
Carson [3]	USA	Prospective	Medical	1996	No	No	No	n/a
Li [4]	USA	Retrospective	Mixed	1984	No	n/a	Yes, 0.01[a]	n/a
Reynolds [5]	USA	Retrospective	Medical	1986–1988	No	No	Yes, <0.01[a]	n/a
Brown [6]	Canada	Retrospective	Mixed	1984–1986	n/a	n/a	Yes, <0.01[a]	n/a
Manthous [7]	USA	Retrospective	Medical	1992–1994	Yes, <0.05	Yes, <0.05	Yes, 0.002[a]	n/a
Pronovost [8]	USA	Retrospective	Surgical	1994–1996	Yes, <0.05[a]	Yes, <0.05[a]	Yes, 0.05[a]	n/a
Baldock [9]	UK	Prospective	Mixed	1995–1998	n/a	n/a	Yes, 0.001	n/a
Rosenfeld [10]	USA	Prospective	Surgical	1996–1997	Yes, <0.01	No	Yes, 0.008[a]	Yes, 36%
Diringer [11]	USA	Retrospective	Neuro	1996–1999	Yes, <0.05	Yes, <0.05	Yes, 0.001	n/a
Blunt [12]	UK	Retrospective	Medical	2000	No	No	Yes, 0.001[a]	n/a
Hanson [13]	USA	Retrospective	Surgical	1994–1995	Yes, <0.05	Yes, <0.05	No	Yes, not quantified
Ghorra [14]	USA	Retrospective	Surgical	1996	No	n/a	n/a	n/a
Tai [15]	Singapore	Prospective	Medical	1993–1994	Yes, 0.01	No	n/a	n/a

ICU intensive care unit, *LOS* length of stay, *USA* United States of America, *n/a* not applicable

[a]Remains significant after adjustment for baseline disease severity

reduction of costs. Of interest, the reduction of cost was only reported in 3 out of 15 studies and suggested a 36 to 61% reduction. Overall, it can be suggested that a closed format staffing is preferable above a traditional ICU staffing. In line with this, the Critical Care Societies recommend the closed format above the "open format." Although it is recommended, the closed format is still not implemented widely which may be caused by a shortage of intensivists [12, 13].

Twenty-four-hour availability of the intensivist

The positive effect of the closed format intensive care staffing on patient outcome, length of stay, and cost raised the question whether a 24-h availability of an intensivist would even further improve these results compared to having only an in-house intensivist during office hours. This hypothesis was supported by a study on the neonatal ICU showing mortality reduction among premature neonates admitted when they introduced a neonatologist or neonatal fellow in-house [14]. Another supportive finding was that patients with an acute condition admitted during weekends have worse outcomes than patients with the same diagnoses admitted during the week [15]. Other studies showed that having a 24-h mandatory staffing presence in the ICU further improves processes of care and staff satisfaction and decreases ICU complication rate and hospital length of stay (LOS) [16]. A recent study showed, however, that the beneficial impact of 24-h staffing on mortality reduction is only present in an open format ICU and absent in a closed format staffing ICU [17]. This notion is supported in a randomized trial conducted in an academic medical ICU in the USA, showing no significant effect of nighttime staffing on the length of stay or on ICU mortality compared to day and evening time intensivist staffing [18]. One may question whether it is cost-effective for a closed format ICU as mortality reduction was not present and 24-h staffing will increase personnel expenditure.

Intensivist-to-bed ratio

Intensivist specialists are scarce recourses and should be utilized as high as possible. For this reason, Dara et al. looked at the optimal intensivist-to-bed ratio [19]. Four time periods based on intensivist-to-ICU-bed ratios of 1:7.5, 1:9.5, 1:12, and 1:15 were identified. Patients in all time periods did not differ on disease severity. Differences in intensivist-to-ICU-bed ratios, ranging from 1:7.5 to 1:15, were not associated with differences in ICU or hospital mortality. However, a ratio of 1:15 was associated with increased ICU LOS.

The impact of the ICU nurse

What is true for the intensivist-to-bed ratio is probably also true for nurse-to-bed ratio. In many countries, intensive care nurses are specialized nurses with extra training. It is not known what the optimum ratio is. In most counties, the ratio of nurse to patient is between 1:1 and 1:2. For patients after hepatectomy or esophagectomy, there is evidence that less patients per nurse results in a decrease in pulmonary or infectious complications, while mortality was not significantly different [20]. A recent report from the UK showed that higher nurse workload was associated with higher mortality in a general ICU population [21]. We suggest prospective studies are needed to assess the true optimal nurse-to-bed ratio.

The impact of outreach teams

Given the fact that critically ill patients are often admitted to the ICU from general nursing departments, it seemed logical to install teams that reach out to these patients before detoriation begins [22]. The Cochrane Collaborative systemically reviewed the literature on the impact of critical care outreach on patient outcomes [23]. Nearly 5000 studies were identified as being potentially relevant with only two randomized controlled trials meeting the inclusion criteria. The first study was the Medical Early Response Intervention and Treatment (MERIT) study, performed in Australia. This was a randomized cluster-controlled trial to study the effects of the introduction of an outreach team. They found that the introduction did not significantly reduce the incidence of unexpected deaths, cardiac arrests, and unplanned ICU admissions [24]. Priestly et al. introduced a nurse-led outreach service that ran 24 h a day and focused on education, support, and practical help for ward staff. This randomized trial resulted in reduced hospital mortality with a trend towards an increased length of stay [25]. The overall conclusion of the Cochrane Review, however, was that the evidence for effectiveness of these outreach services was inconclusive. In a recent multicenter trial, introduction of nationwide implementation in the Netherlands of rapid response systems was associated with a decrease in the composite end point of cardiopulmonary arrests, unplanned ICU admissions, and mortality in patients in general hospital wards [26]. These findings support the implementation of rapid response systems in hospitals to reduce severe adverse events.

The impact of patient digital management systems

The introduction of patient digital management systems (PDMS) provided intensivists with a fast overview of patient's critical data. Having an interface with the electronic medical record at the unit level was significantly associated with a lower risk of mortality in the ICU [27]. The finding that electronic medical records integrated with ICU information systems are associated with lower in-hospital mortality adds support to existing evidence on organizational characteristics associated with in-hospital mortality among ICU patients. The PDMS may also have a role in risk predictions. Risk prediction can be implemented for adverse effects of treatments performed on the ICU, e.g., onset of ventilator-induced lung injury while patients are on the mechanical ventilation. An algorithm can easily been built and screen all electronic records and subsequently warn the attending intensivist in case of increased risk [28–31]. The PDMS can also be used to predict risks after ICU discharge. A recent study used the PDMS to validate an automatic risk of unplanned readmission (Stability and Workload Index for Transfer (SWIFT)) calculator in a prospective cohort of consecutive ICU patients [32]. The authors showed and concluded that the PDMS accurately calculates SWIFT score and can facilitate ICU discharge decisions without the need for manual data collection. Another area where the PDMS resulted in increased patient safety is medication prescription. Electronic prescribing results in increased medication safety [33]. In conclusion, the introduction of the PDMS has resulted in a better patient outcome and reduction of the intensivist task load by which the utilization of intensivists becomes optimized.

Possible future improvements

Pooling of ICU departments

In manufacturing and business, one source of competitive advantage is consolidation of separate units which results in increase of scale and reduction of overhead. Within the service industry, consolidation or pooling also results in improvement of service capacity, hence reduction of wait time. The positive effect of pooling or consolidation might be a future improvement within the ICU. The formation of a mixed closed format ICU model: one central ICU in a hospital instead of several small ones (traditional closed format ICU model), to which all patients independent of their underlying conditions are admitted. This is illustrated in Figs. 1 and 2. We hypothesize that, overall, a mixed closed format ICU model improves patient outcome, increased admission capacity, and reduces at the same time costs, compared to a traditional closed format ICU model; however, data to support this hypothesis is lacking. Studies should aim to obtain data on both patient outcome and cost, before and after introduction of a mixed closed format ICU model.

Step down unit

The main purpose of a step down unit on an ICU is to bridge the differences between the ICU and a general ward (but not to function as a medium care, where "step-up" is also allowed) and therefore to reduce the readmission ratio. Readmission is known to be associated with adverse outcomes [34]. Caregivers and patients experience a substantial gap in monitoring and level of care which may lead to a reduction of the threshold for readmission. Respiratory insufficiency remains one of the most important reasons for readmission. A prospective study is needed to determine whether a step down unit is able to decrease readmission rates.

The mobile intensive care unit

Inter-hospital transport of critically ill patients may have a positive effect on resource utilization by pooling admission capacity of the medical centers or creating focus clinics for certain patient categories. Furthermore, transportation enables the distribution of the most severe patients to large referral medical centers and the less severe patients to more rural centers. In this way, you optimize the utilization by level of care and it may improve the overall patient outcome [35]. For instance, the transportation of patients with very severe respiratory failure, which was considered to preclude conventional ventilation for safe transfer to tertiary centers, was managed by an extra corporal membrane oxygenation referral and retrieval program in New South Wales and had a high rate of survival [36]. The possible downside of these inter-hospital transports is the exposure to adverse events and the cost. However, when using a mobile intensive care unit (MICU) compared to a normal ambulance, a reduction of adverse events during inter-hospital transport from 34 to 12.5% was achieved [37]. Furthermore, it is suggested that the condition of the patient does not predict the risk of adverse events but the formation of the team and equipment available [38]. Unfortunately, data on patient outcome and cost are lacking to support the possible upside on resource utilization improvement as mentioned above.

Distant monitoring—telemedicine

The closed format model of ICU is a superior clinical practice as discussed above, but shortage of intensivists and financial reasons led to the development of telemedicine. In one study [39], they showed that the implementation of telemedicine resulted in a relative risk reduction of mortality of 0.73 (95%CI 0.55–0.95) and reduction of ICU stay from 4.35 to 3.63 days. Furthermore, this resulted in lower variable cost per patient and higher hospital revenues from increased case volumes. Although not all other studies [40–43] have shown similar effects, in general, the results suggest that telemedicine might be a solution to bridge the shortage of intensivists while still improving quality of care and reducing health-care cost in rural areas [44]. Of note, there is no data providing evidence that implementing telemedicine in rural areas is superior to transporting the

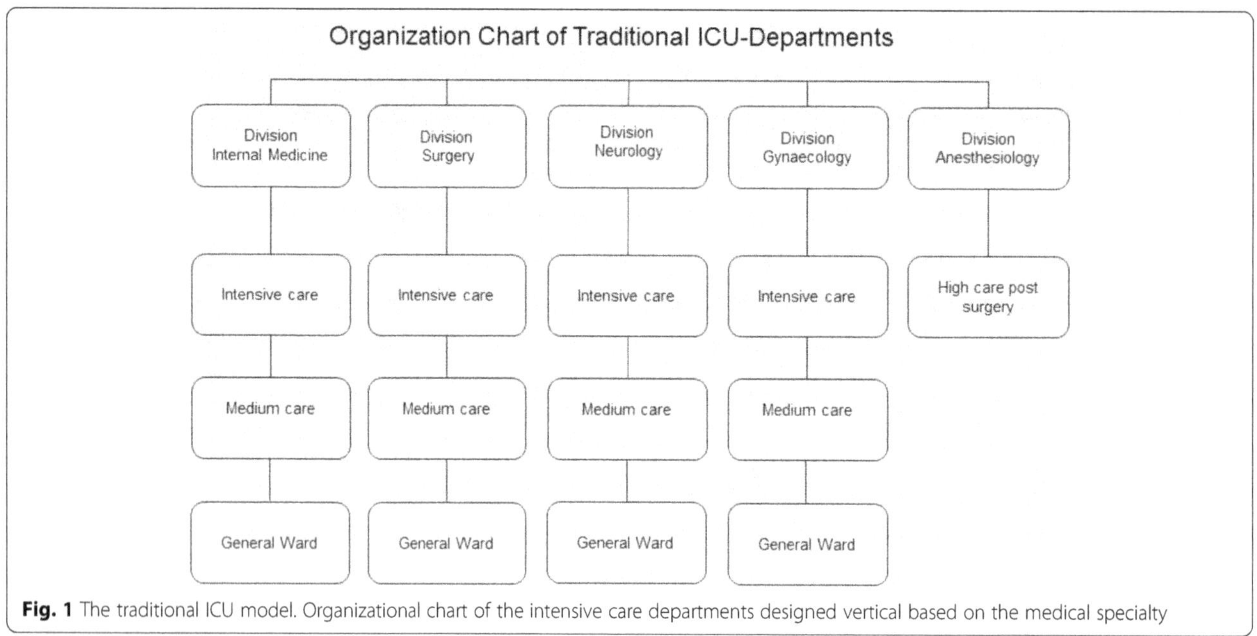

Fig. 1 The traditional ICU model. Organizational chart of the intensive care departments designed vertical based on the medical specialty

critically ill patients to appropriate staffed ICUs. Furthermore, no studies are available to support telemedicine for ICUs located in high-density populations.

Total quality management and quality indicators

Total quality management (TQM) is a philosophy of management for continuously improving the quality of products and processes. According to TQM, quality is a process that can be managed and requires ongoing evaluation and change (continuous quality improvement (CQI)). Before we can apply TQM and CQI in the ICU, we need specific quality indicators. A few of these indicators have been identified for the ICU: (1) percentage of patients with central venous catheter infections, (2) percentage of patients with ventilator-associated pneumonia, (3) percentage of patients with vancomycin-resistant enterococcus, (4) number of complications per patient, (5) rate of gastrointestinal bleeding, (6) average days of mechanical ventilation, (7) average ICU length of stay, and (8) patient satisfaction [45]. Other interesting performance measures for both the health-care provider and the patient are hospital mortality and ICU mortality, corrected for expected mortality (standardized mortality ratio (SMR)) and readmission rates. Obviously, some

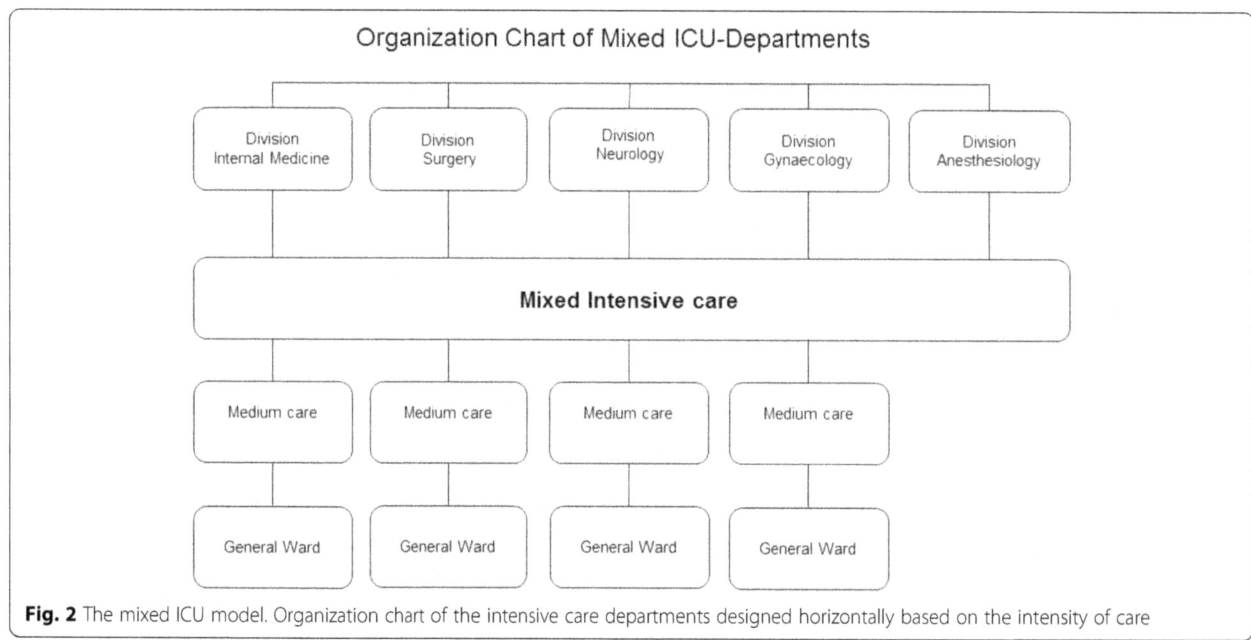

Fig. 2 The mixed ICU model. Organization chart of the intensive care departments designed horizontally based on the intensity of care

indicators may influence other ones, e.g., LOS and readmission rate or duration of mechanical ventilation and number of reintubations. Recently, it is recognized that quality indicators (QIs) should be actionable. They should be developed in such a way that they can be influenced by, in the case of use in intensive care medicine, intensivists. By developing new QIs that are actionable, reliable, valid, and easy to register, quality improvement in intensive cares will be supported. Using a modified RAND technique, new QIs for blood use at Dutch ICUs were developed [45]. The set of QIs will be part of the National Intensive Care Evaluation [46]. To apply TQM and QI, it cannot be neglected to mention evidence-based practice. Indeed, nowadays, quality improvements need to be shown to be effective in clinical studies before they become widely adopted. Although TQM and CQI work in the business environment, it may not be optimal for the health-care industry. A critique on both TQM and CQI is the narrow focus on outcome and not the underlying process.

Use of safety management systems in the ICU and risk assessment

From recent studies in ICU patients, we know that improving patient safety has impact on the safety climate as well as on mortality and length of stay [47, 48]. Risk management is an important part of the safety management system. Retrospective risk analysis focuses on incidents that have taken place; prospective risk analysis has the advantage of its true preventive nature. Retrospective methods that can be used are, for instance, root cause analysis and tripod beta analysis. For prospective risk analysis, there are several other methods. Examples are the bow-tie method and the health-care failure mode and effect analysis (HFMEA) [49–51].

Lean management/Toyota Production System

The processes in an ICU can partly be seen as a manufacturing process. A future improvement could be identifying processes which work in the manufacturing industry which are also applicable for the ICU. One of the possible processes could be lean management. Lean management is a philosophy which is mainly derived from the Toyota Production System (TPS). The original seven "wastes" also known as "muda" were identified by Taiichi Ohno, the Toyota executive felt to be the main developer of the Toyota Production System [52]. Later, on the eighth waste, "talent" has been added. These eight manufacturing terms are presented in Table 2 and can easily be translated into health-care organizations which were done by John Toussaint and Roger Gerard, in their book, *On the Mend* [53]. They have identified "the eight wastes of lean healthcare." Lean is not a "fix it and forget it" approach. It takes a constant commitment from leadership to allow the culture and the processes to create better approaches and more efficient pathways. Lean is not easy to implement and sustain as there is not one common recipe. Lean has succeeded in a number of health-care circumstances [54] but failed in many [55]. Evidence for lean management in the ICU is scarce; only a few projects have been published specifically targeting the ICU department [56, 57]. Whether lean will become

Table 2 Comparison of application of lean management in manufacturing and health-care organization

Type of problem	Manufacturing organization	Health-care organization	Implication for intensive care
Overproduction	Producing ahead of need	Unnecessary treatment and overuse of diagnostic testing	Clear treatment goals and end-of-life decision guidelines
Waiting	Operators standing idle waiting for other workers or machines to finish	Patient waits for an appointment, for test results, for a bed, for discharge paperwork	Clear admission and discharge guidelines
Transport	Moving parts and products unnecessarily	Taking patients to and from tests, moving patients from one room to another	Diagnostic tests being performed at bed side
Over Processing	Performing unnecessary or incorrect activities	Unnecessary forms, asking the same patient the same question more than once, charting everything instead of charting by exception	Digital system Preventing re-enter of patient data Patient centric rounding
Inventory	Having more than the minimum stock necessary	Overstocked drugs that expire, under stocked surgical supplies that lead to delays while staff search for them	Pooling of inventories within the hospital or even within the region just in time
Motion	Making workers look for parts, tools, documents, etc	Searching for supplies, forms, drugs	Correct and logic labelling of all supplies, forms, and drugs
Defects	Inspection, rework, and scrapping parts that do not meet standards	Making and correcting errors, checking for errors	Clear protocols including feedback mechanisms and e-alerts
Talent Waste	Failure to listen to employee ideas for improvement	Using highly trained individuals to do jobs that could be performed by less expensive personnel, failure to listen to employee ideas for improvement	Focus on ICU physician and ICU nurse specific tasks and outsource tasks such as washing patients, paperwork, and move tasks down from ICU physician to ICU nurse when possible

important in ICU organizations will depend mainly on the willingness to let lean enter the ICU and the ability to implement and keep improving lean processes.

Compliance

The evidence that changes in organizational structures in the intensive care department are able to have significant impact on patient outcome and cost is straightforward and sound. However, the implementation and compliance with these recommendations can be difficult. Pronovost et al. showed [58] that the closed format was not implemented in all hospitals and, when so, the intensivists were often not empowered to make decisions. Hence, on paper, the hospitals fulfil the criteria but, in practice, not much has changed. This study underlines the importance of clearly defining guidelines and the importance of implementing processes. Although evidence exists, hospitals and physicians may be reluctant to implement these processes. Explanations for this may be reluctance to change, disbelief of the results of studies, and local factors making it impossible to extrapolate the results in the hospital. In the future, resources should not only be devoted to identifying new process improvements but also to implementing proven processes. Whether this is a role for the physicians, the government, or external companies remains to be determined.

Conclusions

The organization of the intensive care department has been changed over the past decades resulting in better patient outcome and reduction of cost. Major changes are the implementation of the closed format and electronic patient record. Challenges are ahead as the ICU is taking up the largest share of national health-care expenditure, and with the aging of the population, this will continue to increase. We would like to advocate for standard inclusion of cost analysis into future study reports, as financial constraints within the health-care industry have become an important issue nowadays and cost-effectiveness may influence decision-making whether or not to implement an intervention. Besides future improvements of organizational structures within the ICU, the focus should also be on implementation of and compliance with proven beneficial organizational structures.

Abbreviations

HFMEA: Health-care failure mode and effect analysis; ICU: Intensive care unit; LOS: Length of stay; MERIT: Medical early response intervention and treatment; MICU: Mobile intensive care unit; PDMS: Patient digital management systems; QI: Quality indicators; SMR: Standardized mortality ratio; SWIFT: Stability and workload index for transfer; TPS: Toyota Production System; TQM: Total quality management

Acknowledgements

Stephen E. Chick acknowledges the support of the EU through the MSCA-ESA-ITN project (676129).

Funding

Not applicable.

Authors' contributions

AV, MV, DD, and SC designed the paper. AV, SS, and ES wrote the paper. All authors critically reviewed the paper.

Competing interests

The authors declare that they have no competing interests.

Author details

[1]Department of Intensive Care Medicine, Academic Medical Center, Room C3-343, Meibergdreef 9, Amsterdam 1105 AZ, The Netherlands. [2]Department of Intensive Care Medicine, Ter Gooi Ziekenhuizen, Hilversum, The Netherlands. [3]INSEAD Healthcare Management Initiative, INSEAD, Fontainebleau, France.

References

1. Carson SS, Stocking C, Podsadecki T, Christenson J, Pohlman A, MacRae S, Jordan J, Humphrey H, Siegler M, Hall J. Effects of organizational change in the medical intensive care unit of a teaching hospital: a comparison of 'open' and 'closed' formats. Jama. 1996;276:322–8.
2. Dimick JB, Pronovost PJ, Heitmiller RF, Lipsett PA. Intensive care unit physician staffing is associated with decreased length of stay, hospital cost, and complications after esophageal resection. Crit Care Med. 2001;29:753–8.
3. Multz AS, Chalfin DB, Samson IM, Dantzker DR, Fein AM, Steinberg HN, Niederman MS, Scharf SM. A "closed" medical intensive care unit (MICU) improves resource utilization when compared with an "open" MICU. Am J Respir Crit Care Med. 1998;157:1468–73.
4. Nguyen YL, Angus DC, Boumendil A, Guidet B. The challenge of admitting the very elderly to intensive care. Ann Intensive Care. 2011;1:29.
5. Quach S, Hennessy DA, Faris P, Fong A, Quan H, Doig C. A comparison between the APACHE II and Charlson Index Score for predicting hospital mortality in critically ill patients. BMC Health Serv Res. 2009;9:129.
6. Halpern NA, Pastores SM. Critical care medicine in the United States 2000-2005: an analysis of bed numbers, occupancy rates, payer mix, and costs. Crit Care Med. 2010;38:65–71.
7. Halpern NA, Pastores SM. Critical care medicine beds, use, occupancy, and costs in the United States: a methodological review. Crit Care Med. 2015;43:2452–9.
8. Geitona M, Androutsou L, Theodoratou D. Cost estimation of patients admitted to the intensive care unit: a case study of the Teaching University Hospital of Thessaly. J Med Econ. 2010;13:179–84.
9. Tan SS, Bakker J, Hoogendoorn ME, Kapila A, Martin J, Pezzi A, Pittoni G, Spronk PE, Welte R, Hakkaart-van Roijen L. Direct cost analysis of intensive care unit stay in four European countries: applying a standardized costing methodology. Value Health. 2012;15:81–6.
10. Milstein A, Galvin RS, Delbanco SF, Salber P, Buck Jr CR. Improving the safety of health care: the leapfrog initiative. Eff Clin Pract. 2000;3:313–6.
11. Pronovost PJ, Angus DC, Dorman T, Robinson KA, Dremsizov TT, Young TL. Physician staffing patterns and clinical outcomes in critically ill patients: a systematic review. Jama. 2002;288:2151–62.
12. Siegal EM, Dressler DD, Dichter JR, Gorman MJ, Lipsett PA. Training a hospitalist workforce to address the intensivist shortage in American hospitals: a position paper from the Society of Hospital Medicine and the Society of Critical Care Medicine. Crit Care Med. 2012;40:1952–6.
13. Lois M. The shortage of critical care physicians: is there a solution? J Crit Care. 2014;29:1121–2.
14. Lee SK, Lee DS, Andrews WL, Baboolal R, Pendray M, Stewart S. Higher mortality rates among inborn infants admitted to neonatal intensive care units at night. J Pediatr. 2003;143:592–7.

15. Bell CM, Redelmeier DA. Mortality among patients admitted to hospitals on weekends as compared with weekdays. N Engl J Med. 2001;345:663–8.
16. Gajic O, Afessa B, Hanson AC, Krpata T, Yilmaz M, Mohamed SF, Rabatin JT, Evenson LK, Aksamit TR, Peters SG, et al. Effect of 24-hour mandatory versus on-demand critical care specialist presence on quality of care and family and provider satisfaction in the intensive care unit of a teaching hospital. Crit Care Med. 2008;36:36–44.
17. Wallace DJ, Angus DC, Barnato AE, Kramer AA, Kahn JM. Nighttime intensivist staffing and mortality among critically ill patients. N Engl J Med. 2012;366:2093–101.
18. Kerlin MP, Small DS, Cooney E, Fuchs BD, Bellini LM, Mikkelsen ME, Schweickert WD, Bakhru RN, Gabler NB, Harhay MO, et al. A randomized trial of nighttime physician staffing in an intensive care unit. N Engl J Med. 2013;368:2201–9.
19. Dara SI, Afessa B. Intensivist-to-bed ratio: association with outcomes in the medical ICU. Chest. 2005;128:567–72.
20. Amaravadi RK, Dimick JB, Pronovost PJ, Lipsett PA. ICU nurse-to-patient ratio is associated with complications and resource use after esophagectomy. Intensive Care Med. 2000;26:1857–62.
21. West E, Barron DN, Harrison D, Rafferty AM, Rowan K, Sanderson C. Nurse staffing, medical staffing and mortality in intensive care: an observational study. Int J Nurs Stud. 2014;51:781–94.
22. Bristow PJ, Hillman KM, Chey T, Daffurn K, Jacques TC, Norman SL, Bishop GF, Simmons EG. Rates of in-hospital arrests, deaths and intensive care admissions: the effect of a medical emergency team. Med J Aust. 2000;173:236–40.
23. McGaughey J, Alderdice F, Fowler R, Kapila A, Mayhew A, Moutray M: Outreach and early warning systems (EWS) for the prevention of intensive care admission and death of critically ill adult patients on general hospital wards. Cochrane Database Syst Rev 2007;18:Cd005529.
24. Hillman K, Chen J, Cretikos M, Bellomo R, Brown D, Doig G, Finfer S, Flabouris A. Introduction of the medical emergency team (MET) system: a cluster-randomised controlled trial. Lancet. 2005;365:2091–7.
25. Priestley G, Watson W, Rashidian A, Mozley C, Russell D, Wilson J, Cope J, Hart D, Kay D, Cowley K, Pateraki J. Introducing critical care outreach: a ward-randomised trial of phased introduction in a general hospital. Intensive Care Med. 2004;30:1398–404.
26. Ludikhuize J, Brunsveld-Reinders AH, Dijkgraaf MG, Smorenburg SM, de Rooij SE, Adams R, de Maaijer PF, Fikkers BG, Tangkau P, de Jonge E. Outcomes associated with the nationwide introduction of rapid response systems in The Netherlands. Crit Care Med. 2015;43:2544–51.
27. Sales AE, Lapham GG, Squires J, Hutchinson A, Almenoff P, Sharp ND, Lowy E, Li YF. Organizational factors associated with decreased mortality among veterans affairs patients with an ICU stay. Comput Inform Nurs. 2011;29:496–501.
28. Chbat NW, Chu W, Ghosh M, Li G, Li M, Chiofolo CM, Vairavan S, Herasevich V, Gajic O. Clinical knowledge-based inference model for early detection of acute lung injury. Ann Biomed Eng. 2012;40:1131–41.
29. Herasevich V, Tsapenko M, Kojicic M, Ahmed A, Kashyap R, Venkata C, Shahjehan K, Thakur SJ, Pickering BW, Zhang J, et al: Limiting ventilator-induced lung injury through individual electronic medical record surveillance. Crit Care Med 2011, 39:34–39.
30. Ahmed A, Kojicic M, Herasevich V, Gajic O. Early identification of patients with or at risk of acute lung injury. Neth J Med. 2009;67:268–71.
31. Herasevich V, Yilmaz M, Khan H, Hubmayr RD, Gajic O. Validation of an electronic surveillance system for acute lung injury. Intensive Care Med. 2009;35:1018–23.
32. Chandra S, Agarwal D, Hanson A, Farmer JC, Pickering BW, Gajic O, Herasevich V. The use of an electronic medical record based automatic calculation tool to quantify risk of unplanned readmission to the intensive care unit: a validation study. J Crit Care. 2011;26:634. e639-634.e615.
33. Warrick C, Naik H, Avis S, Fletcher P, Franklin BD, Inwald D. A clinical information system reduces medication errors in paediatric intensive care. Intensive Care Med. 2011;37:691–4.
34. Kareliusson F, De Geer L, Tibblin AO. Risk prediction of ICU readmission in a mixed surgical and medical population. J Intensive Care. 2015;3:30.
35. Gebremichael M, Borg U, Habashi NM, Cottingham C, Cunsolo L, McCunn M, Reynolds HN. Interhospital transport of the extremely ill patient: the mobile intensive care unit. Crit Care Med. 2000;28:79–85.
36. Forrest P, Ratchford J, Burns B, Herkes R, Jackson A, Plunkett B, Torzillo P, Nair P, Granger E, Wilson M, Pye R. Retrieval of critically ill adults using extracorporeal membrane oxygenation: an Australian experience. Intensive Care Med. 2011;37:824–30.
37. Wiegersma JS, Droogh JM, Zijlstra JG, Fokkema J, Ligtenberg JJ. Quality of interhospital transport of the critically ill: impact of a mobile intensive care unit with a specialized retrieval team. Crit Care. 2011;15:R75.
38. van Lieshout EJ, de Vos R, Binnekade JM, de Haan R, Schultz MJ, Vroom MB. Decision making in interhospital transport of critically ill patients: national questionnaire survey among critical care physicians. Intensive Care Med. 2008;34:1269–73.
39. Breslow MJ, Rosenfeld BA, Doerfler M, Burke G, Yates G, Stone DJ, Tomaszewicz P, Hochman R, Plocher DW. Effect of a multiple-site intensive care unit telemedicine program on clinical and economic outcomes: an alternative paradigm for intensivist staffing. Crit Care Med. 2004;32:31–8.
40. Franzini L, Sail KR, Thomas EJ, Wueste L. Costs and cost-effectiveness of a telemedicine intensive care unit program in 6 intensive care units in a large health care system. J Crit Care. 2011;26:329. e321-326.
41. Morrison JL, Cai Q, Davis N, Yan Y, Berbaum ML, Ries M, Solomon G. Clinical and economic outcomes of the electronic intensive care unit: results from two community hospitals. Crit Care Med. 2010;38:2–8.
42. Rosenfeld BA, Dorman T, Breslow MJ, Pronovost P, Jenckes M, Zhang N, Anderson G, Rubin H. Intensive care unit telemedicine: alternate paradigm for providing continuous intensivist care. Crit Care Med. 2000;28:3925–31.
43. Willmitch B, Golembeski S, Kim SS, Nelson LD, Gidel L. Clinical outcomes after telemedicine intensive care unit implementation. Crit Care Med. 2012;40:450–4.
44. Kumar S, Merchant S, Reynolds R. Tele-ICU: efficacy and cost-effectiveness of remotely managing critical care. Perspect Health Inf Manag. 2013;10:1f.
45. McMillan TR, Hyzy RC. Bringing quality improvement into the intensive care unit. Crit Care Med. 2007;35:S59–65.
46. van de Klundert N, Holman R, Dongelmans DA, de Keizer NF. Data resource profile: the Dutch National Intensive Care Evaluation (NICE) Registry of Admissions to Adult Intensive Care Units. Int J Epidemiol. 2015;44:1850–1850h.
47. Fanara B, Manzon C, Barbot O, Desmettre T, Capellier G. Recommendations for the intra-hospital transport of critically ill patients. Crit Care. 2010;14:R87.
48. Sexton JB, Berenholtz SM, Goeschel CA, Watson SR, Holzmueller CG, Thompson DA, Hyzy RC, Marsteller JA, Schumacher K, Pronovost PJ. Assessing and improving safety climate in a large cohort of intensive care units. Crit Care Med. 2011;39:934–9.
49. Kerckhoffs MC, van der Sluijs AF, Binnekade JM, Dongelmans DA. Improving patient safety in the ICU by prospective identification of missing safety barriers using the bow-tie prospective risk analysis model. J Patient Saf. 2013;9:154–9.
50. Duwe B, Fuchs BD, Hansen-Flaschen J. Failure mode and effects analysis application to critical care medicine. Crit Care Clin. 2005;21:21–30. vii.
51. Habraken MM, Van der Schaaf TW, Leistikow IP, Reijnders-Thijssen PM. Prospective risk analysis of health care processes: a systematic evaluation of the use of HFMEA in Dutch health care. Ergonomics. 2009;52:809–19.
52. Marchwinski C. Lean lexicon. Cambridge: Lean Enterprise Institute; 2008.
53. Toussaint J. On the mend. Cambridge: Lean Enterprise Institute; 2010.
54. Cima RR, Brown MJ, Hebl JR, Moore R, Rogers JC, Kollengode A, Amstutz GJ, Weisbrod CA, Narr BJ, Deschamps C. Use of lean and six sigma methodology to improve operating room efficiency in a high-volume tertiary-care academic medical center. J Am Coll Surg. 2011;213:83–92. discussion 93-84.
55. DelliFraine JL, Langabeer 2nd JR, Nembhard IM. Assessing the evidence of Six Sigma and lean in the health care industry. Qual Manag Health Care. 2010;19:211–25.
56. Ackerman A. What is lean and what is it doing in my pediatric intensive care unit? Pediatr Crit Care Med. 2011;12:472–4.
57. Muder RR, Cunningham C, McCray E, Squier C, Perreiah P, Jain R, Sinkowitz-Cochran RL, Jernigan JA. Implementation of an industrial systems-engineering approach to reduce the incidence of methicillin-resistant Staphylococcus aureus infection. Infect Control Hosp Epidemiol. 2008;29:702–8. 707 p following 708.
58. Pronovost PJ, Thompson DA, Holzmueller CG, Dorman T, Morlock LL. The organization of intensive care unit physician services. Crit Care Med. 2007;35:2256–61.

5

Usefulness of plasminogen activator inhibitor-1 as a predictive marker of mortality in sepsis

Kota Hoshino*, Taisuke Kitamura, Yoshihiko Nakamura, Yuhei Irie, Norihiko Matsumoto, Yasumasa Kawano and Hiroyasu Ishikura

Abstract

Background: Sepsis is one of the most significant causes of mortality in intensive care units. It indicates crosstalk between inflammation and coagulation. In this study, we aimed to identify prognostic markers among sepsis biomarkers and coagulation/fibrinolysis markers.

Methods: Patients with sepsis according to the Sepsis-3 criteria were enrolled from January 2013 to September 2015. Univariate and multivariate logistic regression analyses were performed to identify an independent predictive marker of 28-day mortality among sepsis biomarkers and coagulation/fibrinolysis markers on ICU admission. Receiver operating characteristic analysis was performed; the optimal cutoff value of 28-day mortality was calculated using the predictive marker. Patients were classified into two groups according to the cutoff level of the predictive marker. Patient characteristics were compared between the groups.

Results: A total of 186 patients were enrolled in this study; the 28-day mortality was 19.4% (36/186). PAI-1 was identified as the only independent predictive marker of 28-day mortality by univariate and multivariate logistic regression. The area under the curve was 0.72; the optimal cutoff level was 83 ng/ml (sensitivity, 75%; specificity, 61%). Patients were classified into a higher group (PAI-1 level ≥83 ng/ml; $n = 85$) and a lower group (PAI-1 level <83 ng/ml; $n = 101$). All disseminated intravascular coagulation (DIC) scores and Sequential Organ Failure Assessment score were significantly higher in the higher group than in the lower group.

Conclusions: PAI-1 can predict prognosis in sepsis patients. PAI-1 reflects DIC with suppressed fibrinolysis and organ failure, with microthrombi leading to microcirculatory dysfunction.

Keywords: Disseminated intravascular coagulation, Fibrinolysis, Pathogen-associated molecular patterns, Sepsis-3

Background

Sepsis is one of the most significant causes of mortality in intensive care units [1], and mortality among septic shock patients has been reported to be 30–50% [2, 3]. To improve the prognosis of sepsis patients, it is important to diagnose and immediately treat sepsis. The usefulness of sepsis biomarkers, such as procalcitonin (PCT) and presepsin (PSEP), has been reported; PCT and PSEP have been reported to be superior to C-reactive protein (CRP) and interleukin-6 for sepsis diagnosis and assessment of sepsis severity [4–6].

The defensive role of thrombosis is referred to as immunothrombosis [7]. Immunothrombosis designates an innate immune response induced by the formation of thrombi in microvessels. However, if left uncontrolled, immunothrombosis can eventually lead to disseminated intravascular coagulation (DIC) [8, 9]. Previous studies reported that the frequency of DIC in sepsis patients was 20–40% [10–13]. Therefore, it is important to measure coagulation/fibrinolysis markers as well as sepsis biomarkers in sepsis to assess the presence of crosstalk between inflammation and coagulation.

In this study, we aimed to identify prognostic markers among sepsis biomarkers and coagulation/fibrinolysis markers.

* Correspondence: hoshinoqq@yahoo.co.jp
Department of Emergency and Critical Care Medicine, Faculty of Medicine, Fukuoka University, 7-45-1 Nanakuma, Jonan-ku, Fukuoka 814-0180, Japan

Methods

Patient selection

This retrospective single-center study was approved by the ethics committee of Fukuoka University Hospital (No. 16-3-14). The criteria for admission to the ICU in patients with sepsis include one or more organ failures including shock or disturbance of consciousness. Patients with sepsis were enrolled from January 2013 to September 2015. The diagnosis of sepsis was based on the definition of Sepsis-3 [14]. The exclusion criteria were age <18 years, presence of leukemia, liver cirrhosis, and cardiopulmonary arrest on admission and occurrence of death within 24 h of ICU admission. Patients were classified into non-survivor and survivor groups on day 28 of ICU admission (Fig. 1).

Patient characteristics

The two groups of patients were compared in terms of age, sex, infection focus, vital signs, the Japanese Association for Acute Medicine DIC score [15] along with the positive rate, the Sequential Organ Failure Assessment (SOFA) score [16] on ICU admission, and therapeutic agents. Moreover, sepsis biomarkers and coagulation/fibrinolysis markers were compared between non-survivor and survivor groups.

Identification of predictive markers

In this study, we examined sepsis biomarkers and coagulation/fibrinolysis markers in blood samples on ICU admission. First, univariate logistic regression analyses were performed. The explanatory variables were CRP, PCT, and PSEP as sepsis biomarkers and platelet counts, prothrombin time international normalized ratio (PT-INR), activated partial thromboplastin time, antithrombin, D-dimer, thrombin-antithrombin complex (TAT), plasmin-α2 plasmin inhibitor complex, protein C (PC), thrombomodulin (TM), soluble fibrin (SF), and plasminogen activator inhibitor-1 (PAI-1) as coagulation/fibrinolysis markers. The response variable was 28-day mortality. Subsequently, multivariate logistic regression analysis was performed to identify the independent predictive marker of 28-day mortality using the markers that were identified as significant in univariate logistic regression.

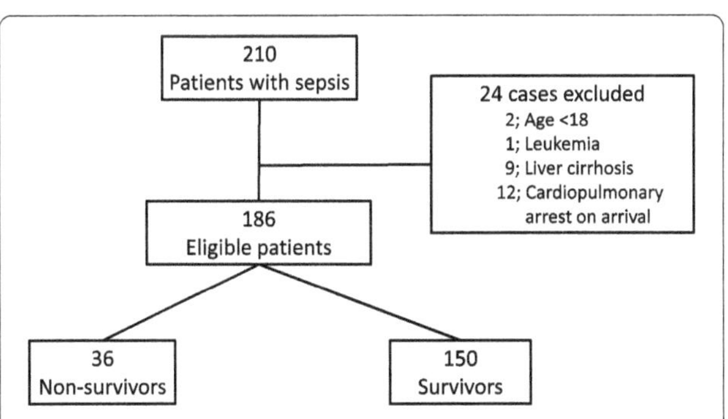

Fig. 1 Flow chart. Flow diagram of patients who met the inclusion/exclusion criteria for the study population

Cutoff value of the predictive marker and relationship with each score

Receiver operating characteristic (ROC) analysis was performed and the optimal cutoff value of 28-day mortality was calculated using the marker that was selected in multivariate logistic regression.

Relationship between the predictive marker and sepsis severity

We divided patients into the following two groups considering the optimal cutoff value: the higher group and the lower group. Patient characteristics were compared between these two groups. The correlations of the predictive marker with DIC and SOFA scores were examined to evaluate the relationship between the predictive marker and each score. In addition, the 28-day survival rate was compared between the higher and the lower groups using the Kaplan–Meier analysis.

Time course of sepsis biomarkers and coagulation/fibrinolysis markers

Time course of sepsis biomarkers and coagulation/fibrinolysis markers that were significantly different according to the univariate analyses were compared between the non-survivor and survivor groups.

Assay of sepsis biomarkers and coagulation/fibrinolysis markers

Blood samples were routinely collected for measuring markers, and there were no lack of data on ICU admission in this study. CRP levels were measured by CRP-LATEX (II) *X2* "SEIKEN" (Denka Seiken Co., Ltd, Tokyo, Japan) using EDTA plasma as a sample. PCT levels were measured by the Elecsys BRAHMS PCT assay (Roche Diagnostics, Tokyo, Japan) using EDTA plasma as a sample. PSEP levels were measured using a compact-automated immunoanalyzer, PATHFAST, based on a chemiluminescent enzyme immunoassay (CLEIA) (Mitsubishi Chemical Medience Corp., Japan). Platelet counts were measured in whole blood using an XT-1800i (Sysmex Co., Kobe, Japan). PT, APTT, AT, D-dimer, PIC, PC, and SF levels were measured in the plasma using a Coapresta 2000 (Sekisui Medicak, Tokyo, Japan). TAT, TM, and PAI-1 levels were measured using a STACIA (Mitsubishi Chemical Medience Corp., Tokyo, Japan). Total PAI-1 including active PAI-1 and tPA-PAI-1 complex was defined as PAI-1 in this study.

Statistical analysis

Continuous variables are presented as median (interquartile range). Comparisons between groups were performed using the chi-square test for dichotomous variables and Mann–Whitney *U* test for continuous variables. ROC analysis, including determination of the area under the curve (AUC), was performed to determine the significance of the marker level for predicting 28-day mortality. The Youden index was used to identify the cutoff value. Correlations between the predictive marker and each score were evaluated using Spearman's rank test. A P value of <0.05 was considered statistically significant. All statistical analyses were performed using JMP version 12 (SAS institute Japan, Tokyo, Japan).

Results

Patient selection

Patient enrollment into the study and exclusion from the study are shown in Fig. 1. Twenty-four of the 210 patients were excluded according to exclusion criteria. A total of 186 patients were enrolled in this study, and the 28-day mortality rate was 19.4% (36/186). Of the 186 patients, 36 patients were classified in the non-survivor group and 150 in the survivor group.

Patient characteristics

Patient characteristics are presented in Table 1. There were significant differences in age, infection focus, SOFA score (in particular, cardiovascular and renal SOFA scores), and continuous renal replacement therapy; however, there was no significant difference among other patient characteristics. With respect to the comparison of sepsis biomarkers and coagulation/fibrinolysis markers, PCT, PT-INR, APTT, TAT, SF, and PAI-1 levels were significantly higher in the non-survivor group than in the survivor group. On the other hand, AT and PC levels were significantly lower in the non-survivor group than in the survivor group (Table 2).

Identification of predictive markers

PSEP ($P < 0.05$) as a sepsis biomarker, TAT ($P < 0.05$), PC ($P < 0.01$), SF ($P < 0.01$), and PAI-1 ($P < 0.01$) as coagulation/fibrinolysis markers, and SOFA score ($P < 0.01$) were selected in univariate logistic regression (Table 3). Subsequently, multivariate logistic regression was performed using PSEP, TAT, PC, SF, PAI-1, and SOFA score as explanatory variables. PAI-1 was found to be the only independent predictive marker of 28-day mortality ($P <$ 0.05; Table 3).

Cutoff value of the predictive marker and relationship with each score

With regard to the accuracy of predicting 28-day mortality based on the level of PAI-1 in the ROC analysis, the AUC was 0.72 and the optimal cutoff value was 83 ng/ml (sensitivity, 75%; specificity, 61%).

Relationship between the predictive marker and sepsis severity

Patients were classified into the higher group (PAI-1 level ≥83 ng/ml; $n = 85$) and the lower group (PAI-1 level <83 ng/ml; $n = 101$). DIC, SOFA scores (in particular, cardiovascular and coagulation SOFA scores), and 28-day mortality were significantly higher in the higher group than those in the lower group (all $P < 0.01$; Table 4). To determine which scores affect the PAI-1 level the most, correlations between the PAI-1 level and DIC or SOFA score were evaluated using Spearman's rank test. We noted positive correlations between the PAI-1 level and DIC score ($r = 0.18$, $P < 0.05$) or SOFA score ($r = 0.32$, $P < 0.01$), in particular, cardiovascular ($r = 0.35$, $P < 0.01$) and renal ($r = 0.22$, $P < 0.01$; Table 5). The 28-day survival rate according to Kaplan–Meier analysis was significantly lower in the higher group than that in the lower group (log-rank test, $P < 0.01$; Fig. 2).

Time course of sepsis biomarkers and coagulation/fibrinolysis markers

Figure 3 shows the time courses of PSEP, TAT, PC SF, and PAI-1 that were significantly different according to univariate analyses. PC and PAI-1 levels were significantly different between the non-survivor and survivor groups on days 0, 3, and 7 ($P < 0.05$). In particular, PAI-1 levels at all time courses were significantly higher in the non-survivor group than those in the survivor group ($P < 0.01$).

Discussion

In this study, we used the new sepsis definition "Sepsis-3" and identified the predictive marker of 28-day mortality among sepsis biomarkers and coagulation/fibrinolysis markers. This study revealed that PAI-1 was the most predictive marker according to the multivariate analysis, and the cutoff value was 83 ng/ml. Morbidities of DIC and organ dysfunctions were significantly higher in the higher PAI-1 group. Moreover, PAI-1 was correlated with SOFA score, in particular cardiovascular and renal scores. PAI-1 levels were significantly higher in the non-survivor group than those in the survivor group during the time course as well as on admission.

The first definition of septic syndrome established in 1992 was based on the concomitant presence of presumed/confirmed infection and at least two of the four Systemic Inflammatory Response Syndrome criteria [17]. The new sepsis definition "Sepsis-3" mentions life-threatening organ dysfunction caused by a dysregulated host response to infection [14]. Therefore, it is important to assess organ dysfunction that is caused by

Table 1 Comparison of patient characteristics

	Total $n = 186$	Non-survivors $n = 36$	Survivors $n = 150$	*P* value
Age (years old)	72 (62–79)	76 (68–81)	71 (61–78)	<0.05
Male	115 (62)	20 (56)	95 (63)	0.39
Infection focus				<0.05
Lung	77 (41)	8 (22)	69 (46)	
Abdomen	61 (33)	21 (58)	40 (27)	
Skin and soft tissue	13 (7)	3 (8)	10 (7)	
Urinary tract	11 (6)	2 (6)	9 (6)	
Others	11 (6)	1 (3)	10 (7)	
Unknown	13 (7)	1 (3)	12 (8)	
Mean blood pressure (mmHg)	78 (67–97)	74 (63–92)	79 (67–97)	0.13
Heart rate (bpm)	110 (95–120)	111 (95–120)	110 (95–121)	0.77
Respiratory rate (bpm)	23 (19–28)	24 (20–28)	22 (18–28)	0.28
Body temperature (°C)	36.9 (36.3-37.9)	36.7 (36.0-37.4)	36.9 (36.4-38.1)	0.06
JAAM DIC score	3 (2–5)	4 (2–6)	3 (2–5)	0.13
JAAM DIC positive rate	87 (47)	21 (58)	66 (44)	0.12
SOFA score	8 (5–11)	11 (8–13)	8 (5–11)	<0.01
Respiratory	2 (2–3)	2 (1–3)	2 (2–3)	0.87
Cardiovascular	1 (0–4)	4 (0–4)	1 (0–4)	<0.01
Liver	0 (0–1)	0 (0–1)	0 (0–1)	0.95
Renal	1 (0–3)	3 (1–4)	1 (0–3)	<0.01
Coagulation	1 (0–2)	0 (0–2)	1 (0–2)	0.85
CNS	1 (0–2)	1 (0–3)	1 (0–2)	0.95
rhs TM	46 (25)	11 (31)	35 (23)	0.37
AT III	28 (15)	6 (17)	22 (15)	0.76
IVIG	92 (49)	21 (58)	71 (47)	0.24
CRRT	44 (24)	17 (47)	27 (18)	<0.01
PMX-DHP	28 (15)	9 (25)	19 (13)	0.06

Data are presented as median (interquartile range) or number (percentage)

JAAM Japanese Association for Acute Medicine, *DIC* disseminated intravascular coagulation, *SOFA* sequential organ failure assessment, *CNS* central nervous system, rhs TM recombinant human soluble thrombomodulin, *AT* antithrombin, *IVIG* intravenous immunoglobulin, *CRRT* continuous renal replacement therapy, *PMX-DHP* direct hemoperfusion with polymyxin B-immobilized fiber

coagulo-fibrinolytic abnormalities in sepsis. This is the first study to evaluate the prognostic value of sepsis biomarkers and coagulation/fibrinolysis markers using the Sepsis-3 definition.

There are some reports that sepsis biomarkers are useful for predicting mortality in patients with sepsis. Clec'h et al. [18] reported that PCT was able to predict mortality in patients with septic shock. Jensen et al. [19] reported that PCT level increase denoted a high risk of mortality. In the multicenter, retrospective, case–control study, PSEP was the only predictive marker of mortality according to multivariate analysis including PCT and PSEP [20]. In this study, PSEP was significant according to the univariate analysis; however, PSEP was not the predictive marker according to the multivariate analysis.

In sepsis, innate immune responses start following the identification of pathogen-associated molecular patterns or damage-associated molecular patterns by pattern-recognition receptors, such as Toll-like receptors expressed on immunocompetent cells and the endothelium. The sensed danger signals activate both intracellular signal transduction pathways and plasma cascades, which together produce pro-inflammatory cytokines, further stimulating the production of inflammatory biomarkers. The actions of inflammatory cytokines trigger the production of large amounts of tissue factor from monocytes/macrophages and the vascular endothelium, thus leading to marked coagulation activation. PAI-1 is synthesized by endothelial cells and hepatocytes. It is the main inhibitor of tissue-type plasminogen activator and

Table 2 Comparison of sepsis biomarkers and coagulation/fibrinolysis markers

	Total $n = 186$	Non-survivors $n = 36$	Survivors $n = 150$	P value
CRP (mg/dl)	12 (5–20)	15 (9–21)	12 (4–20)	0.21
PCT (ng/ml)	7 (1–42)	18 (2–89)	6 (1–33)	<0.05
PSEP (pg/ml)	839 (440–1597)	905 (546–1811)	815 (422–1562)	0.12
Platelet count (×104/μl)	14.8 (8.6–23.0)	16.6 (5.8–25.3)	14.4 (9.0–22.3)	0.81
PT-INR	1.3 (1.2–1.6)	1.5 (1.3–2.1)	1.3 (1.2–1.5)	<0.05
APTT (s)	35 (30–42)	39 (33–45)	34 (30–41)	<0.05
AT (%)	70 (56–87)	63 (48–77)	73 (58–87)	<0.05
D-dimer (μg/ml)	6.8 (2.9–15.7)	8.4 (3.3–18.2)	6.7 (2.8–14.6)	0.27
TAT (ng/ml)	6.9 (3.7–16.5)	8.9 (5.5–34.8)	6.5 (3.2–13.0)	<0.05
PIC (μg/ml)	1.7 (1.0–3.3)	1.5 (0.8–3.2)	1.7 (1.1–3.4)	0.19
PC (%)	47 (33–70)	38 (26–56)	52 (34–70)	<0.01
TM (U/ml)	33 (23–47)	40 (25–52)	32 (23–45)	0.12
SF (μg/ml)	21 (12–62)	45 (17–80)	20 (12–43)	<0.01
PAI-1 (ng/ml)	66 (29–191)	154 (73–527)	51 (26–154)	<0.01

Data are presented as median (interquartile range)
CRP C-reactive protein, *PCT* procalcitonin, *PSEP* presepsin, *PT-INR* prothrombin time-international normalized ratio, *APTT* activated partial thromboplastin time, *AT* antithrombin, *TAT* thrombin-antithrombin complex, *PIC* plasmin α2-plasmin inhibitor complex, *PC* protein C, *TM* thrombomodulin, *SF* soluble fibrin, *PAI-1* plasminogen activator inhibitor-1

plays an important role in the regulation of fibrinolysis. Elevated levels of PAI-1 result in deficient plasminogen activation and are a risk factor for thrombosis, including DIC. It is already known that PAI-1 level is markedly increased in sepsis, fibrinolysis is strongly suppressed, and dissolution of multiple microthrombi is more difficult [21], and because of microcirculatory impairment, severe organ dysfunction may occur [22, 23]. On the other hand, PAI-1 is not involved in malignant tumors such as acute leukemia and solid cancers [23].

Koyama et al. [24] reported that TAT, PC, and PAI-1 were predictive markers of mortality in patients with sepsis. TAT, PC, and PAI-1 were significant according to the univariate analysis as well as a previous study [24],

Table 3 Logistic regression analyses of the coagulation/fibrinolysis markers for 28-day mortality

	Univariate analyses			Multivariate analyses		
Markers	OR	95% CI	P value	OR	95% CI	P value
CRP (mg/dl)	1.020	0.986–1.054	NS			
PCT (ng/ml)	1.000	0.993–1.003	NS			
PSEP (pg/ml)	1.000	1.000–1.000	<0.05	1.000	0.999–1.000	NS
Platelet count (×10^4/μl)	1.003	0.973–1.028	NS			
PT-INR	0.993	0.834–1.034	NS			
APTT (s)	1.013	0.992–1.033	NS			
AT (%)	0.983	0.966–1.000	NS			
D-dimer (μg/ml)	1.005	0.995–1.015	NS			
TAT (ng/ml)	1.015	1.003–1.027	<0.05	0.999	0.982–1.014	NS
PIC (μg/ml)	1.021	0.940–1.094	NS			
PC (%)	0.977	0.959–0.993	<0.01	0.986	0.967–1.004	NS
TM (U/ml)	1.005	0.996–1.014	NS			
SF (μg/ml)	1.021	1.008–1.034	<0.01	1.014	0.997–1.031	NS
PAI-1 (ng/ml)	1.002	1.001–1.003	<0.01	1.002	1.000–1.003	<0.05
SOFA score	1.200	1.078–1.348	<0.01	1.075	0.943–1.231	NS

OR odds ratio, *CI* confidence interval, *CRP* C-reactive protein, *PCT* procalcitonin, *PSEP* presepsin, *PT-INR* prothrombin time-international normalized ratio, *APTT* activated partial thromboplastin time, *AT* antithrombin, *TAT* thrombin-antithrombin complex, *PIC* plasmin α2-plasmin inhibitor complex, *PC* protein C, *TM* thrombomodulin, *SF* soluble fibrin, *PAI-1* plasminogen activator inhibitor-1, *SOFA* sequential organ failure assessment

Table 4 Patient characteristics of the PAI-1 higher and lower groups

	PAI-1 ≥83 ng/ml $n = 85$	PAI-1 <83 ng/ml $n = 101$	*P* value
Age	74 (63–80)	71 (61–78)	0.14
Male	50 (59)	65 (64)	0.44
JAAM DIC score	4 (2–6)	2 (1–5)	<0.01
JAAM DIC positive rate	52 (61)	35 (35)	<0.01
SOFA score	10 (8–12)	7 (4–10)	<0.01
Respiratory	2 (2–3)	2 (1–3)	0.42
Cardiovascular	4 (0–4)	0 (0–3)	<0.01
Liver	0 (0–1)	0 (0–0)	0.09
Renal	2 (0–3)	1 (0–3)	0.18
Coagulation	1 (0–2)	0 (0–1)	<0.01
CNS	1 (1–3)	1 (0–2)	0.12
28-day mortality	27 (32)	9 (9)	<0.01

Data are presented as median (interquartile range) or number (percentage)
PAI-1 plasminogen activator inhibitor-1, *JAAM* Japanese Association for Acute Medicine, *DIC* disseminated intravascular coagulation, *SOFA* sequential organ failure assessment, *CNS* central nervous system

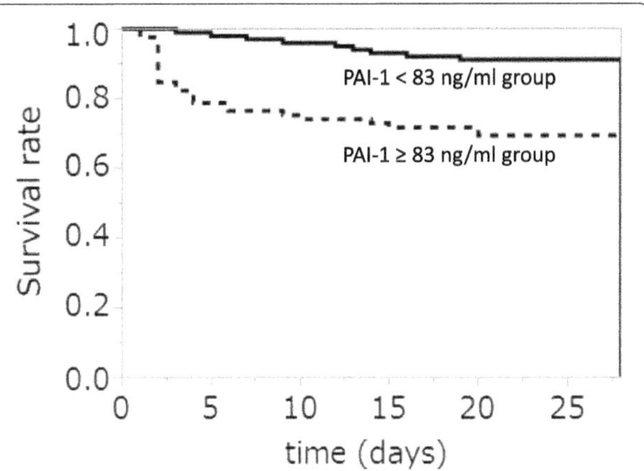

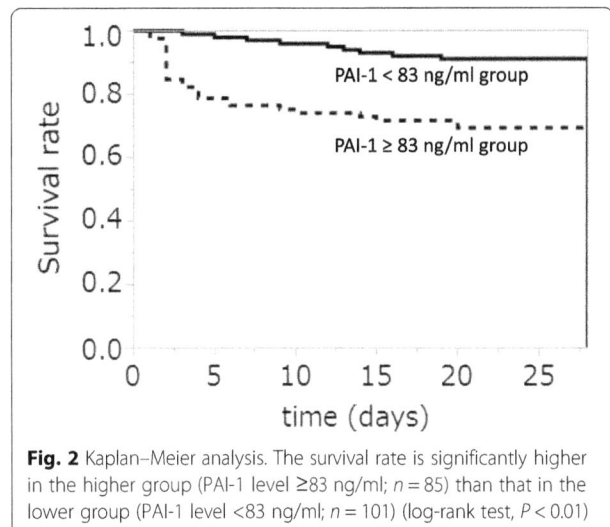

Fig. 2 Kaplan–Meier analysis. The survival rate is significantly higher in the higher group (PAI-1 level ≥83 ng/ml; $n = 85$) than that in the lower group (PAI-1 level <83 ng/ml; $n = 101$) (log-rank test, $P < 0.01$)

and PAI-1 was finally the only predictive marker in this study. Madoiwa et al. [25] examined 117 patients with sepsis-induced DIC and reported that the hazard ratio of 28-day mortality was increasing 23 times with a PAI-1 level of >90 ng/ml. The 90 ng/ml PAI-1 level is similar to the PAI-1 cutoff value of 83 ng/ml in this study. A previous study [24] revealed that the PAI-1 cutoff value was 269 ng/ml; however, the PAI-1 cutoff value in this study was 83 ng/ml. There was a huge difference in the PAI-1 cutoff value between the two studies. Although there is no unified method for PAI-1 level measurement, there are a few reagents for this measurement. The difference in PAI-1 cutoff values may be affected by reagents.

When considering the PAI-1 cutoff level, DIC and SOFA scores were significantly higher in patients with a PAI-1 level of ≥83 ng/ml than in those with a PAI-1 level of <83 ng/ml (all $P < 0.01$). The 28-day survival rate was significantly lower in patients with a level of ≥83 ng/ml than in those with a PAI-1 level of <83 ng/ml ($P < 0.01$). These results suggest that patients with a PAI-1 level of ≥83 ng/ml tend to develop DIC with suppressed fibrinolysis and multiple organ dysfunction. Madoiwa et al. [25] reported that the PAI-1 level correlated with the SOFA score. The results of this previous study are compatible with our results that there was a positive correlation between PAI-1 and the SOFA score in sepsis patients ($r = 0.32$, $P < 0.01$).

Table 5 Correlations between PAI-1 and each score

	Correlation coefficient	*P* value
JAAM DIC score	0.18	<0.05
SOFA score	0.32	<0.01
Respiratory	−0.01	0.90
Cardiovascular	0.35	<0.01
Liver	0.06	0.40
Renal	0.22	<0.01
Coagulation	0.13	0.08
CNS	0.13	0.08

PAI-1 plasminogen activator inhibitor-1, *JAAM* Japanese Association for Acute Medicine, *DIC* disseminated intravascular coagulation, *SOFA* sequential organ failure assessment, *CNS* central nervous system

Vincent et al. [26] studied the relationship of this dysfunction with the outcome. Increased cardiovascular, central nervous system, or renal SOFA score was related to high mortality. Furthermore, both cardiovascular and renal failures cause the highest mortality. In this study, cardiovascular and renal SOFA scores were significantly higher in the non-survivors' group than in the survivors' group. PAI-1 levels were significantly correlated with cardiovascular and renal scores in each SOFA scores. PAI-1 levels reflect the process that sepsis causes organ failures, resulting in death. Moreover, PAI-1 level is superior to SOFA score for predicting mortality.

Fibrinolysis is suppressed in sepsis and multiple microthrombi impair microcirculation, resulting in organ failure. The PAI-1 level reflects this process and can predict mortality in sepsis. In this study, sepsis was diagnosed according to the new definition of "Sepsis-3." PAI-1 reflects coagulo-fibrinolytic abnormalities, particularly suppressed fibrinolysis and organ failure along with microthrombi, leading to microcirculatory dysfunction in sepsis. Therefore, PAI-1 may be a useful marker to assess sepsis severity according to the Sepsis-3 definition.

The present study has some limitations. This was a small, retrospective, single-center study. The sampling timing in the course of sepsis was not detected. Some

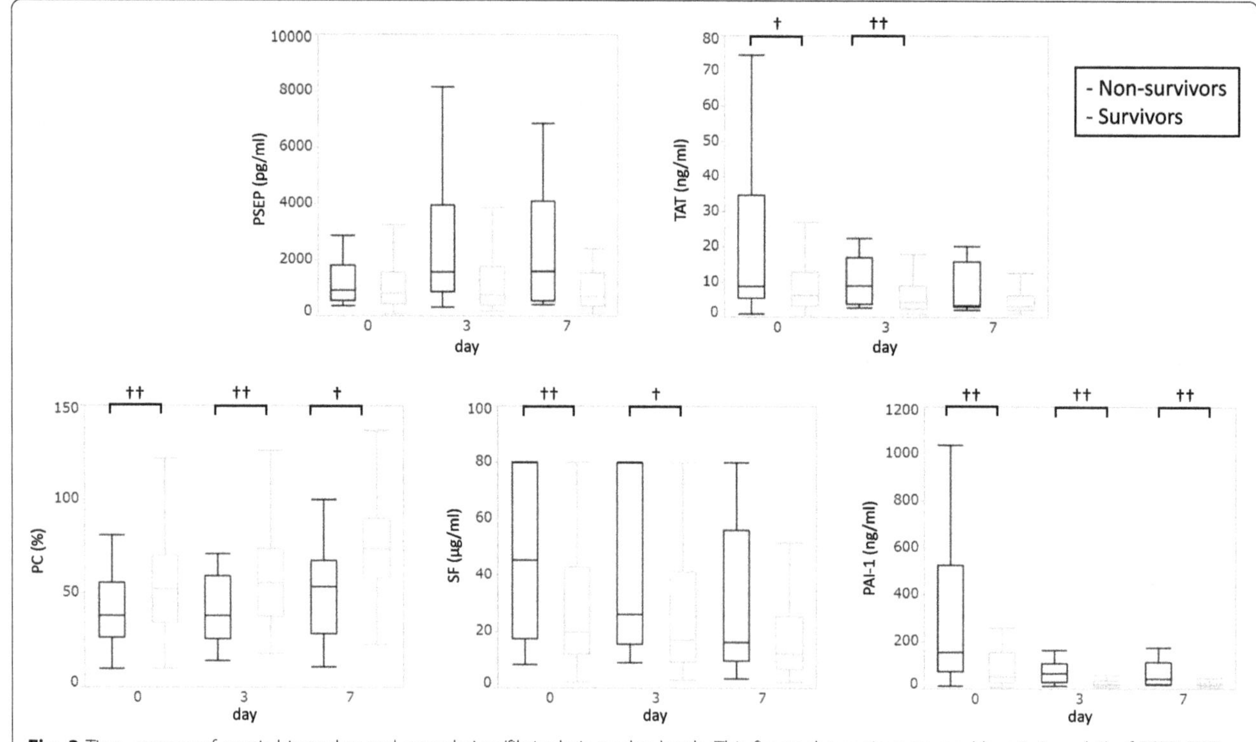

Fig. 3 Time courses of sepsis biomarker and coagulation/fibrinolysis marker levels. This figure shows time course (days 0, 3, and 7) of PSEP, TAT, PC, SF, and PAI-1 levels that were significantly different according to univariate analyses. †$P < 0.05$, ††$P < 0.01$ according to Mann–Whitney U test

patient characteristics between non-survivors and survivors were different; therefore, further studies are required to make sure of the efficacy of PAI-1. Additionally, only sepsis biomarkers and coagulation/fibrinolysis markers that could be examined in our center were used.

Conclusion

PAI-1 can predict prognosis in sepsis patients. In addition, PAI-1 reflects DIC with suppressed fibrinolysis and organ failure, with microthrombi leading to microcirculatory dysfunction.

Acknowledgements

We sincerely thank Ms. Kanae Misumi of the Department of Emergency and Critical Care Medicine, Faculty of Medicine, Fukuoka University for her help in data encoding.

Funding

We had no external funding sources; each author has funded the research with their own funds.

Authors' contributions

KH drafted the manuscript, participated in the study design, and performed the statistics analysis. TK, YN, YI, NM, YK, and HI helped draft the manuscript. All authors read and approved the final manuscript.

Competing interests

The authors declare that they have no competing interests.

References

1. Vincent JL, Rello J, Marshall J, Silva E, Anzueto A, Martin CD, et al. International study of the prevalence and outcomes of infection in intensive care units. JAMA. 2009;302:2323–9.
2. Vincent JL, Sakr Y, Sprung CL, Ranieri VM, Reinhart K, Gerlach H, et al. Sepsis in European intensive care units: results of the SOAP study. Crit Care Med. 2006;34:344–53.
3. Wittebole X, Castanares-Zapatero D, Laterre PF. Toll-like receptor 4 modulation as a strategy to treat sepsis. Mediators Inflamm. 2010;2010: 568396.
4. Endo S, Suzuki Y, Takahashi G, Shozushima T, Ishikura H, Murai A, et al. Usefulness of presepsin in the diagnosis of sepsis in a multicenter prospective study. J Infect Chemother. 2012;18:891–7.
5. Shozushima T, Takahashi G, Matsumoto N, Kojika M, Okamura Y, Endo S. Usefulness of presepsin (sCD14-ST) measurements as a marker for the diagnosis and severity of sepsis that satisfied diagnostic criteria of systemic inflammatory response syndrome. J Infect Chemother. 2011;17:764–9.
6. Ulla M, Pizzolato E, Lucchiari M, Loiacono M, Soardo F, Forno D, et al. Diagnostic and prognostic value of presepsin in the management of sepsis in the emergency department: a multicenter prospective study. Crit Care. 2013;17:R168.
7. Ito T. PAMPs and DAMPs as triggers for DIC. J Intensive Care. 2014;2:67.
8. Engelmann B, Massberg S. Thrombosis as an intravascular effector of innate immunity. Nat Rev Immunol. 2013;13:34–45.
9. Gando S, Otomo Y. Local hemostasis, immunothrombosis, and systemic disseminated intravascular coagulation in trauma and traumatic shock. Crit Care. 2015;19:72.

10. Rangel-Frausto MS, Pittet D, Costigan M, Hwang T, Davis CS, Wenzel RP. The natural history of the systemic inflammatory response syndrome (SIRS). A prospective study. JAMA. 1995;273:117–23.
11. Dhainaut JF, Yan SB, Joyce DE, Pettilä V, Basson B, Brandt JT, et al. Treatment effects of drotrecogin alfa (activated) in patients with severe sepsis with or without overt disseminated intravascular coagulation. J Thromb Haemost. 2004;2:1924–33.
12. Kienast J, Juers M, Wiedermann CJ, Hoffmann JN, Ostermann H, Strauss R, et al. KyberSept investigators: treatment effects of high-dose antithrombin without concomitant heparin in patients with severe sepsis with or without disseminated intravascular coagulation. J Thromb Haemost. 2006;4:90–7.
13. Beale R, Reinhart K, Brunkhorst FM, Dobb G, Levy M, Martin G, et al. Promoting global research excellence in severe sepsis (PROGRESS): lessons from an international sepsis registry. Infection. 2009;37:222–32.
14. Singer M, Deutschman CS, Seymour CW, Shankar-Hari M, Annane D, Bauer M, et al. The Third International Consensus Definitions for Sepsis and Septic Shock (Sepsis-3). JAMA. 2016;315:801–10.
15. Gando S, Iba T, Eguchi Y, Ohtomo Y, Okamoto K, Koseki K, et al. A multicenter, prospective validation of disseminated intravascular coagulation diagnostic criteria for critically ill patients: comparing current criteria. Crit Care Med. 2006;34:625–31.
16. Vincent JL, de Mendonça A, Cantraine F, Moreno R, Takala J, Suter PM, et al. Use of the SOFA score to assess the incidence of organ dysfunction/failure in intensive care units: results of a multicenter, prospective study. Working group on "sepsis-related problems" of the European Society of Intensive Care Medicine. Crit Care Med. 1998;26:1793–800.
17. Bone RC, Balk RA, Cerra FB, Dellinger RP, Fein AM, Knaus WA, et al. Definitions for sepsis and organ failure and guidelines for the use of innovative therapies in sepsis. The ACCP/SCCM Consensus Conference Committee. American College of Chest Physicians/Society of Critical Care Medicine Chest. 1992;101:1644–55.
18. Clec'h C, et al. Diagnostic and prognostic value of procalcitonin in patients with septic shock. Crit Care Med. 2004;32:1166–9.
19. Jensen JU, et al. Procalcitonin increase in early identification of critically ill patients at high risk of mortality. Crit Care Med. 2006;34:2596–602.
20. Masson S, et al. Presepsin (soluble CD14 subtype) and procalcitonin levels for mortality in sepsis: data from the Albumin Italian Outcome Sepsis trial. Crit Care. 2014;18:R6.
21. Sprengers ED, Kluft C. Plasminogen activator inhibitors. Blood. 1987;69:381–7.
22. Fujishima S, Gando S, Saitoh D, Mayumi T, Kushimoto S, Shiraishi S, et al. A multicenter, prospective evaluation of quality of care and mortality in Japan based on the Surviving Sepsis Campaign guidelines. J Infect Chemother. 2014;20:115–20.
23. Asakura H. Classifying types of disseminated intravascular coagulation: clinical and animal models. J Intensive Care. 2014;2:20.
24. Koyama K, Madoiwa S, Nunomiya S, Koinima T, Wada M, Sakata A, et al. Combination of thrombin-antithrombin complex, plasminogen activator inhibitor-1, and protein C activity for early identification of severe coagulopathy in initial phase of sepsis: a prospective observational study. Crit Care. 2014;18:R13.
25. Madoiwa S, Nunomiya S, Ono T, Shintani Y, Ohmori T, Mimuro J, et al. Plasminogen activator inhibitor 1 promotes a poor prognosis in sepsis-induced disseminated intravascular coagulation. Int J Hematol. 2006;84: 398–405.
26. Vincent JL, Moreno R, Takala J, Willatts S, De Mendonça A, Bruining H, et al. The SOFA (Sepsis-related Organ Failure Assessment) score to describe organ dysfunction/failure. On behalf of the Working Group on Sepsis-Related Problems of the European Society of Intensive Care Medicine. Intensive Care Med. 1996;22(7):707–10.

6

Early mobilization of mechanically ventilated patients in the intensive care unit

Shunsuke Taito[1], Nobuaki Shime[2*], Kohei Ota[2] and Hideto Yasuda[3]

Abstract

Several recent studies have suggested that the early mobilization of mechanically ventilated patients in the intensive care unit is safe and effective. However, in these studies, few patients reached high levels of active mobilization, and the standard of care among the studies has been inconsistent. The incidence of adverse events during early mobilization is low. Its importance should be considered in the context of the ABCDE bundle. Protocols of early mobilization with strict inclusion and exclusion criteria are needed to further investigate its contributions.

Keywords: Early mobilization, Mechanically ventilated patients, Intensive care unit, Adverse event, Rehabilitation

Background

Early mobilization includes activities such as sitting, standing and ambulation, as well as passive exercises, like range of motion exercises and ergometry [1–3]. The term "early" has yet to be defined, since among the various studies, the onset of interventions may vary by as much as 1 week [1–7]. Mobilization in the intensive care unit (ICU) is generally considered early.

After the report by Schweickert et al., in 2009, of the effectiveness of early rehabilitation interventions on the physical and mental functions of mechanically ventilated patients [2], several studies have reported similar results in patients hospitalized in the ICU. However, studies of active mobilization beyond the sitting position are few [8, 9], and a consensus has been reached with respect to neither the timing of "early mobilization" [10, 11] nor the prescription of standardized interventions.

This review examines the protocols, the inclusion and exclusion criteria, the effectiveness and safety, and the obstacles to the implementation of early mobilization of mechanically ventilated patients in the ICU.

* Correspondence: shime@koto.kpu-m.ac.jp
[2]Department of Emergency and Critical Care Medicine, Institute of Biomedical and Health Sciences, Hiroshima University, 1-2-3, Kasumi, Minami-ku, Hiroshima 734-8553, Japan
Full list of author information is available at the end of the article

Functional prognosis of mechanically ventilated patients

In a recent worldwide epidemiological survey, the survival rate of patients hospitalized in the ICU who met the diagnostic criteria of acute respiratory distress syndrome (ARDS) was increased up to 66 % by mechanical ventilation [12]. Another study found that nearly 70 % of patients presenting with acute respiratory failure who used mechanical ventilators were discharged from the ICU alive [13]. This increase in survival rate raised the issues of functional prognosis and quality of life (QOL) of the survivors. At 5 years after their discharge from the ICU, the exercise capacity of patients with ARDS remained lower than that of healthy controls, and approximately one fourth had difficulty returning to work [14].

The long-term use of mechanical ventilators may be a risk factor and a cause of ICU-acquired weakness [15], which has been observed in one fourth of patients requiring >7 days of mechanical ventilation [16]. Excessive immobilization is a major cause of ICU-acquired weakness [17], and a relationship between muscle weakness and duration of immobilization has been observed in patients with acute lung injury, whose muscle strength at the time of hospital discharge and 2 years later was reduced by 3 and 11 %, respectively, per each day of immobilization [18]. Therefore, patients mechanically ventilated in the ICU are likely to benefit from early mobilization to prevent ICU-acquired weakness, maintain long-term function, and preserve QOL.

Effectiveness of early mobilization

While early mobilization has become easier to implement, few randomized trials have examined its effectiveness in mechanically ventilated patients (Table 1). In a landmark study, Schweickert et al. randomly assigned 104 mechanically ventilated patients to early physical and occupational therapy versus usual care, and compared the proportions of patients in each group who returned to independent functional status at the time of discharge from the hospital [2]. An independent functional status at hospital discharge was regained by 59 % of patients in the intervention group, in whom early mobilization began at a mean of 1.5 days after the onset of mechanical ventilation, compared with 35 % of patients in the control group in whom early mobilization began at a mean of 7.4 days ($P = 0.02$). Patients in the early mobilization group also suffered from shorter periods of delirium and required fewer days of recurrent mechanical ventilation than the control group during 28 days of follow-up. Burtin et al. evenly assigned 90 mechanically ventilated patients to (a) a 20-min session of bicycle ergometer exercise daily, 5 days/week, in addition to standard care, versus (b) standard care only, and compared the outcomes of 6-min walk tests at the time of discharge from the hospital [3]. In the intervention group, the median 196 m covered in 6 min was significantly longer than the median 143 m covered in the control group. Furthermore, physical function ascertained by the 36-item Short-Form Health Survey were significantly greater in the intervention than in the control group, and the quadriceps femoris strength at discharge were significantly increased in the intervention group, but not in the control group.

Other studies, however, have not confirmed the efficacy of early mobilization. Two randomized trials including >100 mechanically ventilated, critically ill patients, observed insignificant improvements in physical function after intensive physical therapy [4, 5]. More recent, single-center randomized controlled trial, including 300 patients cared in ICU with acute respiratory failure requiring mechanical ventilation, has reported that daily standardized rehabilitation therapy consisting of passive range of motion, physical therapy, and progressive resistance exercise did not result in decreased duration of mechanical ventilation, hospital or ICU length of stay, and long-term physical function in comparison with usual care [7]. Another small, randomized pilot trial reported a significant increase in activity level in an intervention group after undergoing gait training in the ICU, though the length of stay in the ICU and the activity level 6 months later were similar in both study groups [6].

Differences in the interventions imposed in both groups may explain the insignificant effect of early mobilization. In one "negative" study, only 52 % of the planned participants in the intervention group were mobilized early, and 52 % of the patients assigned to the usual care group were mobilized early out of bed [19]. In addition, the time to first intervention or the interventions performed before randomization may influence the study results. In another negative study, the interventions began after eight ventilator days and detailed information regarding the intensity of physical therapy before randomization was not specified [5, 20].

Further studies and analyses are needed to accurately measure the effectiveness of early mobilization, where the contents of "standard care" and the length of the intervention are clearly defined.

Early mobilization in the ABCDE bundle

The "ABCDE bundle" is a strategy incorporated awakening and breathing coordination, delirium monitoring/management, and early exercise/mobility. It was proposed by Vasilevskis et al. in 2010, aiming at improving the prognosis of mechanically ventilated patients in the ICU by preventing delirium and ICU-acquired weakness [21]. The application of all steps, from A to E, to critically ill patients facilitates early mobilization as a voluntary activity during optimal sedation and analgesia. The implementation of the ABCDE bundle shortens the time spent on the ventilator, decreases the incidence of delirium, and increases the rate of early ambulatory mobilization practice [22]. A survey submitted in the state of Michigan in the USA revealed that early mobilization was adopted by 64 % of hospitals, though only 12 % included the whole ABCDE bundle [23]. Standing, walking, and gait exercises can reach higher levels of performance when whole ABCDE bundles are practiced. It is noteworthy that performing the A to D bundle is a prerequisite in order to effectively achieve early mobilization.

Adverse events

The incidence of adverse events during early mobilization is shown in Table 2. Although the majority of studies reported a <5 % incidence of adverse events [2–6, 24–28], it reached 16 % in one study [29], perhaps because of differences in the definitions of adverse events. Some studies have reported fatal adverse events, including extubation or desaturation; however, early mobilization is generally safe.

Inclusion and exclusion criteria and protocols

Each study of early mobilization in the ICU chooses independently its inclusion/exclusion criteria. In addition, protocols of early mobilization are inexistent, including in hospitals where it is being practiced [30]. Consensus statements regarding the performance of exercise by mechanically ventilated patients [31], or risk categories and safety criteria have been proposed in clinical guidelines of physical therapy and rehabilitation for patients in ICU [32]. Since 2014, the Early Rehabilitation Committee

Table 1 Randomized studies of the effects of early mobilization

Reference #	*n*	Study group		Days between intubation and onset of		Outcomes
		Intervention	Control	Intervention	Control	
[2]	104	Exercise and mobilization	Standard care	1.5	7.4	Primary: number of patients returning to independent functional status (ability to perform 6 daily activities and walking independently) at time of discharge from hospital. Secondary: (1) number of hospital days with delirium (2) number of ventilator-free days during first 28 days of hospitalization (3) length of stay in ICU and in hospital
[3]	90	Usual care + bicycle ergometer, 20 min/day, at an intensity level adjusted individually ×5 days/week	Respiratory therapy adjusted to the individual needs + standardized sessions of upper and lower extremities mobilization 5 days/week	14	10	Primary: distance covered in 6 min at time of discharge from the hospital Secondary: isometric quadriceps strength and functional status
[4]	150	Mechanically ventilated patient: physical therapy 15 min/day Non-mechanically ventilated patients: physical therapy 2 × 15 min Exercises: walking in place, moving from sitting to standing, arm and leg active and active resistance motion	Physical therapists provided respiratory and mobility management, based upon individual patient assessment according to unit protocols Usual care was available 7 days/week, 12 h/day	5	5	Primary: distance covered in 6 min at 12 months Secondary: Timed Up and Go Test, physical function in ICU test, assessment of QOL Instrument utility and short form 36 health survey
[5]	120	Delivered for 30 min/day, 7 days/week, while in ICU. Intensive physical therapy program included: 1. Proper breathing techniques during exercise 2. Progressive range of motion; 3. Muscle strengthening exercises 4. Exercises to increase core mobility and strength 5. Retraining of functional mobility	Standard of care physical therapy programs based on national survey Range of motion exercises, positioning, and functional mobility retraining 3 days/week for 20 min in ICU	8	8	Primary: short form of the continuous scale physical functional performance test at 4 weeks Secondary: number of ICU- and hospital-free days on day 28; discharged home, all-cause mortality on day 28, and institution-free days on days 90 and 180
[6]	50	Early goal-directed mobilization comprised functional rehabilitation treatment at the highest level of activity possible for that patient assessed by the ICU mobility scale while receiving mechanical ventilation.	Not based on protocol All usual unit practices were continued, without restrictions to physical therapy or sedation practice	3	3	Primary: higher maximum level of activity measured using the ICU mobility scale, increased duration of activity measured in min/day during the ICU stay compared with standard care Secondary: time from admission to first mobilization; duration of mechanical ventilation, ICU and hospital length of stay, and overall duration of hospitalization;

Table 1 Randomized studies of the effects of early mobilization *(Continued)*

						serious adverse events, number of ventilator- and ICU-free days on day 28; measurement of physical function with the physical function in ICU, the functional status score in ICU, and the Medical Research Council Manual Muscle Tests; ICU-acquired weakness
[7]	300	Standardized rehabilitation therapy 7 days a week from enrollment through hospital discharge protocol contained 3 exercise types: passive range of motion, physical therapy, and progressive resistance exercises	Usual care; received routine care as dictated by the patient's attending physician from Monday through Friday	1	7	Primary: hospital length of stay Secondary: Short Performance Physical Battery score, muscular strength, short form Functional Performance Inventory score, 36-Item Short Form Health Survey physical health survey and mental health survey, mini-mental state examination score (measure of physical function were obtained at ICU discharge, hospital discharge and 2, 4, and 6 months after enrollment, health-related quality-of-life measures were obtained at hospital discharge and 2,4, and 6 months after enrollment)

Table 2 Adverse events during early mobilization

Reference #	*n*	Early mobilization intervention	Incidence of adverse events	Adverse events
[24]	103	Active mobilization: 1449 sessions: sitting on bed and in chair, ambulation	0.96 %	Fall, systolic blood pressure <90 mmHg, oxygen desaturation, feeding tube extraction, systolic blood pressure >200 mmHg
[3]	90	Passive and active therapy, bicycle ergometer exercise	3.76 %	SpO_2 < 90 %, systolic blood pressure >180 mmHg, >20 % decrease in diastolic blood pressure
[2]	104	Passive and active range of motion, sitting, balance exercises, activities of daily living, transfer training, walking	4.0 %	Patient instability (most often because of perceived patient-ventilator asynchrony), 0.2 % serious (desaturation <80 %)
[29]	99	Active mobilization: 498 sessions	16 %	Desaturation ≧5 %, heart rate increase >20 %, ventilator asynchrony/tachypnea, agitation/discomfort, device removal
[25]	20	Active mobilization: 424 sessions: chair sitting, head up tilt, walking	3 %	Decreased muscle tone, hypoxemia, extubation, orthostatic, hypotension
[4]	150	Walking in place, sit to stand transfers, arm and leg active range of motion	None major	–
[26]	1110	Active mobilization: 5267 session: in-bed exercise, in-bed bicycling, sitting, transfer, standing, walking	0.6 %	Arrhythmia, MAP > 140 mmHg, MAP < 55 mmHg, oxygen desaturation, fall, feeding tube extraction, radial artery catheter removal, chest tube removal
[27]	637	16-level early progressive mobility protocol	Not validated	–
[28]	99	Active mobilization: 520 sessions	5 %	Respiratory distress, desaturation, tachypnea or bradycardia, patient's intolerance, tracheostomy removal
[5]	120	Proper breathing techniques during exercise, progressive range of motion, muscle strengthening exercises, exercises designed to improve core mobility and strength, functional mobility retraining	0.16 %	Syncopal episode during a PT session, readmitted to the hospital with polyarthralgia
[6]	50	Early goal-directed mobilization	0.96 %	Fall, systolic blood pressure <90 mmHg, oxygen desaturation, feeding tube extraction, systolic blood pressure >200 mmHg
[7]	300	Passive range of motion, physical therapy, and progressive resistance exercises	6.0 %	Deaths, device removals, reintubations, and patient falls during physical therapy

of the Japanese Society of Intensive Care Medicine has developed an "evidence-based expert consensus" early rehabilitation manual. To date, only 16 % of healthcare providers have prepared protocols of early mobilization, and 36 % are planning to develop a protocol [10, 11]. A survey submitted in the USA found that the adoption of early mobilization protocols shortens the time needed to regain a higher level of ambulatory mobility [1, 33].

Furthermore, a 2013 survey conducted in 12 ICU in Australia and New Zealand found that among 1395 sessions of physical therapy in 192 patients, active mobilization during mechanical ventilation was used only 315 times in the absence of protocol [34]. Based on these observations, Hodgson et al. conducted a randomized trial with a preliminary protocol intervention program, called early goal-directed mobilization, in order to promote the active mobilization of mechanically ventilated patients. This program aimed at conducting the highest level of 30–60 min interventions based on the evaluation of ICU mobility scale [6]. Compared to the usual care, the intervention group reached higher levels of active mobilization and longer duration of active mobilization. Secondary endpoints, such as health-related QOL, anxiety, depression, activity of daily living levels, and rates of return to work were similar in both groups. A study including >500 participants is needed to evaluate patient-centered measures as primary outcome. Hospitals which had already implemented early mobilization found no significant differences in frequency of early mobilization regardless of early mobilization protocols [30], suggesting that, in hospitals that are already practicing early mobilization, protocols are of uncertain efficacy.

Current status and further studies

Although early mobilization is a safe and effective procedure (Table 2), surveys performed at multiple sites have revealed that active mobilization beyond sitting is not commonly practiced, and that it varies among countries.

A survey conducted in 38 Australian and New Zealander ICU in 2009 and 2010 revealed that exercise was limited to the bed in 28 % of 514 patients, and that 25 and 18 %, respectively, performed standing and walking exercises, while no standing and walking exercises were performed by mechanically ventilated patients [9]. Another survey conducted in 2010 and 2011, reported that only 60 % of patients in Australian and 40 % in Scottish ICU reached a level of active mobilization higher than sitting [35], while in 116 German ICU in 2011, 185 of 783 mechanically ventilated (24 %) and only 8 % of tracheally intubated patients reached a level of early mobilization higher than sitting [8]. In the American state of Washington, a questionnaire submitted in 2012 and 2013 revealed that a wide range of motion exercises was routinely practiced in >70 % of hospitals, while only approximately 10 % conducted sitting and standing exercises routinely [33]. In contrast, a survey submitted to Japanese providers of intensive care revealed that range of motion exercises are often practiced, including sitting and standing exercises in 60 and 40 % of patients, respectively [10, 11]. Further studies are warranted to evaluate the effects of early mobilization in Japanese ICU, where extensive exercises are widely practiced.

Impediments and strategies

Based on 40 previous studies, Dubb et al. identified 28 obstacles in the way of early mobilization, including 14 (50 %) related to patients; five structural barriers (18 %), five related to the cultures of ICU (18 %); and four process-related impediments (14 %) [36]. They offered >70 solutions or strategies to deal with each barrier. The obstacles to early mobilization may vary depending on the physician(s), nurse(s), and physical therapist(s) involved in the care of each patient [37, 38]. Inter-professional collaboration needs to be developed with a view to create educational programs and research projects to address the challenges represented by the early mobilization of mechanically ventilated patients in the ICU.

Conclusions

Despite multiple recent studies claiming the safety and effectiveness of early mobilization of mechanically ventilated patients, convincing trials remain few. Early has not been accurately defined, and the differences between intervention and standard care vary among studies. The methods and frequency of standardized early mobilization of mechanically ventilated patients remain unsettled. In addition, the number of the studies included is not big enough and their sample sizes are limited. The generalizability of the findings in this review would therefore be open to question. Additional clinical trials are needed to confirm the efficacy of early mobilization of mechanically ventilated patients in the ICU.

Abbreviations

ARDS, acute respiratory distress syndrome; ICU, intensive care unit; QOL, quality of life

Acknowledgements

There are no acknowledgements to be declared.

Funding

There is no funding to be declared.

Authors' contributions

ST and NS wrote the manuscript. KO and HY critically reviewed and revised the manuscript. All authors have read and approved the final version of the manuscript.

Competing interests

The corresponding author states that NS had been received speaking fees from Pfizer.

Author details

[1]Division of Rehabilitation, Department of Clinical Practice and Support, Hiroshima University Hospital, 1-2-3, Kasumi, Minami-ku, Hiroshima 734-8551, Japan. [2]Department of Emergency and Critical Care Medicine, Institute of Biomedical and Health Sciences, Hiroshima University, 1-2-3, Kasumi, Minami-ku, Hiroshima 734-8553, Japan. [3]Department of Intensive Care Medicine, Kameda Medical Center, 929, Higashi-cho, Kamogawa, Chiba 296-8602, Japan.

References

1. Morris PE, Goad A, Thompson C, Taylor K, Harry B, Passmore L, et al. Early intensive care unit mobility therapy in the treatment of acute respiratory failure. Crit Care Med. 2008;36:2238–43.
2. Schweickert WD, Pohlman MC, Pohlman AS, Nigos C, Pawlik AJ, Esbrook CL, et al. Early physical and occupational therapy in mechanically ventilated, critically ill patients: a randomised controlled trial. Lancet. 2009;373:1874–82.
3. Burtin C, Clerckx B, Robbeets C, Ferdinande P, Langer D, Troosters T, et al. Early exercise in critically ill patients enhances short-term functional recovery. Crit Care Med. 2009;37:2499–505.
4. Denehy L, Skinner EH, Edbrooke L, Haines K, Warrillow S, Hawthorne G, et al. Exercise rehabilitation for patients with critical illness: a randomized controlled trial with 12 months of follow-up. Crit Care. 2013;17:R156.
5. Moss M, Nordon-Craft A, Malone D, Van Pelt D, Frankel SK, Warner ML, et al. A randomized trial of an intensive physical therapy program for acute respiratory failure patients. Am J Respir Crit Care Med. 2016;193:1101–10.

6. Hodgson CL, Bailey M, Bellomo R, Berney S, Buhr H, Denehy L, et al. A binational multicenter pilot feasibility randomized controlled trial of early goal-directed mobilization in ICU. Crit Care Med. 2016;44:1145–52.
7. Morris PE, Berry MJ, Files DC, Thompson JC, Hauser J, Flores L, et al. Standardized rehabilitation and hospital length of stay among patients with acute respiratory failure: a randomized clinical trial. JAMA. 2016;315:2694–702.
8. Nydahl P, Ruhl AP, Bartoszek G, Dubb R, Filipovic S, Flohr HJ, et al. Early mobilization of mechanically ventilated patients: a 1-day point-prevalence study in Germany. Crit Care Med. 2014;42:1178–86.
9. Berney SC, Harrold M, Webb SA, Seppelt I, Patman S, Thomas PJ, et al. Intensive care unit mobility practices in Australia and New Zealand: a point prevalence study. Crit Care Resusc. 2013;15:260–5.
10. Japanese Society for Physicians and Trainees in Intensive Care Clinical Trial Group. 49th brief questionnaire: current rehabilitation practice in intensive care unit in Japan. 2016 January. http://www.jseptic.com/rinsho/questionnaire_490225.pdf (in Japanese). Accessed 13 June 2016.
11. Yasuda H. Current rehabilitation practice in intensive care unit in Japan. Intensivist. 2016;8:508–17 (in Japanese).
12. Bellani G, Laffey JG, Pham T, Fan E, Brochard L, Esteban A, et al. Epidemiology, patterns of care, and mortality for patients with acute respiratory distress syndrome in intensive care units in 50 countries. JAMA. 2016;315:788–800.
13. Esteban A, Anzueto A, Frutos F, Alía I, Brochard L, Stewart TE, et al. Characteristics and outcomes in adult patients receiving mechanical ventilation: a 28-day international study. JAMA. 2002;287:345–55.
14. Herridge MS, Tansey CM, Matté A, Tomlinson G, Diaz-Granados N, Cooper A, et al. Functional disability 5 years after acute respiratory distress syndrome. N Engl J Med. 2011;364:1293–304.
15. Stevens RD, Marshall SA, Cornblath DR, Hoke A, Needham DM, de Jonghe B, et al. A framework for diagnosing and classifying intensive care unit-acquired weakness. Crit Care Med. 2009;37:S299–308.
16. De Jonghe B, Sharshar T, Lefaucheur JP, Authier FJ, Durand-Zaleski I, Boussarsar M, et al. Paresis acquired in the intensive care unit: a prospective multicenter study. JAMA. 2002;288:2859–67.
17. Kress JP, Hall JB. ICU-acquired weakness and recovery from critical illness. N Engl J Med. 2014;370:1626–35.
18. Fan E, Dowdy DW, Colantuoni E, Mendez-Tellez PA, Sevransky JE, Shanholtz C, et al. Physical complications in acute lung injury survivors: a two-year longitudinal prospective study. Crit Care Med. 2014;42:849–59.
19. Berney S, Haines K, Skinner EH, Denehy L. Safety and feasibility of an exercise prescription approach to rehabilitation across the continuum of care for survivors of critical illness. Phys Ther. 2012;92:1524–35.
20. Taito S, Ota K, Shime N. Is earlier and more intensive physical therapy program better? Am J Respir Crit Care Med. 2016 (in press)
21. Vasilevskis EE, Ely EW, Speroff T, Pun BT, Boehm L, Dittus RS. Reducing iatrogenic risks: ICU-acquired delirium and weakness—crossing the quality chasm. Chest. 2010;138:1224–33.
22. Balas MC, Vasilevskis EE, Olsen KM, Schmid KK, Shostrom V, Cohen MZ, et al. Effectiveness and safety of the awakening and breathing coordination, delirium monitoring/management, and early exercise/mobility bundle. Crit Care Med. 2014;42:1024–36.
23. Miller MA, Govindan S, Watson SR, Hyzy RC, Iwashyna T. ABCDE, but in that order? A cross-sectional survey of Michigan intensive care unit sedation, delirium, and early mobility practices. Ann Am Thorac Soc. 2015;12:1066–71.
24. Bailey P, Thomsen GE, Spuhler VJ, Blair R, Jewkes J, Bezdjian L, et al. Early activity is feasible and safe in respiratory failure patients. Crit Care Med. 2007;35:139–45.
25. Bourdin G, Barbier J, Burle JF, Durante G, Passant S, Vincent B, et al. The feasibility of early physical activity in intensive care unit patients: a prospective observational one-center study. Respir Care. 2010;55:400–7.
26. Sricharoenchai T, Parker AM, Zanni JM, Nelliot A, Dinglas VD, Needham DM. Safety of physical therapy interventions in critically ill patients: a single-center prospective evaluation of 1110 intensive care unit admissions. J Crit Care. 2014;29:395–400.
27. Klein K, Mulkey M, Bena JF, Albert NM. Clinical and psychological effects of early mobilization in patients treated in a neurologic ICU: a comparative study. Crit Care Med. 2015;43:865–73.
28. Lee H, Ko YJ, Suh GY, Yang JH, Park CM, Jeon K, et al. Safety profile and feasibility of early physical therapy and mobility for critically ill patients in the medical intensive care unit: beginning experiences in Korea. J Crit Care. 2015;30:673–7.
29. Pohlman MC, Schweickert WD, Pohlman AS, Nigos C, Pawlik AJ, Esbrook CL, et al. Feasibility of physical and occupational therapy beginning from initiation of mechanical ventilation. Crit Care Med. 2010;38:2089–94.
30. Bakhru RN, Wiebe DJ, Mcwilliams DJ, Spuhler VJ, Schweickert WD. An environmental scan for early mobilization practices in U.S. ICUs. Crit Care Med. 2015;43:2360–9.
31. Hodgson CL, Stiller K, Needham DM, Tipping CJ, Harrold M, Baldwin CE, et al. Expert consensus and recommendations on safety criteria for active mobilization of mechanically ventilated critically ill adults. Crit Care. 2014;18:658.
32. Sommers J, Engelbert RH, Dettling-Ihnenfeldt D, Gosselink R, Spronk PE, Nollet F, et al. Physical therapy in the intensive care unit: an evidence-based, expert driven, practical statement and rehabilitation recommendations. Clin Rehabil. 2015;29:1051–63.
33. Jolley SE, Dale CR, Hough CL. Hospital-level factors associated with report of physical activity in patients on mechanical ventilation across Washington State. Ann Am Thorac Soc. 2015;12:209–15.
34. TEAM Study Investigators, Hodgson C, Bellomo R, Berney S, Bailey M, Buhr H, et al. Early mobilization and recovery in mechanically ventilated patients in ICU: a bi-national, multi-centre, prospective cohort study. Crit Care. 2015;19:81.
35. Harrold ME, Salisbury LG, Webb SA, Allison GT. Australia and Scotland ICU Physiotherapy Collaboration. Early mobilisation in intensive care units in Australia and Scotland: a prospective, observational cohort study examining mobilisation practises and barriers. Crit Care. 2015;19:336.
36. Dubb R, Nydahl P, Hermes C, Schwabbauer N, Toonstra A, Parker AM, et al. Barriers and strategies for early mobilization of patients in intensive care units. Ann Am Thorac Soc. 2016;13:724–30.
37. Garzon-Serrano J, Ryan C, Waak K, Hirschberg R, Tully S, Bittner EA, et al. Early mobilization in critically ill patients: patients' mobilization level depends on health care provider's profession. PM R. 2011;3:307–13.
38. Jolley SE, Regan-Baggs J, Dickson RP, Hough CL. Medical intensive care unit clinician attitudes and perceived barriers towards early mobilization of critically ill patients: a cross-sectional survey study. BMC Anesthesiol. 2014;14:84.

7

Early versus late tracheostomy after decompressive craniectomy for stroke

Michael P. Catalino[1], Feng-Chang Lin[2], Nathan Davis[1], Keith Anderson[3], Casey Olm-Shipman[1,4] and J. Dedrick Jordan[1,4*]

Abstract

Background: Stroke patients requiring decompressive craniectomy are at high risk of prolonged mechanical ventilation and ventilator-associated pneumonia (VAP). Tracheostomy placement may reduce the duration of mechanical ventilation. Predicting which patients will require tracheostomy and the optimal timing of tracheostomy remains a clinical challenge. In this study, the authors compare key outcomes after early versus late tracheostomy and develop a useful pre-operative decision-making tool to predict post-operative tracheostomy dependence.

Methods: We performed a retrospective analysis of prospectively collected registry data. We developed a propensity-weighted decision tree analysis to predict tracheostomy requirement using factors present prior to surgical decompression. In addition, outcomes include probability functions for intensive care unit length of stay, hospital length of stay, and mortality, based on data for early (≤ 10 days) versus late (> 10 days) tracheostomy.

Results: There were 168 surgical decompressions performed on patients with acute ischemic or spontaneous hemorrhagic stroke between 2010 and 2015. Forty-eight patients (28.5%) required a tracheostomy, 35 (20.8%) developed VAP, and 126 (75%) survived hospitalization. Mean ICU and hospital length of stay were 15.1 and 25.8 days, respectively. Using GCS, SOFA score, and presence of hydrocephalus, our decision tree analysis had 63% sensitivity and 84% specificity for predicting tracheostomy requirement. The early group had fewer ventilator days (7.3 versus 15.2, $p < 0.001$) and shorter hospital length of stay (28.5 versus 44.4 days, $p = 0.014$). VAP rates and mortality were similar between the two groups. Withdrawal of treatment interventions shortly post-operatively confounded mortality outcomes.

Conclusion: Early tracheostomy shortens duration of mechanical ventilation and length of stay after surgical decompression for stroke, but it did not impact mortality or VAP rates. A decision tree is a practical tool that may be helpful in guiding pre-operative decision-making with patients' families.

Keywords: Decompression, Ischemic stroke, Hemorrhagic stroke, Tracheostomy timing, Ventilator-associated pneumonia

Background

Mechanically ventilated stroke patients are at risk for ventilator-associated pneumonia (VAP) and prolonged stay in intensive care units (ICU) [1–3]. Recent reviews cite the incidence of VAP to be 1–9 occurrences per 1000 ventilator days and suggest its pathogenesis to be multifactorial with timing, duration of endotracheal ventilation, host factors, and virulence of invading bacteria all contributing [4]. Patients with ischemic and hemorrhagic stroke can often wean rapidly from the ventilator after tracheostomy [5]. There is little evidence to guide timing of tracheostomy in patients with large hemispheric infarctions [6]. Generally, tracheostomy may be considered after 7–14 days if extubation is not feasible. Studies have looked at tracheostomy performed as early as hospital day 4 [7], but the definition of "early" and "late" varies widely in the literature [7–11]. Studies have shown a linear relationship between tracheostomy timing and ICU length of stay [3]. Furthermore, delayed tracheostomy may place patients at undue risk of pneumonia from prolonged mechanical ventilation [11–14].

* Correspondence: dedrick@unc.edu
[1]Department of Neurosurgery, University of North Carolina School of Medicine, 170 Manning Drive, Campus Box 7025, Chapel Hill, NC 27599-7025, USA
[4]Department of Neurology, University of North Carolina, 170 Manning Drive, Campus Box 7025, Chapel Hill, NC, USA
Full list of author information is available at the end of the article

The TRACH score [14] and SETscore [15] are two of the most comprehensive tools, among many that are used for predicting tracheostomy in patients with cerebrovascular injury [16]. The reported sensitivity of the TRACH score is 94% and has a specificity of 83% to predict extubation. Furthermore, the SETscore looks at neurological function, brain lesion factors, and general organ function to assess likelihood requiring greater than 2 weeks of ventilator support in stroke patients in the ICU [15]. A SETscore of 8 returned an optimum sensitivity of 65.4% and specificity of 73.5%. These are two helpful tools within a growing body of literature on this topic. In critically ill patients, studies are inconclusive but suggest a decrease in mortality and ICU length of stay and lower sedative requirement after early tracheostomy. [8, 17] The SETPOINT pilot study decreased ICU and 6-month mortality after tracheostomy placement 1–3 days after intubation in patients with all strokes, including subarachnoid hemorrhage, but indicated no change in ICU length of stay [9], although half of the patients randomized to standard tracheostomy died prior to receiving the intervention. We are critical in our interpretation of current literature as large well-controlled studies are still lacking, and those present are considerably heterogeneous. In one trial, about half of the patients assigned to late tracheostomy did not require the intervention at all [7]. Our objectives were to use our robust database and propensity weight methods to identify which factors predicted the need for tracheostomy in stroke patients requiring surgical decompression, as well as to analyze the relationship between the timing of tracheostomy, incidence of VAP, rate of in-hospital mortality, and ICU and hospital length of stay.

Methods

Data registry

The University of North Carolina (UNC) Neuroscience Intensive Care Unit (NSICU) patient registry is a prospectively collected database of all NSICU patients. Institutional Review Board approval was obtained to access the database for research purposes (IRB no. 15-2372). The database was queried. Inclusion criteria were as follows: adult patients, presentation between May 2010 and September 2015, ischemic or hemorrhagic stroke, and decompressive craniectomy. Data was extracted directly from the database, and patient records were reviewed for additional variables as needed. There were no exclusion criteria, and thus, all patients meeting the inclusion criteria were included in the initial analysis. Patients with missing variables were still included; however, specific missing variables excluded patients from the denominator of analyses where data was not available. In the final mortality analysis, patients who died on comfort care were excluded.

Data analysis

Timing of tracheostomy was expressed in terms of post-stroke day or hospital day if the date of injury was indeterminate. A 10-day cutoff was preselected based on previous literature from a recent Cochrane Review [8]. It fell between the routine tracheostomy timing at our institution (7–14 days) and thus was also feasible to study using our database. The treatment group (early) included all patients receiving tracheostomy at or before stroke/hospital day 10, and the control group (late) was those who received a tracheostomy after day 10.

The primary objectives were to develop a predictive model for tracheostomy and compare outcomes for early versus late tracheostomy. Primary outcomes included mortality, ICU length of stay, hospital length of stay, and ventilator-associated pneumonia. Propensity weighting was used to predict the probability of tracheostomy after identifying crude predictors through bivariate analysis. We used propensity scores to control for differences in measured covariates between early and late tracheostomy cohorts by first estimating the probability of receiving tracheostomy based on crude bivariate analysis in Table 2. After weighting, this process leads to a pseudo-population, whose covariate distribution can be matched between early and late tracheostomy cohorts. This not only removes confounding by measured covariates, but also allows us to estimate the association between timing of tracheostomy and outcomes. We report percentages only in the final analysis because the actual counts are based on the pseudo-population. Variables considered for inclusion in the propensity weights were Glasgow Coma Score (GCS), time to surgery, hydrocephalus, location of stroke, and Sequential Organ Failure Assessment (SOFA) score. Time to surgery was not a clinically meaningful predictor after sensitivity analyses, and thus, it was not used in the final weights. GCS has been described as a predictor for tracheostomy after craniectomy for traumatic brain injury, but not for stroke, and thus, we felt it was a meaningful variable to include [18]. Hydrocephalus was defined as any neurological deterioration attributable to elevated ICP, which subsequently required cerebrospinal fluid diversion via a ventriculostomy drain. All primary outcomes were compared using propensity weights. Sensitivity analysis was performed for tracheostomy timing and primary outcomes.

Results

There were 168 patients who received surgical decompression following a stroke (Fig. 1). Descriptive patient characteristics are reported in Table 1. Average GCS on admission was 9.3, average time to surgery was 1.7 days, and average SOFA score was 6.5. There were 131 hemorrhagic and 37 ischemic strokes, of which 37 (28.2%) and 11 (29.7%), respectively, required a tracheostomy. Indications for tracheostomy included failure to wean mechanical ventilation for

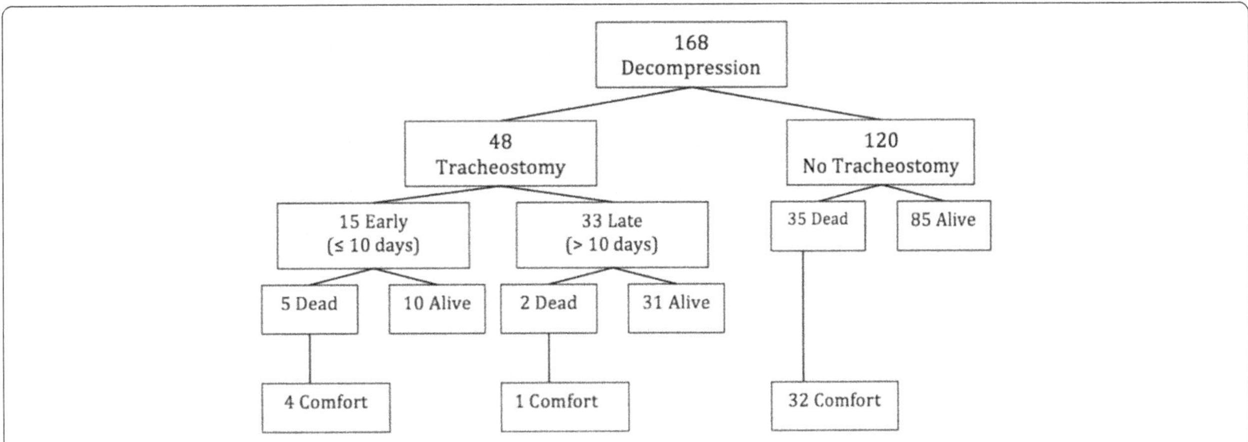

Fig. 1 Flow chart showing the number of patients who underwent decompression for stroke (ischemic or hemorrhagic), those who received a tracheostomy, and survival, including those who were excluded from the final analysis due to death while on comfort-measures-only status

a prolonged period, neurological status that precludes extubation, and multiple failed extubation. Additionally, 35 (20.8%) patients developed VAP. On average, patients contracted VAP 2 days prior to receiving their tracheostomy and 9 days after admission (Table 1). Patients who required tracheostomy had longer ICU length of stay (27.8 versus 10.0 days, $p < 0.001$) and a longer duration of mechanical ventilation (13.0 versus 6.3 days, $p < 0.001$); however, these patients did not demonstrate a significantly longer mean length of hospital stay.

Bivariate analysis comparing covariates among those who received a tracheostomy and those who did not are shown in Table 2. These covariates were used to build propensity weights as shown in Tables 3 and 4. Duration of mechanical ventilation was the only significant variable that correlated with VAP in multivariate regression modeling. Lower GCS, higher SOFA, and hydrocephalus all were associated with higher likelihood of receiving tracheostomy (Tables 3 and 4), and these variables were included in the decision tree analysis (Fig. 2).

Decision tree analysis

GCS was the most important predictor for tracheostomy. Patients with a GCS less than 8, SOFA greater than 5, and hydrocephalus had the highest likelihood of requiring tracheostomy. Combining these classification criteria, the sensitivity is 63% and the specificity is 84%. Figure 2 shows the decision tree analysis, and the caption provides a detailed explanation of its interpretation.

Primary outcomes and tracheostomy timing

Fifteen patients (31.2%) received a tracheostomy prior to hospital day 10, and 33 patients received a tracheostomy after day 10 (68.8%). Propensity-weighted outcomes comparing no tracheostomy versus tracheostomy were reviewed. Patients who received a tracheostomy had comparable mortality (after excluding those who transitioned to comfort measures), higher VAP incidence, and longer ICU length of stay (Additional file 1: Table S2). Early tracheostomy significantly predicted mortality compared to late tracheostomy [10/15 (33.3%) versus 2/33 (6.1%), respectively, $p = 0.006$; Table 3] although this was completely explained by early withdrawal of treatment and death while on comfort care (Table 4). Early tracheostomy did not protect against VAP compared to late tracheostomy (40.0% versus 36.4%, $p = 0.614$). Early tracheostomy did lead to less overall duration of ventilator dependence. Mean ventilator days for early tracheostomy was 7.3 versus 15.2 days for late tracheostomy ($p < 0.001$). Early tracheostomy was associated with a trend toward reducing the ICU length of stay, 20.1 versus 31.5 days, although this difference was not significantly different ($p = 0.073$; Table 3). Early tracheostomy significantly reduced hospital length of stay from 44.4 to 28.5 days ($p = 0.014$; Table 3).

VAP incidence rate was similar for both groups, 40% for early versus 36% for late tracheostomy ($p = 0.614$). If the cutoff is changed to day 7 or earlier, the VAP is much lower for the early group (20 versus 40%, $p = 0.821$), but statistical significance is not reached due to too few patients in this group. For discharge location, early tracheostomy showed a trend toward more favorable discharge locations (40.0 versus 29.0%, $p = 0.192$; Table 4). According to propensity-weighted probability functions for hospital discharge, the early tracheostomy group had a significantly shorter hospital length of stay (Fig. 3). However, propensity-adjusted mortality rate analysis resulted in a significantly higher mortality rate in patients who received an early tracheostomy (33.3 versus 6.1%, $p = 0.006$; Table 3 and Fig. 4a). In addition, patients with early tracheostomies still trended toward favorable discharge (home or to rehab) compared to those with late tracheostomies (40.0% versus 29.0%, respectively) with similar VAP rates (36.4% versus 37.5%, respectively; Table 4).

Table 1 Patient demographics and clinical factors by primary stroke etiology (hemorrhagic or ischemic)

	Total	ICH	Ischemic	*p* value
N	168	131 (78%)	37 (22%)	
Age, mean (SD)	55.3 (15.3)	55.3 (16.2)	55.2 (12.0)	0.116
Male	91 (54%)	65 (50%)	26 (70%)	0.039
Race				
White	86 (57%)	68 (59%)	18 (53%)	0.547
African American	51 (34%)	37 (32%)	14 (41%)	
Other	13 (9%)	11 (9%)	2 (6%)	
BMI, mean (SD)	28.1 (7.4)	27.6 (7.6)	29.7 (6.2)	0.148
Myocardial infarction	8 (5%)	6 (5%)	2 (5%)	1.000
Congestive heart failure	9 (5%)	3 (2%)	6 (16%)	0.004
Peripheral vascular disease	11 (7%)	6 (5%)	5 (13%)	0.067
Dementia	1 (1%)	1 (1%)	0 (0%)	1.000
Cerebrovascular disease	23 (14%)	19 (15%)	4 (11%)	0.787
Chronic lung disease	17 (10%)	14 (11%)	3 (8%)	0.766
Ulcer	3 (2%)	3 (2%)	0 (0%)	1.000
Chronic liver disease	6 (4%)	6 (5%)	0 (0%)	0.340
Diabetes	30 (18%)	18 (14%)	12 (32%)	0.015
Moderate–severe kidney disease	13 (8%)	13 (10%)	0 (0%)	0.074
Diabetes with organ damage	4 (2%)	4 (3%)	0 (0%)	0.577
Tumor	10 (6%)	9 (7%)	1 (3%)	0.461
Leukemia	3 (2%)	3 (2%)	0 (0%)	1.000
Lymphoma	0 (0%)	0 (0%)	0 (0%)	NA
Moderate–severe liver disease	1 (1%)	1 (1%)	0 (0%)	1.000
Malignant tumor	9 (5%)	8 (6%)	1 (3%)	0.685
Metastasis	5 (3%)	5 (4%)	0 (0%)	0.588
AIDS	3 (2%)	1 (1%)	2 (5%)	0.124
Hosp. LOS, mean (SD)	25.8 (27.0)	27.1 (29.2)	21.2 (16.2)	0.246
Discharge location				
SNF	35 (27.8%)	26 (26.8%)	9 (31.0%)	0.560
AIR	54 (42.9%)	40 (41.2%)	14 (48.3%)	
Home	25 (19.8%)	22 (22.7%)	3 (10.3%)	
LTAC	10 (7.9%)	7 (7.2%)	3 (10.3%)	
Hospice	2 (1.6%)	2 (2.1%)	0 (0.0%)	
Discharge condition				
Alive	126 (75.0%)	97 (74.0%)	29 (78.4%)	0.671
Dead without comfort care	5 (3.0%)	4 (3.1%)	1 (2.7%)	
Dead with comfort care	37 (22.0%)	30 (22.9%)	7 (18.9%)	
ICU LOS, mean (SD)	15.1 (16.2)	16.0 (17.7)	11.9 (8.8)	0.190
Readmission to ICU	37 (22.2%)	26 (20.0%)	11 (29.7%)	0.261
GCS on adm., mean (SD)	9.3 (3.7)	8.9 (3.8)	10.6 (3.2)	0.012
Admission mRS, mean (SD)	4.9 (0.4)	4.9 (0.5)	5.0 (0.0)	0.068
SOFA score, mean (SD)	6.5 (2.8)	6.6 (2.8)	6.1 (2.7)	0.331
NIHSS, mean (SD)	18.3 (7.2)	–	18.3 (7.2)	NA

Table 1 Patient demographics and clinical factors by primary stroke etiology (hemorrhagic or ischemic) *(Continued)*

	Total	ICH	Ischemic	*p* value
Location				
Bilateral supratentorial	8 (4.8%)	8 (6.1%)	0 (0.0%)	0.456
Infratentorial	32 (19.0%)	24 (18.3%)	8 (21.6%)	
Left supratentorial	57 (33.9%)	45 (34.4%)	12 (32.4%)	
Right supratentorial	71 (42.3%)	54 (41.2%)	17 (45.9%)	
ICH score, mean (SD)	1.81 (0.95)	1.81 (0.95)	–	NA
IVH	62 (48.1%)	62 (48.1%)	–	NA
Hydrocephalus	88 (68.8%)	88 (68.8%)	–	
Time to surgery, mean (SD)	1.70 (3.6)	1.70 (3.9)	1.68 (2.4)	0.969
Time to ventilator, mean (SD)	0.65 (2.4)	0.63 (2.7)	0.73 (1.3)	0.821
Duration of ventilator, mean (SD)	8.1 (7.7)	8.8 (8.1)	5.9 (5.4)	0.051
# failed weans, mean (SD)	0.37 (0.56)	0.36 (0.57)	0.38 (0.55)	0.873
Tracheostomy	48 (28.6%)	37 (28.2%)	11 (29.7%)	0.840
Hosp tracheostomy day, mean (SD)	13.8 (7.2)	14.4 (7.9)	11.8 (4.0)	0.301
Duration tracheostomy, mean (SD)	29.8 (28.3)	30.2 (27.2)	28.3 (33.3)	0.912
Tracheostomy at discharge	39 (81.3%)	28 (75.7%)	11 (100%)	0.070
Total TRACH score	2.3 (2.4)	2.3 (2.4)	–	NA
Number of VAP, mean (SD)	0.56 (1.22)	0.59 (1.27)	0.46 (1.04)	0.574
Hospital VAP day, mean (SD)	9.5 (11.2)	9.2 (11.6)	10.3 (10.6)	0.826
Tracheostomy VAP day, mean (SD)	− 2 (16.6)	− 4.2 (17.8)	3.2 (13.4)	0.421

AIR acute inpatient rehabilitation, *GCS* Glasgow Coma Score, *ICU* intensive care unit, *LOS* length of stay, *LTAC* long-term acute care, *SD* standard deviation, *SNF* skilled nursing facility, *SOFA* Sequential Organ Failure Assessment

Discussion

Predicting who will require a tracheostomy after decompressive surgery for ischemic stroke or intracerebral hemorrhage remains a challenge. Furthermore, we, and others, have shown that the risk of ventilator-associated pneumonia is strongly associated with duration of mechanical ventilation [2]. Predicting which of these critically brain-injured patients will ultimately need a tracheostomy would be helpful when discussing treatment options with families. We have developed a decision tree, based on key variables present on admission (GCS, SOFA score, and presence of hydrocephalus; Fig. 2), which can help guide clinical judgment as to who may be a candidate for tracheostomy. This adds to the repertoire of clinical decision-making tools available to help expedite tracheostomy placement and free patients from the ventilator. Here, we argue that early tracheostomy may expedite ICU and hospital discharge, but its impact on reducing the risk of ventilator-associated pneumonia and mortality is still unclear.

In the initial TRACH score study, all patients with TRACH score > 2.0 required a tracheostomy, while none with a score < 0.7 required a tracheostomy. In our data, ICH patients requiring decompressive surgery and no tracheostomy had a mean TRACH score of 2.2 and 3.2 for those who did have a tracheostomy ($p = 0.041$). Thus, if using the TRACH score cutoff of 2, as in the original study, many of our patients would have received a tracheostomy that did not ultimately need one [14].

Our decision analysis shows that, in patients with a GCS less than 8, SOFA greater than 5, and hydrocephalus requiring a ventriculostomy, the sensitivity is 63% and the specificity is 84% for predicting tracheostomy requirement. This results in a positive predictive value of 61.2% and a negative predictive value of 85%. Our primary outcome data is similar to the results of a recent meta-analysis by McCredie and colleagues looking at early tracheostomy in patients with severe acute brain injury [19]. They found that although early tracheostomy reduced length of ICU stay, it did not have a significant mortality benefit. These results are in contrast to another study from Brazil which showed a drastically reduced 28-day mortality rate in early tracheostomy patients (9 versus 46%, $p = 0.049$) even with a small sample size ($n = 28$) [20]. Notably, GCS and SOFA score were similar in the two groups, serving as an internal control. However, they also noted an extremely high rate of VAP in the late group (54% in the early group and 70% in the late group), whereas our VAP rate was 40.0% in the early group and 36.4% in the late group. This may help explain the mortality benefit in their population, since higher VAP rates combined with rapid weaning

Table 2 Bivariate analysis for receiving a tracheostomy

	No trach	Trach	*p* value
N	120	48	
Diagnosis			
ICH	94 (78.3%)	37 (77.1%)	0.860
Ischemic	26 (21.7%)	11 (22.9%)	
Age, mean (SD)	56.4 (14.6)	52.4 (16.9)	0.129
Male	65 (54%)	26 (54%)	1.000
Race			
White	61 (58%)	25 (56%)	0.740
African American	34 (32%)	17 (38%)	
Other	10 (10%)	3 (7%)	
BMI, mean (SD)	27.5 (5.9)	29.4 (10.1)	0.133
GCS on adm., mean (SD)	9.7 (3.7)	8.2 (3.6)	0.023
Adm. mRS, mean (SD)	4.92 (0.50)	5.0 (0)	0.246
SOFA score, mean (SD)	6.2 (2.7)	7.1 (2.9)	0.055
NIHSS, mean (SD)	18.1 (6.8)	18.7 (8.7)	0.853
Location			
Bilateral supratentorial	5 (4.2%)	3 (6.3%)	0.638
Infratentorial	23 (19.2%)	9 (18.8%)	
Left supratentorial	38 (31.7%)	19 (39.6%)	
Right supratentorial	54 (45.0%)	17 (35.4%)	
ICH score, mean (SD)	1.77 (1.00)	1.91 (0.82)	0.458
IVH	41 (44.6%)	21 (56.8%)	0.210
Hydrocephalus	58 (63.7%)	30 (81.1%)	0.055
Time to surgery, mean (SD)	1.23 (2.19)	2.85 (5.77)	0.009
VAP	17 (14.2%)	18 (37.5%)	0.001
Number of VAP, mean (SD)	0.38 (1.00)	1.02 (1.56)	0.002

after tracheostomy will reduce total exposure to risk of VAP. Even though the VAP rates were not significantly different, as was true in our study, we suspect this was due to inadequate study power. Despite lack of direct evidence, we still believe early tracheostomy likely reduces total ventilator time eliminating the primary risk

Table 3 Propensity-weighted outcomes for timing of tracheostomy

	Early	Late	*p* value
Mortality	33.3%	6.1%	0.006
VAP	40.0%	36.4%	0.614
Duration of ventilation, mean days (SD)	7.3 (7.2)	15.2 (6.6)	< 0.001
ICU stay, mean days (SD)	20.1 (10.6)	31.5 (28.1)	0.073
Hospital stay, mean days (SD)	28.5 (12.5)	44.4 (33.7)	0.014
Discharge location			
Home/rehabilitation	40.0%	29.0%	0.192
Skilled nursing facility/LTAC	60.0%	71.0%	

Table 4 Propensity-weighted outcomes for timing of tracheostomy (excluding those who died on comfort care)

	Early	Late	*p* value
Mortality	9.1%	3.1%	0.780
VAP	36.4%	37.5%	0.652
Duration of ventilation, mean days (SD)	5.5 (3.4)	15.2 (6.7)	< 0.001
ICU stay, mean days (SD)	20.2 (10.2)	32.0 (28.4)	0.153
Hospital stay, mean days (SD)	31.3 (11.7)	45.3 (33.8)	0.075
Discharge location			
Home/rehabilitation	40.0%	29.0%	0.192
Skilled nursing facility/LTAC	60.0%	71.0%	

factor for VAP, the ventilator itself. Given the reduction in ICU length of stay, there are likely economic benefits from early tracheostomy as well. This was not explicitly studied here. Ongoing prospective controlled trials are needed to ultimately provide sound evidence for true early tracheostomy in these patients.

The trend in mortality was unexpected, so we reviewed all deaths after our final analysis to try and understand this

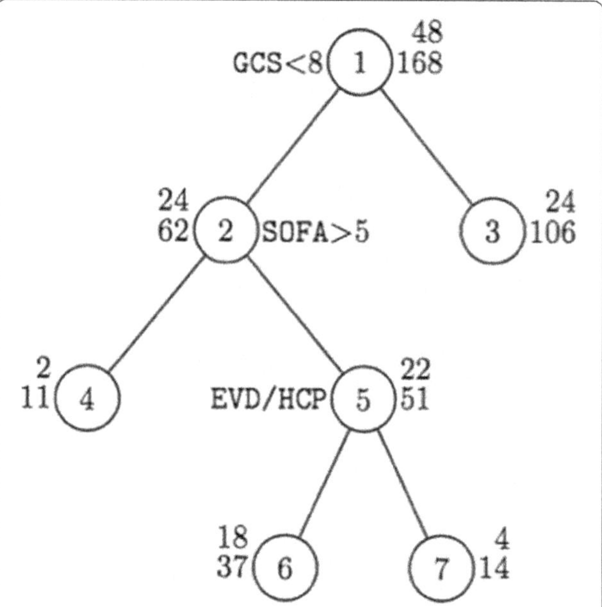

Fig. 2 Decision tree for the prediction of tracheostomy. At each split, a patient goes to the left branch when the left-side condition is satisfied and goes to the right branch when the right-side condition is satisfied. The top number (numerator) is the number of patients who received a tracheostomy. The bottom number (denominator) is the sample size for that group. Assessing 2 and 3 results in odds ratio 2.14 with 95% CI 1.03–4.52 and *p* value = 0.034, 50% sensitivity, and 68% specificity. Assessing 4 and 5 results in odds ratio 3.35 with 95% CI 0.61–35.0 and *p* value = 0.178; sensitivity improves to 54% and specificity to 76%. Finally, assessing 6 and 7 results in odds ratio 2.33 with 95% CI 0.54–12.1 and *p* value = 0.225; combining three classification criteria, the sensitivity is 63% and the specificity is 84%

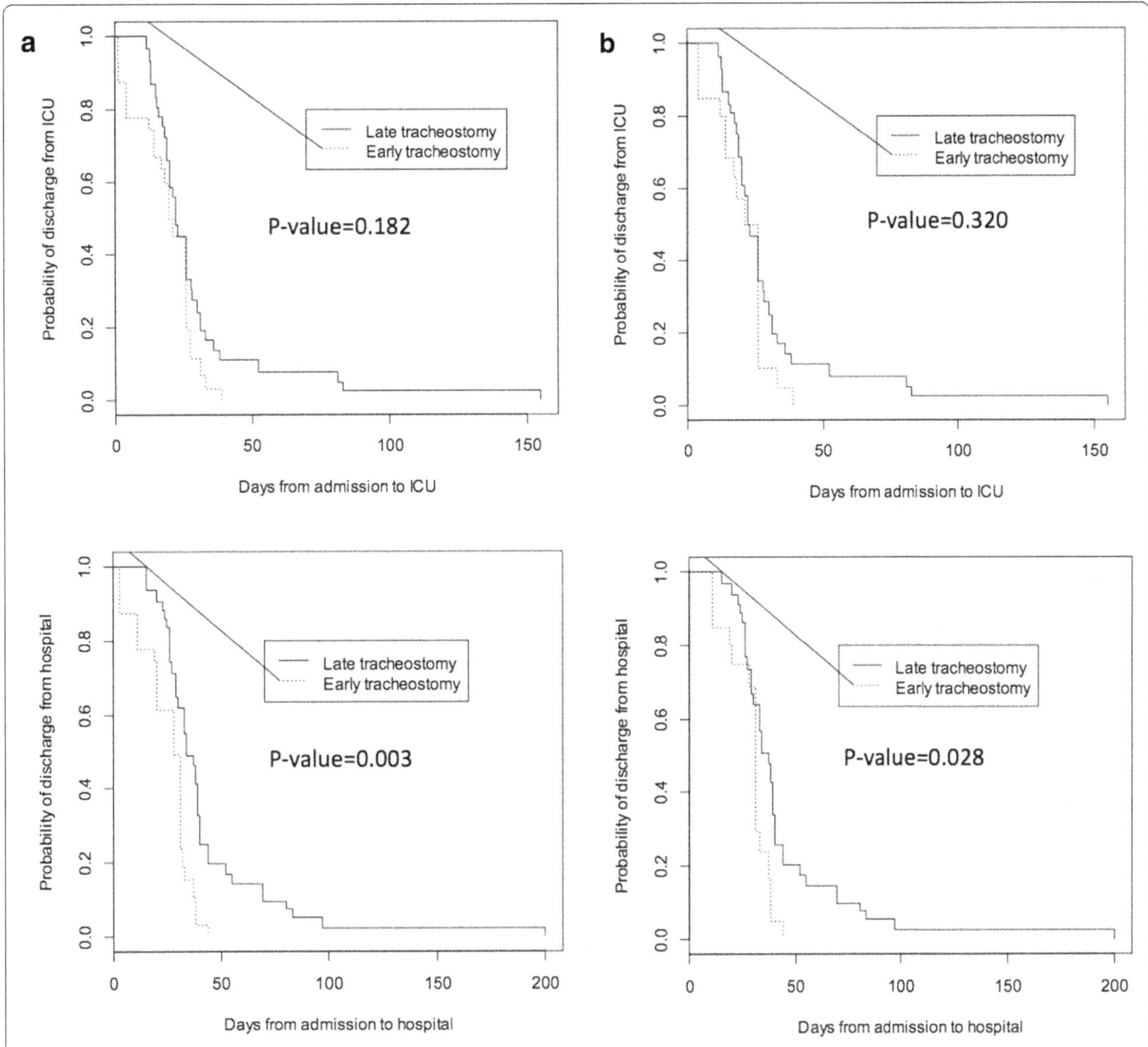

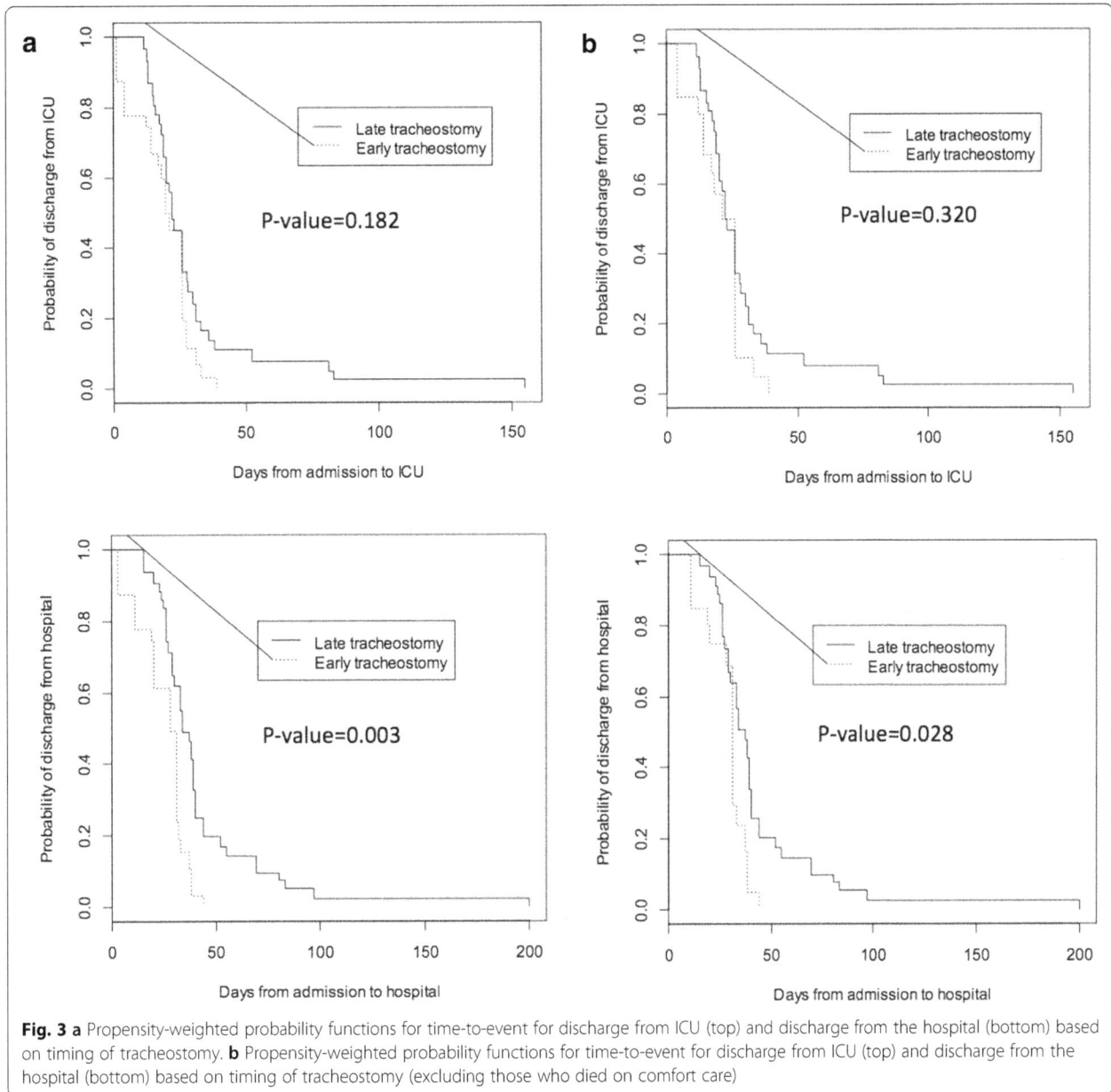

Fig. 3 **a** Propensity-weighted probability functions for time-to-event for discharge from ICU (top) and discharge from the hospital (bottom) based on timing of tracheostomy. **b** Propensity-weighted probability functions for time-to-event for discharge from ICU (top) and discharge from the hospital (bottom) based on timing of tracheostomy (excluding those who died on comfort care)

early mortality phenomenon. We found that a large number of patients died after the family decided to withdraw treatment and transition to comfort care. A total of 42 patients died after decompression, and 37 (88.1%) of them died after transitioning to comfort measures. Among the five others, only two had tracheostomies making the sample too small to draw conclusions on timing of tracheostomy and mortality (Tables 3 and 4 and Fig. 4). However, even after excluding patients who died on comfort care, duration of mechanical ventilation and ICU and hospital length of stay were still significantly shorter in patients with early tracheostomies (Table 4 and Fig. 3b). In conclusion, our propensity-adjusted dataset shows that those who received an early tracheostomy actually trended toward a higher mortality rate (Table 3; Fig. 4a), but this was completely explained by early transition to comfort measures.

The basis of transition to comfort measures is usually a failure to see measurable improvement combined with a poor expected prognosis. This can materialize in various forms in patients with severe brain injuries. It may result in a "prognostic pessimism" [21] or "self-fulfilling prophecy" [22] in patients who are young and have a reasonable chance of survival. In older patients, where withdrawal of support is unlikely to change the outcome, it may be a reasonable decision based on prolonged suffering without clear long-term benefit. The decision to undergo emergent neurosurgery can be even more challenging, as there is often inadequate time and data to make a decision of such

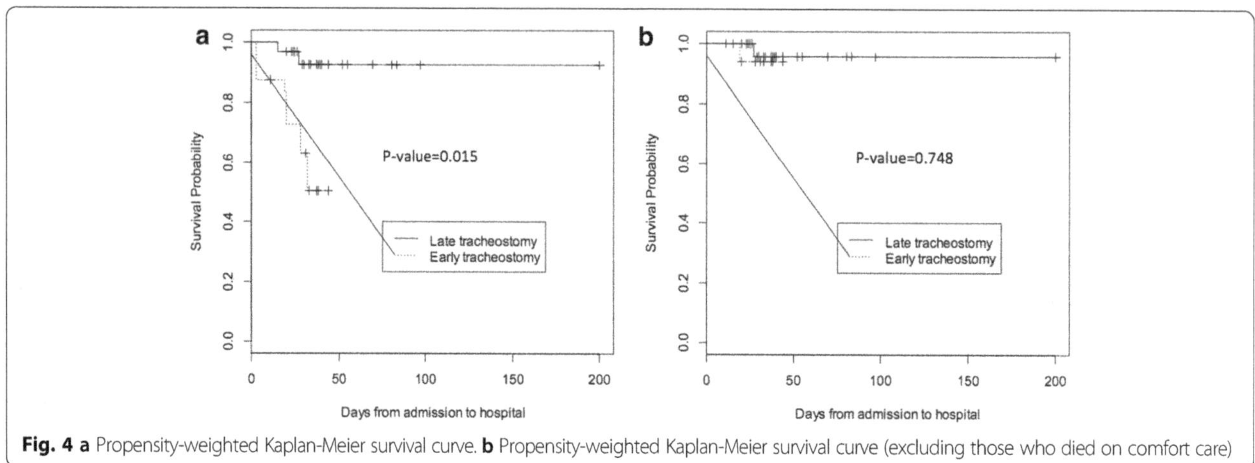

Fig. 4 a Propensity-weighted Kaplan-Meier survival curve. **b** Propensity-weighted Kaplan-Meier survival curve (excluding those who died on comfort care)

importance. Furthermore, prognostic models ideally would have perfect discrimination, with a 0% false positive rate for poor outcome [21]. However, this is currently only available for patients with anoxic brain injury after cardiopulmonary resuscitation, and oftentimes, families just need time under aggressive treatment to cope with the finality of the patient's condition [21].

Our mean patient age was 55 years old, which puts the majority of our patients within the data-supported range for mortality benefit from decompression for ischemic stroke [23–25]. For intracranial hemorrhage, the benefit of surgical decompression is less clear and is often a last resort in the face of cerebral herniation and brainstem compression. When asked about the maximum age compatible with meaningful survival in patients with intracerebral hemorrhage, responders quoted about 70 years [4]. These same authors found that medical support was ultimately withdrawn in about 76.7% of patients who died, which is close to our finding of 88.1%. The decision of medical futility will ultimately fall on the surgeon and intensivist providing the treatment. Predicting tracheostomy dependence may help families with the surgical decision as well, although, even with our decision tree analysis, models remain imperfect. Sometimes, even after maximal intervention and attempts sustain the life of stroke patients, the lack of measureable improvement and small setbacks breach the threshold families have for continuing with the treatment they once desired for their loved one.

Conclusions

The natural history of acute ischemic and hemorrhagic stroke requiring surgical decompression carries a grim prognosis. Early tracheostomy seems to have a few measurable benefits, namely shorter duration of mechanical ventilation and shorter length of stay. These may, however, be significant enough to families, and early tracheostomy may be reasonable to consider. We developed a decision tree analysis that can be used by neurosurgeons and neurointensivists to aid families in their decision-making prior to surgery. Upon ICU admission, surrogate decision-makers often have little time to process these tragic circumstances, and committing someone to a major operation, even if life saving, is often a difficult choice to make. An artificial airway is a concrete outcome laypersons can understand. We believe that these types of tools are useful to inform surrogates, guide appropriate care, and limit unnecessarily aggressive interventions leading to early post-operative withdrawal of treatment and early death.

Additional file

Additional file 1: Table S1. Bivariate analysis for ventilator associated pneumonia. **Table S2.** Outcome analysis with and without tracheostomy using proposed propensity score. (DOCX 15 kb)

Abbreviations

GCS: Glasgow Coma Score; ICU: Intensive care unit; SOFA: Sequential Organ Failure Assessment; VAP: Ventilator-associated pneumonia

Acknowledgements

Not applicable

Funding

The authors provided all the financial support for this study.

Authors' contributions

MPC and JDJ contributed to the study design, data collection, and data analysis; wrote and reviewed the manuscript; and submitted the manuscript. FCL contributed to data analysis and reviewed the manuscript. ND contributed to the study design and data collection and reviewed the manuscript. KA contributed to data collection and reviewed the manuscript. COS contributed to the study design and reviewed the manuscript. All authors read and approved the final manuscript.

Competing interests

The authors declare that they have no competing interests.

Author details
[1]Department of Neurosurgery, University of North Carolina School of Medicine, 170 Manning Drive, Campus Box 7025, Chapel Hill, NC 27599-7025, USA. [2]Department of Biostatistics, Gillings School of Global Public Health, Chapel Hill, NC, USA. [3]School of Medicine, University of North Carolina School of Medicine, Chapel Hill, NC, USA. [4]Department of Neurology, University of North Carolina, 170 Manning Drive, Campus Box 7025, Chapel Hill, NC, USA.

References

1. Alsumrain M, Melillo N, Debari VA, Kirmani J, Moussavi M, Doraiswamy V, et al. Predictors and outcomes of pneumonia in patients with spontaneous intracerebral hemorrhage. J Intensive Care Med. 2013;28(2):118–23.
2. Cocoros NM, Klompas M. Ventilator-associated events and their prevention. Infect Dis Clin N Am. 2016;30(4):887–908.
3. Rabinstein AA, Wijdicks EF. Outcome of survivors of acute stroke who require prolonged ventilatory assistance and tracheostomy. Cerebrovasc Dis. 2004;18:325–31.
4. Kalanuria AA, Zai W, Mirski M. Ventilator-associated pneumonia in the ICU. Crit Care. 2014;18(2):208.
5. van der Lely AJ, Veelo DP, Dongelmans DA, Korevaar JC, Vroom MB, Schultz MJ. Time to wean after tracheotomy differs among subgroups of critically ill patients: retrospective analysis in a mixed medical/surgical intensive care unit. Respir Care. 2006;51(12):1408–15.
6. Torbey MT, Bösel J, Rhoney DH, Rincon F, Staykov D, Amar AP, et al. Evidence-based guidelines for the management of large hemispheric infarction. Neurocrit Care. 2015;22(1):146–64.
7. Young D, Harrison DA, Cuthbertson BH, Rowan K. Effect of early vs late tracheostomy placement on survival in patients receiving mechanical ventilation. JAMA. 2013;309(20):2121–9.
8. Andriolo BN, Andriolo RB, Saconato H, Atallah ÁN, Valente O. Early versus late tracheostomy for critically ill patients (review). Cochrane Database Syst Rev. 2015;(1):1–67. Art. No.: CD007271.
9. Bösel J, Schiller P, Hook Y, Andes M, Neumann JO, Poli S, et al. Stroke-related Early Tracheostomy versus Prolonged Orotracheal Intubation in Neurocritical Care Trial (SETPOINT): a randomized pilot trial. Stroke. 2012;44(1):21–8.
10. Lee YC, Kim TH, Lee JW, Oh IH, Eun YG. Comparison of complications in stroke subjects undergoing early versus standard tracheostomy. Respir Care. 2015;60(5):651–7.
11. Villwock JA, Villwock MR, Deshaies EM. Tracheostomy timing affects stroke recovery. J Stroke Cerebrovasc Dis. 2014;23(5):1069–72.
12. Alshekhlee A, Horn C, Jung R, Alawi AA, Cruz-Flores S. In-hospital mortality in acute ischemic stroke treated with hemicraniectomy in US hospitals. J Stroke Cerebrovasc Dis. 2011;20(3):196–201.
13. Qureshi AI, Suarez JI, Parekh PD, Bhardwaj A. Prediction and timing of tracheostomy in patients with infratentorial lesions requiring mechanical ventilatory support. Crit Care Med. 2000;28(5):1383–7.
14. Szeder V, Ortega-Gutierrez S, Ziai W, Torbey MT. The TRACH score: clinical and radiological predictors of tracheostomy in supratentorial spontaneous intracerebral hemorrhage. Neurocrit Care. 2010;13(1):40–6.
15. Schonenberger S, Al-Suwaidan F, Kieser M, Uhlmann L, Bösel J. The SETscore to predict tracheostomy need in cerebrovascular neurocritical care patients. Neurocrit Care. 2016;25(1):94–104.
16. Huttner HB, Kohrmann M, Berger C, Georgiadis D, Schwab S. Predictive factors for tracheostomy in neurocritical care patients with spontaneous supratentorial hemorrhage. Cerebrovasc Dis. 2006;21:159–65.
17. Meng L, Wang C, Li J, Zhang J. Early vs late tracheostomy in critically ill patients: a systematic review and meta-analysis. Clin Respir J. 2015; 10(6):684–92.
18. Huang Y-H, Lee T-C, Liao C-C, Deng Y-H, Kwan A-L. Tracheostomy in craniectomised survivors after traumatic brain injury: a cross-sectional analytical study. Injury. 2013;44(9):1226–31. https://doi.org/10.1016/j.injury.2012.12.029.
19. McCredie VA, Alali AS, Scales DC, Adhikari NK, Rubenfeld GD, Cuthbertson BH, et al. Effect of early versus late tracheostomy or prolonged intubation in critically ill patients with acute brain injury: a systematic review and meta-analysis. Neurocrit Care. 2017;26(1):14–25.
20. Pinheiro Bdo V, Tostes Rde O, Brum CI, Carvalho EV, Pinto SP, Oliveira JC. Early versus late tracheostomy in patients with acute severe brain injury. J Bras Pneumol. 2010;36(1):84–91.
21. Geurts M, Macleod MR, van Thiel GJMW, van Gijn J, Kappelle LJ, van der Worp HB. End-of-life decisions in patients with severe acute brain injury. Lancet Neurol. 2014;13(5):515–24.
22. Becker KJ, Baxter AB, Cohen WA, Bybee HM, Tirschwell DL, Newell DW, et al. Withdrawal of support in intracerebral hemorrhage may lead to self-fulfilling prophecies. Neurology. 2001;56:766–72.
23. Hofmeijer J, Kappelle LJ, Algra A, Amelink GJ, van Gijn J, van der Worp HB. Surgical decompression for space-occupying cerebral infarction (the Hemicraniectomy After Middle Cerebral Artery infarction with Life-threatening Edema Trial [HAMLET]): a multicentre, open, randomised trial. Lancet Neurol. 2009;8(4):326–33.
24. Jüttler E, Schwab S, Schmiedek P, Unterberg A, Hennerici M, Woitzik J, et al. Decompressive Surgery for the Treatment of Malignant Infarction of the Middle Cerebral Artery (DESTINY): a randomized, controlled trial. Stroke. 2007;38(9):2518–25.
25. Vahedi K, Vicaut E, Mateo J, Kurtz A, Orabi M, Guichard JP, et al. Sequential-design, multicenter, randomized, controlled trial of early Decompressive Craniectomy in Malignant Middle Cerebral Artery Infarction (DECIMAL trial). Stroke. 2007;38(9):2506–17.

8

C-terminal proendothelin-1 (CT-proET-1) is associated with organ failure and predicts mortality in critically ill patients

Lukas Buendgens[1*], Eray Yagmur[2], Jan Bruensing[1], Ulf Herbers[1], Christer Baeck[1], Christian Trautwein[1], Alexander Koch[1] and Frank Tacke[1]

Abstract

Background: Endothelin 1 (ET-1) is a strong vasoconstrictor, which is involved in inflammation and reduced tissue perfusion. C-terminal proendothelin-1 (CT-proET-1) is the stable circulating precursor protein of ET-1. We hypothesized that CT-proET-1, reflecting ET-1 activation, is involved in the pathogenesis of critical illness and associated with its prognosis.

Methods: Two hundred seventeen critically ill patients (144 with sepsis, 73 without sepsis) were included prospectively upon admission to the medical intensive care unit (ICU), in comparison to 65 healthy controls. CT-proET-1 serum concentrations were correlated with clinical data and extensive laboratory parameters. Overall survival was followed for up to 3 years.

Results: CT-proET-1 serum levels at admission were significantly increased in critically ill patients compared to controls. CT-proET-1 serum levels showed significant correlations to systemic inflammation as well as multiple markers of organ dysfunction (kidney, liver, heart). Patients with sepsis displayed higher circulating CT-proET-1 than ICU patients with non-septic diseases. CT-proET-1 levels >74 pmol/L at ICU admission independently predicted ICU death (adjusted hazard ratio (HR) 2.66, 95% confidence interval (CI) 1.30–5.47) and overall mortality during follow-up (adjusted HR 2.19, 95%-CI 1.21–3.98).

Conclusions: CT-proET-1 serum concentrations at admission are increased in critically ill patients and associated with sepsis, disease severity, organ failure, and mortality.

Keywords: C-terminal proendothelin-1, CT-proET-1, ICU, Prognosis, Sepsis, Biomarker, Critical illness, Endothelin, ET-1

Background

Endothelial dysfunction plays an important role in critical illness, especially in sepsis. It mediates hemodynamic disturbances based on the vasotonus, contributes to the balance of pro- and anti-inflammation, regulates nutrient supply and cell migration into tissue, and plays a key role in host-pathogen interaction [1]. Besides other mediators such as nitric oxide (NO), endothelin-1 (ET-1) is one of the major endogenous factors controlling vasotonus that is released from activated endothelial cells. It is the most prominent member of the endothelin family. It binds to two G-protein-coupled receptors, ET_A and ET_B. ET_A promotes potent vasoconstriction and cell growth, whereas ET_B leads to vasodilation and inhibits cell proliferation [2]. Besides in blood vessels, ET-1-receptors are also found in tissues, e.g., cardiomyocytes and glomerular capillaries [3]. Endothelin release from endothelial cells is known to be stimulated by bacterial endotoxin [4] and various inflammatory cytokines such as TNF-alpha [3] or interleukin-6 [5] as well as mechanical factors like reduced shear stress [6].

Consecutively, increased levels of endothelin were found both in animal models of sepsis [7, 8] and human patients with sepsis [9–11]. Moreover, the function of many organs (e.g., liver, lung, heart, or kidney) worsens severely after infusion of ET-1 in animal models [12, 13]. In the past,

* Correspondence: lbuendgens@ukaachen.de
[1]Department of Medicine III, RWTH-University Hospital Aachen, Pauwelsstrasse 30, 52074 Aachen, Germany
Full list of author information is available at the end of the article

various smaller studies could relate these findings to the clinical outcome of patients and demonstrated a relation between ET-1 and mortality in sepsis or septic shock in adults [9, 14, 15] and children [16]. ET-1 itself, however, is difficult to measure due to its limited half-life. Consequently, sample sizes of trials investigating ET-1 tend to be relatively small. The precursor peptide C-terminal proendothelin-1 (CT-proET-1) is far more stable and allows a stoichiometric measurement of ET-1 [17]. This facilitates the analysis of larger group of patients as well as the practical use of this potential biomarker in clinical routine. We therefore investigated CT-proET-1 in a large cohort of 217 consecutively enrolled critically ill patients, including 144 subjects with sepsis, in order to identify associations between CT-proET-1 and organ dysfunction, disease severity as well as ICU, and survival during follow-up in critically ill patients.

Methods

Study design

Written informed consent was obtained from the patient, his or her spouse, or the appointed legal guardian. Patients who were expected to have a short (<3 days) intensive care treatment (e.g., due to post-interventional observation or intoxication) were excluded [18]. The long-term course of patients was assessed by directly contacting the patient, the patients' relatives, or their primary care physician. We used the third international consensus definitions for sepsis and septic shock (sepsis-3) as a post hoc definition for sepsis patients, and all others were classified as non-sepsis patients [19]. For identifying and classifying patients with an acute respiratory distress syndrome (ARDS), we used the Berlin definition of ARDS [20].

Sixty-five healthy blood donors with normal values for blood counts, C-reactive protein, and liver enzymes served as controls. The study protocol was approved by the local ethics committee and conducted in accordance with the ethical standards laid down in the 1964 Declaration of Helsinki (ethics committee of the University Hospital Aachen, RWTH-University, Aachen, Germany, reference number EK 150/06). The current study was part of a larger assessment of biomarkers in critically ill patients, conducted between 2006 and 2014 at our center.

CT-proET-1 measurements

Blood samples were collected directly upon admission of the patient to the ICU prior to therapeutic interventions at the ICU. After centrifugation at 4 °C for 10 min, serum aliquots of 1 mL were frozen immediately at −80 °C. CT-proET-1 serum concentrations were measured using a commercially available fluorescent immunoassay (BRAHMS GmbH/ThermoFischer Scientific, Henningsdorf, Germany) following the manufacturer's protocol. The scientist performing laboratory measurements was fully blinded to any clinical or other laboratory data of the patients or controls.

Statistical analysis

Data are displayed as median and range due to the skewed distribution of most of the parameters. Differences between two groups were assessed by Mann-Whitney U test or chi-squared test. Differences between multiple groups were assessed using the Kruskal-Wallis test. To illustrate differences between subgroups, box plot graphics were used displaying a summary of the median, quartiles, range, and extreme values of the given data. Their whiskers range from the minimum to the maximum value excluding outliers displayed as separate points. An outlier was defined as a value that is smaller than the lower quartile minus 1.5 times the interquartile range or larger than the upper quartile plus 1.5 times the interquartile range. A far-out value was defined as a value that is smaller than the lower quartile minus three times the interquartile range or larger than the upper quartile plus three times the interquartile range [21]. Correlations between variables were assessed with Spearman correlation tests. The Cox regression model was used for univariate and multivariate analysis of risk factors. Kaplan-Meier curves were used to illustrate differences in survival [22]. Differences between the groups regarding survival were assessed with the log-rank test. Receiver operating characteristic (ROC) curve analysis were used to evaluate the value of a predictive marker or a composite score. ROC curves were generated by plotting sensitivity against 1-specificity [23]. Differences between ROC curves were assessed using the method described by DeLong et al. [24]. Statistical analyses were performed with SPSS Version 23 (SPSS, Chicago, IL, USA) and MedCalc Version 16 (MedCalc Software, Ostend, Belgium).

Results

CT-proET-1 serum concentrations are increased in critically ill patients and associated with sepsis

In order to investigate the role of CT-proET-1 in critical illness, we measured serum levels in 217 patients at the time of admission to our medical ICU. In comparison to 65 healthy controls, CT-proET-1 levels were strongly elevated in critically ill patients (median 5.8 vs 65.4 pmol/L, $p < 0.001$, U test; Fig. 1a).

Of all 217 patients, 144 were admitted because of sepsis. The most frequent septic focus was pneumonia ($n = 74$), followed by abdominal ($n = 26$) and urogenital infections ($n = 11$) (detailed data not shown). Non-septic ICU patients were admitted due to cardio-pulmonary diseases ($n = 29$), pancreatitis ($n = 12$), decompensated liver cirrhosis ($n = 9$), and other non-septic diseases ($n = 23$). CT-proET-

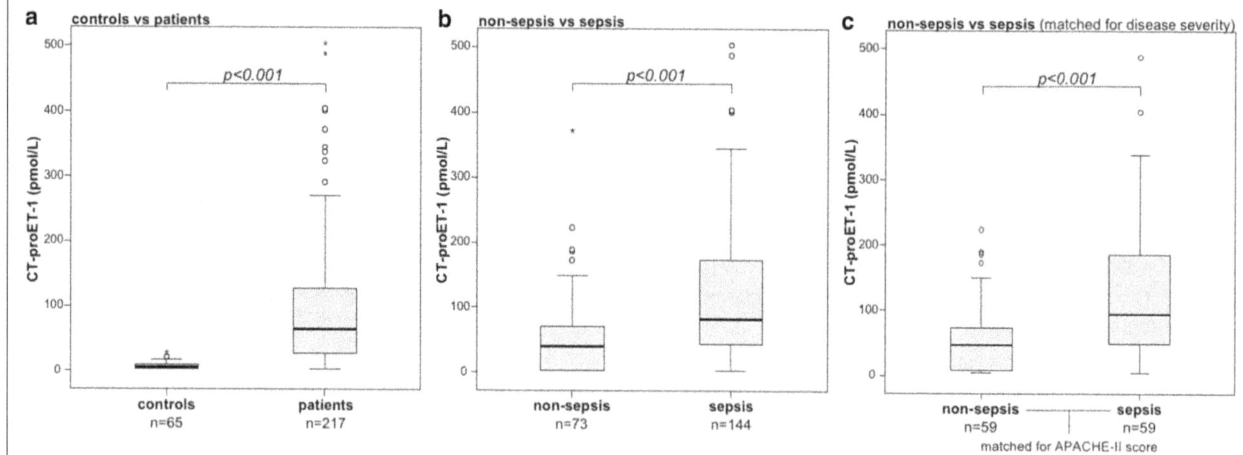

Fig. 1 Serum CT-proET-1 concentrations in critically ill patients and sepsis. **a** Serum levels of CT-proET-1, at the time of admission to the ICU, were significantly higher in critically ill patients than in healthy controls ($p < 0.001$; *U* test). **b** CT-proET-1 levels were significantly higher in patients with sepsis ($p < 0.001$) compared to ICU patients without sepsis. **c** When matched 1:1 with non-sepsis patients for APACHE-II score, age, and sex, CT-proET-1 levels were significantly higher in patients with sepsis compared to ICU patients without sepsis ($p < 0.001$)

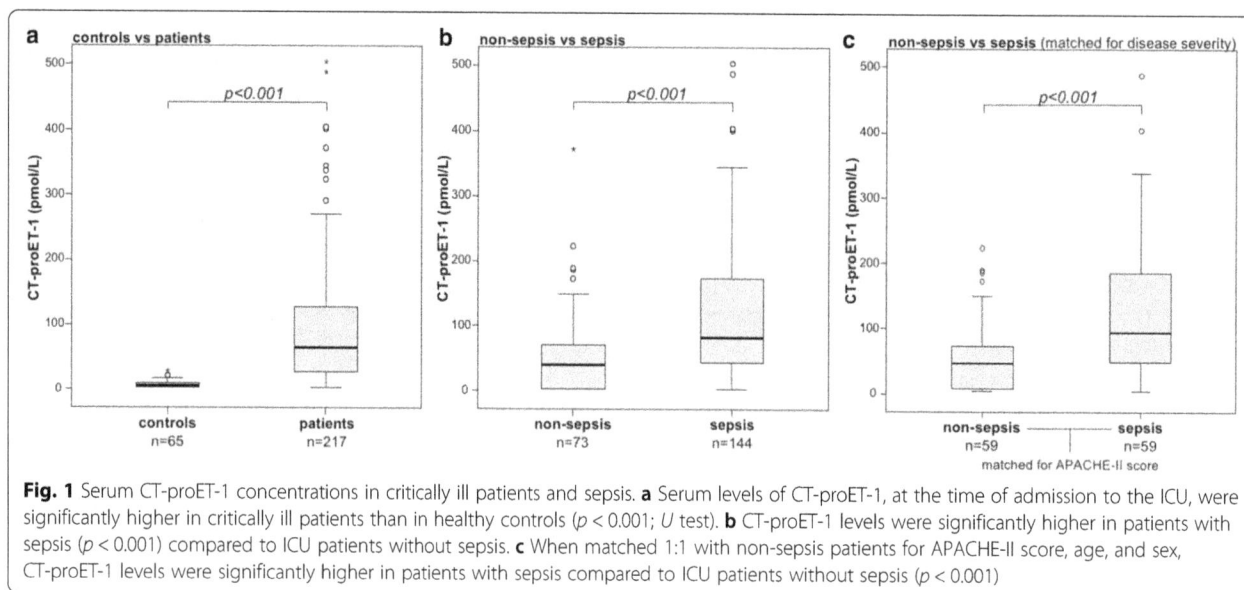

1 levels were significantly higher in patients with sepsis compared to other ICU patients (median 40.9 vs 82.1 pmol/L; $p < 0.001$; Fig. 1b, Table 1). Sepsis and non-sepsis patients did not differ in age or sex, but sepsis patients had significantly higher APACHE-II or SOFA scores, increased mortality, longer stay on the ICU, and an increased vasopressor demand (Table 1). In order to exclude that the difference in CT-pro-ET1 was related to the presence of sepsis and not to disease severity, the non-sepsis ICU patients were matched 1:1 with a patient from the sepsis group for APACHE-II score (disease severity), age, and sex. In this subanalysis, CT-pro-ET1 remained indeed higher in the sepsis group ($p < 0.001$; Fig. 1c).

To investigate a possible use of CT-proET-1 in identifying patients with sepsis, we conducted a ROC curve analysis comparing CT-proET-1 to other, established

Table 1 Baseline patient characteristics and CT-proET-1 serum measurements at ICU admission

Parameter	All patients	Sepsis	Non-sepsis	p^a
Number	217	144	73	
Sex (male/female)	132/85	84/60	48/25	n.s.
Age median, (range) [years]	64 (18–90)	65 (20–90)	61 (18–85)	n.s.
APACHE-II score, median (range)	18 (2–43)	19 (4–43)	14 (2–33)	<0.001
SOFA score, median (range)	9 (0–17)	9 (2–17)	7 (0–17)	0.003
SAPS 2 score, median (range)	41 (0–73)	40 (0–73)	41 (0–73)	0.193
Mechanical ventilation, *n* (%)	144 (69)	98 (63)	46 (63)	n.s.
Ventilation time, median (range) [h]	117 (0–3828)	125.5 (0–2966)	66 (0–2828)	n.s.
Vasopressor demand, *n* (%)	132 (60.8)	99 (68.8)	33 (45.2)	<0.001
ICU days, median (range)	7 (1–137)	8.5 (1–137)	6 (1–45)	0.004
30-day mortality, *n* (%)	41 (18.9)	34 (23.6)	7 (9.6)	0.016
Overall mortality, *n* (%)	86 (41.7)	64 (46.7)	22 (31.9)	0.42
CT-proET-1, median (range) [pmol/L]	43.8 (3–503.6)	82.1 (3–503.6)	40.9 (3–372.9)	<0.001
Leucocytes, median (range) [per nL]	12.9 (0.5–208)	13.8 (0.5–208)	12.5 (1.8–29.6)	0.041
CRP, median (range) [mg/L]	98 (5–230)	160.5 (5–230)	17 (5–230)	<0.001
Cystatin C, median (range) [mg/L]	1.48 (0.39–8.38)	1.69 (0.39–8.38)	1.04 (0.56–2.29)	<0.001
Bilirubin, median (range) [per mg/dL]	0.7 (0.2–20.8)	0.7 (0.2–6.8)	0.7 (0.2–20.8)	n.s.

For quantitative variables, median and range (in parenthesis) are given

Abbreviations: *CRP* C-reactive protein, *CT-proET-1* C-terminal proendothelin-1, *APACHE* Acute Physiology and Chronic Health Evaluation, *SAPS 2* Simplified Acute Physiology Score, *SOFA* Sequential Organ Failure Assessment, *n.s.* not significant

[a]Significance between sepsis and non-sepsis patients was assessed using the Mann-Whitney *U* test or chi-squared test

markers (procalcitonin and C-reactive protein (CRP)). With an AUC of 0.834 (95%-CI 0.768–0.900), CRP was significantly superior to both PCT ($p = 0.046$; DeLong test) and CT-proET-1 ($p = 0.007$; DeLong test). Interestingly, CT-proET-1 was non-inferior to PCT (AUC 0.704 vs 0.757; $p = 0.24$; DeLong test).

CT-proET-1 levels in critically ill patients correlate with clinical disease severity scores and organ dysfunction

Based on the pathogenic role of endothelin-1 for vasoconstriction and impaired tissue perfusion [25], we hypothesized that increased CT-proET-1 might be associated with organ dysfunction in ICU patients. Strikingly, CT-proET-1 levels were strongly associated with markers of renal dysfunction (e.g., creatinine, $r = 0.500$, $p < 0.001$; cystatin C, $r = 0.624$, $p < 0.001$), cholestasis (e.g., bilirubin, $r = 0.148$, $p = 0.031$), impaired hepatic synthesis (e.g., albumin, $r = -0.321$, $p = 0.001$; pseudocholinesterase, $r = -0.438$, $p < 0.001$; prothrombin time, $r = -0.220$, $p = 0.001$) and cardiac failure (e.g., brain natriuretic peptide, $r = 0.505$, $p < 0.001$). Likewise, CT-proET-1 levels correlated with markers of general inflammation (e.g., C-reactive protein, $r = 0.416$, $p < 0.001$, Table 2).

Interestingly, patients with manifest organ failure had significantly elevated CT-proET-1 levels. This was observed for patients with renal failure (defined as a cystatin C-based glomerular filtration rate below 50 mL/min, Fig. 2a), liver failure (defined as prothrombin time <50%, Fig. 2b), or heart failure (defined as a NTproBNP >1000 pg/ml; Fig. 2c). As prior studies reported elevated ET-1 in patients with ARDS compared to controls [26], we further assessed CT-proET-1 serum levels in regard to the degree of an ARDS. However, CT-proET-1 did not differ between ICU patients without ARDS ($n = 22$) and with mild ($n = 29$), moderate ($n = 27$), or severe ($n = 13$) ARDS at the time of admission (Fig. 2d).

Additionally, CT-proET-1 levels were associated with severity of critical illness. Patients with higher APACHE-II (above 18) and SAPS 2 (above the median of the cohort) scores showed significantly increased serum levels of CT-proET-1 (Fig. 3a, b). CT-proET-1 also positively correlated with these disease severity scores (APACHE-II, $r = 0.239$, $p = 0.001$; SAPS 2, $r = 0.400$, $p < 0.001$, Table 2). CT-proET1 did not correlate with the SOFA score, neither for all nor for sepsis patients (detailed data not shown).

CT-proET-1 at admission is an independent predictor of ICU mortality

As CT-proET-1 levels correlate with organ dysfunction and disease severity, we hypothesized that CT-proET-1 serum concentrations at the time of ICU admission might be associated with mortality in critically ill patients. Overall, $n = 41$ (18.9%) of the patients died at the ICU, while $n = 86$ (39.6%) died overall including the follow-up time (of up to 3 years). Remarkably, patients that died at the ICU showed significant higher serum levels of CT-proET-1 at ICU admission than survivors (median 88.3 vs 59.2 pmol/L; $p = 0.029$; Fig. 4a).

By Cox regression analysis, CT-proET-1 levels were found to predict ICU mortality ($p = 0.047$). We used the Youden index (28) to find the best cut-off value regarding sensitivity and specificity. Based on the coordinates of the ROC curve, a CT-proET-1 cut-off value of 74 pmol/L showed the best ratio of sensitivity and specificity in predicting ICU mortality. Interestingly, this value is higher than the measurements of our healthy controls and represents the 99th percentile of a healthy population. Kaplan-Meier survival curve analysis confirmed that high CT-proET-1 levels were strongly associated with 30-day mortality (Fig. 4b; $p = 0.002$). As CT-proET-1 correlates with markers of organ failure, excretion and inflammation, we next tested if CT-proET-1 serum levels can independently predict survival. We performed uni- and multivariate Cox

Table 2 Correlations of CT-proET-1 with clinical scores and other laboratory markers

	All patients	
	r	*p*
Markers of inflammation		
CRP	0.416	<0.001
Procalcitonin	0.343	0.005
IL6	0.172	0.027
Markers of organ dysfunction		
Cystatin C	0.624	<0.001
GFR	−0.534	<0.001
ALT	−0.165	0.016
Bilirubin	0.148	0.031
Prothrombin time	−0.220	0.001
Albumin	−0.321	<0.001
Urea	0.577	<0.001
NTproBNP	0.505	<0.001
Clinical scores		
APACHE-II	0.239	0.001
SOFA	0.136	n.s.
SAPS 2	0.400	<0.001
New and experimental biomarkers		
Resistin	0.449	<0.001
NTproCNP	0.604	<0.001
suPAR	0.529	<0.001

Abbreviations: *ALT* alanine aminotransferase, *APACHE* Acute Physiology and Chronic Health Evaluation, *ALT* alanine aminotransferase, *CRP* C-reactive protein, *GFR* glomerular filtration rate, *IL6* interleukin 6, *NTproBNP* amino-terminal propeptide of brain natriuretic peptide, *NTproCNP*, amino-terminal propeptide of C-type natriuretic peptide, *SAPS* Simplified Acute Physiology Score, *SOFA* sequential organ failure assessment, *suPAR* soluble urokinase plasminogen activator receptor, *n.s.* not significant

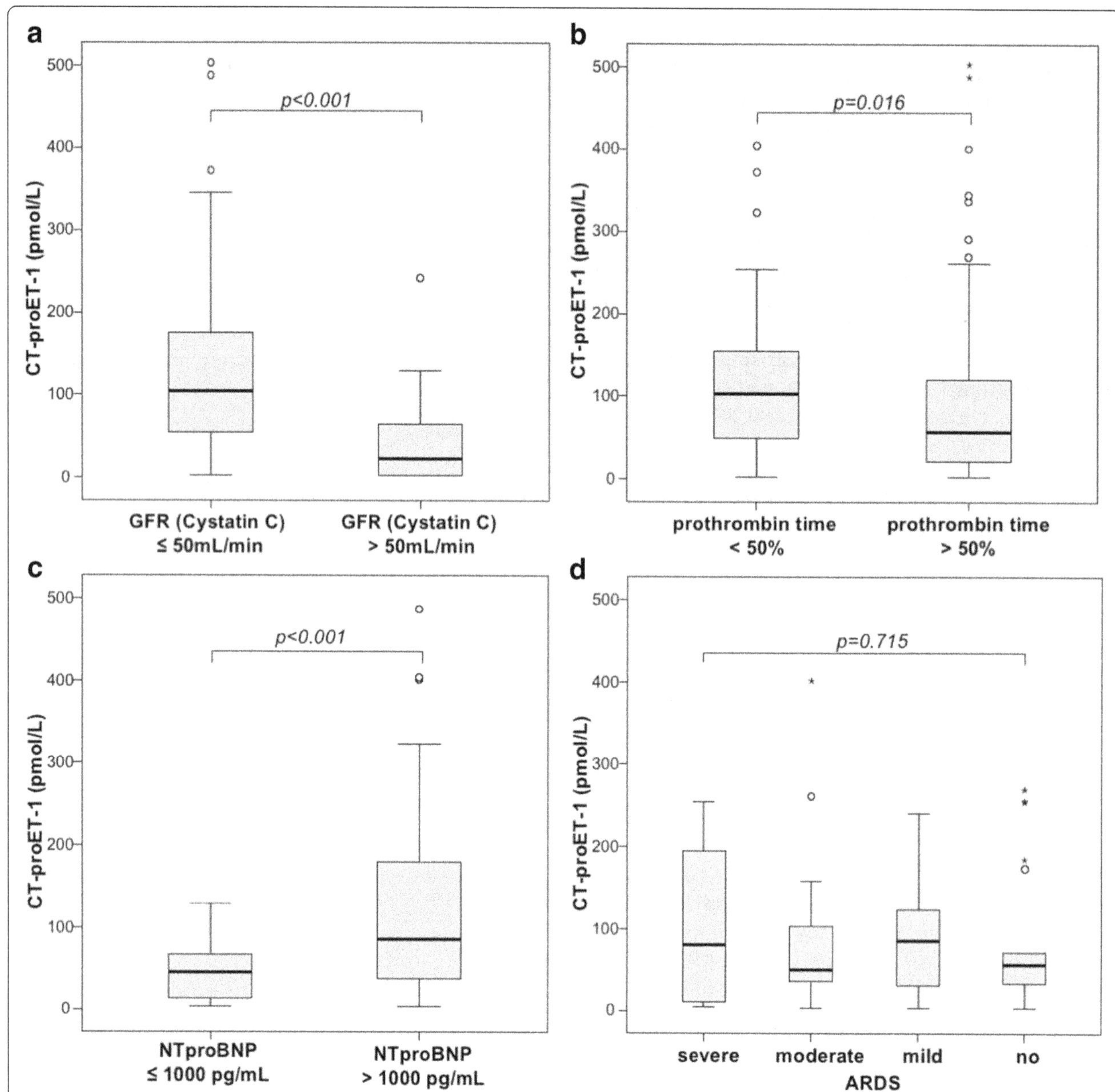

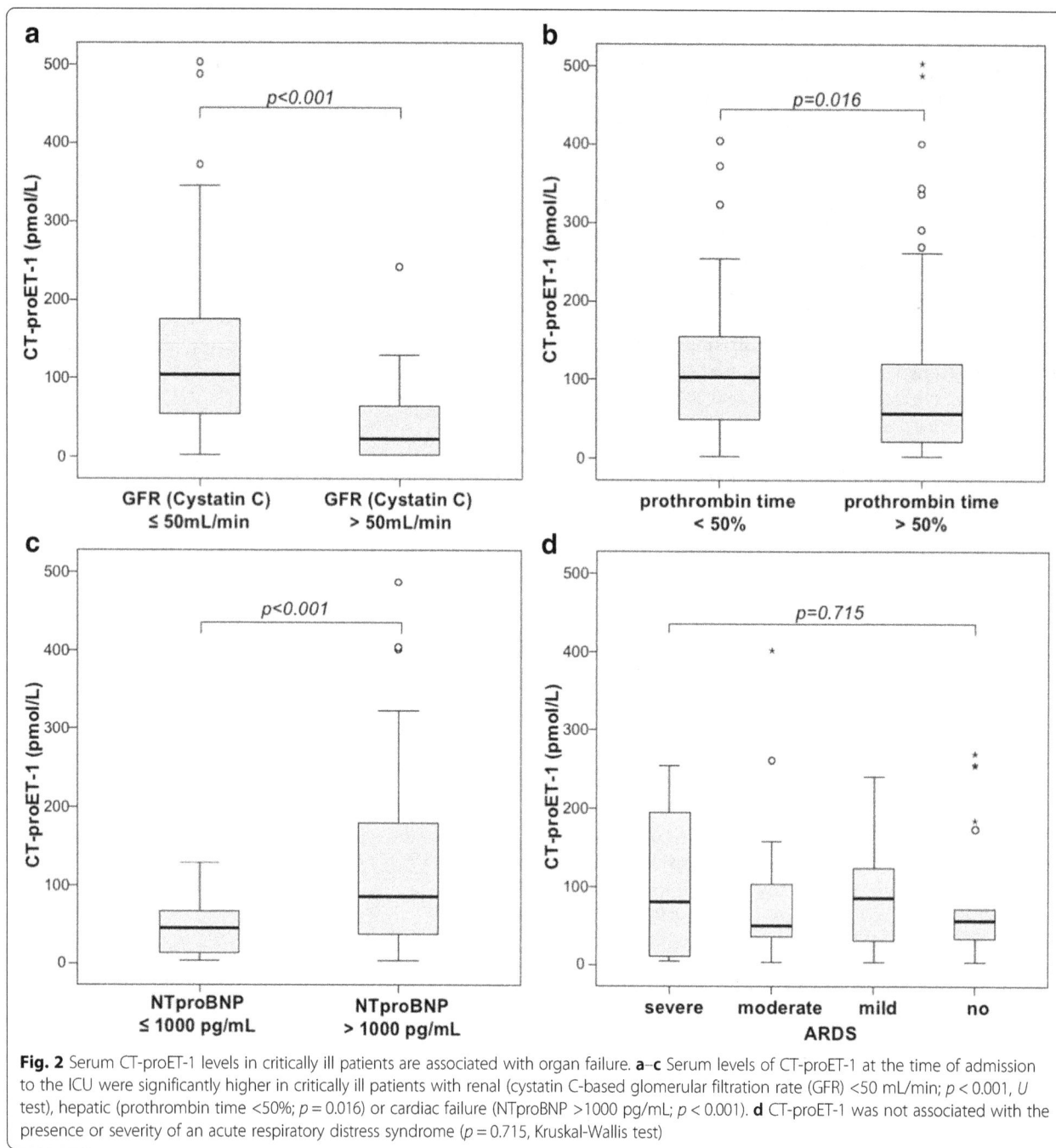

Fig. 2 Serum CT-proET-1 levels in critically ill patients are associated with organ failure. **a**–**c** Serum levels of CT-proET-1 at the time of admission to the ICU were significantly higher in critically ill patients with renal (cystatin C-based glomerular filtration rate (GFR) <50 mL/min; $p < 0.001$, *U* test), hepatic (prothrombin time <50%; $p = 0.016$) or cardiac failure (NTproBNP >1000 pg/mL; $p < 0.001$). **d** CT-proET-1 was not associated with the presence or severity of an acute respiratory distress syndrome ($p = 0.715$, Kruskal-Wallis test)

regression analysis including age, markers of inflammation (i.e., CRP), renal (i.e., creatinine), circulatory (i.e., lactate), and hepatic dysfunction (i.e., bilirubin, prothrombin time). Here, high CT-proET-1 (>74 pmol/L) was an independent predictor of ICU mortality in critically ill patients (adjusted hazard ratio (HR) 2.66 (95% CI 1.30–5.47), Table 3).

High levels of CT-proET-1 at ICU admission are associated with overall survival

Given its association with short-term mortality, we examined if the level of CT-proET-1 at admission to the ICU was also related to long-term outcome. We found that CT-proET-1 levels were significantly higher in patients that died during the follow-up period compared to the overall surviving patients (median 53.7 vs 89.9 pmol/L; $p = 0.003$; Fig. 5a).

Again, Kaplan-Meier analysis showed a good discrimination in terms of long-term survival between the groups with high and low CT-proET-1 values (Fig. 5b, $p < 0.001$).

In addition, we conducted uni- and multivariate Cox regression analyses including age, markers of inflammation (i.e., CRP) and renal (i.e., creatinine), circulatory (i.e., lactate),

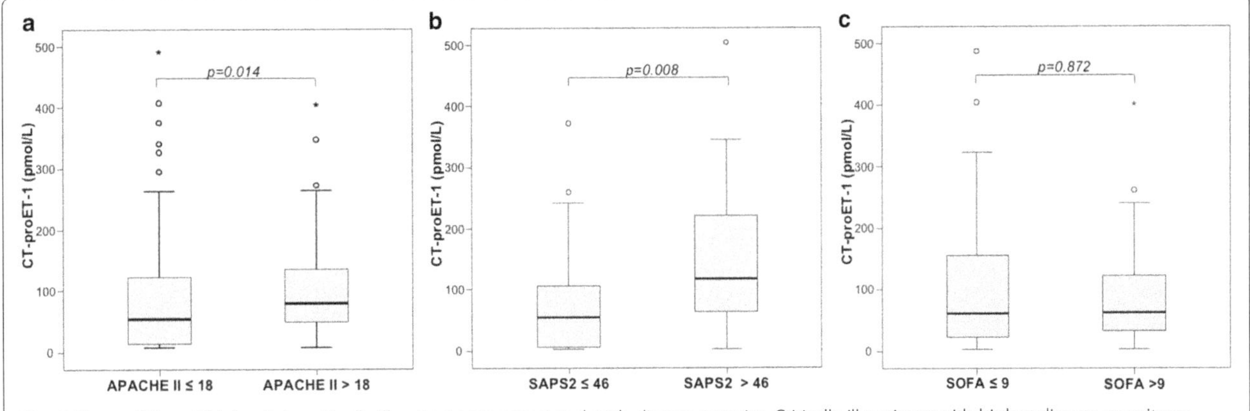

Fig. 3 Serum CT-proET-1 levels in critically ill patients are associated with disease severity. Critically ill patients with higher disease severity as represented by APACHE-II (**a**), SAPS 2 (**b**) showed significantly higher CT-proET-1 levels, while SOFA score (**c**) was unrelated to CT-proET-1

and hepatic dysfunction (i.e., bilirubin, prothrombin time) (Table 4). Adjusted by the factors above high CT-proET-1 (>74 pmol/L) remained an independent predictor of overall survival (adjusted HR 2.19, 95%-CI 1.21–3.98).

Discussion

In this study, we demonstrate striking regulations of circulating CT-proET-1 in a large cohort of critically ill patients, supporting our hypothesis to use this stoichiometric indicator of ET-1 as a diagnostic and prognostic biomarker in intensive care medicine. We could show that CT-proET-1 is significantly elevated in critically ill patients compared to healthy controls, correlates with disease severity and organ failure, and is an independent risk predictor for ICU and overall mortality.

Previous smaller studies [9, 14, 15] had reported an association of CT-proET-1 with short-term mortality in patients with sepsis. In contrast, one study on 99 sepsis patients that measured CT-proET-1 within 48 h after admission did not reproduce the relation between CT-proET-1 and mortality risk [27]. Very recently, Lundberg and colleagues reported that elevated CT-proET-1 levels at ICU admission were associated with 7-day and 28-day mortality in 53 patients with septic shock [14]. Our study now extends these prior findings to a more heterogeneous, larger prospective cohort of medical ICU patients demonstrating a clear prognostic value of circulating CT-

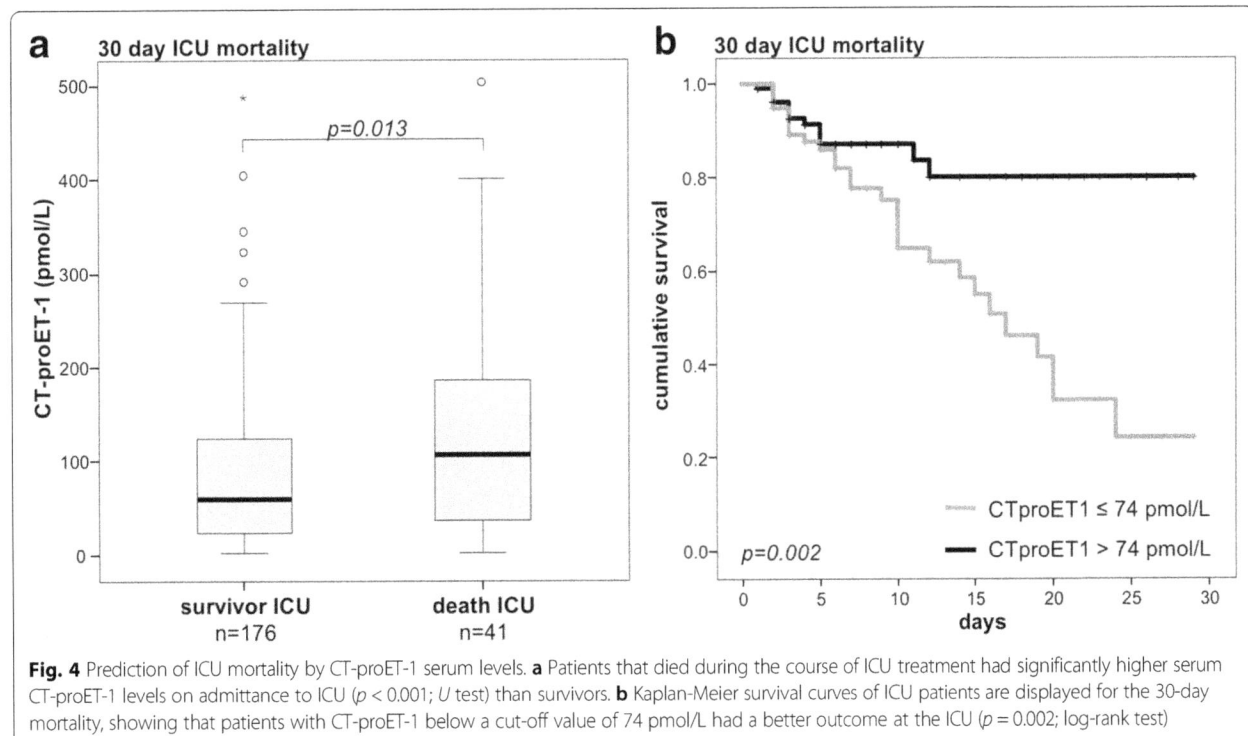

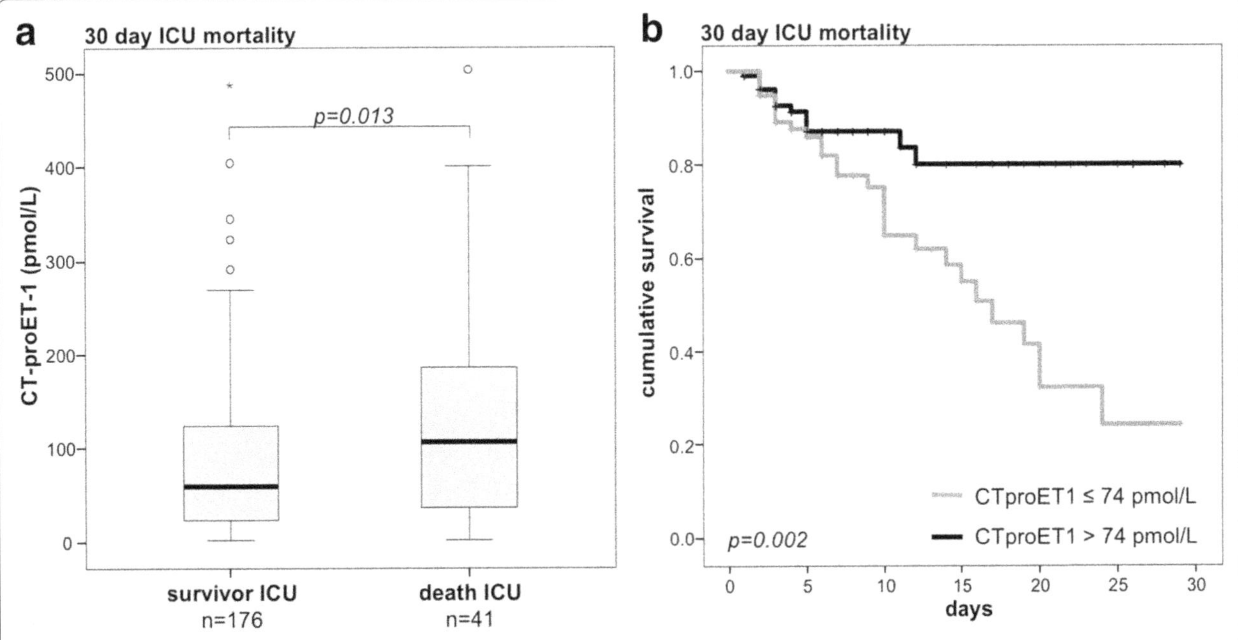

Fig. 4 Prediction of ICU mortality by CT-proET-1 serum levels. **a** Patients that died during the course of ICU treatment had significantly higher serum CT-proET-1 levels on admittance to ICU ($p < 0.001$; *U* test) than survivors. **b** Kaplan-Meier survival curves of ICU patients are displayed for the 30-day mortality, showing that patients with CT-proET-1 below a cut-off value of 74 pmol/L had a better outcome at the ICU ($p = 0.002$; log-rank test)

Table 3 Uni- and multivariate Cox regression analyses for CT-proET-1 levels at ICU admission to predict ICU mortality

	Unadjusted HR (95%-CI)	*p*	Adjusted HR (95%-CI)	*p*
CT-proET-1 > 74 pmol/L	2.658 (1.375–5.137)	0.004	2.663 (1.296–5.470)	0.008
Creatinine (per mg/dL)	–	n.s.		
CRP (per mg/L)	–	n.s.		
Bilirubin (per mg/dL)	1.129 (1.021–1.249)	0.018	–	n.s.
Prothrombin time (per %)	0.988 (0.977–1)	0.045	–	n.s.
Lactate (per mmol/L)	1.115 (1.03–1.207)	0.007	1.20 (1.109–1.298)	<0.001
Age (per year)	1.034 (1.011–1.058)	0.003	1.045 (1.019–1.71)	0.003

Variables with an univariate $p < 0.25$ were included in the multivariate model
Abbreviations: *95%-CI*, 95% confidence interval, *CRP* C-reactive protein, *CT-proET-1* C-terminal proendothelin-1, *n.s.* not significant

proET-1. While patients with sepsis had higher CT-proET-1 levels than ICU patients with non-septic disease, CT-proET-1 at ICU admission predicted 30-day mortality for the total patient cohort as well as for sepsis or non-sepsis patients. Moreover, we found that CT-proET-1 levels at ICU admission were even indicative of the long-term mortality risk, based on follow-up observations of about 3 years. This effect of CT-proET-1 on ICU and overall mortality was independent from single markers of organ failure or inflammation, indicating that CT-proET-1 could be useful in clinical algorithms or scores aiming at identifying high-risk patients upon ICU admission.

A prior study by Druml et al. found an association between ET-1 and the presence of an ARDS [26]. We did not observe such an association, but our study population was considerably different. While our cohort included a rather heterogeneous population of medical ICU patients with and without sepsis, Druml et al. specifically investigated ARDS patients in comparison to healthy controls, presumably with fewer confounding comorbidities than in our patient population.

Moreover, our findings might also provide important insights into the role of ET-1 (measured by CT-proET-1) in the pathogenesis of critical illness. The serum levels of CT-proET1 correlated with organ dysfunction and disease severity, but not with lactate, a marker of shock and circulatory failure. Thus, CT-proET1 reflects not a just mere hypoperfusion of tissues due to circulatory failure, but a more complex endothelial activation or dysfunction related to organ failure.

Nonetheless, our exploratory study has several limitations. These include the single center setting with the retrospective assessment of CT-proET1 in a prospectively enrolled study cohort. Moreover, we do not have

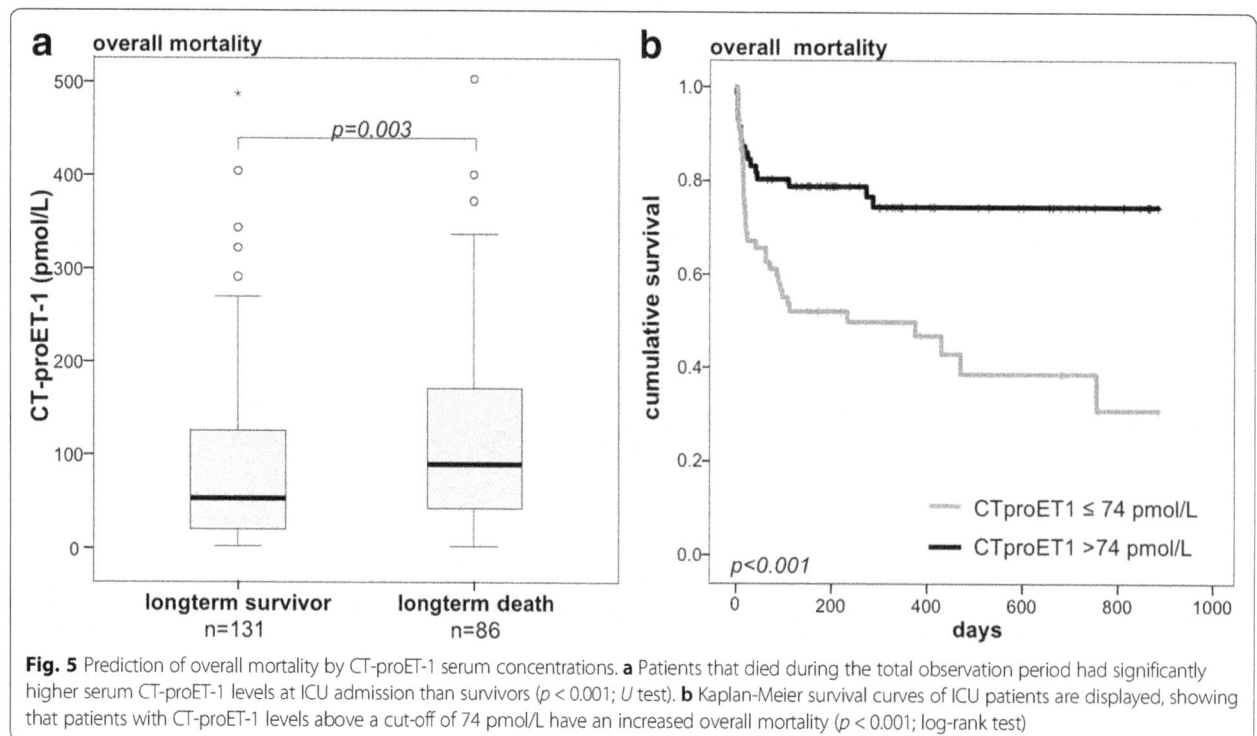

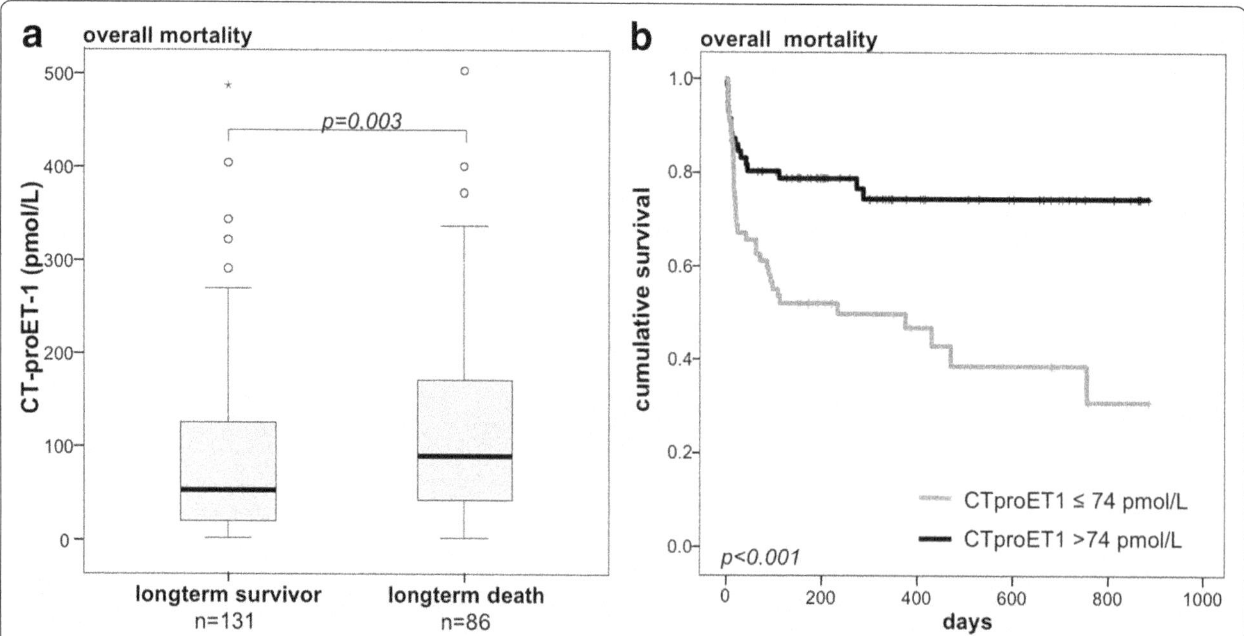

Fig. 5 Prediction of overall mortality by CT-proET-1 serum concentrations. **a** Patients that died during the total observation period had significantly higher serum CT-proET-1 levels at ICU admission than survivors ($p < 0.001$; *U* test). **b** Kaplan-Meier survival curves of ICU patients are displayed, showing that patients with CT-proET-1 levels above a cut-off of 74 pmol/L have an increased overall mortality ($p < 0.001$; log-rank test)

Table 4 Uni- and multivariate Cox regression analyses for CT-proET-1 levels at ICU admission to predict overall mortality

	Unadjusted HR (95%-CI)	p	Adjusted HR (95%-CI)	p
CT-proET-1 > 74 pmol/L	2.731 (1.535–4.858)	0.001	2.193 (1.209–3.975)	0.01
Creatinine (per mg/dL)	1.034 (0.946–1.129)	0.461	–	n.s.
CRP (per mg/L)	1.002 (0.999–1.006)	0.129	–	n.s.
Bilirubin (per mg/dL)	1.16 (0.935–1.16)	0.176	–	n.s.
Prothrombin time (per %)	0.99 (0.979–1)	0.052	–	n.s.
Lactate (per mmol/L)	1.082 (0.949–1.234)	0.239	–	n.s.
Age (per year)	1.036 (1.014–1.059)	<0.001	1.028 (1.005–1.051)	0.04

Variables with a univariate $p < 0.25$ were included in the multivariate model
Abbreviations: 95%-CI 95% confidence-interval, *CRP* C-reactive protein, *CT-proET-1* C-terminal proendothelin-1, *n.s.* not significant

longitudinal measurements of CT-proET1, which could potentially improve the prognostic validity of this marker. Also, organ failure assessment was solely based on laboratory parameters, but no functional tests (like echocardiography or liver biopsy).

However, the hyperactivation of ET-1 in our cohort of ICU patients and the strong association of ET-1 with organ dysfunction and mortality indicate that ET-1 might be a potential drug target in critical illness and sepsis. It is tempting to speculate that antagonizing systemic supra-physiological ET-1 levels holds therapeutic potential to improve tissue perfusion. In fact, the endothelin receptor antagonist bosentan has shown positive effects on tissue perfusion [28, 29] and cardiac output [30, 31] in animal models of septic shock. Moreover, the application of bosentan in a rodent model of septic shock was even able to improve survival [32]. Interestingly, this effect was more pronounced, if bosentan was given in the hypodynamic stage after fluid resuscitation, a disease stage where specific treatment options are currently scarce. Our data corroborate to further investigate ET-1-antagonistic approaches in the ICU setting, in order to define the efficacy as well as optimal dose and timing for such an intervention.

Conclusions

Our study shows that CT-proET-1 is elevated in critically ill patients and in sepsis. It is associated with organ dysfunction and poses an independent risk factor for ICU and overall mortality. The potential as a drug treatment target in critically ill patients requires further investigations.

Abbreviations

95%-CI: 95% confidence interval; APACHE: Acute Physiology and Chronic Health Evaluation; ARDS: Acute respiratory distress syndrome; AUC: Area under the curve; CRP: C-reactive protein; CT-proET-1: C-terminal proendothelin-1; ET-1: Endothelin-1; HR: Hazard ratio; ICU: Intensive care unit; NTproBNP: N-terminal B-type natriuretic peptide; ROC: Receiver operating characteristics; SAPS 2: Simplified acute physiology score; SOFA: Sequential Organ Failure Assessment

Acknowledgements

This work was supported by the German Research Foundation (DFG; Ta434/5-1 and SFB/TRR57) and the Interdisciplinary Center for Clinical Research (IZKF) Aachen.

Funding

This work was supported by the German Research Foundation (DFG Ta434/5-1 & SFB/TRR57) and the Interdisciplinary Centre for Clinical Research (IZKF) within the faculty of Medicine at the RWTH Aachen University.

Authors' contributions

LB, FT, and AK designed the study, analyzed data, and wrote the manuscript. EY performed the laboratory measurements. UH, CB, and JB collected the data and assisted in patient recruitment. CT revised the manuscript. All authors took part in the manuscript writing and approved the final manuscript.

Competing interests

The authors declare that they have no competing interests.

Key messages

CT-proET-1 is a stoichiometric surrogate of the potent endogenous vasoconstrictor endothelin-1 (ET-1).
CT-proET-1 is significantly elevated in critically ill patients ($n = 217$) at admission to the ICU compared with healthy controls ($n = 65$).
CT-proET-1 is elevated in sepsis compared to non-septic ICU patients and is associated with systemic inflammation as well as organ failure.
High CT-proET-1 is an independent risk predictor for ICU and overall mortality.
These data imply that CT-proET-1 is a promising prognostic biomarker in critical illness and that ET-1 could be a novel drug target in the pathogenesis of sepsis and septic shock.

Author details

[1]Department of Medicine III, RWTH-University Hospital Aachen, Pauwelsstrasse 30, 52074 Aachen, Germany. [2]Medical Care Center, Dr. Stein and Colleagues, 41061 Mönchengladbach, Germany.

References

1. Aird WC, Rangel-Frausto M, Pittet D, Costigan M, Bone R, Balk R, et al. The role of the endothelium in severe sepsis and multiple organ dysfunction syndrome. Blood. 2003;101:3765–77.
2. Barton M, Yanagisawa M. Endothelin: 20 years from discovery to therapy. Can J Physiol Pharmacol. 2008;86:485–98.
3. Hynynen MM, Khalil RA. The vascular endothelin system in hypertension—recent patents and discoveries. Recent Pat Cardiovasc Drug Discov. 2006;1:95–108.
4. Sugiura M, Inagami T, Kon V. Endotoxin stimulates endothelin-release in vivo and in vitro as determined by radioimmunoassay. Biochem Biophys Res Commun. 1989;161:1220–7.
5. Yamashita J, Ogawa M, Nomura K, Matsuo S, Inada K, Yamashita S, et al. Interleukin 6 stimulates the production of immunoreactive endothelin 1 in human breast cancer cells. Cancer Res. 1993;53:464–7.
6. Yoshizumi M, Kurihara H, Sugiyama T, Takaku F, Yanagisawa M, Masaki T, et al. Hemodynamic shear stress stimulates endothelin production by cultured endothelial cells. Biochem Biophys Res Commun. 1989;161:859–64.

7. Kaddoura S, Curzen NP, Evans TW, Firth JD, Poole-Wilson PA. Tissue expression of endothelin-1 mRNA in endotoxaemia. Biochem Biophys Res Commun. 1996;218:641–7.
8. Kaszaki J, Wolfárd A, Boros M, Baranyi L, Okada H, Nagy S. Effects of antiendothelin treatment on the early hemodynamic changes in hyperdynamic endotoxemia. Acta Chir Hung. 1997;36:152–3.
9. Brauner JS, Rohde LE, Clausell N. Circulating endothelin-1 and tumor necrosis factor-α: early predictors of mortality in patients with septic shock. Intensive Care Med. 2000;26:305–13.
10. Weitzberg E, Lundberg JM, Rudehill A. Elevated plasma levels of endothelin in patients with sepsis syndrome. Circ Shock. 1991;33:222–7.
11. Pittet JF, Morel DR, Hemsen A, Gunning K, Lacroix JS, Suter PM, et al. Elevated plasma endothelin-1 concentrations are associated with the severity of illness in patients with sepsis. Ann Surg. 1991;213:261–4.
12. Fenhammar J, Andersson A, Forestier J, Weitzberg E, Sollevi A, Hjelmqvist H, et al. Endothelin receptor A antagonism attenuates renal medullary blood flow impairment in endotoxemic pigs. PLoS One. 2011;6:e21534.
13. Piechota-Polańczyk A, Gorąca A. Influence of specific endothelin-1 receptor blockers on hemodynamic parameters and antioxidant status of plasma in LPS-induced endotoxemia. Pharmacol Reports. 2012;64:1434–41.
14. Lundberg OHM, Bergenzaun L, Rydén J, Rosenqvist M, Melander O, Chew MS. Adrenomedullin and endothelin-1 are associated with myocardial injury and death in septic shock patients. Crit Care. 2016;20:178.
15. Schuetz P, Christ-Crain M, Morgenthaler NG, Struck J, Bergmann A, Müller B. Circulating precursor levels of endothelin-1 and adrenomedullin, two endothelium-derived, counteracting substances, in sepsis. Endothelium. 2008;14:345–51.
16 Rey C, García-Hernández I, Concha A, Martínez-Camblor P, Botrán M, Medina A, et al. Pro-adrenomedullin, pro-endothelin-1, procalcitonin. C-reactive protein and mortality risk in critically ill children: a prospective study. Crit Care. 2013;17:R240.
17 Papassotiriou J, Morgenthaler NG, Struck J, Alonso C, Bergmann A. Immunoluminometric assay for measurement of the C-terminal endothelin-1 precursor fragment in human plasma. Clin Chem. 2006;52:1144–51.
18 Koch A, Gressner OA, Sanson E, Tacke F, Trautwein C, Van Cromphaut S, et al. Serum resistin levels in critically ill patients are associated with inflammation, organ dysfunction and metabolism and may predict survival of non-septic patients. Crit Care. 2009;13:R95.
19 Singer M, Deutschman CS, Seymour CW, Shankar-Hari M, Annane D, Bauer M, et al. The third international consensus definitions for sepsis and septic shock (sepsis-3). Jama. 2016;315:801–10.
20 The ARDS Definition Task Force. Acute respiratory distress syndrome. J. Am. Med. Assoc. 2012;307:1.
21 Koch A, Sanson E, Voigt S, Helm A, Trautwein C, Tacke F. Serum adiponectin upon admission to the intensive care unit may predict mortality in critically ill patients. J Crit Care. 2011;26:166–74.
22 Koch A, Voigt S, Sanson E, Duckers H, Horn A, Zimmermann HW, et al. Prognostic value of circulating amino-terminal pro-C-type natriuretic peptide in critically ill patients. Crit Care. 2011;15:R45.
23 Koch A, Sanson E, Helm A, Voigt S, Trautwein C, Tacke F. Regulation and prognostic relevance of serum ghrelin concentrations in critical illness and sepsis. Crit Care. 2010;14:R94.
24 DeLong ER, DeLong DM, Clarke-Pearson DL. Comparing the areas under two or more correlated receiver operating characteristic curves: a nonparametric approach. Biometrics. 1988;44:837–45.
25 Wu R, Dong W, Zhou M, Cui X, Simms HH, Wang P. Ghrelin improves tissue perfusion in severe sepsis via downregulation of endothelin-1. Cardiovasc Res. 2005;68:318–26.
26 Druml W, Steltzer H, Waldhausl W, Lenz K, Hammerle A, Vierhapper H, et al. Endothelin-1 in adult respiratory distress syndrome. Am Rev Respir Dis. 1993;148:1169–73.
27 Guignant C, Venet F, Voirin N, Poitevin F, Malcus C, Bohé J, et al. Proatrial natriuretic peptide is a better predictor of 28-day mortality in septic shock patients than proendothelin-1. Clin Chem Lab Med. 2010;48:1813–20.
28 Krejci V, Hiltebrand LB, Erni D, Sigurdsson GH. Endothelin receptor antagonist bosentan improves microcirculatory blood flow in splanchnic organs in septic shock. Crit Care Med. 2003;31:203–10.
29 Oldner A, Wanecek M, Goiny M, Weitzberg E, Rudehill A, Alving K, et al. The endothelin receptor antagonist bosentan restores gut oxygen delivery and reverses intestinal mucosal acidosis in porcine endotoxin shock. Gut. 1998; 42:696–702.
30 Wanecek M, Oldner A, Rudehill A, Sollevi A, Alving K, Weitzberg E. Cardiopulmonary dysfunction during porcine endotoxin shock is effectively counteracted by the endothelin receptor antagonist bosentan. Shock. 1997; 7:364–70.
31 Weitzberg E, Hemsén A, Rudehill A, Modin A, Wanecek M, Lundberg JM. Bosentan-improved cardiopulmonary vascular performance and increased plasma levels of endothelin-1 in porcine endotoxin shock. Br J Pharmacol. 1996;118:617–26.
32 Iskit AB, Senel I, Sokmensuer C, Guc MO. Endothelin receptor antagonist bosentan improves survival in a murine caecal ligation and puncture model of septic shock. Eur J Pharmacol. 2004;506:83–8.

9

Evolved role of the cardiovascular intensive care unit (CICU)

Shunji Kasaoka

Abstract

Cardiovascular intensive care refers to special systemic management for the patients with severe cardiovascular disease (CVD), which consists of heart disease and vascular disease. CVD is one of the leading causes of death in the world. In order to prevent death due to CVDs, an intensive care unit for severe CVD patients, so-called cardiovascular intensive care unit (CICU), has been developed in many general hospitals. The technological developments of clinical cardiology, such as invasive hemodynamic monitoring and intracoronary interventional procedures and devices, have resulted in evolution of intensive care for CVDs. Subsequently, severe CVD patients admitted to CICU are increasing year by year. Dedicated medical staff is required for CICU in order to perform best patient management. It is necessary for optimal patient care to select effective means from various hemodynamic tools and to adjust the usage according to the clinical situation such as cardiogenic shock and acute heart failure. Furthermore, the patients in the CICU often have various complications such as respiratory failure and renal failure. Therefore, medical staffs who work at CICU are required to have the ability to practice systemic intensive care.

Keywords: Acute myocardial infarction, Cardiovascular intensive care, Cardiovascular disease, Coronary care unit, Intensive care unit

Background

Cardiovascular intensive care refers to special systemic management for the patients with severe cardiovascular disease (CVD), which consists of heart disease and vascular disease. The heart diseases include coronary artery diseases (CAD) such as angina and myocardial infarction, cardiomyopathy, myocarditis, heart arrhythmia, hypertensive heart disease, and valvular heart disease. The vascular diseases include aortic dissection, aortic aneurysm, peripheral artery disease, etc.

It is reported that CVD is the second leading cause of mortality worldwide, accounting for 17 million deaths in 2013 [1]. Although the risk factors for the development of CVD are similar throughout the world, improvement of cardiovascular risk factors such as smoking and obesity is effective to reduce the incidence of CVD.

In recent years, in order to prevent death due to CVDs, an intensive care unit for severe CVD patients, so-called cardiovascular intensive care unit (CICU), has been developed in many general hospitals [2]. In this article, I will review the history of the CICU and discuss the recent changes in cardiovascular intensive care.

Correspondence: kasaoka@kuh.kumamoto-u.ac.jp
Department of Emergency and General Medicine, Kumamoto University Hospital, 1-1-1 Honjo, Chuo-ku, Kumamoto 860-8556, Japan

Epidemiology of cardiovascular diseases

CVDs consist of various heart diseases and vascular diseases. The pathogenesis of onset depends on each CVD. There are many risk factors for heart diseases: age, smoking, obesity, hypertension, diabetes mellitus, and hyperlipidemia. These risk factors increased from 12.3 million deaths (25.8%) in 1990 to 17.9 million deaths (32.1%) in 2015 [3]. Many important cardiovascular risk factors are modifiable by lifestyle change and drug treatment such as prevention of hypertension, hyperlipidemia, and diabetes. It is estimated that 90% of CVD is preventable [4].

CVDs are common among elderly people. In the USA, it is reported that 11% of people between 20 and 40 years old have CVD, while 37% between 40 and 60 years, 71% between 60 and 80 years, and 85% over 80 years have CVD [5].

According to vital statistics of the Ministry of Health, Labor and Welfare in Japan, CVD is the second leading cause of death in Japan. About 200,000 people died due to CVDs in 2015. In addition, approximately 60,000

Japanese people have an out-of-hospital cardiac arrest due to CVDs every year and the overall life-saving rate is still low [6].

Since the CVDs contain many fatal emergency diseases, coronary care unit (CCU) was established as a facility responsible for intensive care in the acute phase in order to improve the outcome of the CVDs.

Progress from the coronary care unit to the cardiovascular intensive care unit

The development of CCU in the mid-twentieth century was a major advance in cardiology practice [7]. CCU was developed in the 1960s when it became clear that close monitoring by specially trained staff, cardiopulmonary resuscitation (CPR), and medical interventions can reduce mortality due to CVD complications such as cardiogenic shock and fatal arrhythmias.

CCU, which was initially established as a separate unit for the early detection and treatment of arrhythmias complicating AMI, currently provides the setting for the monitoring and treatment of a wide variety of critical CVD states. Therefore, the CCU has come to be called the CICU. The role of cardiovascular intensive care has evolved with the rapid progress of diagnostic and therapeutic strategies in the practice of clinical cardiology [7]. The technological developments of clinical cardiology, such as invasive hemodynamic monitoring and intracoronary interventional procedures and devices, have resulted in evolution of intensive care for CVDs. Subsequently, severe CVD patients admitted to CICU are increasing year by year.

Figure 1 displays my concept about cardiovascular intensive care. In the era of CCU, the main target patients were acute myocardial infarction (AMI). Percutaneous coronary intervention (PCI) and defibrillation were important treatments. Subsequently, as the target patients spread to heart failure, shock, out-of-hospital cardiac arrest, etc., the need for cardiovascular intensive care including respiratory management and blood purification therapy increased.

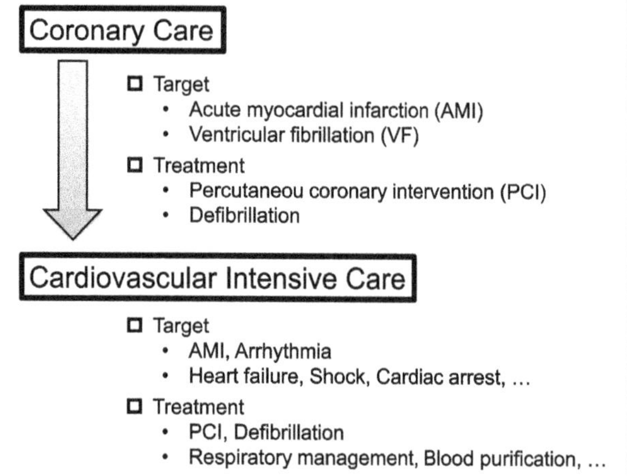

Fig. 1 Evolved role of the cardiovascular intensive care

Features of cardiovascular intensive care

The CICU is a hospital ward specialized in the care of patients with severe heart diseases, such as AMI, cardiomyopathy, and arrhythmias. Those patients often complain of heart failure and cardiogenic shock. Therefore, the severe CVD patients need continuous monitoring and intensive care.

The main feature of CICU is the availability of the continuous monitoring of the cardiac rhythm by electrocardiography (ECG). This allows early intervention with medication, cardioversion, or defibrillation, improving the prognosis of the severe CVD patients. Furthermore, cardiovascular intensive care needs to have various kinds of diagnostic medical equipment as shown in Table 1. Also, therapeutic equipment necessary for cardiovascular intensive care is shown in Table 2. In addition to circulation management, systemic management is required in the CICU. So, it is necessary to prepare a ventilator and a blood purification device as well as the auxiliary circulation devices, such as intra-aortic balloon pump (IABP) and percutaneous cardiopulmonary support system (PCPS) in the CICU. Recently, it is also indispensable to provide the equipment for performing targeted temperature management for the patients resuscitated from cardiogenic out-of-hospital cardiac arrest (OHCA) [8].

A dedicated medical staff is required for cardiovascular intensive care in order to perform best patient management. In Japan, cardiologists certified by the Japan Circulation Society are assigned to CICU. In addition, nurses and technicians who are trained on professional care of CVD patients are also assigned. In order to provide the best patient management, team medical care through cooperation of medical staff in the CICU is indispensable. The CICU physician staff needs the ability to evaluate electrocardiograms and cardiac functions by echocardiography.

Table 1 Diagnostic equipment necessary for cardiovascular intensive care

• Bedside monitoring system: ECG, blood pressure, respiratory rate
• Pulse oximeter (SpO_2)
• Thermometer
• Twelve-lead electrocardiography
• Cardiac ultrasound device
• Cardiac output measurement system: Swan-Ganz catheter
• Portable X-ray imaging equipment
• Doppler blood flow meter
• Blood gas analyzer

Table 2 Therapeutic equipment necessary for cardiovascular intensive care

• Defibrillator
• Cardiac pacemaker
• Noninvasive ventilation system
• Mechanical ventilator
• Blood purification device
• Intra-aortic balloon pump
• Percutaneous cardiopulmonary assist device
• Temperature management system

In recent years, cardiologists have been required not only circulation management but also systemic intensive care practices such as respiratory management and infusion management. Cooperation between cardiologists and intensive care specialists is also important to cope with CVD patients with various complications, such as respiratory failure, renal failure, and sepsis. I believe that systemized training related to general intensive care is necessary so that CICU staff can master the use of diagnostic and therapeutic medical equipments shown in Tables 1 and 2.

In the USA, coronary care units are usually subsets of intensive care units (ICU) dedicated to the care of critically ill cardiac patients. These units are usually present in hospitals that routinely engage in cardiothoracic surgery. It is reported that noncardiovascular disease-related acuity has significantly increased in the CICU and may be influencing mortality [9].

Recently, it is reported that lessons learned from advances in cardiovascular intensive care can be broadly applied to address the urgent need to improve outcomes and efficiency in a variety of health care settings [10]. The CICU is a high-risk environment that admits complex patients suffering from acute conditions that can become life-threatening at any moment. It is reported that simulation-based teaching program yields many benefits for cardiac intensive care units, allowing professionals to acquire not only procedural skills specific to the practice but also confidence and competence as members of an efficient and skilled resuscitation team [11].

Monitoring of the heart and vascular system

The most important monitor in cardiovascular intensive care is an electrocardiogram that evaluates the cardiac rhythm of the CVD patients. In addition, hemodynamic monitoring of invasive arterial pressure and pulmonary artery pressure may be required in the CVD patients complicated with cardiogenic shock or acute heart failure. Hemodynamic evaluation is an important factor in the severity assessment of those patients. For CICU medical staff, it is necessary for optimal patient care to select effective means from various hemodynamic tools and to adjust the usage according to the clinical situation [12].

Since the introduction in the 1970s, pulmonary artery catheter has been commonly utilized for hemodynamic monitoring in the critically ill patient, especially in the adult population [13]. The standard pulmonary artery catheter, as developed by Drs. Swan and Ganz, has four lumens along its length, and these lumens allow for the assessment of hemodynamic data in various places along the right-sided circulation [14]. Data available include right atrium pressure, right ventricle pressure, pulmonary artery pressure, and pulmonary capillary wedge pressure. Using these variables and measured values of heart rate, systemic arterial pressure, and cardiac output, numerous hemodynamic variables can be calculated, including pulmonary and systemic vascular resistance. Cardiac output is most commonly measured with the pulmonary artery catheter using the thermodilution technique. Advantages of the thermodilution method include its validated reliability and its ease of use at the bedside of CCU.

Furthermore, cardiac output can be measured with new technology, which is estimated by analysis of the pulse contour from an arterial waveform, since the systolic portion of the waveform reflects stroke volume (SV) [12]. In recent years, these devices have been used for hemodynamic monitoring in the CICU.

Although the use of invasive hemodynamic monitoring has declined in recent years, it is possible to obtain useful information for assessing the pathology and severity of the CVDs and determining the treatment policy for the critically ill patients.

Targeted temperature management for the patients with out-of-hospital cardiac arrest in the CICU

In patients surviving out-of-hospital cardiac arrest, targeted temperature management (TTM), previously known as mild therapeutic hypothermia, has been reported to significantly improve long-term neurological outcome and may prove to be one of the most important clinical advancements in the resuscitation science [8].

Clinical benefit of therapeutic hypothermia in patients with post-cardiac arrest syndrome (PCAS) has been demonstrated by two randomized control trials since 2002 [15, 16]. However, the term "therapeutic hypothermia" has been replaced with "targeted temperature management (TTM)" since 2011 after the meeting of five major professional physician societies [17]. Subsequently, a large multicenter study comparing TTM between 33 and 36 °C did not show the advantage of 33 °C above 36 °C [18]. Therefore, it is proposed that TTM treatment should be administered to OHCA patients with a shockable initial rhythm. The OHCA patients with ventricular fibrillation (VF) are the main indications for TTM.

Therefore, it is necessary to establish a system to perform the TTM for resuscitated patients admitted to CICU. Doctors and nurses who work at CICU are required to have knowledge and skills on TTM.

Cardiac arrest, a sudden stop in effective blood flow, often happens outside the hospital. It is difficult for many patients who experience out-of-hospital cardiac arrests to survive. The most common cause of cardiac arrest is heart attack, and the most effective treatment for cardiac arrest is immediate cardiopulmonary resuscitation (CPR) and defibrillation by anyone who can do these procedures. The term, "Chain of Survival" is guidelines to help people survive cardiac arrest [19]. The five guidelines in the adult out-of-hospital Chain of Survival that are recommended by the American Heart Association (AHA) are:

1. Recognition of cardiac arrest and activation of the emergency response system
2. Early cardiopulmonary resuscitation with an emphasis on chest compressions
3. Rapid defibrillation
4. Basic and advanced emergency medical services
5. Advanced life support and post-cardiac arrest care

Recently, it is reported that the proportion of OHCA patients with a favorable neurological outcome improved significantly after the implementation of the fifth link [20]. TTM is included in the treatment for post-cardiac arrest syndrome (PCAS) which is on the fifth chain. TTM can be induced and maintained with basic means such as ice packs, fans, cold air blankets, and infusion of cold fluids or with costly advanced systems such as surface cooling pads or endovascular catheters [21]. Recently, a multicenter study comparing the effects of surface cooling and endovascular cooling was conducted [22]. Endovascular cooling appears to be more efficient in rapidly reaching and better controlling the targeted temperature with a decreased workload for nurses during the TTM period. However, endovascular cooling was not significantly superior to basic surface cooling in terms of favorable outcome. CICU medical staff needs to become proficient in using various devices for body temperature management.

Management of cardiogenic shock in the CICU

Cardiogenic shock is a condition in which insufficient organ perfusion occurs due to decreased cardiac output [23]. Causes of cardiogenic shock include severe heart diseases such as AMI, fulminant myocarditis, and cardiomyopathy. This life-threatening emergency condition requires intensive monitoring with aggressive hemodynamic support. In order to survive patients with cardiogenic shock, resuscitation treatment must be performed before irreversible damage to important organs occurs.

The key to good outcome in patients with cardiogenic shock is a systematic approach, with rapid diagnosis and rapid start of pharmacological treatment to maintain blood pressure and cardiac output as well as treatment for the underlying disease. Pulmonary artery catheter is a useful method for evaluating the hemodynamics of shock patients. All shock patients require admission to general ICU or CICU. A multidisciplinary cardiogenic shock team is recommended to guide the rapid and efficient use of these available treatments [23]. All patients with cardiogenic shock require close hemodynamic monitoring, volume support to ensure adequate sufficient preload, and ventilatory support such as tracheal intubation and mechanical ventilation [24]. In mechanical circulatory support such as IABP, PCPS should be considered for patients with shock refractory to conventional medical therapy [23]. Cardiogenic shock is a clinical condition with high mortality rate. Further improvement of cardiovascular intensive care is expected to improve the life-saving rate of cardiogenic shock.

Conclusions

Cardiovascular intensive care unit (CICU) is a hospital ward that specializes in the care of patients who have experienced ischemic heart disease as well as other severe heart disease. Furthermore, the patients in the CICU often have various complications such as respiratory failure and renal failure. Therefore, medical staffs who work at CICU are required to have the ability to practice systemic intensive care.

Abbreviations

AHA: American Heart Association; AMI: Acute myocardial infarction; CAD: Coronary artery disease; CCU: Coronary care unit; CICU: Cardiovascular intensive care unit; CPR: Cardiopulmonary resuscitation; CVD: Cardiovascular disease; ECG: Electrocardiography; IABP: Intra-aortic balloon pump; ICU: Intensive care unit; OHCA: Out-of-hospital cardiac arrest; PCAS: Post-cardiac arrest syndrome; PCI: Percutaneous coronary intervention; PCPS: Percutaneous cardiopulmonary support system; SV: Stroke volume; TTM: Targeted temperature management

Acknowledgements

Not applicable.

Funding

Not applicable.

Competing interests

The author declares that he has no competing interests.

References

1. Bowry AD, Lewey J, Dugani SB, Choudhry NK. The burden of cardiovascular disease in low- and middle-income countries: epidemiology and management. Can J Cardiol. 2015;31:1151–9.
2. Gidwani UK, Kini AS. From the coronary care unit to the cardiovascular intensive care unit: the evolution of cardiac critical care. Cardiol Clin. 2013; 31:485–92.
3. GBD 2015 Mortality and Causes of Death, Collaborators. Global, regional, and national life expectancy, all-cause mortality, and cause-specific mortality for 249 causes of death, 1980-2015: a systematic analysis for the Global Burden of Disease Study 2015. Lancet. 2016;388: 1459–544.
4. McGill HC, McMahan CA, Gidding SS. Preventing heart disease in the 21st century: implications of the Pathobiological Determinants of Atherosclerosis in Youth (PDAY) study. Circulation. 2008;117:1216–27.
5. Go AS, Mozaffarian D, Roger VL, et al. Heart disease and stroke statistics—2013 update: a report from the American Heart Association. Circulation. 2013;127:e6–e245.
6. Kitamura T, Kiyohara K, Sakai T, et al. Public-access defibrillation and out-of-hospital cardiac arrest in Japan. N Engl J Med. 2016;375:1649–59.
7. Walker DM, West NE, Ray SG. British cardiovascular society working group on acute cardiac care. From coronary care unit to acute cardiac care unit: the evolving role of specialist cardiac care. Heart. 2012;98:350–2.
8. Fukuda T. Targeted temperature management for adult out-of-hospital cardiac arrest: current concepts and clinical applications. J Intensive Care. 2016;4:30.
9. Katz JN, Shah BR, Volz EM, et al. Evolution of the coronary care unit: clinical characteristics and temporal trends in healthcare delivery and outcomes. Crit Care Med. 2010;38:375–81.
10. Loughran J, Puthawala T, Sutton BS, et al. The cardiovascular intensive care unit—an evolving model for health care delivery. J Intensive Care Med. 2017;32:116–23.
11. Brunette V, Thibodeau-Jarry N. Simulation as a tool to ensure competency and quality of care in the cardiac critical care unit. Can J Cardiol. 2017;33:119–27.
12. Steven M, Hollenberg MD. Hemodynamic monitoring. Chest. 2013;143: 1480–8.
13. Tsang R. Hemodynamic monitoring in the cardiac intensive care unit. Congenit Heart Dis. 2013;8:568–75.
14. Swan HJ, Ganz W, Forrester J, et al. Catheterization of the heart in man with use of a flow-directed balloon-tipped catheter. N Engl J Med. 1970;283:447–51.
15. Hypothermia after Cardiac Arrest Study Group. Mild therapeutic hypothermia to improve the neurologic outcome after cardiac arrest. N Engl J Med. 2002;346:549–56.
16. Bernard SA, Gray TW, Buist MD, et al. Treatment of comatose survivors of out-of-hospital cardiac arrest with induced hypothermia. N Engl J Med. 2002;346:557–63.
17. Nunnally ME, Jaeschke R, Bellingan GJ, et al. Targeted temperature management in critical care: a report and recommendations from five professional societies. Crit Care Med. 2011;39:1113–25.
18. Nielsen N, Wetterslev J, Cronberg T, Trial Investigators TTM, et al. Targeted temperature management at 33 °C versus 36 °C after cardiac arrest. N Engl J Med. 2013;369:2197–206.
19. Hazinski MF, Nolan JP, Aickin R, et al. Part 1: Executive Summary 2015 International Consensus on Cardiopulmonary Resuscitation and Emergency Cardiovascular Care Science with Treatment Recommendations. Circulation. 2015;132(suppl 1):S2–S39.
20. Tagami T, Hirata K, Takeshige T, et al. Implementation of the fifth link of the chain of survival concept for out-of-hospital cardiac arrest. Circulation. 2012; 126:589–97.
21. Polderman KH, Herold I. Therapeutic hypothermia and controlled normothermia in the intensive care unit: practical considerations, side effects, and cooling methods. Crit Care Med. 2009;37:1101–20.
22. Deye N, Cariou A, Girardie P, et al. Endovascular versus external targeted temperature management for patients with out-of-hospital cardiac arrest. Circulation. 2015;132:182–93.
23. Doll JA, Ohman EM, Patel MR, et al. A team-based approach to patients in cardiogenic shock. Catheter Cardiovasc Interv. 2016;88:424–33.
24. Szymanski FM, Filipiak KJ. Cardiogenic shock—diagnostic and therapeutic options in the light of new scientific data. Anaesthesiology Intensive Therapy. 2014;46:301–6.

10

Damage control resuscitation: a practical approach for severely hemorrhagic patients and its effects on trauma surgery

Yasumitsu Mizobata

Abstract

Coagulopathy observed in trauma patients was thought to be a resuscitation-associated phenomenon. The replacement of lost and consumed coagulation factors was the mainstay in the resuscitation of hemorrhagic shock for many decades. Twenty years ago, damage control surgery (DCS) was implemented to challenge the coagulopathy of trauma. It consists of three steps: abbreviated surgery to control the hemorrhage and contamination, resuscitation in the intensive care unit (ICU), and planned re-operation with definitive surgery. The resuscitation strategy of DCS focused on the rapid reversal of acidosis and prevention of hypothermia through the first two steps. However, direct treatment of coagulopathy was not emphasized in DCS.

Recently, better understanding of the pathophysiology of coagulopathy in trauma patients has led to the logical opinion that we should directly address this coagulopathy during major trauma resuscitation. Damage control resuscitation (DCR), the strategic approach to the trauma patient who presents in extremis, consists of balanced resuscitation, hemostatic resuscitation, and prevention of acidosis, hypothermia, and hypocalcemia. In balanced resuscitation, fluid administration is restricted and hypotension is allowed until definitive hemostatic measures begin. The administration of blood products consisting of fresh frozen plasma, packed red blood cells, and platelets, the ratio of which resembles whole blood, is recommended early in the resuscitation.

DCR strategy is now the most beneficial measure available to address trauma-induced coagulopathy, and it can change the treatment strategy of trauma patients. DCS is now incorporated as a component of DCR. DCR as a structured intervention begins immediately after rapid initial assessment in the emergency room and progresses through the operating theater into the ICU in combination with DCS. By starting from ground zero with the performance of DCS, DCR allows the trauma surgeon to correct the coagulopathy of trauma. The effect of the reversal of coagulopathy in massively hemorrhagic patients may change the operative strategy with DCS.

Keywords: Damage control resuscitation, Acute traumatic coagulopathy, Massive transfusion protocol, Damage control surgery, Balanced resuscitation

Background

Massive bleeding following injury remains the main cause of death in trauma patients. Uncontrolled hemorrhage is reported to be responsible for 40% of trauma deaths [1]. The central measure for controlling such bleeding incorporated physical hemostatic approaches, such as surgery or interventional radiology. Coagulopathy had been thought to be a resuscitation-induced phenomenon, and replacement of the lost and consumed coagulation factors was the mainstay in the resuscitation of hemorrhagic shock. Recently, better understanding of the pathophysiology of coagulopathy in trauma patients has led to the logical opinion that we should directly address coagulopathy during major trauma resuscitation. Damage control resuscitation (DCR) is a strategic approach to the trauma patient who presents in extremis. In this review article, the pathophysiology of the coagulopathy in trauma patients, the theoretical and practical aspects of DCR, and the revolution of damage control surgery (DCS) incorporated with DCR are discussed.

Correspondence: mizobata@med.osaka-cu.ac.jp
Department of Traumatology and Critical Care Medicine, Graduate School of Medicine, Osaka City University, 1-4-3 Asahimachi, Abeno-ku, Osaka City, Osaka 545-8585, Japan

Coagulopathy in trauma

Resuscitation-associated coagulopathy

Traditionally, the coagulopathy observed in trauma patients was thought to be "resuscitation-associated coagulopathy," which is caused by the consumption of coagulation factors, dilution of coagulation factors after massive infusion, hypothermia, and acidosis. An increasing incidence of coagulopathy was observed with increasing amounts of intravenous fluids administered [2]. The administration of large amounts of fluids and blood products, exposure of the body, and surgical intervention performed for resuscitation cause the hypothermia. The alcohol and drugs, which are one of the causes of trauma incident, increase heat loss from the trauma patient. Hypothermia is observed in about 60% of trauma patients who require emergency operative interventions [3]. It is associated with platelet dysfunction and reduced enzyme activities [4] and an increased risk of bleeding and mortality of trauma patients [5]. Inadequate tissue perfusion due to hemorrhagic shock results in anaerobic metabolism and the subsequent production of lactic acid, which causes metabolic acidosis. The high chloride content in crystalloid solutions, such as 0.9% normal saline, exacerbates the metabolic acidosis [6, 7]. The activity of most of the coagulation factors is dependent on the blood pH. For example, the activity of factors VIIa and Xa/Va decreases by over 90% [8] and 70% [9], respectively, when the blood pH decreases from 7.4 to 7.0.

A vicious cycle

In 1982, Kashuk and his colleagues emphasized the importance of coagulopathy in their clinical review of 161 patients with major abdominal vascular injury [10]. They reported that most of the deaths were a result of hemorrhage, and overt coagulopathy was identified in 51% of patients after vascular control was achieved.

The term "lethal triad" was used to describe the physiologic derangement observed in these patients and refers to the triad of the deteriorating status of acute coagulopathy, hypothermia, and acidosis of exsanguinating trauma patients. The lethal triad forms a downward spiral, and further hemorrhage deteriorates the triad. Unless this cycle can be broken, the patient's death is unavoidable. From this aspect, this downward spiral is known as the "vicious cycle of trauma" or the "bloody vicious cycle," which demands as much attention from the physician as the classically emphasized initial resuscitation and operative intervention.

Acute traumatic coagulopathy

Recently, injury itself is reported to cause early coagulopathy [11, 12], which is known as "trauma-induced coagulopathy" [13] or "acute traumatic coagulopathy (ATC)" [14]. ATC is an obvious early coagulopathy and occurs prior to significant dilution [14, 15], within 30 min of injury [12], and affects a quarter of the patients with severe trauma [14]. The patients with this coagulopathy have higher mortality than those with normal clotting function [14].

Although the pathophysiology of ATC is not fully understood, it is thought to occur following injury and concomitant hypoperfusion [16]. ATC is affected primarily through activated protein C, which causes both anticoagulant effects and fibrinolytic effects by inhibiting plasminogen activator inhibitor-1. Instead of the importance of tissue factor, another group has argued that the coagulopathy in trauma is one of disseminated intravascular coagulation with a fibrinolytic phenotype, which is characterized by activation of the coagulation pathways, insufficient anticoagulation mechanisms, and increased fibrinolysis [17, 18].

These recent understandings of ATC have guided the principle and practice of DCR, which directly addresses the hemostatic dysfunction of the severely injured patient.

Damage control resuscitation

Management of coagulopathy in trauma patients

In the severely injured patient, unless the lethal triad of hypothermia, acidosis, and coagulopathy is prevented, death is unavoidable [19]. DCS is a resuscitation strategy that was devised to avoid these physiological disorders. It consists of three steps: abbreviated surgery to control the hemorrhage and contamination, resuscitation in the intensive care unit (ICU), and planned re-operation with definitive surgery [20]. The resuscitation strategy of DCS focused on the rapid reversal of acidosis and the prevention of hypothermia through the first two steps. However, direct treatment of coagulopathy was not emphasized in DCS. The coagulopathy observed in hemorrhagic patients was thought to be a result of resuscitation, acidosis, and hypothermia. Thus, the aim of DCS was to avoid the acidosis and hypothermia resulting from aggressive definitive surgery. Little attention was paid to the early derangement of coagulation function caused by the trauma itself. In contrast, DCR directly addresses the trauma-induced coagulopathy immediately upon patient admission [21] or in the pre-hospital setting [22]. DCR consists of balanced resuscitation, hemostatic resuscitation, and prevention of acidosis, hypothermia, and hypocalcemia.

Balanced resuscitation

The patient's response to the rapid infusion of isotonic fluid or blood is the indicator of the need for surgical or interventional hemostatic procedures. Aggressive fluid resuscitation was the initial fluid therapy recommended for many decades. However, this approach may contribute to increased blood loss and higher mortality [23]. The warning concerning the massive administration of fluid was already reported about 100 years ago by Captain *Cannon* [24]. He commented that, "There is no doubt that in some cases such injections have had definitely beneficial effects, however, the injection of a fluid, that will increase blood pressure, has dangers in itself. If the pressure is raised before the surgeon is ready to check any bleeding, blood needed may be lost."

Increasing evidence has shown that aggressive crystalloid-based resuscitation strategies are associated with cardiac and pulmonary complications [25], gastrointestinal dysfunction, coagulation disturbances, and disorders of immunological and inflammatory mediators [26]. The administration of large volumes of fluids results in imbalances of intracellular and extracellular osmolarity that affect cell volume. Disturbances in cell volume then disrupt numerous regulatory mechanisms responsible for controlling the inflammatory cascade.

For these reasons, an alternative approach to the treatment of hemorrhagic patients was recently proposed and practiced. The approach was introduced as permissive hypotension, delayed resuscitation, or controlled resuscitation. The aim of these resuscitation strategies is not hypotension but rather to balance the risk of decreased tissue perfusion with the benefits from the prevention of coagulopathy.

In 1994, Bickell and colleagues investigated the benefit of delayed fluid resuscitation in a randomized controlled trial. Five hundred eighty-nine adult patients with penetrating injuries and a pre-hospital systolic blood pressure of less than 90 mmHg were enrolled in the trial [27]. The application of delayed fluid resuscitation increased the survival rate of of the patients from 62 to 70%.

After this report, several randomized or retrospective studies concerning balanced resuscitation were reported; however, the benefit to mortality varied among the studies [28–31]. Turner et al. randomized more than 1000 patients to immediate or delayed resuscitation in the prehospital setting but showed no beneficial effects on mortality [28]. Both Dutton et al. and Morrison et al. investigated the effects of hypotensive resuscitation in about 100 patients, but the results varied between these two reports [29, 30]. Duke et al. retrospectively compared cohorts with standard and restricted fluid resuscitation and reported that restricted fluid resuscitation showed a survival benefit [31].

When evaluating the effects of balanced resuscitation, these results should be interpreted cautiously. The patients enrolled in the Bickell et al. and Duke et al. reports were victims of penetrating injury only. In the reports of Morrison et al. and Dutton et al., the rates of patients with penetrating injury were 93 and 51%, respectively. The time from hospital arrival to the emergency operation was very short, and furthermore, the patients were in their 20s or 30s. There are other concerns, such as the low protocol compliance in the Turner et al. report and the difficulty of controlling the blood pressure at the aimed-for level in the Dutton et al. and Morrison et al. reports.

The ninth edition of the Advanced Trauma Life Support emphasizes the concept of balanced resuscitation, and the term "aggressive resuscitation" has been eliminated. The standard use of 2 L of crystalloid resuscitation as the starting point for all resuscitation has been modified to the initiation of 1 L of crystalloid infusion. Early use of blood and blood products for patients in shock is emphasized [32].

The most recent randomized controlled trial to evaluate the efficacy of balanced resuscitation was reported in 2015 [33]. This multicenter study was performed in 19 emergency medical services systems in the USA and Canada. The controlled resuscitation resulted in a reduction of early crystalloid resuscitation volume and an increase in the early transfusion of blood products. Although mortality at 24 h was not different among all patients, it improved in the subgroup with blunt trauma. The controlled resuscitation strategy can be successfully and safely implemented in a civilian environment beginning with the out-of-hospital setting and extending into early hospital care.

Hemostatic resuscitation

In 2007, Borgman and Holcomb et al. reported a survival benefit for the high ratio of plasma to red blood cell (RBC) in patients who received massive transfusions at a combat support hospital [34]. A high plasma to RBC ratio (1:1.4) was independently associated with improved survival, primarily by decreasing death from hemorrhage. Following this article, several studies investigating the survival benefit of a high ratio of fresh frozen plasma (FFP) to RBC were reported [35–40]. Although the ratio of FFP to RBC differed between the studies, a significant decrease in the mortality of the massively transfused patients in the high-ratio population as compared to the low-ratio population was achieved in both the civilian setting and the combat situation.

However, it remains controversial which ratio, 1:1 or 1:2, is beneficial and when the ratio should be achieved. Snyder et al. worried about the survival bias in the beneficial results observed in the retrospective studies [41]. Holcomb and colleagues investigated the relationship between in-hospital mortality and the early transfusion of plasma or platelets, and time variance in the delivery of plasma to RBC or platelet to RBC ratios in a multicenter prospective observational study [42]. The number of patients receiving the higher ratio rose as time passed. In the first 6 h, patients receiving a ratio of less than 1:2 were three to four times more likely to die than patients receiving a ratio of 1:1 or higher. They concluded that the earlier and higher ratio of plasma to RBCs decreased in-hospital mortality, and this beneficial effect was enhanced when the high ratio was achieved in the first 6 h after admission. In the Japan-Observational study for Coagulation and Thrombolysis in Early Trauma (J-OCTET), 189 severe trauma adult patients were registered [43]. Although the area under the curve was not high, the receiver operating characteristic curve analysis showed that the FFP/RBC ratio of 1.0 resulted in maximum sensitivity and specificity for survival. They concluded that a transfusion with an FFP/RBC ratio over 1.0 within the first 6 h reduces the risk of death by about 60% in patients with blunt hemorrhagic trauma.

The most recent randomized trial to evaluate the suitable ratio of plasma to RBCs for patients with severe trauma and major bleeding was performed in the pragmatic, randomized optimal platelet and plasma ratios (PROPPR) study [44], in which 680 patients were randomized to receive either a 1:1:1 or 1:1:2 ratio of plasma, platelets, and RBCs. Although the mortality was not significantly different between the two groups, more patients in the 1:1:1 group achieved hemostasis. Exsanguination, which was the predominant cause of death within the first 24 h, was significantly decreased in the high-ratio group.

Rewarming

In DCR, hypothermia should be managed in conjunction with the efforts to correct the trauma-induced coagulopathy. It is essential to rewarm the torso using passive warming measures, such as insulting foil, blankets, and the removal of wet clothes. The initial fluid resuscitation should be carried out with warmed infusions at a fluid temperature of 40–42 °C [5, 45]. Heated air inhalation, gastric or body cavity lavage with warmed fluids, and heat radiation are widely performed as well as the standardized use of warming measures with rapid infusers. The temperature in the emergency room and the operating room should be raised, at best to a thermally neutral range (28–29 °C) [46]. If the hypothermia persists or quickly relapses despite these maximal rewarming efforts, ongoing hemorrhage and unresolved tissue hypoperfusion and hypoxia should be suspected.

Reversing acidosis

Buffering of metabolic acidosis using drugs not only aggravates the intracellular acidosis but also does not reverse the coagulopathy [47]. Reversal of metabolic acidosis in the trauma patient is better obtained through fluid and blood resuscitation and vasopressor support with surgical control of hemorrhage. Shock should be reversed and end-organ perfusion is restored [48]. Because vital signs such as blood pressure and heart rate are not adequate to evaluate peripheral tissue perfusion, several endpoints of resuscitation are addressed. Base deficit and lactate levels are the reliable indices with which to evaluate the adequacy of the resuscitation and end-organ perfusion. Not only the initial lactate value upon admission but also lactate clearance from plasma within the first few hours of resuscitation correlate with the mortality of trauma patients [49, 50].

Tranexamic acid

Because hyperfibrinolysis was recognized to contribute to the acute coagulopathy in trauma, administration of antifibrinolytic agents had theoretical benefit. The clinical randomization of an antifibrinolytic in significant hemorrhage 2 (CRASH-2) study, a large multi-center randomized controlled trial, investigated the effect of tranexamic acid on mortality and blood product requirements in trauma patients with hemorrhagic shock [51]. The study was undertaken in 274 hospitals in 40 countries. More than 20,000 adult trauma patients were randomized to receive either tranexamic acid or placebo within 8 h of injury. All-cause mortality and the risk of death due to bleeding were significantly decreased with the administration of tranexamic acid. Maximal beneficial effects were achieved if it was given within the first 3 h of injury. However, a recent study indicated that the majority of severely injured patients have fibrinolysis shutdown, and therefore, tranexamic acid may have no effect [52, 53]. The greatest benefit of tranexamic acid may be in patients in whom increased clot lysis is shown to be present using thromboelastography.

Fibrinogen concentrates

Fibrinogen plays a central role in the coagulation process. It bridges activated platelets and works as the key substrate of thrombin to generate a stable fibrin mesh. In patients with blood loss, fibrinogen has been reported to decrease more rapidly under critically low concentrations than the other coagulation factors [54]. Thus, the supplementation of fibrinogen is a measure that makes sense when treating the coagulopathy of trauma patients. The effect of the administration of fibrinogen concentrates on outcome was investigated by matched-pairs analysis using the German Trauma Registry [55]. Although 30-day mortality was comparable, 6-h mortality was significantly lower in the patients receiving fibrinogen. The fibrinogen concentrates might have delayed the cause of death from early hemorrhagic collapse to late multiple organ failure.

Prothrombin complex concentrate

Recently, prothrombin complex concentrate, derived from human plasma and contains variable amounts of factors II, VII, IX, and X, is used to correct coagulopathy [56, 57]. Goal-directed coagulation management using thromboelastometry was used to evaluate requirements of clotting factors [56, 57]. The administration of fibrinogen concentrate alone or in combination with prothrombin complex concentrate resulted in a significant improvement of fibrin polymerization and shorter clotting time [56]. Schochl et al. used fibrinogen concentrate and prothrombin concentrate complex as first-line therapies for coagulopathy based on thromboelastography in a study of 131 severely injured patients [57]. Transfusion of fresh frozen plasma and cryoprecipitate was avoided in the vast majority of these patients and outcomes were better than predicted.

Cryoprecipitate

In the countries, where administration of fibrinogen concentrates is not approved in trauma patients, cryoprecipitate is the alternative treatment option as a source of fibrinogen. However, there are no reports suggesting positive effects of cryoprecipitate administration on the survival of exsanguinating trauma patients [58–60]. Although cryoprecipitate contains high concentrations of fibrinogen, it is hampered by several relevant disadvantages in terms of its availability, allogenicity, and the need for blood type matching and time-consuming thawing. Because the timing and indications for the administration of cryoprecipitate were unclear in the previously reported studies, a prospective randomized trial will be required to evaluate its benefit [59].

Calcium

Calcium acts as an important cofactor in the coagulation cascade. Low levels of ionized calcium at admission are associated with increased mortality and an increased requirement for massive transfusion [61, 62]. Citrate, which is used as an anticoagulant in blood product components, chelates calcium and exacerbates the hypocalcemia, particularly when used in the FFP. The faster the transfusion is given, the faster the reduction of the calcium concentration occurs [63]. An ionized calcium concentration of less than 0.6–0.7 mmol/L could lead to coagulation defects. In addition, contractility of the heart and systemic vascular resistance are diminished under decreased ionized calcium levels. Because of its combined beneficial cardiovascular and coagulation effects, the calcium concentration should be monitored periodically with every ten units of transfusion, and it is recommended that a concentration of at least 0.9 mmol/L be maintained [64, 65].

Massive transfusion protocol

Massive transfusion is typically defined as the transfusion of ten or more units of packed red blood cells within the first 24 h of injury. It is important for the resuscitation staff to identify the patients who might require massive transfusion early in the process of initial resuscitation. Following the prediction of massive transfusion, blood products should be delivered in a quick and timely manner at a high ratio of plasma, RBCs, and platelets. To achieve this quick response, not only the resuscitation staff but also the blood bank staff need to incorporate pre-implemented guidelines and flow charts for massive transfusion protocol (MTP) into their work flow [48, 66–68]. The protocol includes patient selection for activation of the MTP, description of the staff who should declare the activation, and the means by which the resuscitation team and the blood bank are informed of the protocol's activation. In the blood bank, cooled packs of O negative RBCs, type AB FFP, and platelets will be pre-packed for quick delivery. A high-ratio pack is continually delivered each time blood is requested until the protocol is deactivated. Type-specific blood will be delivered as soon as the patient's blood type is determined.

The MTP was implemented in 85% of the trauma centers in the USA as of 2010 [69]. The MTP is bundled with the administration of calcium, factor VIIa, and fibrinogen. The laboratory examination of coagulation function by thromboelastography is included as are other standard blood laboratory tests.

The beneficial effects of the implementation of the MTP have been reported by several authors to be reductions in mortality and in the use of blood products [67, 70, 71]. Furthermore, compliance with the protocol affects patient outcome [66]. Because it is complex to transfuse blood products in a timely and safe manner, implementation of the MTP is essential for institutions caring for severely injured trauma patients. Improved blood bank procedures, effective and efficient rewarming procedures, application of damage control techniques, and aggressive correction of coagulopathy will contribute to the survival benefit [72].

It is important to activate the MTP as quickly as possible; however, it is worth considering that massive transfusion, especially with the administration of FFP, has adverse effects for a subgroup of trauma patients. Inaba and colleagues retrospectively investigated the incidence opportunity following plasma transfusion in patients who did not require massive transfusion [73]. Although there was no improvement in survival with plasma transfusion, the overall rate of complications was significantly higher in the patients receiving plasma products.

Several scores, such as the trauma associated severe hemorrhage (TASH) [74], the scoring system developed by McLaughlin [75], assessment of blood consumption (ABC) [76], and traumatic bleeding severity score (TBSS) [77] scores, are proposed for the prediction of patients who require massive transfusion in the early phase of resuscitation. Each score includes the systolic blood pressure and heart rate on admission or after the initial resuscitation. The focused assessment with sonography for trauma exam, extremity and/or pelvic injury, sex, age, or laboratory data are assessed to calculate these scores. Recently, the TBSS score was modified to predict the need for massive transfusion more quickly [78]. The systolic blood pressure on arrival but after fluid resuscitation was used. The predictive value of the modified TBSS is still high and is reported to be equivalent to that of the TASH score.

Remote DCR

The concept and practice of the DCR is recently applied in the pre-hospital setting and named as remote DCR (RDCR) [79]. Not only the fixed-ratio coagulation therapy using the high ratio of plasma and platelets to pRBC but also the coagulation factor concentrate-based treatment is proposed in the RDCR. It includes three major components to a step-wise approach to achieve hemostasis: (1) stop (hyper)fibrinolysis, tranexamic acid; (2) support clot formation, fibrinogen concentrate; and (3) increase thrombin generation, prothrombin complex concentrate [22]. Although RDCR warrants further investigation concerning its effect on the mortality or the blood products requirement, and the assessment of the patient's coagulation function in the instrument limited environment, the tranexamic acid has been implemented in the RDCR in the US, French, British, and Israeli militaries as well as the British, Norwegian, and Israeli civilian ambulance services. A prospective cohort study in the civilian trauma center demonstrated reduction in mortality and multiple organ failure for patients treated with tranexamic acid in the subgroup of patients with shock [80]. In the report of Wafaisade et al., the propensity score matched analysis using the German trauma database demonstrated the prolonged time to death and reduction in early mortality in the tranexamic acid-administered trauma patients [81]. The updated European guideline suggests the administration of the first dose of tranexamic acid en route to the hospital as a grade 2C recommendation [82].

DCR and DCS

Adverse effects of DCS

After the recognition of the vicious cycle in trauma patients, a paradigm shift in the surgical treatment of severely hemorrhagic patients occurred. DCS was developed to challenge the lethal triad of trauma. It was originally reported by Stone and colleagues in 1983 [83] and named by Rotondo and Schwab in 1993 [20]. Since these reports, DCS has become the standard of care for the most severely injured patients. It has been widely applied not only for abdominal trauma but also for thoracic [84], vascular [85], pelvic [86], and extremity injuries [87, 88]. DCS has led to better outcomes in severely hemorrhagic patients [89]. Ten years of experience have shown that patients who receive DCS for penetrating abdominal trauma have higher survival rates and a decreased incidence of hypothermia in the operating room [90]. In the early decades after DCS was introduced, it was performed in cooperation with aggressive volume resuscitation.

Although DCS was popularized and resulted in reduced mortality, the abbreviated surgical techniques and open abdomen management led to significant increases in sub-acute complications, such as open abdomen, acute respiratory distress syndrome, intra-abdominal infections, and multiple organ failure [91]. In particular, open abdomen management resulted in an increase in severe morbidities, such as anastomotic breakdown, ventral hernias, and enteroatmospheric fistula [92, 93]. Aggressive resuscitation increased the incidence of these complications [26].

Studies have recently warned against the overuse of DCS [94, 95]. Clinical outcomes may be improved with more selective use of DCS accompanied by DCR [96].

Changes of surgical strategy in DCR

The severely hemorrhagic patient has a limited amount of physiologic reserve before irreversible derangement, organ damage, and collapse occur. DCR restores this reserve, allowing more definitive treatment that results in decreased postoperative complications and improved outcomes [40, 68].

DCS is now incorporated as a component of DCR and should not be practiced in isolation [64]. DCR as a structured intervention should begin immediately after rapid initial assessment in the emergency room and progresses through the operating theater into the ICU in combination with DCS [48].

By starting from ground zero with the performance of DCS, DCR allows the trauma surgeon to correct the lethal triad, particularly the coagulopathy of trauma. Definitive therapy can be completed at the first operation in patients who are warm, well perfused, and without coagulopathy [97, 98].

Higa and colleagues reported that DCR increased the administration of blood products with less infusion of crystalloid solution and was associated with a survival advantage and shorter length of stay in the trauma ICU for patients with severe hemorrhage [96]. Although the number of laparotomy patients increased, the number of patients requiring damage control laparotomy decreased from 36 to 9%, and the mortality for patients requiring open laparotomy improved from 22 to 13%. The application of DCR to damage control laparotomy techniques results in an improvement in the ability to achieve primary fascia closure and decreases the requirement for staged laparotomy [99]. In addition, DCR may decrease the surgical hemostatic requirement in severely injured patients. A retrospective study showed an increase in the success rate of nonoperative management from 54 to 74% for grades IV and V severe blunt liver injury after the implementation of DCR [100]. DCR may herald the beginning of the end for DCS [98].

Conclusions

DCR strategy is the measure that directly addresses trauma-induced coagulopathy. Although several concerns, such as the plasma to RBCs ratio, the method of achieving balanced resuscitation, and the administration of other coagulation factors, are not completely resolved, it is now the most beneficial measure for treating trauma-induced coagulopathy, and it can change the treatment strategy of trauma patients. The effect of the reversal of coagulopathy in the massively hemorrhagic patient may shift the operative strategy from one of DCS to definitive surgery.

Abbreviations

ABC: Assessment of blood consumption; ATC: Acute traumatic coagulopathy; CRASH-2: Clinical randomization of an antifibrinolytic in significant hemorrhage 2; DCR: Damage control resuscitation; DCS: Damage control surgery; FFP: Fresh frozen plasma; ICU: Intensive care unit; J-OCTET: Japan-observational study for coagulation and thrombolysis in early trauma; MTP: Massive transfusion protocol; PROPPR: Pragmatic, randomized optimal platelet and plasma ratios; RBC: Red blood cell; RDCR: Remote damage control resuscitation; TASH: Trauma associate severe hemorrhage; TBSS: Traumatic bleeding severity score

Acknowledgements

Not applicable.

Funding

No funding.

Authors' contributions

YM wrote, read, and approved the final manuscript.

Competing interests

The author declares that he/she has no competing interests.

References

1. Sauaia A, Moore FA, Moore EE, Moser KS, Brennan R, Read RA, et al. Epidemiology of trauma deaths: a reassessment. J Trauma. 1995;38(2):185–93.
2. Maegele M, Lefering R, Yucel N, Tjardes T, Rixen D, Paffrath T, et al. Early coagulopathy in multiple injury: an analysis from the German Trauma Registry on 8724 patients. Injury. 2007;38(3):298–304.
3. Gregory JS, Flancbaum L, Townsend MC, Cloutier CT, Jonasson O. Incidence and timing of hypothermia in trauma patients undergoing operations. J Trauma. 1991;31(6):795–8. discussion 798-800.
4. Wolberg AS, Meng ZH, Monroe 3rd DM, Hoffman M. A systematic evaluation of the effect of temperature on coagulation enzyme activity and platelet function. J Trauma. 2004;56(6):1221–8.
5. Beekley AC. Damage control resuscitation: a sensible approach to the exsanguinating surgical patient. Crit Care Med. 2008;36(7 Suppl):S267–74.
6. Besen BA, Gobatto AL, Melro LM, Maciel AT, Park M. Fluid and electrolyte overload in critically ill patients: an overview. World J Crit Care Med. 2015;4(2):116–29.
7. Santi M, Lava SA, Camozzi P, Giannini O, Milani GP, Simonetti GD, et al. The great fluid debate: saline or so-called "balanced" salt solutions? Ital J Pediatr. 2015;41:47.
8. Meng ZH, Wolberg AS, Monroe 3rd DM, Hoffman M. The effect of temperature and pH on the activity of factor VIIa: implications for the efficacy of high-dose factor VIIa in hypothermic and acidotic patients. J Trauma. 2003;55(5):886–91.
9. Martini WZ. Coagulopathy by hypothermia and acidosis: mechanisms of thrombin generation and fibrinogen availability. J Trauma. 2009;67(1):202–8. discussion 208-9.
10. Kashuk JL, Moore EE, Millikan JS, Moore JB. Major abdominal vascular trauma—a unified approach. J Trauma. 1982;22(8):672–9.
11. Hess JR, Brohi K, Dutton RP, Hauser CJ, Holcomb JB, Kluger Y, et al. The coagulopathy of trauma: a review of mechanisms. J Trauma. 2008;65(4):748–54.
12. Floccard B, Rugeri L, Faure A, Saint Denis M, Boyle EM, Peguet O, et al. Early coagulopathy in trauma patients: an on-scene and hospital admission study. Injury. 2012;43(1):26–32.
13. Chang R, Cardenas JC, Wade CE, Holcomb JB. Advances in the understanding of trauma-induced coagulopathy. Blood. 2016;128(8):1043–9.
14. Brohi K, Singh J, Heron M, Coats T. Acute traumatic coagulopathy. J Trauma. 2003;54(6):1127–30.
15. MacLeod JB, Lynn M, McKenney MG, Cohn SM, Murtha M. Early coagulopathy predicts mortality in trauma. J Trauma. 2003;55(1):39–44.
16. Brohi K, Cohen MJ, Ganter MT, Matthay MA, Mackersie RC, Pittet JF. Acute traumatic coagulopathy: initiated by hypoperfusion: modulated through the protein C pathway? Ann Surg. 2007;245(5):812–8.
17. Gando S, Wada H, Kim HK, Kurosawa S, Nielsen JD, Thachil J, et al. Comparison of disseminated intravascular coagulation in trauma with coagulopathy of trauma/acute coagulopathy of trauma-shock. J Thromb Haemost. 2012;10(12):2593–5.
18. Gando S, Wada H, Thachil J. Scientific, Standardization Committee on DICotISoT, Haemostasis. Differentiating disseminated intravascular coagulation (DIC) with the fibrinolytic phenotype from coagulopathy of trauma and acute coagulopathy of trauma-shock (COT/ACOTS). J Thromb Haemost. 2013;11(5):826–35.
19. Moore EE. Staged laparotomy for the hypothermia, acidosis, and coagulopathy syndrome. Am J Surg. 1996;172:405–10.
20. Rotondo MF, Schwab CW, McGonigal MD, Phillips 3rd GR, Fruchterman TM, Kauder DR, et al. 'Damage control': an approach for improved survival in exsanguinating penetrating abdominal injury. J Trauma. 1993;35(3):375–82. discussion 382-3.
21. Ho AM, Karmakar MK, Dion PW. Are we giving enough coagulation factors during major trauma resuscitation? Am J Surg. 2005;190(3):479–84.
22. Maegele M. Coagulation factor concentrate-based therapy for remote damage control resuscitation (RDCR): a reasonable alternative? Transfusion. 2016;56 Suppl 2:S157–65.
23. Rezende-Neto JB, Rizoli SB, Andrade MV, Ribeiro DD, Lisboa TA, Camargos ER, et al. Permissive hypotension and desmopressin enhance clot formation. J Trauma. 2010;68(1):42–50.
24. Cannon WB, Fraser J, Cowell EM. The preventive treatment of wound shock. JAMA. 1918;70:618–21.
25. Brandstrup B, Tonnesen H, Beier-Holgersen R, Hjortso E, Ording H, Lindorff-Larsen K, et al. Effects of intravenous fluid restriction on postoperative complications: comparison of two perioperative fluid regimens: a randomized assessor-blinded multicenter trial. Ann Surg. 2003;238(5):641–8.
26. Cotton BA, Guy JS, Morris Jr JA, Abumrad NN. The cellular, metabolic, and systemic consequences of aggressive fluid resuscitation strategies. Shock. 2006;26(2):115–21.
27. Bickell WH, Wall Jr MJ, Pepe PE, Martin RR, Ginger VF, Allen MK, et al. Immediate versus delayed fluid resuscitation for hypotensive patients with penetrating torso injuries. N Eng J Med. 1994;331(17):1105–9.
28. Turner J, Nicholl J, Webber L, Cox H, Dixon S, Yates D. A randomised controlled trial of prehospital intravenous fluid replacement therapy in serious trauma. Health Technol Assess. 2000;4(31):1–57.

29. Dutton RP. Low-pressure resuscitation from hemorrhagic shock. Int Anesthesiol Clin. 2002;40(3):19–30.
30. Morrison CA, Carrick MM, Norman MA, Scott BG, Welsh FJ, Tsai P, et al. Hypotensive resuscitation strategy reduces transfusion requirements and severe postoperative coagulopathy in trauma patients with hemorrhagic shock: preliminary results of a randomized controlled trial. J Trauma. 2011;70(3):652–63.
31. Duke MD, Guidry C, Guice J, Stuke L, Marr AB, Hunt JP, et al. Restrictive fluid resuscitation in combination with damage control resuscitation: time for adaptation. J Trauma Acute Care Surg. 2012;73(3):674–8.
32. The ATLS subcommittee, American College of Surgeons' Committee on Trauma, and International ATLS working group. Advanced trauma life support (ATLS(R)): the ninth edition. J Trauma Acute Care Surg. 2013;74(5):1363–6.
33. Schreiber MA, Meier EN, Tisherman SA, Kerby JD, Newgard CD, Brasel K, et al. A controlled resuscitation strategy is feasible and safe in hypotensive trauma patients: results of a prospective randomized pilot trial. J Trauma Acute Care Surg. 2015;78(4):687–95. discussion 695-7.
34. Borgman MA, Spinella PC, Perkins JG, Grathwohl KW, Repine T, Beekley AC, et al. The ratio of blood products transfused affects mortality in patients receiving massive transfusions at a combat support hospital. J Trauma. 2007;63(4):805–13.
35. Holcomb JB, Wade CE, Michalek JE, Chisholm GB, Zarzabal LA, Schreiber MA, et al. Increased plasma and platelet to red blood cell ratios improves outcome in 466 massively transfused civilian trauma patients. Ann Surg. 2008;248(3):447–58.
36. Duchesne JC, Hunt JP, Wahl G, Marr AB, Wang YZ, Weintraub SE, et al. Review of current blood transfusions strategies in a mature level I trauma center: were we wrong for the last 60 years? J Trauma. 2008;65(2):272–6. discussion 276-8.
37. Kashuk JL, Moore EE, Johnson JL, Haenel J, Wilson M, Moore JB, et al. Postinjury life threatening coagulopathy: is 1:1 fresh frozen plasma:packed red blood cells the answer? J Trauma. 2008;65(2):261–70. discussion 270-1.
38. Sperry JL, Ochoa JB, Gunn SR, Alarcon LH, Minei JP, Cuschieri J, et al. An FFP: PRBC transfusion ratio >/=1:1.5 is associated with a lower risk of mortality after massive transfusion. J Trauma. 2008;65(5):986–93.
39. Gunter Jr OL, Au BK, Isbell JM, Mowery NT, Young PP, Cotton BA. Optimizing outcomes in damage control resuscitation: identifying blood product ratios associated with improved survival. J Trauma. 2008;65(3):527–34.
40. Duchesne JC, Islam TM, Stuke L, Timmer JR, Barbeau JM, Marr AB, et al. Hemostatic resuscitation during surgery improves survival in patients with traumatic-induced coagulopathy. J Trauma. 2009;67(1):33–7. discussion 37-9.
41. Snyder CW, Weinberg JA, McGwin Jr G, Melton SM, George RL, Reiff DA, et al. The relationship of blood product ratio to mortality: survival benefit or survival bias? J Trauma. 2009;66(2):358–62. discussion 362-4.
42. Holcomb JB, del Junco DJ, Fox EE, Wade CE, Cohen MJ, Schreiber MA, et al. The prospective, observational, multicenter, major trauma transfusion (PROMMTT) study: comparative effectiveness of a time-varying treatment with competing risks. JAMA Surg. 2013;148(2):127–36.
43. Hagiwara A, Kushimoto S, Kato H, Sasaki J, Ogura H, Matsuoka T, et al. Can early aggressive administration of fresh frozen plasma improve outcomes in patients with severe blunt trauma?—a report by the Japanese Association for the Surgery of Trauma. Shock. 2016;45(5):495–501.
44. Holcomb JB, Tilley BC, Baraniuk S, Fox EE, Wade CE, Podbielski JM, et al. Transfusion of plasma, platelets, and red blood cells in a 1:1:1 vs a 1:1:2 ratio and mortality in patients with severe trauma: the PROPPR randomized clinical trial. JAMA. 2015;313(5):471–82.
45. Tieu BH, Holcomb JB, Schreiber MA. Coagulopathy: its pathophysiology and treatment in the injured patient. World J Surg. 2007;31(5):1055–64.
46. Rossaint R, Bouillon B, Cerny V, Coats TJ, Duranteau J, Fernandez-Mondejar E, et al. Management of bleeding following major trauma: an updated European guideline. Crit Care. 2010;14(2):R52.
47. Brohi K, Cohen MJ, Davenport RA. Acute coagulopathy of trauma: mechanism, identification and effect. Curr Opin Crit Care. 2007;13(6):680–5.
48. Kaafarani HM, Velmahos GC. Damage control resuscitation in trauma. Scand J Surg. 2014;103(2):81–8.
49. Husain FA, Martin MJ, Mullenix PS, Steele SR, Elliott DC. Serum lactate and base deficit as predictors of mortality and morbidity. Am J Surg. 2003;185(5):485–91.
50. Vandromme MJ, Griffin RL, Weinberg JA, Rue 3rd LW, Kerby JD. Lactate is a better predictor than systolic blood pressure for determining blood requirement and mortality: could prehospital measures improve trauma triage? J Am Coll Surg. 2010;210(5):861–7.
51. Shakur H, Roberts I, Bautista R, Caballero J, Coats T, Dewan Y, et al. Effects of tranexamic acid on death, vascular occlusive events, and blood transfusion in trauma patients with significant haemorrhage (CRASH-2): a randomised, placebo-controlled trial. Lancet. 2010;376(9734):23–32.
52. Moore HB, Moore EE, Liras IN, Gonzalez E, Harvin JA, Holcomb JB, et al. Acute fibrinolysis shutdown after injury occurs frequently and increases mortality: a multicenter evaluation of 2,540 severely injured patients. J Am Coll Surg. 2016;222(4):347–55.
53. Moore HB, Moore EE, Gonzalez E, Chapman MP, Chin TL, Silliman CC, et al. Hyperfibrinolysis, physiologic fibrinolysis, and fibrinolysis shutdown: the spectrum of postinjury fibrinolysis and relevance to antifibrinolytic therapy. J Trauma Acute Care Surg. 2016;77(6):811–7.
54. Hiippala ST, Myllyla GJ, Vahtera EM. Hemostatic factors and replacement of major blood loss with plasma-poor red cell concentrates. Anesth Analg. 1995;81(2):360–5.
55. Wafaisade A, Lefering R, Maegele M, Brockamp T, Mutschler M, Lendemans S, et al. Administration of fibrinogen concentrate in exsanguinating trauma patients is associated with improved survival at 6 hours but not at discharge. J Trauma Acute Care Surg. 2013;74(2):387–3. discussion 393-5.
56. Ponschab M, Voelckel W, Pavelka M, Schlimp CJ, Schochl H. Effect of coagulation factor concentrate administration on ROTEM(R) parameters in major trauma. Scand J Trauma Resus Emerg Med. 2015;23:84.
57. Schochl H, Nienaber U, Hofer G, Voelckel W, Jambor C, Scharbert G, et al. Goal-directed coagulation management of major trauma patients using thromboelastometry (ROTEM)-guided administration of fibrinogen concentrate and prothrombin complex concentrate. Crit Care. 2010;14(2):R55.
58. Curry N, Rourke C, Davenport R, Beer S, Pankhurst L, Deary A, et al. Early cryoprecipitate for major haemorrhage in trauma: a randomised controlled feasibility trial. Br J Anaesth. 2015;115(1):76–83.
59. Holcomb JB, Fox EE, Zhang X, White N, Wade CE, Cotton BA, et al. Cryoprecipitate use in the Prospective Observational Multicenter Major Trauma Transfusion study (PROMMTT). J Trauma Acute Care Surg. 2013; 75(1 Suppl 1):S31–9.
60. Olaussen A, Fitzgerald MC, Tan GA, Mitra B. Cryoprecipitate administration after trauma. Eur J Emerg Med. 2016;23(4):269–73.
61. Ho KM, Leonard AD. Concentration-dependent effect of hypocalcaemia on mortality of patients with critical bleeding requiring massive transfusion: a cohort study. Anaesth Intensive Care. 2011;39(1):46–54.
62. Magnotti LJ, Bradburn EH, Webb DL, Berry SD, Fischer PE, Zarzaur BL, et al. Admission ionized calcium levels predict the need for multiple transfusions: a prospective study of 591 critically ill trauma patients. J Trauma. 2011;70(2): 391–5. discussion 395-7.
63. Lier H, Bottiger BW, Hinkelbein J, Krep H, Bernhard M. Coagulation management in multiple trauma: a systematic review. Intensive Care Med. 2011;37(4):572–82.
64. Jansen JO, Thomas R, Loudon MA, Brooks A. Damage control resuscitation for patients with major trauma. BMJ. 2009;338:b1778.
65. Perkins JG, Cap AP, Weiss BM, Reid TJ, Bolan CD. Massive transfusion and nonsurgical hemostatic agents. Crit Care Med. 2008;36(7 Suppl):S325–39.
66. Bawazeer M, Ahmed N, Izadi H, McFarlan A, Nathens A, Pavenski K. Compliance with a massive transfusion protocol (MTP) impacts patient outcome. Injury. 2015;46(1):21–8.
67. Riskin DJ, Tsai TC, Riskin L, Hernandez-Boussard T, Purtill M, Maggio PM, et al. Massive transfusion protocols: the role of aggressive resuscitation versus product ratio in mortality reduction. J Am Coll Surg. 2009; 209(2):198–205.
68. Duchesne JC, Kimonis K, Marr AB, Rennie KV, Wahl G, Wells JE, et al. Damage control resuscitation in combination with damage control laparotomy: a survival advantage. J Trauma. 2010;69(1):46–52.
69. Schuster KM, Davis KA, Lui FY, Maerz LL, Kaplan LJ. The status of massive transfusion protocols in United States trauma centers: massive transfusion or massive confusion? Transfusion. 2010;50(7):1545–51.
70. Cotton BA, Gunter OL, Isbell J, Au BK, Robertson AM, Morris Jr JA, et al. Damage control hematology: the impact of a trauma exsanguination protocol on survival and blood product utilization. J Trauma. 2008;64(5): 1177–82. discussion 1182-3.
71. Dente CJ, Shaz BH, Nicholas JM, Harris RS, Wyrzykowski AD, Patel S, et al. Improvements in early mortality and coagulopathy are sustained better in patients with blunt trauma after institution of a massive transfusion protocol in a civilian level I trauma center. J Trauma. 2009;66(6):1616–24.

72. Cinat ME, Wallace WC, Nastanski F, West J, Sloan S, Ocariz J, et al. Improved survival following massive transfusion in patients who have undergone trauma. Arch Surg. 1999;134(9):964–8. discussion 968-70.
73. Inaba K, Branco BC, Rhee P, Blackbourne LH, Holcomb JB, Teixeira PG, et al. Impact of plasma transfusion in trauma patients who do not require massive transfusion. J Am Coll Surg. 2010;210(6):957–65.
74. Yucel N, Lefering R, Maegele M, Vorweg M, Tjardes T, Ruchholtz S, et al. Trauma Associated Severe Hemorrhage (TASH)-Score: probability of mass transfusion as surrogate for life threatening hemorrhage after multiple trauma. J Trauma. 2006;60(6):1228–36. discussion 1236-7.
75. McLaughlin DF, Niles SE, Salinas J, Perkins JG, Cox ED, Wade CE, et al. A predictive model for massive transfusion in combat casualty patients. J Trauma. 2008;64(2 Suppl):S57–63. discussion S63.
76. Nunez TC, Voskresensky IV, Dossett LA, Shinall R, Dutton WD, Cotton BA. Early prediction of massive transfusion in trauma: simple as ABC (assessment of blood consumption)? J Trauma. 2009;66(2):346–52.
77. Ogura T, Nakamura Y, Nakano M, Izawa Y, Nakamura M, Fujizuka K, et al. Predicting the need for massive transfusion in trauma patients: the Traumatic Bleeding Severity Score. J Trauma Acute Care Surg. 2014;76(5):1243–50.
78. Ogura T, Lefor AK, Masuda M, Kushimoto S. Modified traumatic bleeding severity score: early determination of the need for massive transfusion. Am J Emerg Med. 2016;34(6):1097–101.
79. Gerhardt RT, Strandenes G, Cap AP, Rentas FJ, Glassberg E, Mott J, et al. Remote damage control resuscitation and the Solstrand Conference: defining the need, the language, and a way forward. Transfusion. 2013; 53 Suppl 1:9S–16S.
80. Ausset S, Glassberg E, Nadler R, Sunde G, Cap AP, Hoffmann C, et al. Tranexamic acid as part of remote damage-control resuscitation in the prehospital setting: a critical appraisal of the medical literature and available alternatives. J Trauma Acute Care Surg. 2015;78(6 Suppl 1):S70–5.
81. Wafaisade A, Lefering R, Bouillon B, Bohmer AB, Gassler M, Ruppert M. Prehospital administration of tranexamic acid in trauma patients. Crit Care. 2016;20(1):143.
82. Spahn DR, Bouillon B, Cerny V, Coats TJ, Duranteau J, Fernandez-Mondejar E, et al. Management of bleeding and coagulopathy following major trauma: an updated European guideline. Crit Care. 2013;17(2):R76.
83. Stone HH, Strom PR, Mullins RJ. Management of the major coagulopathy with onset during laparotomy. Ann Surg. 1983;197(5):532–5.
84. Vargo DJ, Battistella FD. Abbreviated thoracotomy and temporary chest closure: an application of damage control after thoracic trauma. Arch Surg. 2001;136(1):21–4.
85. Rasmussen TE, Clouse WD, Jenkins DH, Peck MA, Eliason JL, Smith DL. The use of temporary vascular shunts as a damage control adjunct in the management of wartime vascular injury. J Trauma. 2006;61(1):8–12.
86. Henry SM, Tornetta 3rd P, Scalea TM. Damage control for devastating pelvic and extremity injuries. Surg Clin North Am. 1997;77(4):879–95.
87. Scalea TM, Boswell SA, Scott JD, Mitchell KA, Kramer ME, Pollak AN. External fixation as a bridge to intramedullary nailing for patients with multiple injuries and with femur fractures: damage control orthopedics. J Trauma. 2000;48(4):613–21. discussion 621-3.
88. Pape HC, Hildebrand F, Pertschy S, Zelle B, Garapati R, Grimme K, et al. Changes in the management of femoral shaft fractures in polytrauma patients: from early total care to damage control orthopedic surgery. J Trauma. 2002;53(3):452–61. discussion 461-2.
89. Sutton E, Bochicchio GV, Bochicchio K, Rodriguez ED, Henry S, Joshi M, et al. Long term impact of damage control surgery: a preliminary prospective study. J Trauma. 2006;61(4):831–4. discussion 835-6.
90. Johnson JW, Gracias VH, Schwab CW, Reilly PM, Kauder DR, Shapiro MB, et al. Evolution in damage control for exsanguinating penetrating abdominal injury. J Trauma. 2001;51(2):261–9. discussion 269-71.
91. Smith BP, Adams RC, Doraiswamy VA, Nagaraja V, Seamon MJ, Wisler J, et al. Review of abdominal damage control and open abdomens: focus on gastrointestinal complications. J Gastrointestin Liver Dis. 2010;19(4):425–35.
92. Diaz Jr JJ, Dutton WD, Ott MM, Cullinane DC, Alouidor R, Armen SB, et al. Eastern Association for the Surgery of Trauma: a review of the management of the open abdomen—part 2 "Management of the open abdomen". J Trauma. 2011;71(2):502–12.
93. Dubose JJ, Lundy JB. Enterocutaneous fistulas in the setting of trauma and critical illness. Clin Colon Rectal Surg. 2010;23(3):182–9.
94. Cotton BA, Reddy N, Hatch QM, LeFebvre E, Wade CE, Kozar RA, et al. Damage control resuscitation is associated with a reduction in resuscitation volumes and improvement in survival in 390 damage control laparotomy patients. Ann Surg. 2011;254(4):598–605.
95. Roberts DJ, Bobrovitz N, Zygun DA, Ball CG, Kirkpatrick AW, Faris PD, et al. Indications for use of damage control surgery in civilian trauma patients: a content analysis and expert appropriateness rating study. Ann Surg. 2016;263(5):1018–27.
96. Higa G, Friese R, O'Keeffe T, Wynne J, Bowlby P, Ziemba M, et al. Damage control laparotomy: a vital tool once overused. J Trauma. 2010;69(1):53–9.
97. Holcomb JB, Jenkins D, Rhee P, Johannigman J, Mahoney P, Mehta S, et al. Damage control resuscitation: directly addressing the early coagulopathy of trauma. J Trauma. 2007;62(2):307–10.
98. Schreiber MA. The beginning of the end for damage control surgery. Br J Surg. 2012;99 Suppl 1:10–1.
99. Bradley M, Galvagno S, Dhanda A, Rodriguez C, Lauerman M, DuBose J, et al. Damage control resuscitation protocol and the management of open abdomens in trauma patients. Am Surg. 2014;80(8):768–75.
100. Shrestha B, Holcomb JB, Camp EA, Del Junco DJ, Cotton BA, Albarado R, et al. Damage-control resuscitation increases successful nonoperative management rates and survival after severe blunt liver injury. J Trauma Acute Care Surg. 2015;78(2):336–41.

11

Make it SIMPLE: enhanced shock management by focused cardiac ultrasound

Ka Leung Mok

Abstract

Background: Shock is a spectrum of circulatory failure that, if not properly managed, would lead to high mortality. Special diagnostic and treatment strategies are essential to save lives. However, clinical and laboratory findings are always non-specific, resulting in clinical dilemmas.

Main content: Focused cardiac ultrasound (FoCUS) has emerged as one of the power tools for clinicians to answer simple clinical questions and guide subsequent management in hypotensive patients. This article will review the development and utility of FoCUS in different types of shock. The sonographic features and ultrasound enhanced management of hypotensive patients by a de novo "SIMPLE" approach will be described. Current evidence on FoCUS will also be reviewed.

Conclusion: Focused cardiac ultrasound provides timely and valuable information for the evaluation of shock. It helps to improve the diagnostic accuracy, narrow the possible differential diagnoses, and guide specific management. SIMPLE is an easy-to-remember mnemonic for non-cardiologists or novice clinical sonographers to apply FoCUS and interpret the specific sonographic findings when evaluating patients in shock.

Keywords: Shock, Ultrasound, Echocardiography, Emergency department, Critical care, Sepsis

Background

Shock is a clinical syndrome in which there is inadequate cellular and tissue oxygenation due to circulatory failure [1]. The presentation of shock can vary with different causes of shocks and degrees of physiological abnormalities. Shock can be classified into five different categories according to the underlying pathophysiology, namely hypovolemic shock (due to hemorrhage or intravascular volume depletion), cardiogenic shock (e.g., acute myocardial infarction, myocarditis), obstructive shock (e.g., pulmonary embolism, tension pneumothorax, and cardiac tamponade), and distributive shock (e.g., septic, neurogenic, and anaphylactic), and lastly, shock related to cellular poisoning [2]. One of the cardinal features of shock is hypotension. It can be defined as systolic blood pressure lower than 90 mmHg or more precisely mean arterial pressure lower than 65 mmHg as suggested by the latest international consensus definitions for sepsis and septic shock [3]. It is associated with high mortality and adverse hospital outcomes in non-traumatic patients in the emergency department [4, 5].

In order to save our patients in shock, early diagnosis, and timely targeted therapy is vital. To do so in a timely manner is a challenge as clinical presentation of different types of shock may be similar. Point-of-care ultrasound (PoCUS) performed by clinicians providing direct care to the patients is considered an invaluable clinical tool to facilitate diagnosis-making, to rule out potentially fatal conditions, and to provide guidance to life-saving procedures [6]. Among the different applications of PoCUS, focused cardiac ultrasound (FoCUS) is gaining popularity in emergency care settings. It is considered as one of the core emergency ultrasound applications by the American College of Emergency Physicians and the International Federation for Emergency Medicine [7, 8]. Recently, FoCUS has been integrated into scanning protocols together with focused scans in other regions, e.g., lung, abdomen, and lower limb deep vein system to manage

Correspondence: dr.mokkl@gmail.com
Accident and Emergency Department, Ruttonjee Hospital, 266 Queen's Road East, Wanchai, Hong Kong SAR

patients in clinically undifferentiated hypotensive state [9–11]. In the following sessions, the SIMPLE approach, the role of FoCUS in the management of shock, and the current evidence for this application will be discussed.

Essentials of FoCUS and SIMPLE approach

The name "focused cardiac ultrasound" (FoCUS) is interchangeable with "focused echocardiography," "emergency echocardiography," "bedside limited echocardiography," "point-of-care cardiac ultrasound," and "goal-directed echocardiography" [12]. Lately, the term "focused cardiac ultrasound" has been recognized as a more appropriate term to take into account the nature of point-of-care application of ultrasound assessment of cardiac anatomy and physiology, distinct from the formal echocardiographic study done by cardiologists, according to the first international evidence-based recommendations issued by World Interactive Network Focused on Critical UltraSound (WINFOCUS) [13]. FoCUS was first introduced into emergency communities in the 1990s [14, 15]. With the wider availability and miniaturization of ultrasound machines, FoCUS has quickly become standard practice in acute care settings across the globe. In contrast to the conventional comprehensive echocardiography performed in the cardiac laboratory by cardiologists, FoCUS is performed by emergency physicians or intensivists at the bedside. It is essentially a limited evaluation of cardiac function, pericardial space, and intravascular volume in order to answer clinical questions vital to patient management. Contrary to what some may believe, the requirement for the FoCUS is not high. A portable or even pocket-sized handheld ultrasound machine can provide adequate image quality for assessment of left ventricular function, detection of pericardial effusion, and measurement of abdominal aorta size [16–18]. Pocket-sized machines are advantageous in unfavorable environments where full-sized machines will be impractical, e.g., pre-hospital assessment in an ambulance or helicopter [19].

FoCUS makes use of the same five orthodox views as in transthoracic echocardiographic study (TTE), (Fig. 1) to assess cardiac function, namely the left parasternal long and short axis views, apical four-chamber view, apical two-chamber view, and subxyphoid four-chamber view. Besides, subcostal visualization of the inferior vena cava (IVC) is frequently integrated into FoCUS to assess volume status and fluid responsiveness in hypotensive patients (Fig. 2) [9, 10]. 2D imaging and M-mode are employed for assessment in FoCUS. Doppler study is reserved for more sophisticated measurements in the

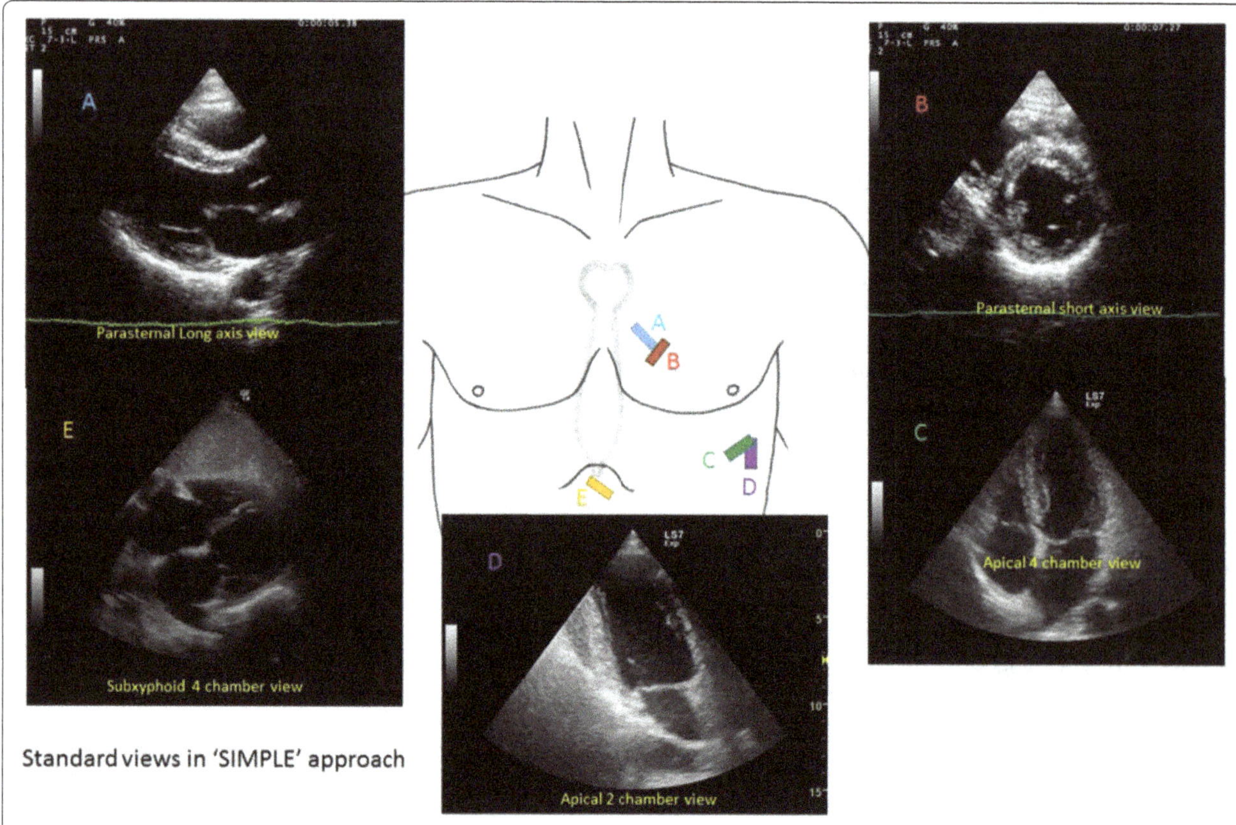

Fig. 1 Five standard views used in focus echocardiography. They include parasternal long axis (**a**), parasternal short axis (**b**), apical four-chamber (**c**), apical two-chamber (**d**), and subxyphoid four-chamber views (**e**)

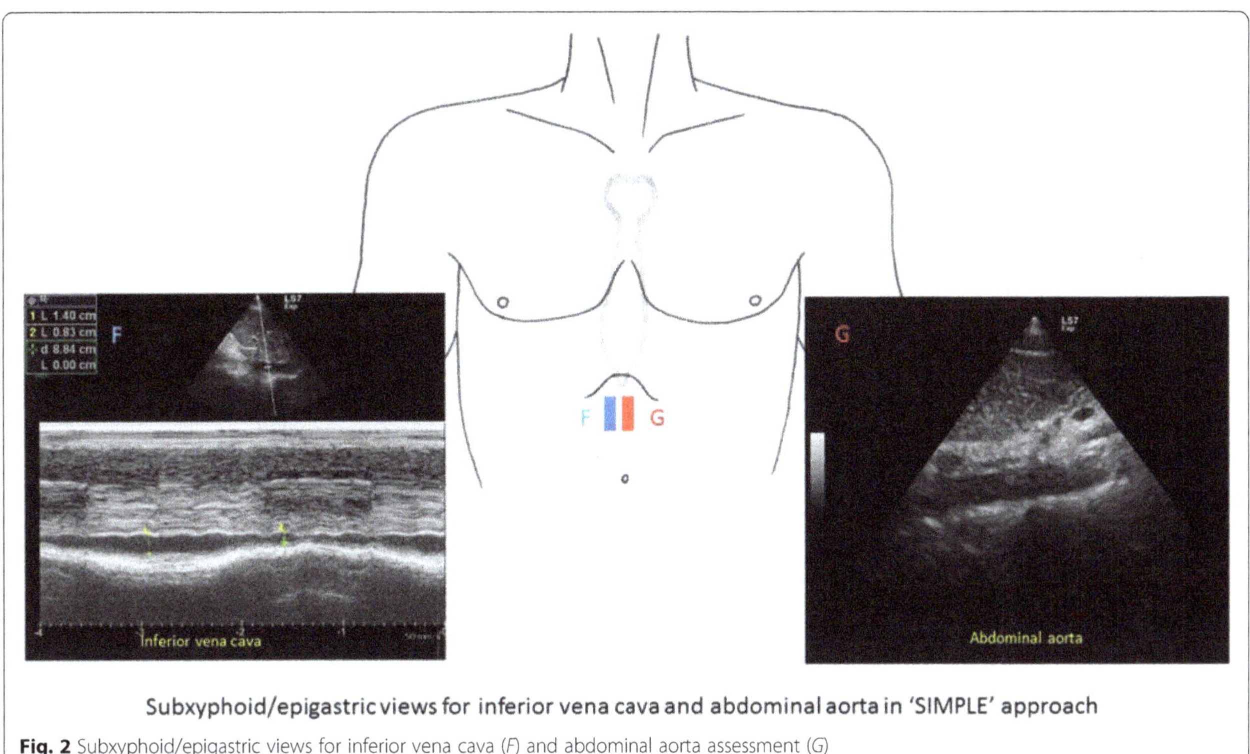

Fig. 2 Subxyphoid/epigastric views for inferior vena cava (*F*) and abdominal aorta assessment (*G*)

cardiac laboratory, such as in assessing valvular dysfunction, calculating stroke volume, and mitral inflow velocity. These measurements would take longer time to achieve and may technically difficult during the initial phase of resuscitation when adequate visualization of the heart cannot be easily obtained. According to the international evidence-based recommendations for FoCUS, Doppler assessment of valvular dysfunction is considered beyond the scope of FoCUS and reserved for evaluation by standard comprehensive echocardiography [13]. Thus, this review will mainly focus on the application of 2D imaging and M-mode study to rapidly assess patients in shock.

In the assessment of hypotensive patients, several key sonographic findings should be evaluated. They include the chamber sizes, in particular the left ventricle (LV) and the right ventricle (RV), the interventricular septum (IVS), the IVC, the presence of intramural mass (commonly blood clots and myxoma), myocardial thickness and motion during systole, the presence of pericardial effusion or pleural effusion, LV systolic function and the abdominal aorta in the epigastrium. All of these can be summarized into a "SIMPLE" approach (Table 1). It will give emergency physicians and intensivists a useful checklist in the evaluation of hypotensive patients.

In addition to the five orthodox TTE views, the subcostal region or epigastrium is included in this SIMPLE scanning protocol to assess the size of IVC and abdominal aorta which may be involved in aortic dissection and aneurysmal rupture (Fig. 2). In this approach, a single ultrasound probe is used to look for the causes for hypotension and guide treatment by means of a focused point-of-care ultrasound study. Concerning the sequence of examination, it would be a good habit to start at the parasternal views then move to the apical view and, finally, the subxyphoid/epigastric regions to assess the IVC and the abdominal aorta. However, in some patients with emphysematous lungs, hyperinflation of the chest and morbid obesity, and on mechanical ventilation, only one to two views can be obtained for evaluation. Cardiac function assessment, although limited, may still be possible in these situations through the remaining one to two views. If FoCUS reveals features of hypovolemia (as will be discussed later), a focused assessment with sonography for

Table 1 SIMPLE approach for evaluation of key elements during focused cardiac ultrasound sound (FoCUS) in shock patients

SIMPLE approach in focused cardiac ultrasound	
S	*C*hamber size and shape, particularly LV and RV size
I	*IV*C size and collapsibility *IV*S movement *In*timal flaps inside the aorta, suggestive of aortic dissection
M	*M*ass in the heart chambers (commonly intramural clots and atrial myxoma) *M*yocardium (motion and thickness)
P	*P*ericardial effusion *P*leural effusion
L	*L*eft ventricular systolic function
E	Abdominal aorta in the *e*pigastrium

trauma (FAST) protocol (i.e., SIMPLE + FAST approach) is warranted to look for intra-abdominal bleeding and hemothorax. Although limited when compared to comprehensive echocardiography carried out in the cardiac laboratory, this approach provides valuable information concerning the pathology, heart function, and physiology to differentiate between different types of shock and guide subsequent management.

Chamber sizes

The size of the heart chambers reflects the preload status (i.e., the intravascular volume) and heart function based on the volume-pressure relationship of a compliant heart chamber, in the absence of pre-existing or concurrent diseases such as cardiomyopathy or massive myocardial infarction. LV end-diastole diameter (LVEDD) and LV end-diastole area (LVEDA) (Fig. 3) can be used to assess the circulatory volume status [20]. A LVEDA of less than 10 cm^2 or a LVEDA index (LVEDA/body surface area) of less than 5.5 cm^2/m^2 indicates significant hypovolemia [21]. Obliteration of the LV cavity would be seen in severe hypovolemia [22]. In contrast, fluid overload can cause dilatation of the left ventricle. An LVEDA of more than 20 cm^2 suggests volume overload [21]. However, in the case of severe RV dysfunction, LV can also be small due to underloading. Concentric LV hypertrophy and constrictive pericarditis may also lead to small LVEDA so caution should be taken for interpretation in these conditions.

The size of the RV can give clues to the right heart function. Normally, it should be smaller than the LV and the apex should be formed by LV, not RV (Fig. 1). It is easily visualized in the apical four-chamber view as a triangular-shaped structure. The normal basal diameter of RV should be less than 4 cm [23]. If it is enlarged acutely in the appropriate clinical setting, the diagnosis of acute right heart failure due to massive pulmonary embolism should be suspected. The end-diastole area ratio of RV/LV should be less than 0.6 in the normal heart. A ratio higher than 0.66 would suggest cor pulmonale [24]. When this happens together with a normal RV wall thickness (<5 mm in parasternal long views), then it is very likely that there is acute right heart failure resulting from massive pulmonary embolism.

IVS movement

Normally, LV appears as a circular or donut-shaped structure (Fig. 1), and the IVS moves towards the center of LV during systole from the parasternal short axis view. When there is acute pulmonary embolism, high right ventricular pressure will cause more forceful and prolonged contracture of RV [24]. The IVS would then be pushed towards the left side, leading to flattening of the IVS or a D-shaped appearance of the LV on parasternal short axis view during end-systole or early-diastole (Fig. 4). In contrast, during systole, the LV contracts and the pressure in LV will become high again, pushing the IVS to the right side. This refers to "paradoxical movement" of the IVS.

IVC size and collapsibility

Traditionally, the central venous pressure (CVP) has been used for fluid status assessment and monitoring. Nonetheless, it is not only invasive but also proven to correlate poorly with the blood volume status in a systematic review [25]. Recent studies suggest the use of echocardiography to assess fluid status and fluid responsiveness by measuring IVC size and its collapsibility [26–30]. The IVC can be seen at the subxyphoid area, slightly off midline to the right of the abdominal aorta on transverse view. IVC size should be measured in

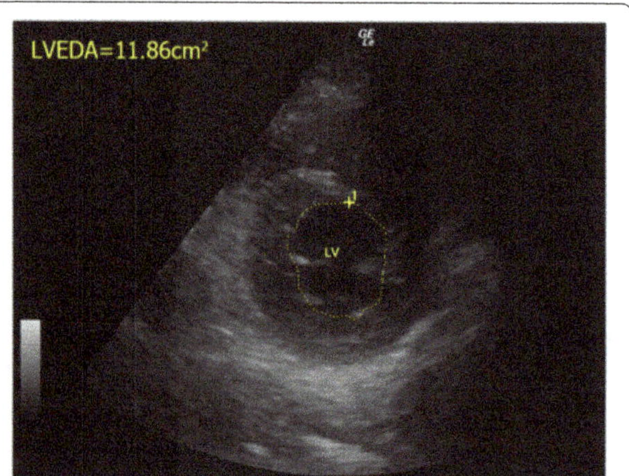

Fig. 3 The normal LVEDA measurement. The LVEDA is measured at the level of mid-papillary level of left parasternal short axis view in a normal human being. (*LVEDA* left ventricular end diastolic area, *LV* left ventricle)

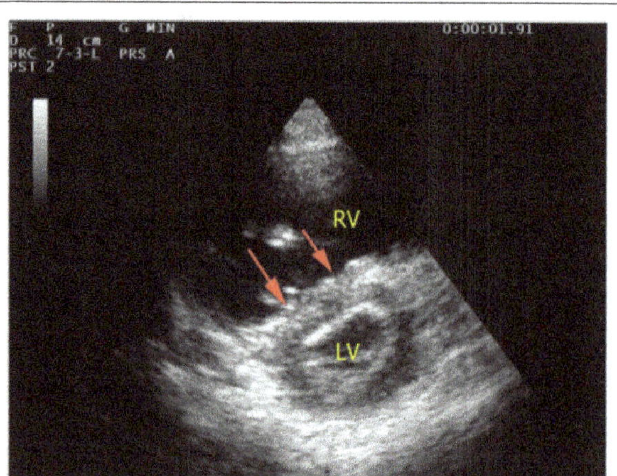

Fig. 4 Acute cor pulmonale due to massive pulmonary embolism. A parasternal short axis view shows a dilated RV and D-shaped LV on parasternal view in a patient with massive pulmonary embolism. The flattened IVS is highlighted by *red arrows*. (*RV* right ventricle; *LV* left ventricle)

longitudinal view around 2 cm caudal to the point where the hepatic vein joins the IVC to the right atrium (RA) [31]. One should bear in mind that incorrect measurement will occur if the longitudinal view of IVC is off axis. M-mode tracing of the size of the IVC throughout the respiratory cycle can be obtained at this point (Fig. 5). In patients with spontaneous breathing effort, the IVC collapses on inspiration but distends on expiration due to change in intrathoracic pressure. The reverse occurs in patients on mechanical ventilation.

IVC size can be used as a surrogate measurement of preload and volume status and therefore right atrial pressure (RAP). IVC diameter can be used to estimate RA pressure. The American Society of Echocardiography suggested the cutoff value of 2.1 cm [32]. IVC diameter <2.1 cm that collapses >50 % with inspiration would correlate with RA pressure of 3 mmHg (range, 0–5 mm Hg) while an IVC diameter >2.1 cm that collapses <50 % with inspiration suggests high RAP of 15 mm Hg (range, 10–20 mmHg). In patients with hypovolemic shock, the IVC diameter will be expected to be <2.1 cm and collapse >50 % with inspiration. In a recent meta-analysis of data from five studies on the sonographic measurement of the IVC in assessing the fluid status in the emergency department (ED), it was evidenced that the maximum IVC diameter is lower (6.3 mm 95 % CI 6–6.5 mm) in patients with hypovolemia than euvolemia [28]. Resuscitation of hypotensive patients usually involves fluid challenge. IVC diameter may give us some clues. The IVC distensibility index where maximum IVC diameter minus minimal IVC diameter divided by minimal IVC diameter times 100 % was found to be useful in predicting fluid responsiveness using the cutoff of 18 % in mechanically ventilated patients [29]. However, for patients with spontaneous breathing, the value of IVC size was less distinguished in predicting fluid responsiveness. With the cutoff of 40 %, the IVC collapsibility index that is maximum IVC diameter minus minimum IVC diameter divided by maximum IVC diameter times 100 % would only give a sensitivity of 70 %, specificity of 80 %, positive predictive value of 72 %, and negative predictive value of 83 % [30]. In trauma patients with hemorrhage, IVC measurement in addition to FAST is also helpful for managing trauma patients with hypovolemia to guide fluid therapy and shorten the time to operation theater [33, 34].

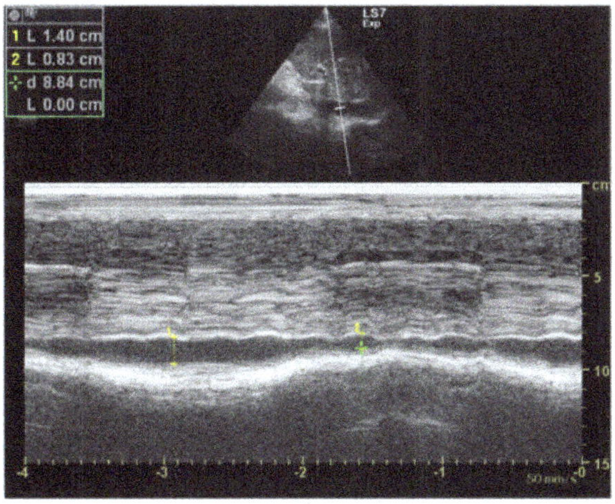

Fig. 5 Normal M-mode tracing of the inferior vena cava throughout the respiratory cycle. Variation of the inferior vena cava diameter throughout the respiratory cycle is shown

Intimal flap in aortic dissection

Aortic dissection is a potentially fatal but challenging vascular emergency. The cardinal feature of this disorder is a tear of the intimal layer of the aorta causing blood to dissect between layers of the aortic wall and propagate along the vessel. Hypotension was found to present in 16.4 % of patients with aortic dissection [35]. However, clinical features and chest X-ray findings are seldom confirmatory. With the availability of FoCUS, we can rule in aortic dissection and detect the associated complications, e.g., pericardial effusion, cardiac tamponade, pleural effusion, myocardial ischemia, and aortic regurgitation. The proximal part of the ascending aorta can be assessed by FoCUS from the parasternal long axis view. The abdominal aorta (as discussed later) should be assessed in suspected cases of aortic dissection. The pathognomonic sonographic feature of aortic dissection is the presence of intimal flap which appears as an echogenic thin linear structure separating the true and false lumens inside the aorta (Fig. 6). Dilatation of the aortic root (>4 cm), aortic regurgitation, and presence of pericardial effusion are auxiliary findings. The sensitivity and specificity of TTE for type A aortic dissection are 78–90 and 87–96 %, respectively [36, 37]. Positive findings can

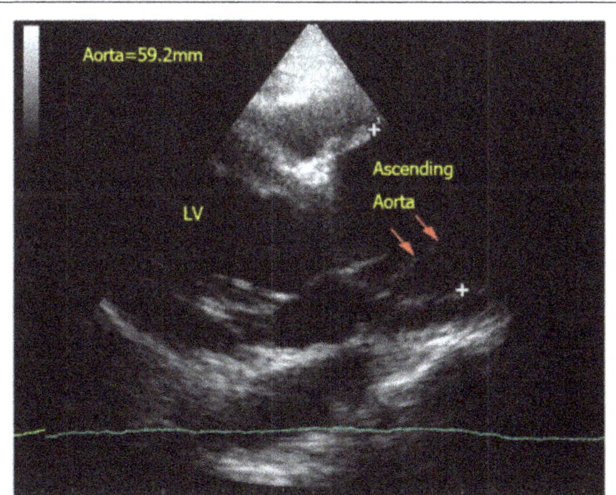

Fig. 6 Aortic dissection. Intimal flap (*red arrow*) is seen in the dilated proximal ascending aorta (5.9 cm) in a confirmed case of type A aortic dissection. (*LV* left ventricle)

speed up management and confirm life-threatening complications. Since only the proximal part of the ascending aorta can be seen in TTE, aortic dissection cannot be ruled out completely and other modality of imaging should be considered in patients with high clinical suspicion.

Mass in cardiac chambers: thrombus/myxoma

Intra-cardiac masses are not commonly seen on sonographic examination. But when present, in the appropriate clinical setting, they help establish the diagnosis of obstructive shock. The presence of intramural thrombus in right-sided cardiac chambers can confirm the clinical suspicion of pulmonary embolism and guide subsequent treatment [38]. Intracardiac thrombi appear as echogenic masses (Fig. 7) in the right atrium, right ventricle, pulmonary arteries, and IVC. The thrombi may be attached to the atrial or ventricular wall or be freely mobile [39]. LV thrombi resulting from causes such as atrial fibrillation, dilated left atrium (LA), and myocardial infarction may cause obstruction if large enough to occlude the left ventricular outflow tract (LVOT) and mitral valve. Another intracardiac mass that can cause obstructive shock is the atrial myxoma. It is the commonest primary cardiac tumor and most commonly involves the left atrium (75 %) [40]. It is often attached to the atrial wall and protrudes between the atrium and ventricle causing obstruction throughout the cardiac cycle, like a pinball machine. Occasionally, metastatic tumors may also cause obstructive shock in a similar manner as atrial myxoma [41].

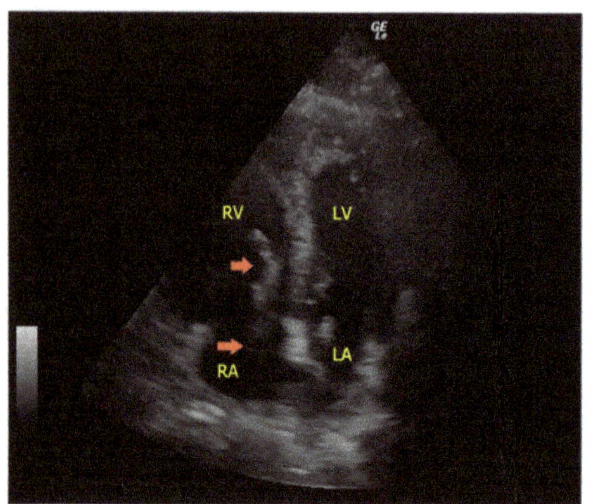

Fig. 7 Pulmonary embolism. In this apical four-chamber view, echogenic blood clots (*red arrows*) in the right atrium protruding into the right ventricle through the tricuspid valve during diastole are seen in a patient with confirmed massive pulmonary embolism(*RA* right atrium, *RV* right ventricle, *LA* left atrium, *LV* left ventricle)

Myocardium

During systole, different parts of the LV thicken in a coordinated fashion to act as a pump to eject blood out of the heart. According to the European society of Cardiology and American Society of Echocardiography, the LV can be divided into 17 segments and each individual segment can then be graded as normal/hyperkinetic, hypokinetic (reduced thickening), akinetic (absent thickening), or dyskinetic (abnormal thinning and stretching especially in aneurysm) according to their motions during systole [23, 42]. This can give clue to myocardial ischemia/infarct and the culprit coronary vessel involved when the areas of abnormal regional wall motion correspond to the territory supplied by the culprit vessel. With compatible sonographic findings and clinical picture, primary percutaneous intervention will be warranted when myocardial ischemia/infarct is believed to be the cause for cardiogenic shock.

Abnormal thickening of the myocardium (LV posterior wall and interventricular septum thickness >1 cm at end-diastole; RV free wall >5 mm) is suggestive of chronic heart conditions resulting from pressure overload (e.g., hypertensive cardiomyopathy, hypertrophic cardiomyopathy, pulmonary hypertension, and aortic stenosis). Together with gross dilatation of ventricle and atrium, detection of myocardial thickening is considered by the latest international consensus to be an essential part of FoCUS [13]. It can help avoiding misdiagnosing pre-existing heart conditions (e.g., chronic cor pulmonale) as an acute one (e.g., acute massive pulmonary embolism) and avoiding inappropriate treatments (e.g., intravenous fibrinolytic).

Pericardial effusion vs pleural effusion

The pericardial sac is a potential space for fluid to collect due to both systemic illness (e.g., connective tissue disease and uremia) and local pathology (e.g., myocardial rupture, aortic dissection, and metastasis). Although difficult to detect by physical exam or chest X-ray, pericardial effusion is easily picked up by FoCUS. Usually, pericardial effusion appears as an anechoic rim surrounding the heart, best seen in the parasternal long axis view or subxyphoid four-chamber view. However, if the effusion is caused by inflammatory condition or hemorrhage (i.e., hemopericardium), there may be echogenicity within the pericardial sac. The pericardium appears as a densely echogenic film-like reflection posterior to the anechoic pericardial effusion (Fig. 8a, b). Sometimes pleural effusion can also be detected by echocardiography, and novice sonographers may find it confusing. Pericardial effusion can be differentiated from pleural effusion as pericardial effusion is located anterior to the descending aorta and does not extend beyond the atrioventricular groove (Fig. 9). Sometimes, pericardial or epicardial fat can also be mistaken as pericardial effusion. Epicardial fat usually appears as an

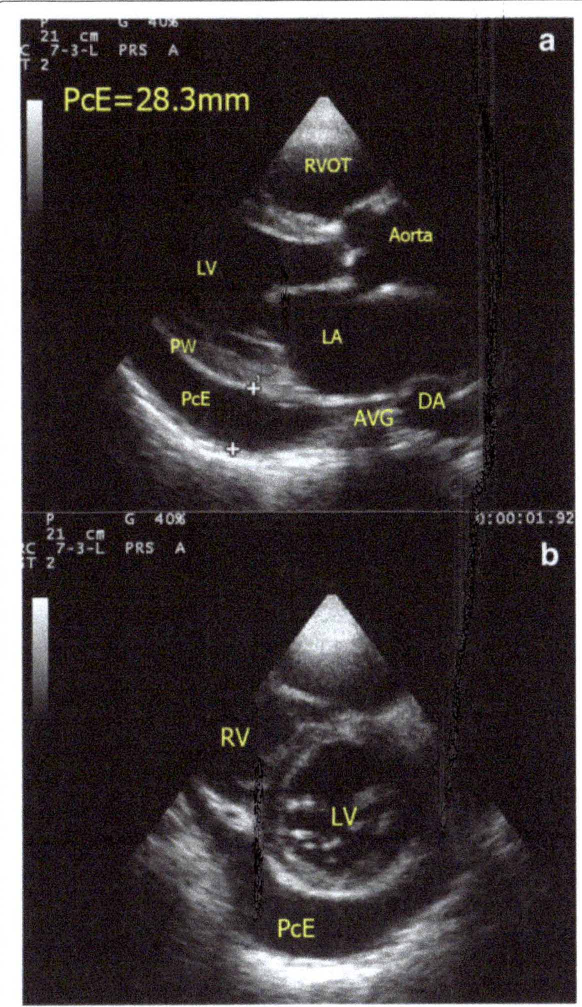

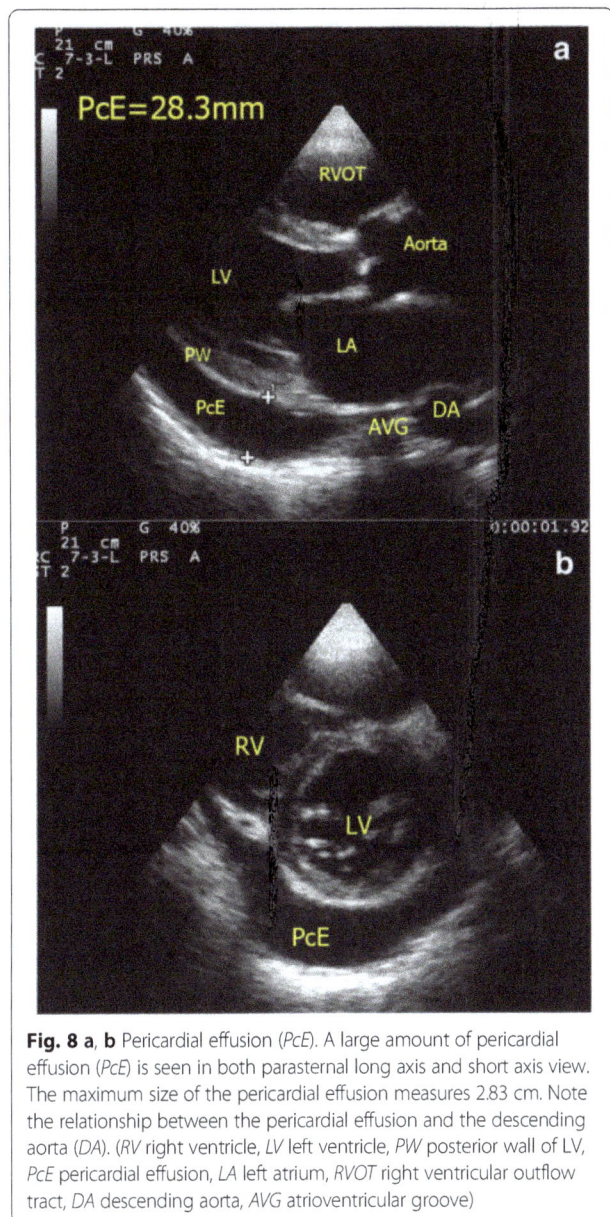

Fig. 8 a, **b** Pericardial effusion (*PcE*). A large amount of pericardial effusion (*PcE*) is seen in both parasternal long axis and short axis view. The maximum size of the pericardial effusion measures 2.83 cm. Note the relationship between the pericardial effusion and the descending aorta (*DA*). (*RV* right ventricle, *LV* left ventricle, *PW* posterior wall of LV, *PcE* pericardial effusion, *LA* left atrium, *RVOT* right ventricular outflow tract, *DA* descending aorta, *AVG* atrioventricular groove)

echogenic structure lying within the pericardial sac just anterior to the heart on the parasternal long axis view [43]. The size of pericardial effusion should be quantified according to its maximum thickness measured during diastole (small <1 cm not circumferential, moderate <1 cm circumferential around the heart, large 1–2 cm circumferential, very large >2 cm with/without evidence of cardiac tamponade) [44]. Acute accumulation of pericardial effusion can lead to impaired right heart filling and, in turn, cardiac tamponade that will be discussed in the next session.

LV systolic function

Echocardiography or cardiac ultrasound can give an accurate assessment of global function of the left ventricle

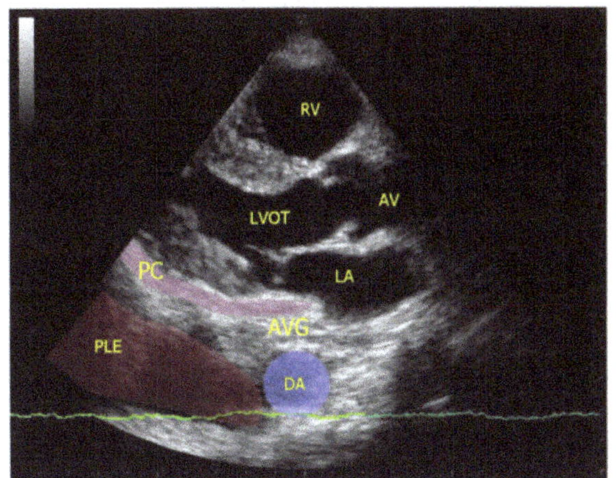

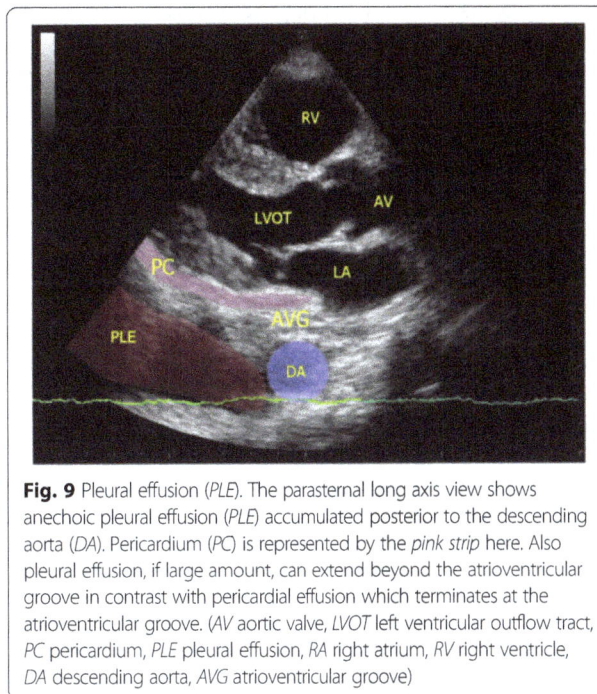

Fig. 9 Pleural effusion (*PLE*). The parasternal long axis view shows anechoic pleural effusion (*PLE*) accumulated posterior to the descending aorta (*DA*). Pericardium (*PC*) is represented by the *pink strip* here. Also pleural effusion, if large amount, can extend beyond the atrioventricular groove in contrast with pericardial effusion which terminates at the atrioventricular groove. (*AV* aortic valve, *LVOT* left ventricular outflow tract, *PC* pericardium, *PLE* pleural effusion, *RA* right atrium, *RV* right ventricle, *DA* descending aorta, *AVG* atrioventricular groove)

and guide subsequent treatment (e.g., inotropic support versus fluid therapy). There are several options to assess the LV systolic function sonographically, including fractional shortening (FS) and LV ejection fraction (LVEF).

In M-mode, FS of the left ventricle can be assessed by placing a cursor just near the tip of the mitral valve leaflets in parasternal long axis view. The M-mode tracing will show the change in LV diameter during the cardiac cycle and FS can be calculated by the following formula:

$$\mathrm{FS} = (\mathrm{LVEDD{-}LVESD})/\mathrm{LVEDD} \times 100\%$$

The normal value should be 25–45 % for adults [42]. If the value falls below <15 %, severe LV systolic dysfunction is present. This measurement is very simple and easy. However, the measurement must be done perpendicular to the axis of the left ventricle, and the ventricle should not be foreshortened. There is also an assumption of no severe dysfunction in other parts of the left ventricle.

In B-mode, the LVEF can be measured by the modified Simpson biplane method. Most modern ultrasound machines have the calculation package pre-installed. The endocardial margins of the LV are traced in systole and diastole from two different views (i.e., two individual planes perpendicular to each other) to calculate the volume change between systole and diastole. The normal LVEF should be >55 %, and <30 % indicates severe left ventricular systolic dysfunction [42]. This is not a simple method compared with the FS, and the endocardial margins have to be traced correctly or under/overestimation of the LVEF may result. In emergency settings, suboptimal images of the LV and inadequate cardiac views would render this method less practical.

Assessment of LVEF by eyeballing appears the most feasible yet reliable method for estimating the LV systolic function. It can be done through assessing the movement and thickening of the LV myocardium, the change in size and shape of the LV chamber as well as the mitral valve anterior leaflet excursion in the cardiac cycle. It was found that the accuracy of eyeballing estimation correlated well with other quantitative methods including Simpson biplane ejection fraction, fractional shortening, wall motion score index, and aortic valve (AV) plane displacement [45, 46]. This advantage is not confined only to the experienced cardiologists. With focused training, the estimation of LV ejection fraction by emergency physicians had a strong agreement with cardiologists [47–49]. Even inexperienced emergency medicine trainees could achieve good agreement on the visual estimation of LV ejection fraction with cardiologists after web-based learning and proctored practical training ($K = 0.79$, 95 % CI 0.773 to 0.842) [49]. Thus, visual estimation of the LV ejection fraction should form an important part of left heart systolic function assessment in FoCUS, in particular when quantitative measurements are not possible due to poor echogenicity of the heart and limited cardiac views in some patients.

Abdominal aortic at the epigastrium

The proximal part of abdominal aorta can be easily visualized by ultrasound. It should be integrated into the scanning protocol of FoCUS in addition to the IVC measurement. It lies along the mid-line of the abdomen, on the left side of the IVC, and anterior to the bony vertebra. The normal size of the abdominal aorta should be less than 3 cm. Abdominal aortic aneurysm (AAA) is diagnosed when the diameter is >3 cm. AAA can rupture and cause profound hypotension due to hypovolemia. Clinical presentation may be subtle, and reliance on physical findings alone may miss this potentially fatal condition as the sensitivity of abdominal palpation is only 68 % [42, 50]. PoCUS has outstanding sensitivity and specificity for AAA approaching 100 % and has been proved to shorten the time to emergency operation [51, 52]. Other arterial catastrophes including rupture of splenic artery aneurysm can also be detected in a similar way to AAA [53]. Echogenic intimal flap seen inside the aortic lumen can confirm the diagnosis of aortic dissection (Fig. 10a, b). This may improve the sensitivity of FoCUS in diagnosing aortic dissection, especially in cases involving the descending aorta.

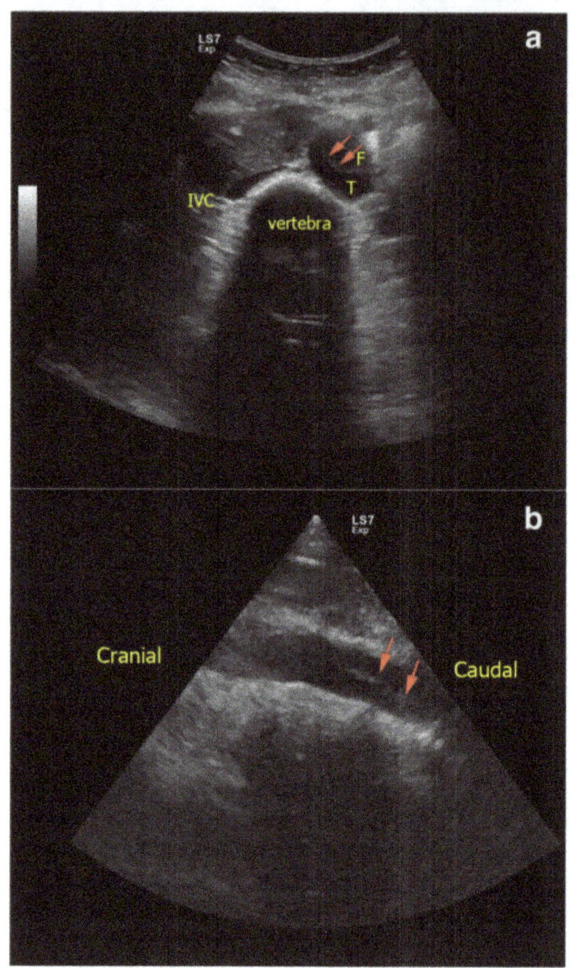

Fig. 10 a, b Aortic dissection of abdominal aorta. In this patient with extensive Stanford type A aortic dissection, intimal flap (*red arrows*) is seen inside the lumen of abdominal aorta as an echogenic film separating the false lumen (*F*) and true lumen (*T*). (*F* false lumen, *T* true lumen, *IVC* inferior vena cava)

Evaluation of undifferentiated shock by SIMPLE approach

Hypovolemic shock

In patients with hypovolemia, the left ventricle becomes small with a smaller LVEDA (<10 cm^2). The lumen of the LV may even be obliterated and the ventricular walls are seen to be “kissing” (Fig. 11a, b) [22]. The IVC collapses, and the size becomes less than 2 cm with >50 % collapsibility (Fig. 12). Hyperdynamic LV with normal or higher than normal ejection fraction and normal myocardial thickening is found. Depending on the source of bleeding, hemothorax may be an incidental finding in FoCUS but it should not be misinterpreted as pericardial effusion. The epigastric area should be screened for the presence of an aortic aneurysm. If an aortic aneurysm is found in a hypotensive patient, aneurysmal rupture should be suspected and urgent surgical consultation is warranted. FAST scan should also be done when no obvious sources of bleeding can be identified in the context of hypovolemic shock. Fluid responsiveness can be predicted by using the IVC collapsibility index in ventilated patients to guide subsequent fluid therapy.

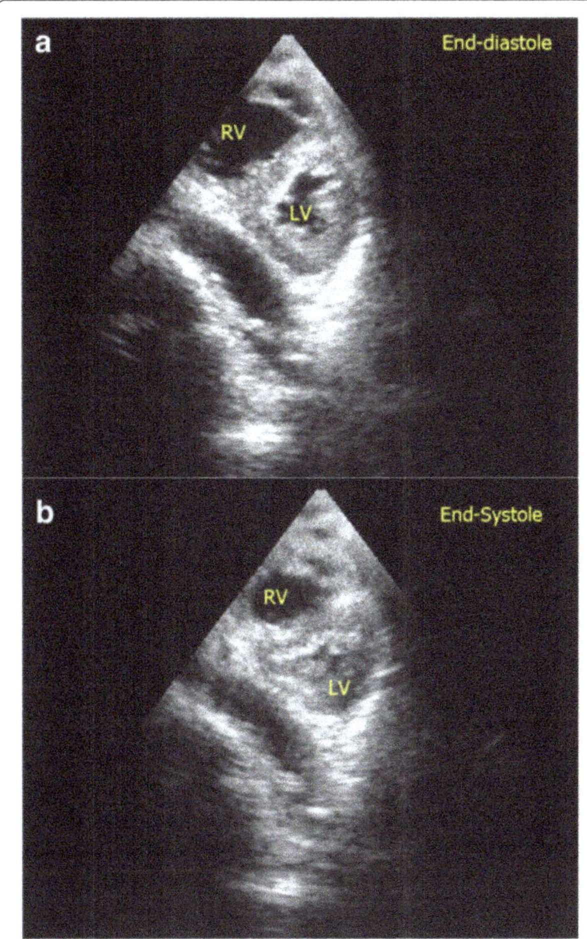

Fig. 11 a, b Severe hypovolemic shock. Kissing walls of left ventricle on parasternal short axis view is shown. The left ventricle is obliterated during systole. This patient suffered from severe hypovolemia due to gastrointestinal bleeding. (*RV* right ventricle, *LV* left ventricle)

Cardiogenic shock

Echocardiography or cardiac ultrasound definitely has a role in managing cardiogenic shock due to LV dysfunction and valvular dysfunction. LV would be dilated, and fractional shortening would be impaired (Fig. 13). Dilated IVC >2.1 cm with the absence of respiratory variability is expected. Regional wall motion abnormality may be seen if the underlying cause for cardiogenic shock is myocardial ischemia. The whole myocardium would be hypokinetic in the case of global systolic dysfunction (e.g., due to myocarditis). As mentioned before, LV systolic function can be assessed by quantitative measurements including FS and LVEF by using the modified Simpson biplane method. However, all these measurements require good visualization of the LV and clear delineation of the endocardium. Errors commonly occur when the optimal image of the LV cannot be obtained in emergency settings. Thus, visual estimation, so called eyeballing, would be more practical in these situations. By obtaining valuable information on pump function, inotropic support and judicious fluid administration is indicated. Emergency transferal of the patients to cardiac catheterization facility for revascularization can also be facilitated in myocardial infarction.

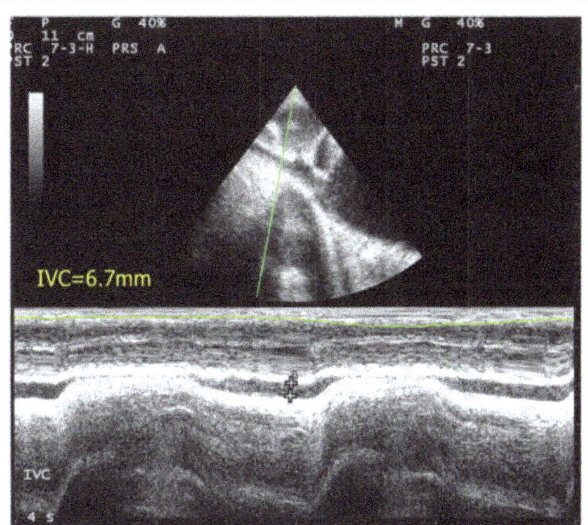

Fig. 12 Collapsed IVC. IVC thickness is markedly reduced (thickness = 6.7 mm) with complete collapse on inspiration in a patient with hypovolemic shock

Obstructive shock

Cardiac tamponade

One of the major causes for obstructive shock is cardiac tamponade. The presence of pericardial effusion and hypotension raises the suspicion of cardiac tamponade. Large amounts of effusion would cause cardiac tamponade, but even small effusions, if accumulated rapidly, can cause

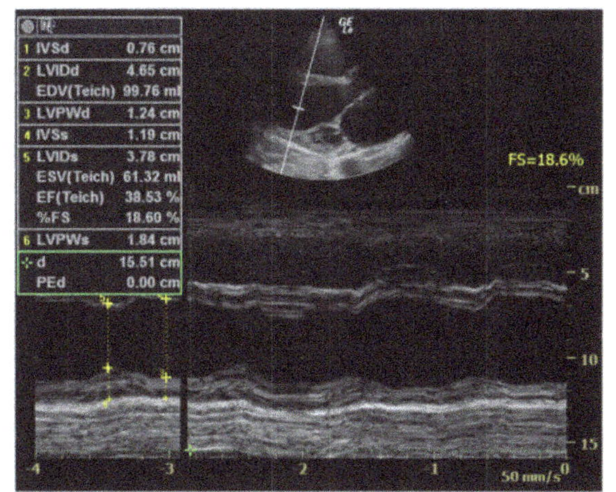

Fig. 13 Poor LV systolic function. This parasternal long axis view shows a dilated LV with poor fractional shortening (FS = 18.6 %) in a patient with dilated cardiomyopathy and hypotension (*FS* = fractional shortening)

cardiac tamponade due to the tough, non-distensible nature of the pericardial sac. Although cardiac tamponade is essentially a clinical diagnosis, FoCUS can help to confirm the presence of pericardial effusion, provide useful real-time hemodynamic information and tamponade physiology, and guide therapeutic pericardiocentesis. Sonographic features of cardiac tamponade include RA collapse, RV diastolic collapse, distended IVC, and respiratory variation of the mitral inflow velocity. The latter is essentially the sonographic version of pulsus paradoxicus. Pulsed wave Doppler is required to detect the variation so it is out of the scope of this SIMPLE approach (Table 2). RA collapse can be easily recognized when the RA inverts during ventricular end-diastole when the pressure inside the atrium becomes lowest (Fig. 14a). RV diastolic collapse is recognized as part of the RV free wall not expanding during early diastole (Fig. 14b). RA collapse is a more sensitive but non-specific sonographic sign of cardiac tamponade while diastolic RV collapse is considered to be more specific. Plethoric IVC without any variation during respiration is an additional sign to look for in cardiac tamponade. When the diagnosis of cardiac tamponade is established, FoCUS-guided pericardiocentesis can then be performed. Ultrasound-guided pericardiocentesis is now considered to be the standard of care because it carries higher successful rate and fewer complications than the blind approach [54, 55]. The apex was identified as the optimal location for pericardiocentesis in 1127 consecutive patients from the Mayo Clinic over 21 years [56].

Massive pulmonary embolism

Massive pulmonary embolism causes acute RV dysfunction. RV is usually dilated with basal diameter >4 cm and RV/LV ratio >0.6. The normal triangular-shaped RV is distorted, and the apex is no longer dominated by the LV on the apical four-chamber view. The IVS shows paradoxical movement, and D-shaped LV chamber would be appreciated in the parasternal short axis view (Fig. 4). The IVC is distended with minimal or absent respiratory variation (Fig. 15). Free flowing echogenic thrombus may occasionally be seen in the right heart and IVC (Fig. 7). McConnell's sign which is defined as mid-RV free wall akinesia with sparing of the apex may occasionally be seen [57]. It is thought to be a specific but not very sensitive sign for acute pulmonary embolism (sensitivity 77 %; specificity 96 %). This specific sign is believed to be caused by tethering of the RV to the hyperdynamic LV apex [57, 58]. LV becomes hyperdynamic as the left heart is trying hard to compensate for the hypotension. The American College of Chest Physicians suggests that fibrinolysis should be warranted in patients with hypotension due to massive pulmonary embolism [59]. When severe right heart dysfunction is confirmed by FoCUS with hypoxia, hypotension, and tachycardia, the diagnosis of massive pulmonary embolism should rank top on the list of differentials. Intravenous fibrinolytic therapy should be prudently considered if there is no contraindication to reverse acute right heart dysfunction due to pulmonary embolism and surgical embolectomy may be needed in patients with contraindication to systemic fibrinolysis.

Aortic dissection

Aortic dissection can be picked up by FoCUS when the intimal flap is in the aorta (Fig. 6). The complications of aortic dissection can also be detected. Retrograde dissection into the pericardial sac can cause pericardial effusion and even cardiac tamponade. Echogenic pericardial effusion and even clots are occasionally seen (Fig. 16). The IVC becomes plethoric when cardiac tamponade is present. Regional wall motion abnormality may also be detected in the case of acute myocardial ischemia secondary to ostial occlusion by the intimal flap, usually involving the right coronary artery [60]. It is often rewarding to scan the abdominal aorta in patients suspicious of distal aortic dissection as sometimes the intimal flap which cannot be seen in the ascending aorta may be seen here and the diagnosis is obvious (Fig. 10a, b).

Septic shock

Septic shock represents a distinctive spectrum of hemodynamic instability. In the early stage, the afterload is reduced and left ventricular dysfunction, although present, is masked by the severely reduced afterload due to sepsis [61, 62]. Thus, FoCUS will find a normal LVEDA but small left ventricular end-systolic area (LVESA) and a hyperdynamic LV. There is a substantial decrease in the size of the LV from diastole to systole in contrast to hypovolemia where the LV size is small throughout the cardiac cycle. The IVC would collapse in this stage with >50 % inspiratory collapse. After the initial phase, myocardial depression occurs in around 60 % septic patients [63]. Once the afterload is restored by vasopressors and fluid therapy, the LV myocardial dysfunction is unmasked. LV would be normal or dilated with myocardial hypocontractility [61–63]. At this stage, the IVC is distended and the respiratory collapsibility is lost similar to the profile in cardiogenic shock. Recognizing these sonographic findings can help clinicians tailoring appropriate treatments to different stages of septic shock.

SIMPLE approach versus other protocols

Since 2001, different protocols for shock assessment have been described in the literature. Table 3 summarizes and compares the current major protocols for undifferentiated shock and cardiac arrest. There is a growing trend towards integrating different aspects of point-of-care ultrasound including focused cardiac ultrasound, IVC and aorta assessment, and lung scan into different protocols [9, 70, 75–77].

Table 2 Summary of typical findings in different types/causes of shock by SIMPLE approach

Type of shock		Hypovolemic	Cardiogenic	Septic	Distributive	Pulmonary embolism	Cardiac Tamponade	Aortic Dissection
S	*Chamber size*	Small LV	Dilated LV	Early: small LVESA Late: normal/dilated	Near normal LVEDA but small LVESA	Dilated RV, small/normal LV	Diastolic collapse of RA and RV; normal LV	Usually normal
I	*IVC thickness*	Collapsed	Distended <50 % respiratory collapse	Early: collapsed Late: distended	Collapsed	Distended and loss of respiratory collapse	Distended and loss of respiratory collapse	Normal when no cardiac tamponade
	IVS movement	Normal	Reduced	Early: normal Late: reduced	Normal	Paradoxical IVS and D-shaped LV	Normal	Normal
	Intimal flap	Absent	Absent	Absent	Absent	Absent	Absent	Present
M	*Myocardial thickening/motion*	Hyperdynamic	Hypokinetic	Early: hyperdynamic Late: hypokinetic	Hyperdynamic or normal	McConell's sign, LV hyperdynamic	Diastolic collapse of RA and RV	Normal if coronary ostia not involved
	Masses in heart	Absent	Intramural thrombi if AF/AMI	Absent	Absent	Thrombi in RA/RV and IVC	Absent	Absent
P	*Pericardial effusion*	Absent	Small amount if inflammatory cause	Absent	Absent	Absent	Moderate to large but can be small if acutely collected	Present if retrograde dissection and echogenic
	Pleural effusion	Absent	Present	Present if pneumonia	Absent	Usually absent	Absent	Present if hemothorax
L	*LV systolic function*	Hyperdynamic	Poor	Early: normal or hyperdynamic Late: impaired	Normal or hyperdynamic	Normal or hyperdynamic	Normal	Normal
E	*Abdominal aorta in epigastrium*	Aneurysmal if due to AAA rupture	Normal	Normal	Normal	Normal	Normal	Intimal flap seen

AF atrial fibrillation, *AMI* acute myocardial infarct, *LV* left ventricle, *LVEDA* left ventricular end-diastolic area, *LVESA* left ventricular end-systolic area, *RA* right atrium, *RV* right ventricle

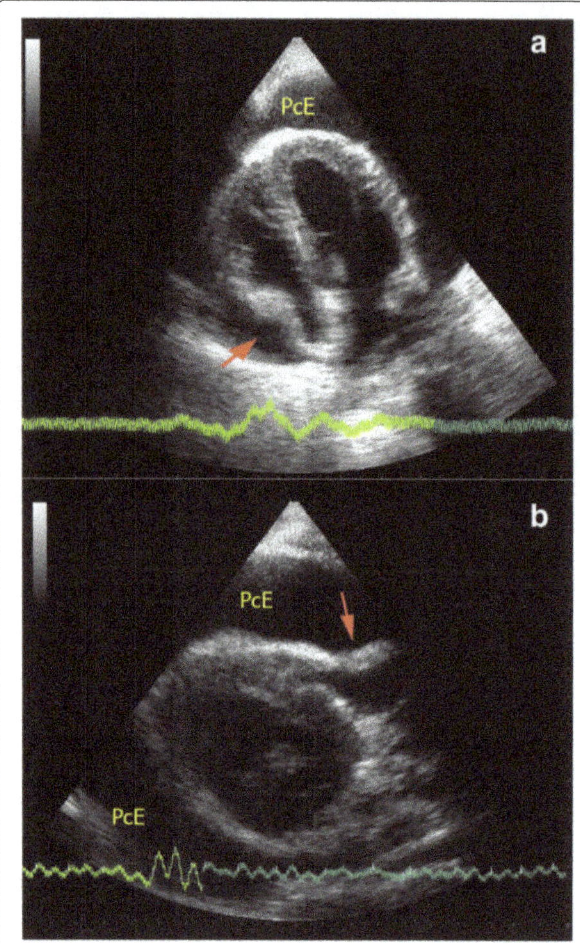

Fig. 14 a, b Cardiac tamponade. These two images show collapsed RA and RV (*red arrows*) on apical four-chamber view and parasternal long axis view in a patient with cardiac tamponade (*PcE* = pericardial effusion)

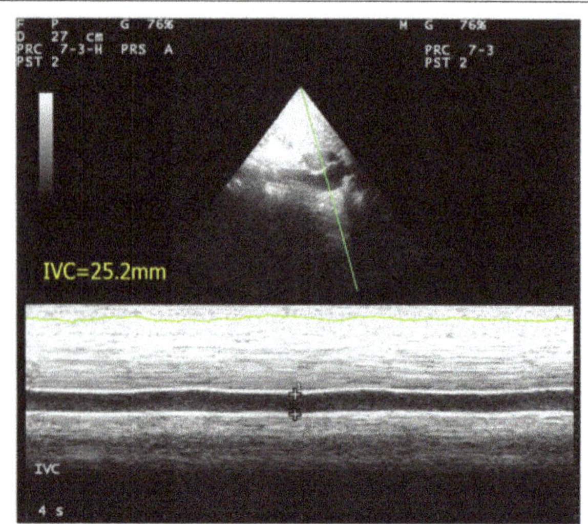

Fig. 15 Distended IVC. This is the M-mode tracing of IVC in a patient with massive PE. The IVC is plethoric of a diameter >2.1 cm with only minimal respiratory variation (*IVC* = inferior vena cava)

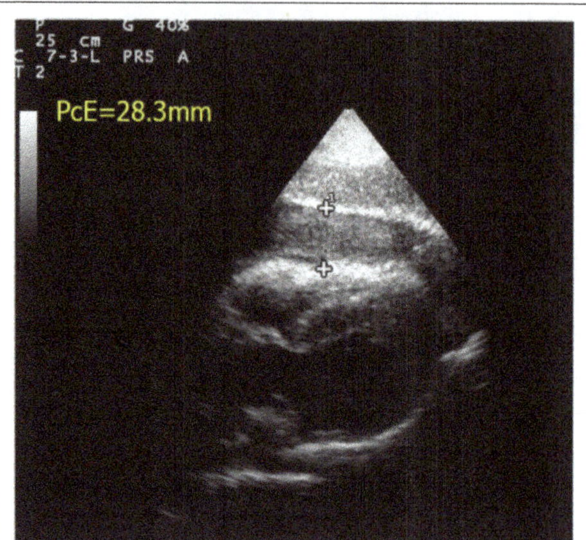

Fig. 16 Hemopericardium and cardiac tamponade. This subxyphoid four-chamber view shows echogenic clots and hemopericardium in a patient with cardiac tamponade due to aortic dissection (*PcE* pericardial effusion; thickness = 28.3 mm)

The goal is to find a systematic and practical way to classify the challenging but non-specific clinical syndrome of circulatory failure into four more specific and manageable types of shock.

In contrast to existing protocols like rapid ultrasound for shock and hypotension (RUSH) [9], abdominal and cardiac evaluation with sonography in shock (ACES) [10], undifferentiated hypotension patient (UHP) [11], Trinity [64], or focused assessed transthoracic echocardiography (FATE) [65], every single letter in the SIMPLE approach represents a specific assessment in cardiac ultrasound. This simple mnemonic provides clinicians with a simple and easy-to-remember, yet valuable checklist of sonographic findings to look for when managing patients in shock. Unlike the RUSH protocol, physiology is not emphasized in the SIMPLE approach but systematic interpretation of sonographic findings can help the clinicians narrow down the differential diagnosis of shock and guide initial therapy (e.g., small and kissing LV with flat IVC already warrants fluid resuscitation and hypovolemia is suspected, while dilated and hypokinetic LV would suggest cardiogenic shock and inotropic support is needed). It can also help avoiding complications associated with indiscriminate use of fluid therapy and inotropes.

To my knowledge, this is the first protocol to include two specific findings explicitly: intramural mass and intimate flap so as to improve the diagnostic power of two challenging and lethal conditions, namely massive pulmonary embolism and aortic dissection. Although abdominal assessment is not routinely included in the SIMPLE approach, combination with FAST to look for the source of intra-abdominal bleeding is indicated when

Table 3 Summary of current major protocols of point-of-care ultrasound for undifferentiated shock/cardiac arrest

Protocols	Year of publication	Cardiac views	IVC size	Abdominal aorta	Lung scan	Remarks
UHP [11]	2001	SXP+/−PLX, PSX	No	Yes	No	Simplified version of extended FAST
Trinity [64]	2002	PLX, PSX	No	Yes	Pleural effusion only	Similar to extended FAST
FATE [65]	2004	PLX, PSX, AP4, SXP	No	No	Pleural effusion only	Chronic pathologies included
BLEEP [66]	2004	SXP, PSX	Yes	No	No	Pediatric patients only
CAUSE [67]	2007	4 views	Yes	Yes	Yes	Cardiac arrest
FEER [68]	2007	SXP, PLX, PSX, AP4	No	No	No	Integrated into ACLS protocol for cardiac arrest
BEAT [69]	2008	PLX, PSX, AP4, SXP	Yes	No	No	Surgical patients; SV and CI included
ACES [10]	2008	SXP, PLX, AP4	Yes	Yes	Pleural effusion only	
RUSH-HIMAP [70]	2009	PLX, AP4	Yes	Yes	Yes	
RUSH-pump, pipe, tank [9]	2010	PLX, PSX, SXP, AP4	Yes	Yes	Yes	Physiological model of pump, pipe, tank
FEEL [71]	2010	SXP, PLX. AP4 (any one of them)	No	No	Pleural effusion only	Cardiac arrest and peri-arrest state
EGLS [72]	2011	PLX, PSX, AP4, SXP	Yes	No	Yes	Lung scan first approach
FREE [73]	2011	PLX, PSX, AP4, SXP	Yes	No	No	Trauma patients
FALLS [74]	2012	Not specifically mentioned	No	No	Yes	Mainly lung scan
FAST and RELIABLE [75]	2012	PLX, PSX, AP4, SXP	Yes	Yes	Yes	Ectopic pregnancy included
Volpicelli et al. [76]	2013	PLS, SXP, AP4	Yes	Yes	Yes	Similar to RUSH [9]
Shokoohi et al. [77]	2015	SXP, PLX, PSX, AP4	Yes	Yes	Yes	FAST included
SIMPLE	2016	PLX, PSX, AP4, AP2, SXP	Yes	Yes	No	Easy-to-remember checklist of sonographic findings; intracardiac mass and intimal flap included; can be combined with FAST

PSX parasternal short axis view, *PLX* parasternal long axis view, *SXP* subxyphoid view, *AP4* apical four-chamber view, *AP2* apical two-chamber view, *IVC* inferior vena cava, *ACLS* advanced cardiac life support, *ICU* intensive care unit, *FAST* focused assessment with sonography for trauma, *SV* stroke volume, *CI* cardiac index

FoCUS reveals features of hypovolemia. As most emergency physicians and intensivists have been using FAST scan routinely in trauma assessment, a combination of SIMPLE with FAST (SIMPLE + FAST) would easily be incorporated into their daily practices. SIMPLE + FAST suggests cardiac assessment first before abdominal assessment in order to detect obstructive and cardiogenic shock, in contrast to the FAST + RELIABLE protocol suggested by Liteplo et al. [75]. This allows early specific treatment such as pericardiocentesis and inotropes to correct the circulatory failure and prevent indiscriminative fluid challenge which is detrimental in cardiogenic shock.

Current evidence of FoCUS for evaluation of shock

Among the literature, there is growing evidence demonstrating that FoCUS could improve the diagnostic accuracy and change the clinical management. Although the results of this evidence may not necessarily prove that FoCUS can lead to better patient survival and shorten the hospital stay, it can logically be assumed that with more accurate diagnostic capability for various types of shock, implementation of FoCUS could lead to a better clinical outcome in patients with circulatory failure.

FoCUS is helpful in confirming the correct diagnoses and detecting the etiology of shock. In a randomized trial in 184 patients by Jones et al. in the emergency department, early goal-directed ultrasound at 0 min was found to correctly diagnose the etiology of shock in 80 % of patients compared 50 % of patients in the group only received standard care at the initial 15 min of presentation in the emergency department [78]. This trial can be concluded into two important points. Firstly, it was the first study to prove that early focused ultrasound can allow the emergency physicians to narrow the differential diagnoses of shock. Secondly, it proved that early focused ultrasound at the initial presentation is feasible and can be combined with standard care interventions, e.g., venous access establishment, electrocardiography, blood sample analysis, and chest radiography.

Subsequent trials on protocol-driven ultrasound for diagnosis of shock further confirmed the role of FoCUS to diagnose and differentiate different types of shock in the emergency department. Volpicelli et al. did a prospective study on 108 ED patients in undifferentiated shock by comparing the sonographic diagnosis with the final clinical diagnosis [76]. The ultrasound assessment in this study included FoCUS and IVC assessment, lung scan, abdominal scan for free fluid, and leg scan for deep vein thrombosis. They found a very good concordance between the ultrasound diagnosis and the final clinical diagnosis ($k = 0.710$). Ghane et al. also found similar finding in a study in 52 ED patients by using RUSH protocol ($k = 0.7$) [79]. It was also found that ultrasound achieved 100 % sensitivity for hypovolemic and obstructive shock, 91.7 % sensitivity for cardiogenic shock, and 94.6–100 % specificity for all types of shock. However, in distributive and mixed type of shock, the sensitivity was found to be lower only 70–75 %. The same group also found similar results in another study on 77 patients [80]. The common limitation of the above three studies is that ultrasound assessments were done by either radiologist or emergency physicians experienced in PoCUS, and so the results may not be generalizable to other inexperienced clinicians from other specialties.

Apart from correct diagnosis and differentiation of shock, the other major role of FocUS for shock is to tailor the treatment according to the underlying etiology and improve the clinical outcome of patients. In an observational study conducted on 220 patients in intensive care unit, use of FoCUS by hand-held ultrasound device was found to be associated with significantly lower fluid prescription (49 vs 66 mL/kg, $p = 0.01$) and more dobutamine use (22 vs 12 %, $p = 0.01$) than the historical control group which was managed in a standard fashion [81]. More importantly, this study found that FoCUS group had better 28-day survival (66 vs 56 %, $p = 0.04$) and a reduction in acute kidney injury (20 vs 39 %). These findings are supportive of using FoCUS to guide the resuscitation of hypotensive patients. The limitations of this study include no randomization, use of historical control, and a significant number of patients (14 %) with significant valvular pathologies. Another recent study performed in ED also confirmed the impact of FoCUS findings on management plan (in 24.6 % of patients), including the use of intravenous fluid, vasoactive agents, or blood products. This study also found an excellent concordance of protocol-driven ultrasound diagnostic protocol in undifferentiated hypotension with the final diagnosis ($k = 0.80$). Moreover, ultrasound was also found to influence the diagnostic imaging, consultation, and patient disposition in this study. Again, the limitations are the lack of randomization and use of single ultrasound operator.

Conclusions

Managing patients in profound shock poses a very great challenge to clinicians. Correct diagnosis and timely specific treatment to restore the otherwise jeopardized circulation are vital to the survival of hypotensive patients. Throughout the past 10 years, FoCUS has emerged as one of the important allies of emergency physicians and intensivists to provide crucial answers to challenging clinical conditions. In properly trained hands, FoCUS can provide real-time valuable information on the pathology and physiology of circulation to differentiate between different types of shocks. Through the suggested SIMPLE approach, different types of shocks can be characterized according to 2D ultrasound findings and simple measurements (Table 2). This approach is not only simple and practical but also provides an easy-to-remember checklist of ultrasound findings for clinicians to focus on when managing patients with undifferentiated shock. Integrating SIMPLE approach with FAST scan (i.e., SIMPLE + FAST) can be feasible and particularly helpful in identifying intraperitoneal bleeding and initiating fluid resuscitation in hypovolemic shock. Current evidence supports the role of FoCUS in undifferentiated shock to improve the diagnostic accuracy, narrow the possible differential diagnoses, and guide specific management. More high-quality clinical trials are warranted to further look into the impact of FoCUS on the clinical outcomes, patient survival, and financial implication in future.

Abbreviations

AAA, abdominal aortic aneurysm; ACES, abdominal and cardiac evaluation with sonography in shock [10]; ACLS, advanced cardiac life support; AF, atrial fibrillation; AMI, acute myocardial infarction; AP2, apical two-chamber view; AP4, apical four-chamber view; AV, aortic valve; AVG, atrioventricular groove; BEAT, bedside echocardiographic assessment in trauma/critical care [69]; BLEEP, bedside limited echocardiography by emergency physician [66]; CAUSE, cardiac arrest ultrasound exam [67]; CI, cardiac index; CVP, central venous pressure; DA, descending aorta; ED, emergency department; EGLS, echo-guided life support [72]; FALLS, fluid administration limited by lung sonography [74]; FAST, focused assessment with sonography for trauma; FATE, focused assessed transthoracic echocardiography [12]; FEEL, focused echocardiographic evaluation in life support and peri-resuscitation of emergency patients [71]; FEER, focused echocardiographic evaluation in resuscitation [73]; FoCUS, focused cardiac ultrasound; FS, fractional shortening; ICU, intensive care unit; IVC, inferior vena cava; IVS, interventricular septum; LA, left atrium; LV, left ventricle; LVEDA, left ventricle end-diastole area; LVEDD, left ventricle end-diastole diameter; LVEF, left ventricular ejection fraction; LVESA, left ventricular end-systolic area; LVOT, left ventricular outflow tract; PC, pericardium; PcE, pericardial effusion; PLE, pleural effusion; PLX, parasternal long axis view; PoCUS, point-of-care ultrasound; PSX, parasternal short axis view; PW, posterior wall of left ventricle; RA, right atrium; RAP, right atrial pressure; RUSH, rapid ultrasound for shock and hypotension [9]; RUSH-HIMAP, rapid ultrasound for shock and hypotension-heart, inferior vena cava, Morrison pouch with FAST exam view and hemothorax windows, aorta, and pneumothorax [70]; RV, right ventricle; RVOT, right ventricular outflow tract; SV, stroke volume; SXP, subxyphoid view; TTE, transthoracic echocardiography; UHP, undifferentiated hypotension patient [11]; WINFOUCS, World Interactive Network Focused on Critical UltraSound

Acknowledgements

Not applicable.

Funding

The author received no funding in writing up this article.

Authors' contributions

There is only one author who drafted the manuscript, read, and approved the final manuscript.

Competing interests

The author declares that he has no competing interests in writing up this article.

References

1. Vincent JL, De Backer D. Circulatory shock. N Engl J Med. 2013;369:1726–34.
2. Jones AE, Kline JE: S. In: Marx JA, Hockberger RS, Walls RM, editors. Rosen's emergency medicine: concepts and clinical practice. Volume 1. 8th ed. Philadelphia: Saunders; 2014. p. 67–71.
3. Singer M, Deutschman CS, Seymour C, et al. The Third International Consensus definitions for sepsis and septic shock (sepsis-3). JAMA. 2016;315(8):801–10.
4. Jones AE, Aborn LS, Kline JA. Severity of emergency department hypotension predicts adverse hospital outcome. Shock. 2004;22(5):410–4.
5. Holler JG, Bech CN, Henriksen DP, Mikkelsen S, Pedersen C, Lassen AT. Nontraumatic hypotension and shock in the emergency department and the prehospital setting, prevalence, etiology, and mortality: a systematic review. Calvert J, ed. PLoS One. 2015;10(3):e0119331. doi:10.1371/journal.pone.0119331.
6. Moore CL, Copel JA. Point-of-care ultrasonography. N Engl J Med. 2011; 364:749–57.
7. American College of Emergency Physicians. ACEP emergency ultrasound guidelines—2008. Ann Emerg Med. 2009;53:550–70.
8. International Federation for Emergency Medicine. Point-of-care ultrasound curriculum guidelines. http://www.ifem.cc/wp-content/uploads/2016/03/IFEM-Point-of-Care-Ultrasound-Curriculum-Guidelines-2014-2.pdf. Accessed on 7 Mar 2016.
9. Perera P, Mailhot T, Diley D, The MD, RUSH. Exam: rapid ultrasound in shock in the evaluation of the critically ill. Emerg Med Clin N Am. 2010;28:29–56.
10. Atkinson PRT, McAulety DJ, Kendall RJ, Abeyakoon O, Reid CG, Connolly J, Lewis D. Abdominal and Cardiac Evaluation with Sonography in Shock (ACES): an approach by emergency physicians for the use of ultrasound in patients with undifferentiated hypotension. Emerg Med J. 2009;26(2):87–91. doi:10.1136/emj.2007.056242.
11. Rose JS, Bair AE, Mandavia D, The KDJ, UHP. Ultrasound protocol: a novel ultrasound approach to the empiric evaluation of the undifferentiated hypotensive patient. Am J Emerg Med. 2001;19:299–302.
12. Manasia AR, Nagaraj HM, Kodali RB, Croft LB, Oropello JM, Kohi-Seth R, et al. Feasibility and potential clinical utility of goal-directed transthoracic echocardiography performed by noncardiologist intensivists using a small hand-carried device (SonoHeart) in critically ill patients. J Cardiothorac Vasc Anesth. 2005;19(2):155–9.
13. Via G, Hussain A, Wells M, Reardon R, ElBarbary M, et al. International evidence-based recommendations for focused cardiac ultrasound. J Am Soc Echocardiogr. 2014;27(7):683. doi:10.1016/j.echo.2014.05.001. e1-683.e33.
14. Oh JK, Meloy TD, Seward JB. Echocardiography in the emergency room: is it feasible, beneficial, and cost-effective? Echocardiography. 1995;12:163–70.
15. Plummer D. Principles of emergency ultrasound and echocardiography. Ann Emerg Med. 1989;18:1291–7.
16. Frederiksen CA, Juhl-olsen P, Larsen UT, Nielsen DG, Eika B, Sloth E. New pocket echocardiography device is interchangeable with high-end portable system when performed by experienced examiners. Acta Anaesthesiol Scand. 2010;54:1217–23. doi:10.1111/j.1399-6576.2010.02320.
17. Andersen GN, Haugen BO, Graven T, Salvesen Ø, Mjølstad OC, Dalen H. Feasibility and reliability of point-of-care pocket-sized echocardiography. Eur J Echocardiogr. 2011;12(9):665–70. doi:10.1093/ejechocard/jer108.
18. Mjølstad OC, Andersen GN, Dalen H, et al. Feasibility and reliability of point-of-care pocket-size echocardiography performed by medical residents. Eur Heart J Cardiovasc Imaging. 2013;14(12):1195–202. doi:10.1093/ehjci/jet062.
19. Darocha T, Gatazkowski R, Sobczyk D, Zyla Z, Drwila R. Point-of-care ultrasonography during rescue operations on board a Polish Medical Air Rescue helicopter. J Ultrason. 2014;14:414–20.
20. Cheung AT, Savino JS, Weiss SJ, Aukburg SJ, Berlin JA. Echocardiographic and hemodynamic indexes of left ventricular preload in patients with normal and abnormal ventricular function. Anesthesiology. 1994;81:376–87.
21. Vermeiren G, Malbrain M, Walpot J. Cardiac ultrasonography in the critical care setting: a practical approach to assess cardiac function and preload for the "non-cardiologist". Anaesthesiol Intensive Ther. 2015;47:s89–s104.
22. Leung JM, Levine EH. Left ventricular end-systolic cavity obliteration as an estimate of intraoperative hypovolemia. Anesthesiology. 1994;81:1102–9.
23. Lang RM, Bierig M, Devereux RB, Flachskampf FA, Foster E, Pellikka PA, Picard MH, American Society of Echocardiography's Nomenclature and Standards Committee, Task Force on Chamber Quantification, American College of Cardiology Echocardiography Committee, American Heart

Association, European Association of Echocardiography, European Society of Cardiology, et al. Recommendations for chamber quantification. Eur J Echocardiogr. 2006;7(2):79–108. doi:10.1016/j.euje.2005.12.014.
24. Jardin F, Dubourg O, Bourdarias JP. Echocardiographic pattern of acute cor pulmonale. Chest. 1997;111(1):209–17.
25. Marik PE, Baram M, Vahid B. Does the central venous pressure predict fluid responsiveness? A systematic review of the literature and the tale of seven mares. Chest. 2008;134:172–8.
26. Feissel M, Michard F, Faller JP, Teboul JL. The respiratory variation in inferior vena cava diameter as a guide to fluid therapy. Intensive Care Med. 2004;30(9):1834–7.
27. Yanagawa Y, Sakamoto T, Okada Y. Hypovolemic shock evaluated by sonographic measurement of the inferior vena cava during resuscitation in trauma patients. J Trauma. 2007;63:1245–8.
28. Dipti A, Soucy Z, Surana A, Chandra S. Role of inferior vena cava diameter in assessment of volume status: a meta-analysis. Am J Emerg Med. 2012;30:1414–9. e1.
29. Barbier C, Loubieres Y, Schmit C, Hayon J, Ric^ome JL, et al. Respiratory changes in inferior vena cava diameter are helpful in predicting fluid responsiveness in ventilated septic patients. Intensive Care Med. 2004;30:1740–6.
30. Muller L, Bobbia X, Toumi M, Louart G, Molinari N, et al. Respiratory variations of inferior vena cava diameter to predict fluid responsiveness in spontaneously breathing patients with acute circulatory failure: need for a cautious use. Crit Care. 2012;16(5):R188. doi:10.1186/cc11672.
31. Wallace DJ, Allison M, Stone MB. Inferior vena cava percentage collapse during respiration is affected by the sampling location: an ultrasound study in healthy volunteers. Acad Emerg Med. 2010;17:96–9. doi:10.1111/j.1553-2712.2009.00627.x.
32. Rudski LG, Lai WW, Afilalo J, Hua L, Hanschumacher MD, et al. Guidelines for the echocardiographic assessment of the right heart in adults: a report from the American Society of Echocardiography endorsed by the European Association of Echocardiography, a registered branch of the European Society of Cardiology, and the Canadian Society of Echocardiography. J Am Soc Echocardiogr. 2010;23:685.
33. Ferrada P, Vanguri P, Anand RJ, Whelan J, Duane T, et al. A, B, C, D, echo: limited transthoracic echocardiogram is a useful tool to guide therapy for hypotension in the trauma bay—a pilot study. J Trauma Acute Care Surg. 2013;74(1):220–3. doi:10.1097/TA.0b013e318278918a.
34. Ferrada P, Evans D, Wolfe L, Anand RJ, Vanguri P, et al. Findings of a randomized controlled trial using limited transthoracic echocardiogram (LTTE) as a hemodynamic monitoring tool in the trauma bay. J Trauma Acute Care Surg. 2014;76(1):31–7.
35. Hagan PG, Nienaber CA, Isselbacher EM, Bruckman D, Karavite DJ, Russman PL, et al. International Registry of Acute Aortic Dissection (IRAD): new insights from an old disease. JAMA. 2000;283:897–903.
36. Nienaber CA, von Kodolitsch Y, Nicolas V, Siglow V, Piepho A, Jaup T, et al. The diagnosis of thoracic aortic dissection by noninvasive imaging procedures. N Engl J Med. 1993;328:1–9.
37. Evangelista A, Flachskamp FA, Erbel R, Antonini-Canterin F, Vlachopoulos C, Rocchi G, et al. Echocardiography in aortic diseases: EAE recommendations for clinical practice. Eur J Echocardiogr. 2010;11:645–58.
38. Brodmanna M, Starka G, Pabsta E, Luegerb A, Pilger E. Pulmonary embolism and intracardiac thrombi—individual therapeutic procedures. Vascular Med. 2000;5:27–31.
39. Cohen R, Loarte P, Navarro V, Mirrer B. Echocardiographic findings in pulmonary embolism: an important guide for the management of the patient. World J Cardiovas Diseases. 2012;2:161–4. doi:10.4236/wjcd.2012.23027.
40. Reynen K. Cardiac myxoma. N Engl J Med. 1995;333(24):1610–7.
41. Wilson SP, Suszanski J, Goyal N. Prompt diagnosis of an unusual cause of obstructive shock using point-of-care ultrasound. J Emerg Med. 2015;49(5): e151–2. doi:10.1016/j.jemermed.2015.06.033.
42. Lang RM, Badano LP, Mor-Avi V, Afilalo J, Armstrong A, Ernade L, et al. Recommendations for cardiac chamber quantification by echocardiography in adults: an update from the American Society of Echocardiography and the European Association of Cardiovascular Imaging. J Am Soc Echocardiogr. 2015;28:1–39.
43. Perera P, Lobo V, Williams SR, Gharahbaghian L. Cardiac echocardiography. Crit Care Clin. 2014;30:47–92.
44. Kendall JL, Bahner DP, Blavias M, Budhram G, Dean AJ, Fox CJ et. Al. American College of Physician Policy Statement: Emergency Ultrasound Imaging Criteria Compendium 2014. http://www.acep.org/workarea/downloadasset.aspx?id=32886 Accessed on March 29, 2016.
45. Gudmundsson P, Rydberg E, Winter R, Wilenheimer R. Visually estimated left ventricular ejection fraction by echocardiography is closely correlated with formal quantitative methods. Int J Cardiol. 2005;101:209–12.
46. Shaghgaldi K, Gudmundsson P, Manouras A, Brodin LA, Winter R. Visually estimated ejection fraction by two dimensional and triplane echocardiography is closely correlated with quantitative ejection fraction by real-time three dimensional echocardiography. Cardiovascular Ultrasound. 2009;7:41. doi:10.1186/1476-7120-7-41.
47. Unluer EE, Karagoz A, Akoglu H, Bayata S. Visual estimation of bedside echographic ejection fraction by emergency physicians. West J Emerg Med. 2014;15(2):221–6.
48. Randazzo MR, Snoey ER, Levitt A, Binder K. Accuracy of emergency physician assessment of left ventricular ejection fraction and central venous pressure using echocardiography. Acad Emerg Med. 2003;10(9):973–7.
49. Bustam A, Noor Azhar M, Singh Veriah R, Arumugam K, Loch A. Performance of emergency physicians in point-of-care echocardiography following limited training. Emerg Med J. 2014;31:369–73.
50. Fink HA, Lederle FA, Roth CS, Bowles CA, Nelson DB, Haas MA. The accuracy of physical examination to detect abdominal aortic aneurysm. Arch Intern Med. 2000;160(6):833–6.
51. Tayal VS, Graf CD, Gibbs MA. Prospective study of accuracy and outcome of emergency ultrasound for abdominal aortic aneurysm over two years. Acad Emerg Med. 2003;10:867–71.
52. Plummer D, Clinton J, Matthew B. Emergency department ultrasound improves time to diagnosis and survival in ruptured abdominal aortic aneurysm. Acad Emerg Med. 1998;5:417.
53. Lo WL, Mok KL. Ruptured splenic artery aneurysm detected by emergency ultrasound—a case report. Crit Ultrasound J. 2015;7:9. doi:10.1186/s13089-015-0026-4.
54. Callahan JA, Seward JB, Nishimura RA, Miller Jr FA, Reeder GS, Shub C, et al. Two-dimensional echocardiographically guided pericardiocentesis: experience in 117 consecutive patients. Am J Curdiol. 1985;55:476–9.
55. Kopecky SL, Callahan JA, Tajik AJ, Seward JB. Percutaneous pericardial catheter drainage: report of 42 consecutive cases. Am J Curdiol. 1986;58:633–5.
56. Tsang T, Enriquez-Sarano M, Freeman WK. Consecutive 1127 therapeutic echocardiographically guided pericardiocenteses: clinical profile, practice patterns and outcomes spanning 21 years. Mayo Clin Proc. 2002;77:429–36.
57. McConnell MV, Solomon SD, Rayan ME, Come PC, Goldhaber SZ, Lee RT. Regional right ventricular dysfunction detected by echocardiography in acute pulmonary embolism. Am J Cardiol. 1996;78:469–73.
58. López-Candales A, Edelman K, Candales MD. Right ventricular apical contractility in acute pulmonary embolism: the McConnell sign revisited. Echocardiography. 2010;27:614–20.
59. Guyatt GH, Akl EA, Crowther M, Gutterman DD, Schunemann HJ, American College of Chest Physicians Antithrombotic Therapy and Prevention of Thrombosis Panel. Executive Summary: antithrombotic therapy and prevention of thrombosis, 9th ed: American College of Chest Physicians evidence-based clinical practice guidelines. Chest. 2012;141(2 Suppl):7S–47S.
60. Spittell PC, Spittell Jr JA, Joyce JW, Tajik AJ, Edwards WD, Schaff HV, et al. Clinical features and differential diagnosis of aortic dissection: experience with 236 cases (1980 through 1990). Mayo Clin Proc. 1993;68:642–51.
61. Repessé X, Charron C, Vieillard-Baroncorresponding A. Evaluation of left ventricular systolic function revisited in septic shock. Crit Care. 2013;17(4):164.
62. Via G, Price S, Storti E. Echocardiography in the sepsis syndromes. Crit Ultrasound J. 2011;3(2):71–85.
63. Vieillard-Baron CV, Charron C, et al. The actual incidence of global left ventricular hypokinesia in adult septic shock. Crit Care Med. 2008;36:1701–6.
64. Bahner DP. Trinity: a hypotensive ultrasound protocol. JDMS. 2002;18:193–8.
65. Jensen MB, Sloth E, Larsen KM, Schmidt MB. Transthoracic echocardiography for cardiopulmonary monitoring in intensive care. Eur J Anaesthsiol. 2004;21:700–7.
66. Pershad J, Myers S, Plouman C, Rosson C, Elam K, et al. Bedside limited echocardiography by the emergency physician is accurate during evaluation of the critically ill patient. Pediatrics. 2004;114:e667–671.
67. Hernandez C, Shuler K, Hannan H, Sonyika C, Likourezos A, et al. C.A.U.S.E.: cardiac arrest ultra-sound exam—a better approach to managing patients in primary non-arrhythmogenic cardiac arrest. Resuscitation. 2008;76(2):198–206.
68. Breitkreutz R, Walcher F, Seeger FH. Focused echocardiographic evaluation in resuscitation management: concept of an advanced life support-conformed algorithm. Crit Care Med. 2007;35(5 Suppl):S150–61.
69. Gunst M, Ghaemmaghami V, Sperry J, Robinson M, O'Keeffe T, et al. Accuracy of cardiac function and volume status estimates using the

bedside echocardiographic assessment in trauma/critical care. J Trauma. 2008;65(3):509–16. doi:10.1097/TA.0b013e3181825bc5.
70. Weingart SD, Duque D, and Nelson B. Rapid ultrasound for shock and hypotension (RUSH-HIMAPP), 2009, http://emcrit.org/rush-exam/original-rush-article/.
71. Breitkreutz R, Price S, Steiger HV, Seeger FH, Ilper H, et al. Focused echocardiographic evaluation in life support and peri-resuscitation of emergency patients: a prospective trial. Resuscitation. 2010;81(11):1527–33. doi:10.1016/j.resuscitation.2010.07.013.
72. Lanctot JF, Valois M, Beaulieu Y. EGLS: echo-guided life support. Crit Ultrasound J. 2011;3:123–9.
73. Ferrada P, Murthi S, Anand RJ, Bochicchio GV, Scalea T. Transthoracic focused rapid echocardiographic examination: real-time evaluation of fluid status in critically ill trauma patients. J Trauma. 2011;70(1):56–62. doi:10.1097/TA.0b013e318207e6ee. discussion 62-4.
74. Lichtenstein D. FALLS-protocol: lung ultrasound in hemodynamic assessment of shock. Heart Lung and Vessels. 2013;5(3):142–7.
75. Liteplo A, Noble V, Atkinson P. My patient has no blood pressure: point-of-care ultrasound in the hypotensive patient—FAST and RELIABLE. Ultrasound. 2012; 20:64–8. doi:10.1258/ult.2011.011044.
76. Volpicelli G, Lamorte A, Tullio M, Cardinale L, Giraudo M, et al. Point-of-care multiorgan ultrasonography for the evaluation of undifferentiated hypotension in the emergency department. Intensive Care Med. 2013;39(7):1290–8. doi:10.1007/s00134-013-2919-7.
77. Shokoohi H, Boniface KS, Pourmand A, Liu YT, Davison DL, et al. Bedside ultrasound reduces diagnostic uncertainty and guides resuscitation in patients with undifferentiated hypotension. Crit Care Med. 2015;43(12): 2562–9. doi:10.1097/CCM.0000000000001285.
78. Jones AE, Tayal Suilivan DM, Kline JA. Randomized controlled trial of immediate versus goal directed ultrasound to identify the cause of nontraumatic hypotension in emergency department patients. Crit Care Med. 2004;32:1703–8.
79. Ghane MR, Gharib M, Ebrahimi A, Saeedi M, Akbari-Kamrani M, et al. Accuracy of early rapid ultrasound in shock (RUSH) examination performed by emergency physician for diagnosis of shock etiology in critically ill patients. J Emerg Trauma Shock. 2015;8(1):5–10. doi:10.4103/0974-2700.145406.
80. Ghane MR, Gharib MH, Ebrahimi A, Samimi K, Rezaee M, et al. Accuracy of rapid ultrasound in shock (rush) exam for diagnosis of shock in critically ill patients. Trauma Monthly. 2015;20(1):e20095. doi:10.5812/traumamon.20095.
81. Kanji HD, McCallum J, Sirounis D, MacRedmond R, Moss R, et al. Limited echocardiography-guided therapy in subacute shock is associated with changes in management and improved outcome. J Crit Care. 2014;29(5): 700–5. doi:10.1016/j.jcrc.2014.04.008.

12

Predicting contrast-induced nephropathy after CT pulmonary angiography in the critically ill: a retrospective cohort study

Kwok M. Ho[1,2,4*] and Yusrah Harahsheh[1,3]

Abstract

Background: It is uncertain whether we can predict contrast-induced nephropathy (CIN) after CT pulmonary angiography (CTPA). This study compared the ability of a validated CIN prediction score with the Pulmonary Embolism Severity Index (PESI) in predicting CIN after CTPA.

Methods: This cohort study involved critically ill adult patients who required a CTPA to exclude acute pulmonary embolism (PE). Patients with end-stage renal failure requiring dialysis were excluded. CIN was defined as an elevation in plasma creatinine concentrations > 44.2μmol/l (or 0.5 mg/dl) within 48 h after CTPA.

Results: Of the 137 patients included, 77 (51%) were hypotensive, 54 (39%) required inotropic support, and 68 (50%) were mechanically ventilated prior to the CTPA. Acute PE was confirmed in 21 patients (15%) with 14 (10%) being bilateral. CIN occurred in 56 patients (41%) with 35 (26%) required dialysis subsequent to CTPA. The CIN prediction score had a good ability to discriminate between patients with and without developing CIN (Area under the receiver-operating-characteristic (AUROC) curve 0.864, 95% confidence interval [CI] 0.795–0.916) and requiring subsequent dialysis (AUROC 0.897, 95% CI 0.833–0.942) and was better than the PESI in predicting both outcomes (AUROC 0.731, 95% CI 0.649–0.804 and 0.775, 95% CI 0.696–0.842, respectively). A CIN risk score > 10 and 12 had an 82.1 and 85.7% sensitivity and 81.5 and 78.4% specificity to predict subsequent CIN and dialysis, respectively. The CIN prediction model tended to underestimate the observed risks of dialysis, but this was improved after recalibrating the slope and intercept of the original prediction equation.

Conclusions: The CIN prediction score had a good ability to discriminate between critically ill patients with and without developing CIN after CTPA. Used together for critically ill patients with suspected acute PE, the CIN prediction score and PESI may be useful to inform clinicians when the benefits of a CTPA scan will outweigh its potential harms.

Keywords: Acute kidney injury, Complications, Contrast, Prediction, Venous thromboembolism

Background

Venous thromboembolism (VTE), including deep vein thrombosis (DVT) and pulmonary embolism (PE), is one of the most preventable causes of death and morbidity in hospitalised patients [1, 2]. The incidence of asymptomatic VTE, including PE, in critically ill or injured patients is very high despite anticoagulant prophylaxis [3]. In one cohort study, up to 10% of the patients already had unsuspected DVT at the time of ICU admission [4] and PE accounted for about 1% of all emergency intensive care unit (ICU) admissions [5].

For patients presenting with non-specific symptoms and signs of PE, including chest pain, respiratory failure, or hypotension, a computed tomography pulmonary angiography (CTPA) is often needed to confirm or exclude a life-threatening acute PE. In addition to a small risk of anaphylaxis, use of radiocontrast can induce acute kidney injury or contrast-induced nephropathy (CIN), especially in patients with pre-existing renal impairment. Although

* Correspondence: kwok.ho@health.wa.gov.au
[1]Department of Intensive Care Medicine, Royal Perth Hospital, 4th Floor, North Block, Wellington Street, Perth, Western Australia 6000, Australia
[2]School of Population and Global Health, University of Western Australia, Perth, Western Australia, Australia
Full list of author information is available at the end of the article

some retrospective observational studies have suggested that CIN may have been overemphasised or may not even exist in patients without multiple risk factors for CIN [6, 7], recent randomised controlled trials did demonstrate that risk of CIN in patients at extreme risk for CIN can be attenuated with aggressive interventions [8, 9]. While most patients who develop CIN will not require dialysis and will recover without permanent complications, there is an increasing evidence to suggest that CIN can induce long-term renal damage and mortality in high-risk patients. In the study by Mehran et al., the risks of requiring dialysis for CIN and 1-year mortality were 13 and 33% for those with multiple risk factors for CIN compared to only < 0.5 and 2% for those with the lowest risk of developing CIN, respectively [10]. The clinical significance of CIN was further confirmed by a recent study which showed that nearly one third of the in-hospital mortality after percutaneous coronary intervention was attributable to CIN, and one death could be potentially prevented by preventing nine cases of CIN [11].

The decision to proceed with a CTPA to exclude a life-threatening acute PE in patients with multiple risk factors for CIN is difficult. Theoretically, a CTPA will be justifiable provided its benefits outweigh its harms. In practice, to balance the benefits and risks of a radiocontrast study for critically ill patients is challenging. Firstly, in critically ill patients presenting with symptoms and signs of a life-threatening PE, opportunities to use prophylactic measures against CIN, including aggressive intravenous hydration, are limited [12–15]. Secondly, many risk factors for CIN, including heart failure, hypotension, and increasing age, are also risk factors for mortality in acute PE [10, 16, 17], suggesting that patients who are most at risk of dying from acute PE are, perhaps, also most at risk of developing CIN after a CTPA scan [18, 19].

Data on prediction of CIN are largely derived from cardiology patients who undergo radiological interventions [10]; whether any existing CIN prediction models can reliably predict CIN after a CTPA, especially when applied to the critically ill, remains uncertain. We hypothesised that in critically ill patients with suspected acute PE, their risk of CIN after CTPA can be estimated by the CIN prediction model developed by Mehran et al. [10]. In this study, we assessed the accuracy of the CIN risk prediction score in a cohort of critically ill patients who needed a CTPA to exclude acute PE. In addition, because Pulmonary Embolism Severity Index (PESI) shares a number of predictors with the CIN risk prediction score, we also wanted to compare the ability of these two prediction models in predicting CIN, as well as mortality, in critically ill patients with suspected acute PE requiring a CTPA scan [16].

Methods

All critically ill adult patients at Royal Perth Hospital intensive care unit who required an urgent CTPA scan to exclude acute PE, between January 2013 and September 2017, were included. The data analysed included age, gender, with factors that were needed to estimate risks of CIN and dialysis, including hypotension, use of intra-aortic balloon pump, congestive heart failure, anaemia, diabetes mellitus, and baseline renal function before the CTPA (http://tools.farmacologiaclinica.info/index.php) [10]. In addition, the information needed to calculate the PESI include underlying cancer, chronic lung disease, hypoxaemia, tachypnoea, hypothermia, altered mental state, and tachycardia were also collected and analysed [16]. In this study, patients with end-stage renal failure requiring long-term dialysis or patients who had a contrast CT chest scan not specifically tailored to look for acute PE were excluded.

Similar to other studies on CIN, CIN was defined as an elevation in plasma creatinine concentrations > 44.2μmol/l (or 0.5 mg/dl) within 48 h after the CTPA in this study—the same time frame used in the original study by Mehran et al. [10] which was not significantly different from the time frame (1 to 4 days) used in most recent interventional and observational studies on CIN [6–9]. As for the requirement for dialysis, this was captured until hospital discharge. The study centre used between 50 and 75 ml of intravenous radiocontrast (either Ultraject Optiray®350: active ingredient ioversol or Omnipaque-350: active ingredient iohexol) for all CTPA scans. All data used in this retrospective cohort study were already collected for administrative purposes, and the clinicians who made the decision to initiate dialysis for the study patients were blinded to the Mehran's predicted risk of CIN but not the clinical risk factors for CIN. All procedures performed in this study were in accordance with the ethical standards of the institutional and national research committee and with the 1964 Helsinki declaration and its later amendments or comparable ethical standards. Because the study only used clinical data that were already collected for administrative purposes, formal patient consent was considered not necessary, and this study was registered with the Royal Perth Hospital Clinical Safety and Quality Unit (No: 22233) with an intention for peer-review publication.

Statistical analyses

Categorical and continuous variables with skewed distributions were analysed by Chi-square and Mann Whitney tests, respectively. Area under the receiver-operating-characteristic (AUROC) curve was used to assess whether the existing CIN prediction score and PESI were useful in discriminating between patients with and without CIN and, similarly, for requiring subsequent dialysis. In this study, an AUROC > 0.8, between 0.7 and 0.8, and < 0.7 were defined as good, satisfactory, and unsatisfactory, respectively. Sample size ($N = 124$) was determined by assuming (a) 95% power, (b) the Mehran's CIN prediction model had an AUROC of 0.8 to predict CIN and the AUROC for PESI was 0.7, and (c) the risk of CIN was 25% after CTPA in the critically ill.

Calibration of the CIN prediction score and PESI was assessed by the Hosmer-Lemeshow Chi-square statistics and by comparing the observed and predicted risks in a calibration plot. If the CIN prediction score was not well-calibrated, an attempt was made to recalibrate the prediction equation's slope and intercept using logistic regression to see if this could improve the calibration of the score without using different or additional covariates. Missing data for any of the predictors needed for both prediction models were considered as normal to avoid over-inflating the prediction ability of the models. All statistical analyses were performed by SPSS for Windows (version 24.0, IBM, USA) and MedCalc for Windows (version 12.5, Ostend, Belgium), and a two-tailed α-error of < 5% was taken as significant. The TRIPOD Checklist for this study is listed in Additional file 1: Table S1, and non-identifiable data will be available by contacting the corresponding author.

Results

Characteristics of the study patients

Of the 141 patients who required a CTPA to exclude acute PE during the study period, 137 patients who did not have end-stage renal failure were included for further analysis. Prior to the CTPA, 77 patients (51%) were hypotensive, 54 (39%) required inotropic support, and 68 (50%) were mechanically ventilated. Acute PE was confirmed in 21 patients (15%) with 14 (10%) being bilateral. Pneumonia was diagnosed in 66 (48%) patients by the CTPA scan. CIN within 48 h after CTPA occurred in 56 patients (41%), with 35 patients (26%) required subsequent dialysis during the same hospital stay. The characteristics and outcomes of the study cohort are described in detail in Table 1, and no patients had missing data on the risk factors needed to estimate the CIN prediction score and PESI, occurrence of CIN, and requirement for dialysis.

Predicting CIN, dialysis, and mortality

The CIN prediction score (median 9, interquartile range 4–16) had a good ability to discriminate between patients with and without developing CIN within 48 h after the CTPA (AUROC 0.864, 95% confidence interval [CI]

Table 1 Characteristics and outcomes of the study patients ($N = 137$)

Variables	Median (interquartile range) unless stated otherwise
Age, years	53 (43–69)
Male, no. (%)	97 (70.8)
Comorbidities, no. (%):	
- Diabetes mellitus	41 (30)
- Cancer	28 (20)
- Chronic lung disease	33 (24)
- Congestive heart failure	56 (41)
Baseline organ support therapy, no. (%):	
- Inotropes	54 (39)
- Mechanical ventilation	68 (50)
- Intra-aortic balloon pump	2 (2)
Baseline physical signs, no. (%):	
- Tachycardia (> 110 bpm)	68 (50)
- Hypotension (< 100 mmHg)	70 (51)
- Tachypnoea (> 30 breaths/min)	77 (56)
- Hypothermia (< 36C°)	19 (14)
- Altered mental state	38 (28)
- Hypoxaemia (SaO_2 < 90%)	104 (76)
Haemoglobin concentrations, d/L	110 (89–131)
Haematocrit, %	33 (27–40)
Plasma creatinine conc., μmol/L	89 (64–137)
CIN risk score	9 (4–16)
Pulmonary Embolism Severity Index	144 (99–190)
APACHE II score	23 (17–31)
Outcomes:	
Maximum creatinine conc. within 48 h after CTPA, μmol/L	92 (65–178)
CIN within 48 h of CTPA, no. (%)	56 (41)
Required subsequent dialysis, no. (%)	35 (26)
Acute pulmonary embolism (PE), no. (%)	21 (15)
Bilateral PE, no. (%)	14 (10)
Pneumonia on CTPA, no. (%)	66 (48)
Hospital mortality, no. (%)	69 (50)
Length of ICU stay, days	6 (3–16)
Length of hospital stay, days	13 (7–26)
CIN prediction score > 10: PPV for CIN, %	75.5
CIN prediction score > 10: NPV for CIN, %	86.6
CIN prediction score > 12: PPV for dialysis, %	58.2
CIN prediction score > 12: NPV for dialysis, %	94.0

APACHE Acute Physiology and Chronic Health Evaluation, *CTPA* CT pulmonary angiography, *CIN* contrast-induced nephropathy: defined as an elevation in plasma creatinine concentrations > 44.2μmol/l (or 0.5 mg/dl) within 48 h after CTPA, *ICU* intensive care unit, *NPV* negative predictive value, *PPV* positive predictive value, *SaO_2* arterial oxygen saturation

0.795–0.916), which was better than the PESI (AUROC 0.731, 95% CI 0.649–0.804; difference in AUROC 0.133, $p = 0.001$) (Fig. 1) or using baseline plasma creatinine concentrations alone without the other components of the CIN score (AUROC 0.732, 95% CI 0.641–0.823) (Fig. 2). A CIN risk score > 10 and 12 had an 82.1 and 85.7% sensitivity and 81.5 and 78.4% specificity to predict subsequent CIN (Youden index J 0.64, 95% CI 0.50–0.74) and dialysis (Youden index J 0.64, 95% CI 0.44–0.74), respectively.

Similarly, the CIN prediction score was also better than the PESI in discriminating between patients who required subsequent dialysis and those who did not (AUROC 0.897, 95% CI 0.833–0.942 vs. 0.775, 95% CI 0.696–0.842, respectively; difference in AUROC 0.121, $p = 0.009$) (Fig. 3).

The calibration plots showed that the CIN prediction score underestimated both the observed risks of CIN (Hosmer-Lemeshow Chi-square = 9.4, $p = 0.009$) and dialysis (Hosmer-Lemeshow Chi-square = 15.3, $p = 0.001$) (Figs. 4 and 5). After recalibration of the slope and intercept of the prediction equation, the CIN predicted risks of requiring dialysis after a CTPA were more closely related to the observed risks of dialysis (recalibrated CIN risk = $1/(1 + e^{4.888-\text{CIN score} \times 0.297})$) (Fig. 6).

Despite not all study patients had a confirmed acute PE, the PESI still had a satisfactory ability and indeed far

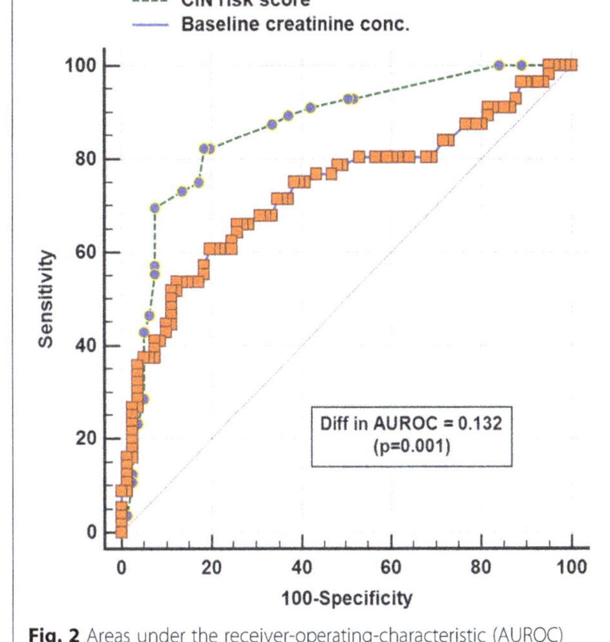

Fig. 2 Areas under the receiver-operating-characteristic (AUROC) curve of the contrast-induced nephropathy (CIN) prediction score and baseline plasma creatinine concentration to predict risk of CIN. CIN was defined as an elevation in plasma creatinine concentrations > 44.2μmol/l (or 0.5 mg/dl) within 48 h after computed tomography pulmonary angiography

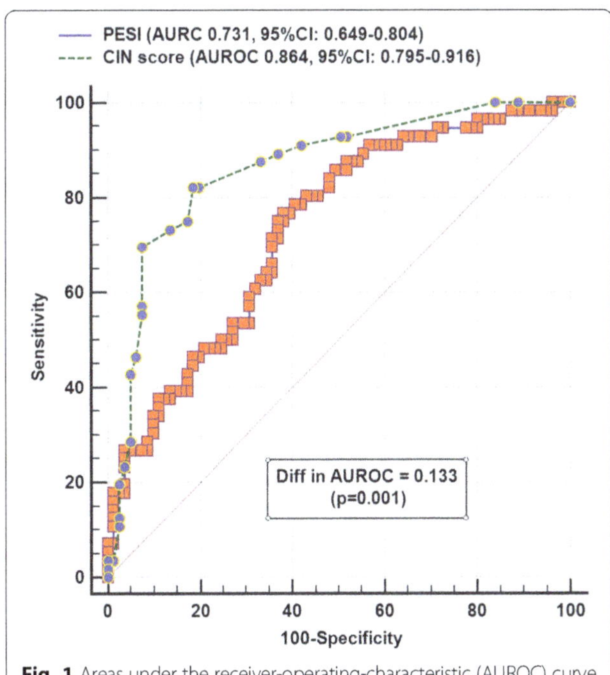

Fig. 1 Areas under the receiver-operating-characteristic (AUROC) curve of the Pulmonary Embolism Severity Index (PESI) and contrast-induced nephropathy (CIN) prediction score to predict risk of CIN. CIN was defined as an elevation in plasma creatinine concentrations > 44.2μmol/l (or 0.5 mg/dl) within 48 h after computed tomography pulmonary angiography

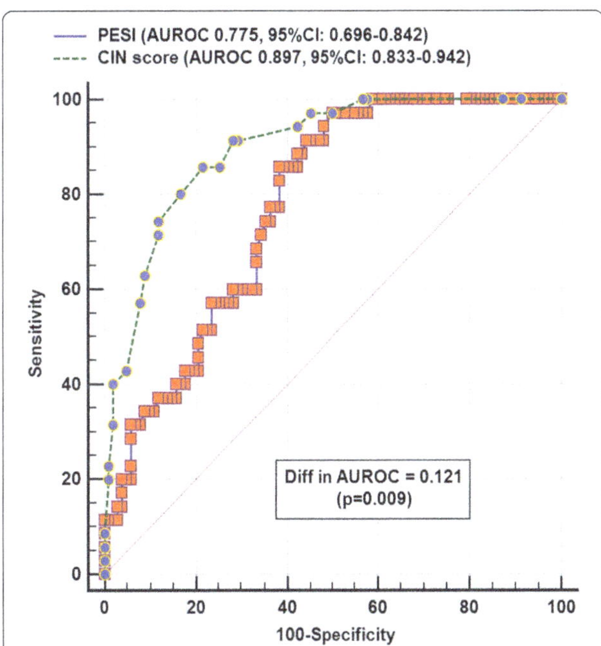

Fig. 3 Areas under the receiver-operating-characteristic (AUROC) curve of the Pulmonary Embolism Severity Index (PESI) and contrast-induced nephropathy (CIN) prediction score to predict risk of requiring dialysis

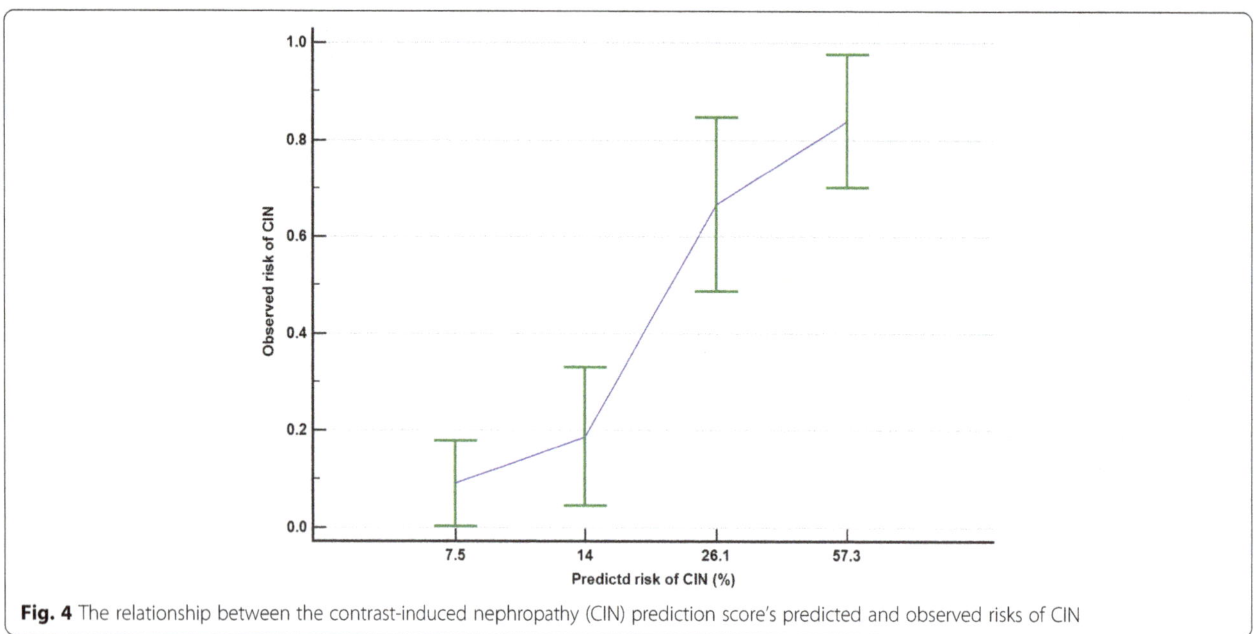

Fig. 4 The relationship between the contrast-induced nephropathy (CIN) prediction score's predicted and observed risks of CIN

better ability than the CIN prediction score to discriminate between survivors and non-survivors (AUROC 0.794, 95% CI 0.716–0.858 vs. 0.625, 95% CI 0.538–0.706; difference in AUROC 0.169, $p = 0.001$) (Fig. 7). CIN prediction score and PESI were, however, both unsatisfactory in predicting the presence of PE on the CTPA (both AUROC < 0.6).

Discussion

This study showed that CIN (41%) and dialysis (26%) after a CTPA scan were not rare in the critically ill with a suspected life-threatening acute PE. In patients with unstable vital signs and physiology requiring multiple organ support, the CIN prediction score had a good ability to discriminate between patients with and without developing CIN (AUROC 0.864) and requiring dialysis (AUROC 0.897) subsequently and was better than the PESI in predicting both outcomes. A CIN risk score > 10 and 12 had an 82.1 and 85.7% sensitivity and 81.5 and 78.4% specificity to predict subsequent CIN and dialysis, respectively. However, the CIN prediction score tended to underestimate the risks of CIN and dialysis and was also inferior to the PESI in predicting mortality in the critically ill with suspected PE. These results have some clinical implications and require further discussion.

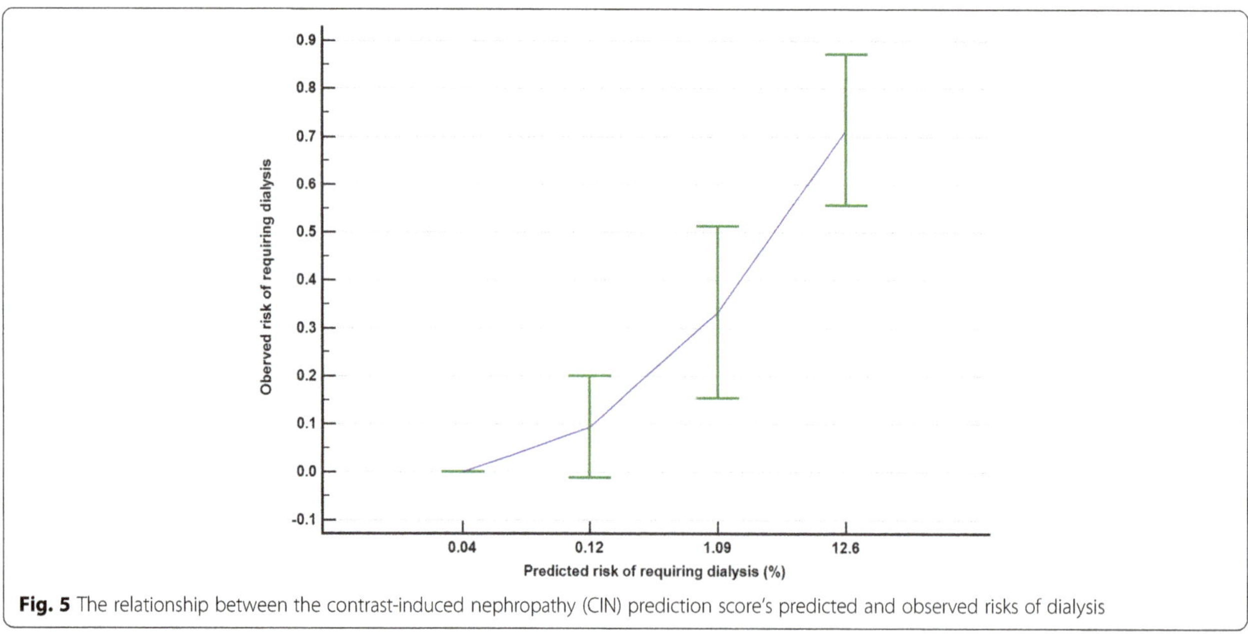

Fig. 5 The relationship between the contrast-induced nephropathy (CIN) prediction score's predicted and observed risks of dialysis

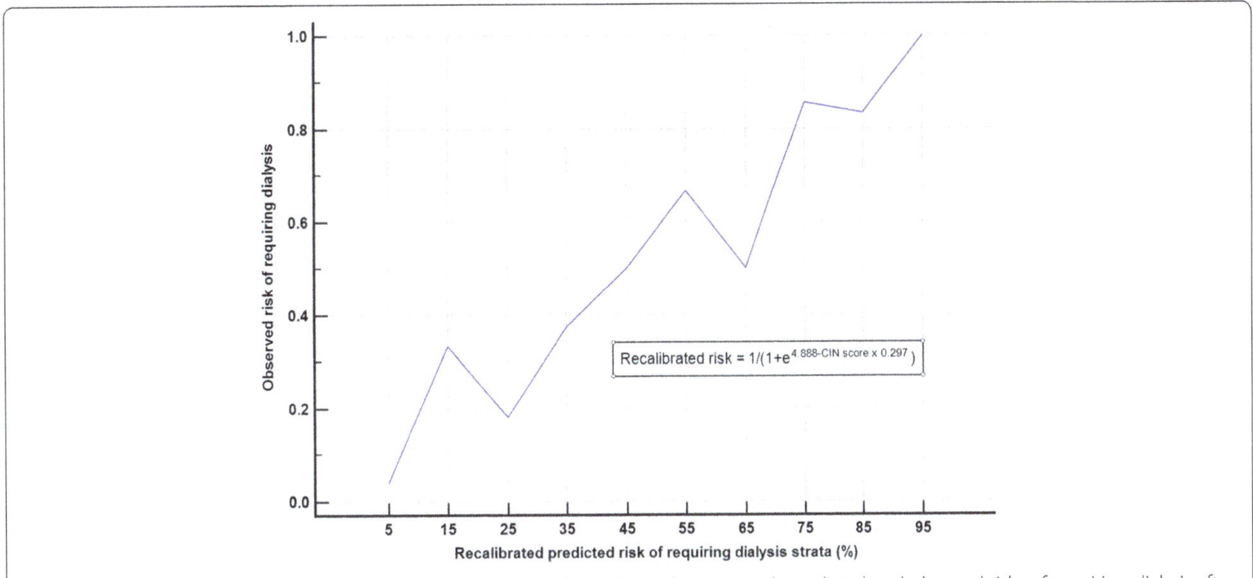

Fig. 6 The relationship between the contrast-induced nephropathy (CIN) prediction score's predicted and observed risks of requiring dialysis after recalibrating the prediction equation's slope and intercept

First, despite an increasing awareness of the importance of VTE in the critically ill, PE remains as one of the frequently missed diagnoses—identified only in autopsies [20–23]. Because the pre-test probability of VTE in the critically ill is high, d-dimers are not useful and CTPA has practically become the gold standard to confirm or exclude a life-threatening acute PE [20]. This practice is further supported by the fact that a CTPA can also evaluate the right ventricular size, which reflects the severity of acute PE. In addition, a CTPA may provide important information on alternative differential diagnoses such as pneumonia. Nevertheless, our results suggest that there is a risk of CIN associated with any radiocontrast studies, including a CTPA scan, in the critically ill. It is possible that the deteriorations in renal function after a CTPA in some of our patients could occur regardless of whether radiocontrast had been used, or at least in part, if not purely due to the natural progression of a life-threatening illness. The differential ability of the CIN prediction score and PESI in predicting CIN and mortality suggests that the severity of illness alone may not fully explain the risks of renal dysfunction and dialysis after a CTPA scan. PESI and CIN prediction score do share some similar risk factors (such as age, congestive heart failure, and hypotension), but there are also factors in the CIN prediction score that are distinct from the PESI, including diabetes mellitus, anaemia, and pre-existing renal impairment [10, 18, 19]. As such, we can argue that radiocontrast was likely to play a contributing role in inducing the increases in plasma creatinine concentrations in our patients, especially in those with multiple risk factors for CIN [10, 18, 19].

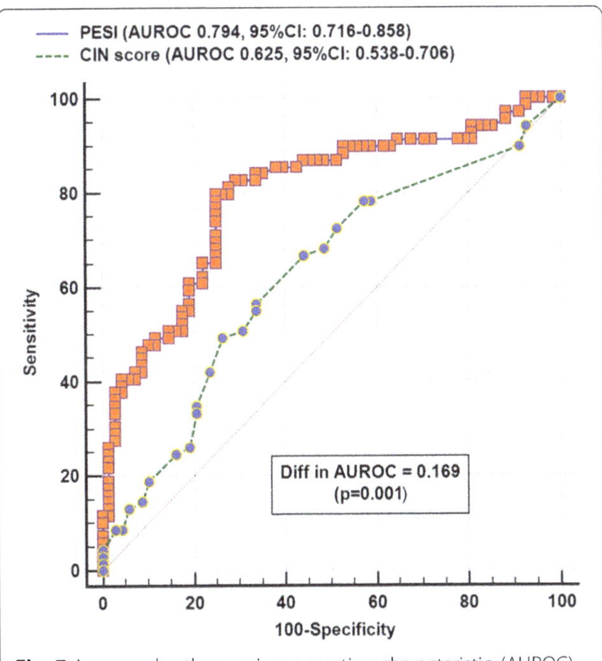

Fig. 7 Areas under the receiver-operating-characteristic (AUROC) curve of the Pulmonary Embolism Severity Index (PESI) and contrast-induced nephropathy (CIN) prediction score to predict risk of hospital mortality

Our results also suggest that the CIN prediction score and PESI may also have complementary roles in determining the balance between benefits and harms of a CTPA in a patient with suspected acute PE. Theoretically, a CTPA will be justifiable if the predicted risk of mortality by the PESI is higher than the predicted risk of requiring dialysis by the CIN prediction score in any patients with symptoms and signs of acute PE. Conversely, if the CIN prediction score's predicted risk of requiring dialysis is much higher than the predicted risk of mortality by the PESI (when the CIN risk score is >16 and PESI is <126) (Fig. 8), perhaps an alternative way to diagnose or exclude an acute PE, possibly by a combination of tests—such as transoesophageal echocardiography, lower limb venous ultrasonography, and ventilation-perfusion scan—should be seriously considered in reducing the long-term consequences of CIN [10, 24]. However, a delay in doing a CTPA scan to allow aggressive intravenous hydration or other forms of CIN prophylaxis does not confer substantial benefits in reducing CIN after CTPA in an acute care setting [25, 26].

Second, our study showed that the CIN prediction score had a good discriminative ability but was not well-calibrated in predicting both CIN and dialysis after a CTPA in the critically ill. It should be noted that our primary results—AUROC, sensitivity, and specificity—are known to be not affected by prevalence (or pre-test probability) of the outcome of interest. In addition, after recalibration of the intercept and slope of the existing CIN prediction equation, the predicted risks of requiring dialysis appeared to match the observed risks much better (Fig. 7). This result suggests that the covariates used in the CIN prediction are largely 'good or valid' predictors for CIN in the critically ill, even though they are derived from cardiology patients. Hence, further refinement and recalibration of the CIN prediction score for patients who require a CTPA will be feasible, and relatively straightforward, by a prospective multicentre cohort study. Using a conservative rule of one covariate per ten outcomes and assuming an incidence (or pre-test probability) of CIN is 20% (or 10%), a sample size >600 (or 1200) patients will be needed to develop a CIN prediction model with 12 predictors for the critically ill which can then be validated with a similar or larger size study.

Finally, we need to acknowledge the limitations of this study. Although the CIN prediction score has included a number of risk factors for renal dysfunction after administration of radiocontrast, there are other risk factors that might also be important, including use of nephrotoxic drugs and presence of infection. The significance of these risk factors in predicting CIN should be considered in developing a CIN prediction model for patients undergoing a CTPA scan. With a relatively small sample size, we were unable to test the relative importance of each risk factor contained in the CIN prediction score, both in predicting CIN as well as the presence of PE and its associated mortality. As such, a large prospective multicentre study will be essential to improve our understanding on when, and in whom, a CTPA will be most beneficial.

Conclusions

In summary, CIN and dialysis were not rare in critically ill patients who had unstable vital signs after using CTPA scan to exclude a life-threatening acute PE. Despite only derived from cardiology patients, the CIN prediction score had a good ability to discriminate between patients with and without developing CIN and requiring dialysis after an urgent CTPA scan and indeed was better than the PESI in predicting both adverse renal outcomes. Further research is, however, needed to improve the calibration of the current CIN prediction score or reconstruct an even

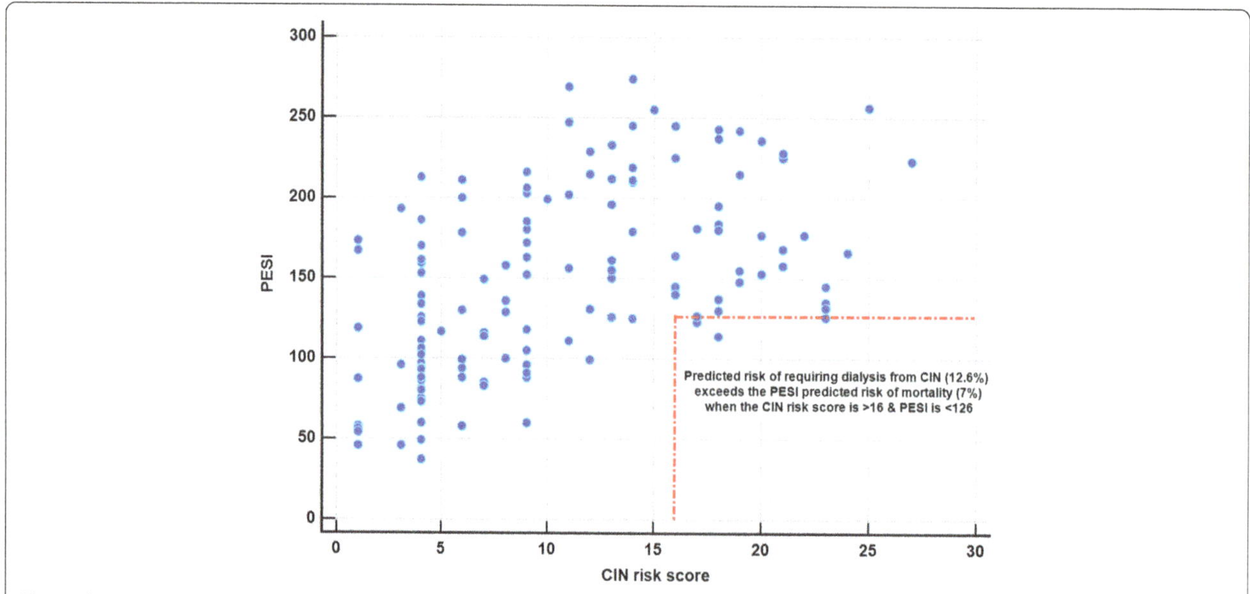

Fig. 8 The situations when contrast-induced nephropathy (CIN) prediction score's predicted risk of dialysis exceeds the Pulmonary Embolism Severity Index (PESI)'s predicted risk of mortality

more accurate prediction score in predicting CIN and dialysis in the critically ill who require different types of radiocontrast study. Used together for critically ill patients with suspected acute PE, the CIN prediction score and PESI may be useful to inform clinicians when the benefits of a CTPA scan will outweigh its potential harms.

Abbreviations

AUROC: Area under the receiver-operating-characteristic; CIN: Contrast-induced nephropathy; CTPA: Computed tomography pulmonary angiography; PE: Pulmonary embolism; PESI: Pulmonary Embolism Severity Index

Acknowledgements

KMH is funded by the Raine Medical Research Foundation and WA Health through the Raine Clinical Research Fellowship. The authors would like to thank Dr. Swithin Song for his advice on the dose of radiocontrast needed for a CT pulmonary angiography.

Funding

None.

Authors' contributions

KMH contributed to the design of the study, data collection, analysis, and drafting of the manuscript. YH contributed to the design of the study, interpretation of the data, and drafting the manuscript. Both authors read and approved the final manuscript.

Competing interests

The authors declare that they have no competing interests.

Author details

[1]Department of Intensive Care Medicine, Royal Perth Hospital, 4th Floor, North Block, Wellington Street, Perth, Western Australia 6000, Australia. [2]School of Population and Global Health, University of Western Australia, Perth, Western Australia, Australia. [3]School of Medicine and Pharmacology, University of Western Australia, Perth, Western Australia, Australia. [4]School of Veterinary and Life Sciences, Murdoch University, Perth, Western Australia, Australia.

References

1. Galson SK. The Surgeon General's Call to Action to Prevent Deep Vein Thrombosis and Pulmonary Embolism. https://www.ncbi.nlm.nih.gov/books/NBK44178/. Accessed 30 Nov 2017.
2. National Quality Forum. National Voluntary Consensus Standards for Prevention and Care of Venous Thromboembolism: additional performance measures. 2008. http://www.qualityforum.org/Publications/2008/10/National_Voluntary_Consensus_Standards_for_prevention_and_Care_of_Venous_Thromboembolism__Additional_Performance_Measures.aspx. Accessed 30 Nov 2017.
3. Schultz DJ, Brasel KJ, Washington L, Goodman LR, Quickel RR, Lipchik RJ, et al. Incidence of asymptomatic pulmonary embolism in moderately to severely injured trauma patients. J Trauma. 2004;56:727–31.
4. Cook DJ, Crowther MA. Thromboprophylaxis in the intensive care unit: focus on medical-surgical patients. Crit Care Med. 2010;38:S76–82.
5. Ho KM, Chavan S. Prevalence of thrombocytosis in critically ill patients and its association with symptomatic acute pulmonary embolism. A multicentre registry study. Thromb Haemost. 2013;109:272–9.
6. RJ MD, JS MD, Carter RE, Hartman RP, Katzberg RW, Kallmes DF, et al. Intravenous contrast material exposure is not an independent risk factor for dialysis or mortality. Radiology. 2014;273:714–25.
7. Wilhelm-Leen E, Montez-Rath ME, Chertow G. Estimating the risk of radiocontrast-associated nephropathy. J Am Soc Nephrol. 2017;28:653–9.
8. Briguori C, Visconti G, Focaccio A, Airoldi F, Valgimigli M, Sangiorgi GM, et al. REMEDIAL II investigators. Renal insufficiency after contrast media administration trial II (REMEDIAL II): RenalGuard system in high-risk patients for contrast-induced acute kidney injury. Circulation 2011; 124:1260-1269.
9. Brar SS, Aharonian V, Mansukhani P, Moore N, Shen AY, Jorgensen M, et al. Haemodynamic-guided fluid administration for the prevention of contrast-induced acute kidney injury: the POSEIDON randomised controlled trial. Lancet. 2014;383:1814–23.
10. Mehran R, Aymong ED, Nikolsky E, Lasic Z, Iakovou I, Fahy M, et al. A simple risk score for prediction of contrast-induced nephropathy after percutaneous coronary intervention: development and initial validation. J Am Coll Cardiol. 2004;44:1393–9.
11. Kooiman J, Seth M, Nallamothu BK, Heung M, Humes D, Gurm HS. Association between acute kidney injury and in-hospital mortality in patients undergoing percutaneous coronary interventions. Circ Cardiovasc Interv. 2015;8:e002212.
12. Liu Y, Chen JY, Tan N, Zhou YL, Yu DQ, Chen ZJ, et al. Safe limits of contrast vary with hydration volume for prevention of contrast-induced nephropathy after coronary angiography among patients with a relatively low risk of contrast-induced nephropathy. Circ Cardiovasc Interv. 2015;8(6).
13. Ho KM, Morgan DJ. Use of isotonic sodium bicarbonate to prevent radiocontrast nephropathy in patients with mild pre-existing renal impairment: a meta-analysis. Anaesth Intensive Care. 2008;36:646–53.
14. Subramaniam RM, Suarez-Cuervo C, Wilson RF, Turban S, Zhang A, Sherrod C, et al. Effectiveness of prevention strategies for contrast-induced nephropathy: a systematic review and meta-analysis. Ann Intern Med. 2016; 164:406–16.
15. Ho KM. Pitfalls in haemodynamic monitoring in the postoperative and critical care setting. Anaesth Intensive Care. 2016;44:14–9.
16. Aujesky D, Obrosky DS, Stone RA, Auble TE, Perrier A, Cornuz J, et al. Derivation and validation of a prognostic model for pulmonary embolism. Am J Respir Crit Care Med. 2005;172:1041–6.
17. Ho KM. Balancing the risks and benefits of using emergency diagnostic radiocontrast studies to diagnose life-threatening illness in critically ill patients: a decision analysis. Anaesth Intensive Care. 2016;44:724–8.
18. Yazıcı S, Kırış T, Emre A, Ceylan US, Akyüz Ş, Uzun AO, et al. Relation of contrast nephropathy to adverse events in pulmonary emboli patients diagnosed with contrast CT. Am J Emerg Med. 2016;34:1247–50.
19. Mitchell AM, Jones AE, Tumlin JA, Kline JA. Prospective study of the incidence of contrast-induced nephropathy among patients evaluated for pulmonary embolism by contrast-enhanced computed tomography. Acad Emerg Med. 2012;19:618–25.
20. Minet C, Potton L, Bonadona A, Hamidfar-Roy R, Somohano CA, Lugosi M, et al. Venous thromboembolism in the ICU: main characteristics, diagnosis and thromboprophylaxis. Crit Care. 2015;19:287.
21. Perkins GD, McAuley DF, Davies S, Gao F. Discrepancies between clinical and postmortem diagnoses in critically ill patients: an observational study. Crit Care. 2003;7:R129–32.
22. McLeod AG, Geerts W. Venous thromboembolism prophylaxis in critically ill patients. Crit Care Clin. 2011;27:765–80.
23. Ho KM, Burrell M, Rao S, Baker R. Incidence and risk factors for fatal pulmonary embolism after major trauma: a nested cohort study. Br J Anaesth. 2010;105:596–602.
24. Mitchell AM, Kline JA, Jones AE, Tumlin JA. Major adverse events one year after acute kidney injury after contrast-enhanced computed tomography. Ann Emerg Med. 2015;66:267–74.
25. Kooiman J, Sijpkens YW, van Buren M, Groeneveld JH, Ramai SR, van der Molen AJ, et al. Randomised trial of no hydration vs. sodium bicarbonate hydration in patients with chronic kidney disease undergoing acute computed tomography-pulmonary angiography. J Thromb Haemost. 2014; 12:1658–66.
26. Turedi S, Erdem E, Karaca Y, Tatli O, Sahin A, Turkmen S, et al. The high risk of contrast-induced nephropathy in patients with suspected pulmonary embolism despite three different prophylaxis: a randomized controlled trial. Acad Emerg Med. 2016;23:1136–45.

13

Monitoring the coagulation status of trauma patients with viscoelastic devices

Yuichiro Sakamoto*, Hiroyuki Koami and Toru Miike

Abstract

Coagulopathy is a physiological response to massive bleeding that frequently occurs after severe trauma and is an independent predictive factor for mortality. Therefore, it is very important to grasp the coagulation status of patients with severe trauma quickly and accurately in order to establish the therapeutic strategy. Judging from the description in the European guidelines, the importance of viscoelastic devices in understanding the disease condition of patients with traumatic coagulopathy has been widely recognized in Europe. In the USA, the ACS TQIP Massive Transfusion in Trauma Guidelines proposed by the American College of Surgeons in 2013 presented the test results obtained by the viscoelastic devices, TEG® 5000 and ROTEM®, as the standard for transfusion or injection of blood plasma, cryoprecipitate, platelet concentrate, or anti-fibrinolytic agents in the treatment strategy for traumatic coagulopathy and hemorrhagic shock. However, some studies have reported limitations of these viscoelastic devices. A review in the Cochrane Library published in 2015 pointed out the presence of biases in the abovementioned reports in trauma patients and the absence of a quality study in this field thus far. A quality study on the relationship between traumatic coagulopathy and viscoelastic devices is needed.

Background

Two of the major causes of coagulopathy in trauma patients are coagulopathy secondary to hemorrhagic shock due to massive bleeding and coagulopathy due to severe head injury [1]. The release of tissue factor from the damaged brain tissue is postulated as the cause of coagulopathy due to severe head injury. The fundamental treatment for shock due to bleeding is treatment to achieve hemostasis, but fluid infusion and blood transfusion for long periods of time under insufficient hemostasis may lead to the derangement of hemostasis and the impairment of hemostasis due to hypothermia [2–4]. Therefore, it is important to achieve hemostasis quickly without missing the timing in which the patient is able to cope with physiological changes in the early stage of massive bleeding such as tachycardia, wetness, and coldness in the extremities, and anxiety, rather than cope with hypotension that is a physiological response to massive bleeding. It is also important to perform blood transfusion quickly and appropriately as well as obtain immediate hemostasis for the treatment of hemorrhagic shock that accounts for 90% of incidents of traumatic shock. Since coagulation abnormality which is a physiological response to massive bleeding frequently occurs after severe trauma and is an independent predictive factor for mortality, it is very important to grasp the coagulation status of the patient quickly and accurately in order to establish the therapeutic strategy [1, 5].

It has been recognized that trauma patients are more likely to die from intraoperative metabolic failure than from a failure to complete operative repairs. Damage control surgery (DCS) is surgery that is designed to restore normal physiology prior to normal anatomy in critically ill patients. DCS is important for the treatment of trauma because the development of coagulopathy due to radical hemostasis is fatal [5, 6]. DCS is a therapeutic concept in which hemostasis is achieved in as short a time as possible, physiological function is normalized by postoperative intensive care, and then injury repair is completed by planned reoperation if necessary [7].

For this purpose, the status and degree of coagulopathy must be determined quickly with objective indicators. For example, it is possible that continuation of a surgical operation in a patient with a defect in coagulability fails to save the life of the patient because of uncontrollable bleeding. To avoid such a situation, the criteria known

* Correspondence: sakamoy@cc.saga-u.ac.jp
Department of Emergency and Critical Care Medicine, Faculty of Medicine, Saga University, 5-1-1 Nabeshima, Saga City, Saga 849-8501, Japan

as the trauma triad of death (deadly triad) consisting of hypothermia, metabolic acidosis, and coagulopathy have been proposed for the introduction of DCS [7]. In actual clinical practice, body temperature and acid-base equilibrium can be quickly measured. However, measurement of prothrombin time (PT) that is commonly used as the indicator of coagulability requires more than 60 min before the result is obtained [8]. In addition, it has been said that these indicators reflect the early stage of the coagulation process and that the amount of thrombin produced in this period is only 4% of the total prothrombin [9]. Furthermore, the PT and activated partial thromboplastin time (APTT) do not necessarily reflect the in vivo status of coagulability such as the influence of platelets, because the tests are carried out by adding a blood clotting accelerant to plasma separated from whole blood. The activated clotting time (ACT) that uses whole blood may not reflect the in vivo status of coagulability either, because the test also only reflects the early stage of coagulation similar to PT and APTT [10]. We review the principles of measurement by viscoelastic devices and guidelines for the treatment of traumatic coagulopathy.

Principle of measurement by viscoelastic devices

TEG5000 system

The Thrombelastograph (TEG®) is a device that measures the change in viscoelasticity of whole blood without separating out the plasma. The TEG was developed based on a concept reported by Hartert in 1948 [11]. The TEG® was reported as the most rapid available test for providing reliable information on coagulopathy in patients with multiple injuries [12]. Since the usefulness of the TEG® for monitoring coagulability during liver transplantation surgery was reported in 1985 [13], this instrument has been widely used in clinical settings. In addition to the TEG®, the rotational thromboelastometer (ROTEM®) has been used as a common viscoelastic device. A new device has been developed in Japan, and it has a completely different principle of measurement from that of conventional point-of-care (POC) devices to assess coagulation and hemostatic function. This device is the Total Thrombus-Formation Analysis System (T-TAS®) whose measurement principle will be explained elsewhere in this article.

As for the principle of measurement by POC devices, the TEG®5000 and ROTEM® delta optically measure changes in mechanical impedance to a sensor pin generated by clotting-induced change in elasticity of whole blood in a cuvette after the addition of a coagulation accelerant [14, 15].

ROTEM system

In the ROTEM® system, the results are displayed in a graph in which the horizontal axis is time (min) and the vertical axis is clot amplitude (mm) which represents the firmness of the clot (Fig. 1). Various parameters can be measured with the ROTEM® system such as the duration from the start of measurement to the beginning of clotting time, duration from the start of clotting to the time when the clot amplitude representing clot firmness reaches 20 mm (clot formation time, CFT) and its angle (α angle), the clot amplitude every 5 min after the beginning of clotting (A 5–30) and its maximum (maximum clot firmness, MCF), the lysis index at 30, 45, and 60 min after the beginning of clotting (LI 30, 45, and 60), and the maximum lysis index (ML) which can be monitored in real time. The results in a normal healthy person are shown in Fig. 2, and the results in representative patients with a clotting abnormality are shown in Fig. 3. In clinical practice, we observe complicated findings in quite a lot of patients with some types of coagulation abnormalities. Case 1 was an 80-year-old woman who complained of vertigo (Fig. 4). She was referred to

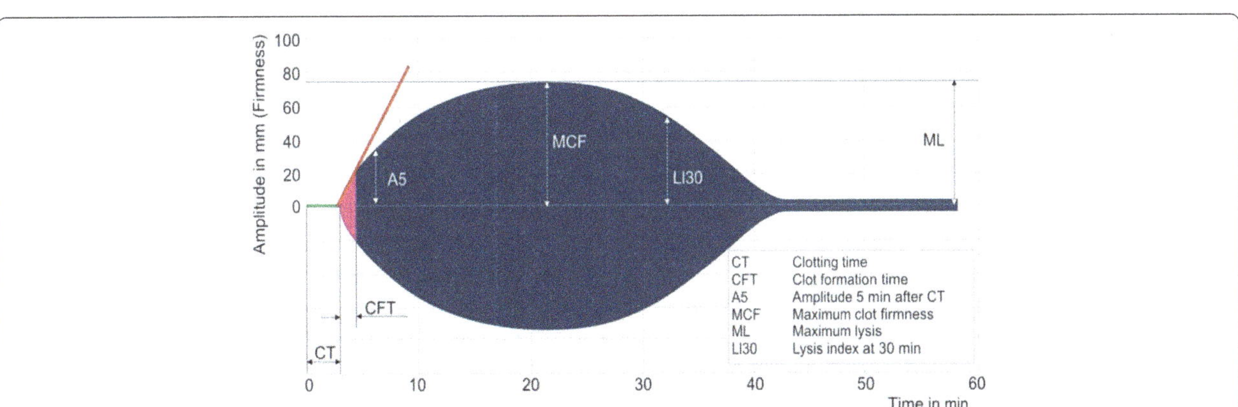

Fig. 1 An example of results obtained using the ROTEM system. In the ROTEM® system, the results are displayed in a graph in which the horizontal axis is time (min) and the vertical axis is clot amplitude (mm) based on the firmness of the clot. Various parameters can be measured in real time such as clotting time (CT), clot formation time (CFT), the amplitude at 5 min (A5), maximum clot firmness (MCF), maximum lysis (ML), and lysis index at 30 min (LI30)

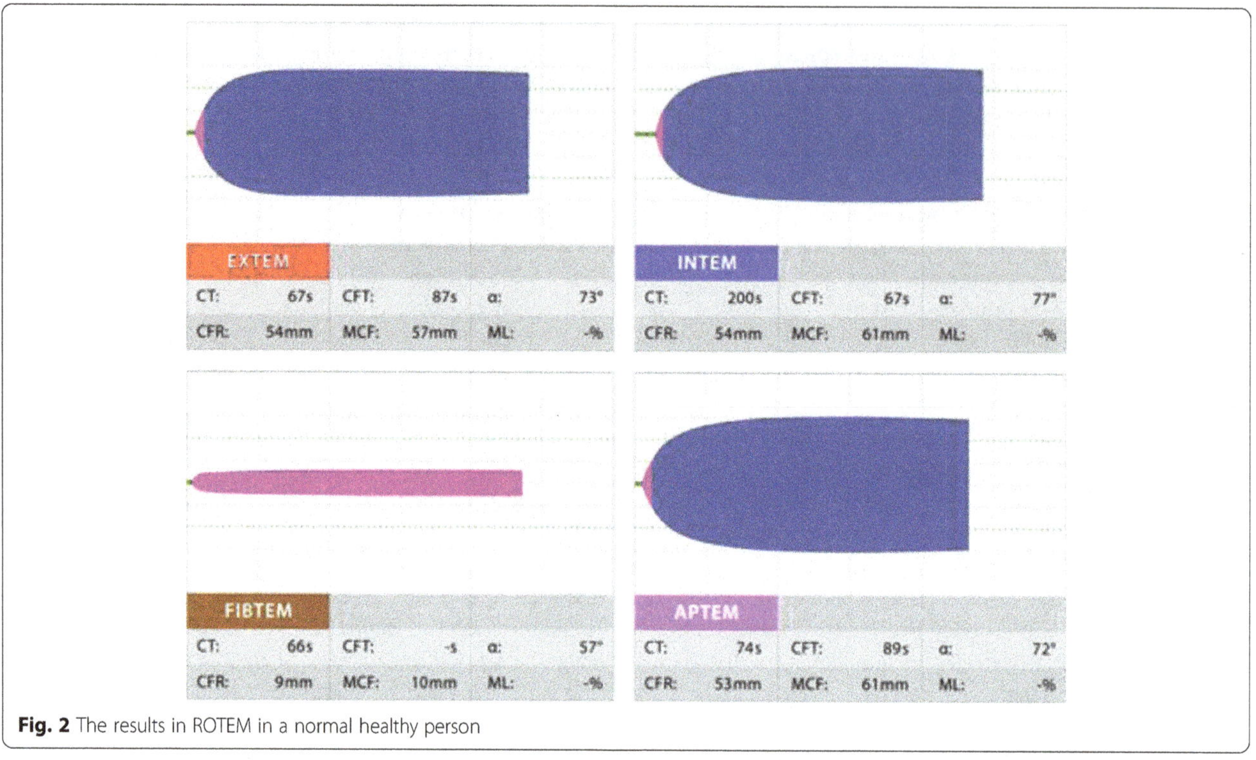

Fig. 2 The results in ROTEM in a normal healthy person

our hospital because of suspicion of cerebral bleeding. Her past medical history showed that she underwent artificial blood vessel replacement surgery for thoracoabdominal aortic aneurysm 8 years previously, and she had chronic hepatitis C, liver cirrhosis (Child-Pugh class B), and chronic atrial fibrillation. On admission to our emergency department (ED), her consciousness was alert and her vital signs were nearly stable except for slight hypertension. Her blood profiles showed significantly reduced platelet count ($3.5 \times 10^4/\mu L$) and fibrinogen level (72.6 mg/dL), prolonged PT-international normalized ratio (INR) (1.47), prolonged aPTT (41.0 s), elevated D dimer level (23.89 μg/mL), and significantly elevated thrombin-antithrombin complex (TAT) level (31.6 ng/mL).We considered that her reduced platelet count also indicated platelet dysfunction. In these data, the parameters of fibrinolysis implied not hyperfibrinolysis but clot retraction because the ML in EXTEM and APTEM was 15% or more [16]. This patient was not diagnosed with any acute cerebrovascular disease, and she was discharged on the same day.

In the TEG®5000 system, tests are carried out by adding premanufactured reagents to a citrated or heparinized whole blood sample in a cuvette. Reagents for TEG®5000 are as follows: kaolin, which is the basic reagent for activating the intrinsic pathway; heparinase that excludes the effect of heparin; tissue factor that activates the extrinsic pathway; batroxobin that induces abnormal fibrin formation; activated factor XIII that promotes fibrin cross-linkage; arachidonic acid (AA) and adenosine diphosphate (ADP) that activate the respective receptor on platelets; and a platelet aggregation inhibitor, abciximab [14]. The TEG®5000 system allows us to conduct six different tests by using different combinations of these reagents. Kaolin TEG is the basic test in TEG® and measures the clotting activity of the intrinsic pathway. Kaolin TEG + heparinase which consists of kaolin and heparinase can detect the influence of heparin. Rapid TEG® that uses kaolin and tissue factor enables the rapid measurement of clot-forming capacity. TEG functional fibrinogen that uses tissue factor and abciximab assesses fibrin-polymerizing activity. Measurement of platelet function is a characteristic function of TEG®, so-called TEG® platelet mapping. The combination of batroxobin, activated factor XIII and AA or the combination of batroxobin, activated factor XIII and ADP can assess the influence of acetylsalicylic acid or a P2Y12 inhibitor, respectively.

Figure 5 shows the typical presentation of measurement data obtained by TEG®.

The TEG® and ROTEM® systems are based on the same basic principle of measurement. The results that can be obtained from the two systems are summarized in Table 1.

We introduced the ROTEM® delta in the emergency room of our hospital in January 2013. Clotting time measured in the EXTEM test was a significantly reliable predictor of sepsis-induced disseminated intravascular coagulation (DIC) among 13 sepsis patients [17].

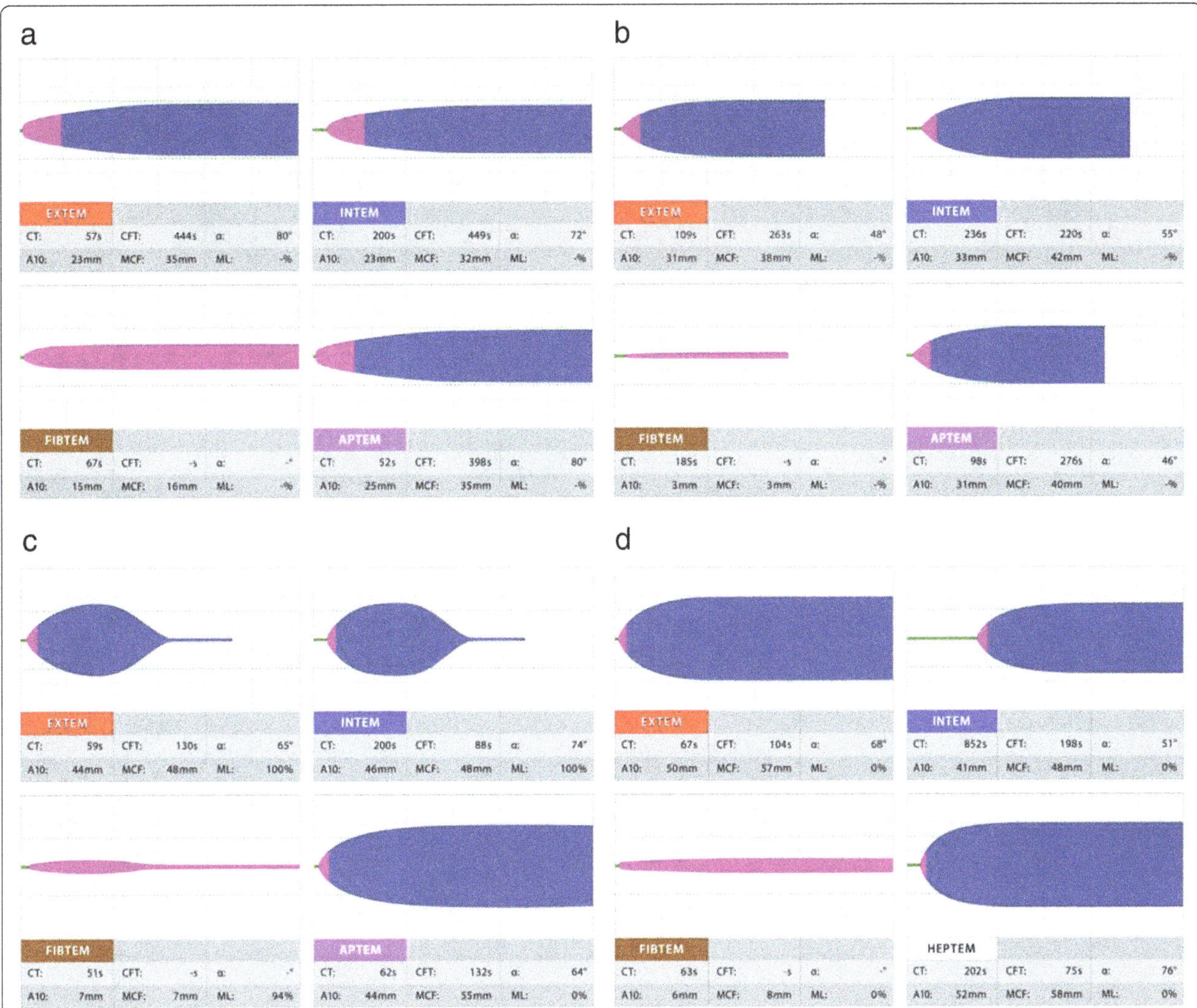

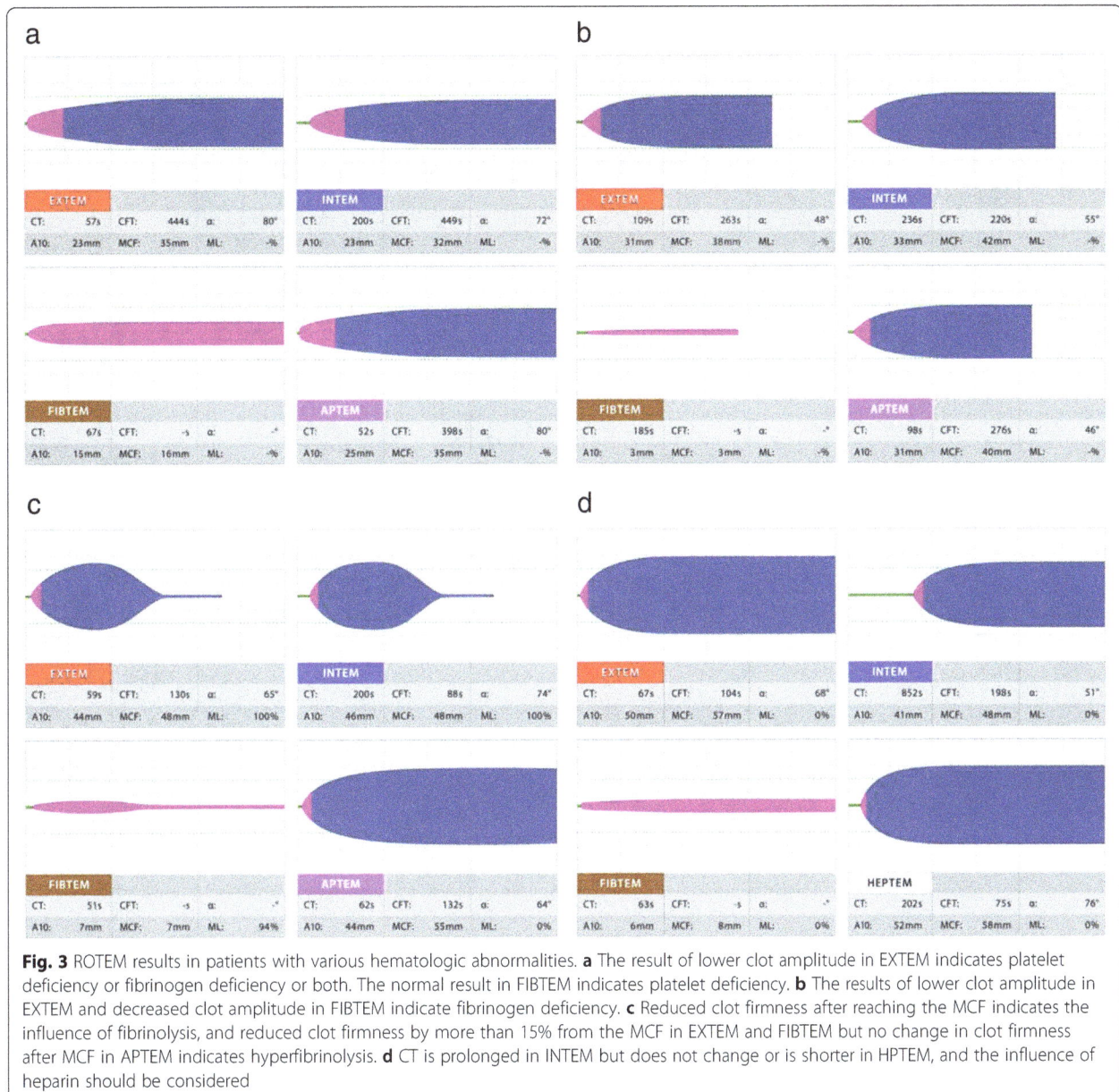

Fig. 3 ROTEM results in patients with various hematologic abnormalities. **a** The result of lower clot amplitude in EXTEM indicates platelet deficiency or fibrinogen deficiency or both. The normal result in FIBTEM indicates platelet deficiency. **b** The results of lower clot amplitude in EXTEM and decreased clot amplitude in FIBTEM indicate fibrinogen deficiency. **c** Reduced clot firmness after reaching the MCF indicates the influence of fibrinolysis, and reduced clot firmness by more than 15% from the MCF in EXTEM and FIBTEM but no change in clot firmness after MCF in APTEM indicates hyperfibrinolysis. **d** CT is prolonged in INTEM but does not change or is shorter in HPTEM, and the influence of heparin should be considered

Interestingly, the clotting time measured in EXTEM was strongly correlated with the DIC score of the Japanese Association for Acute Medicine [17]. We assessed the differences in results between traumatized and septic DIC cases that were diagnosed by the same DIC scoring system [18]. This study found that the plasma fibrinogen level and clot firmness measured in the FIBTEM test were significantly different between groups with the same severity. Another paper reported a patient with asymptomatic hyperfibrinolysis diagnosed by ROTEM secondary to anaphylactic shock [19]. In fact, hyperfibrinolysis was significantly associated with elevated serum lactate level (≥4.0 mmol/L) among patients with systemic circulatory insufficiency [20].

T-TAS system

T-TAS® is a device that observes the time course of thrombus formation in whole blood flowing in a simulated blood vessel at a constant rate [21]. Since the pressure curve reflects the rate of thrombus formation and thrombus firmness, coagulability and platelet function can be assessed by reading the pressure curve. There are two types of chips having a built-in simulated blood vessel, called PL-chip and AR-chip [22].

The PL-chip which is specialized for the assessment of platelet function consists of a simulated blood vessel in which the inner surface is coated with collagen [23]. Thrombus formation is observed using whole blood anticoagulated with hirudin, a thrombin inhibitor.

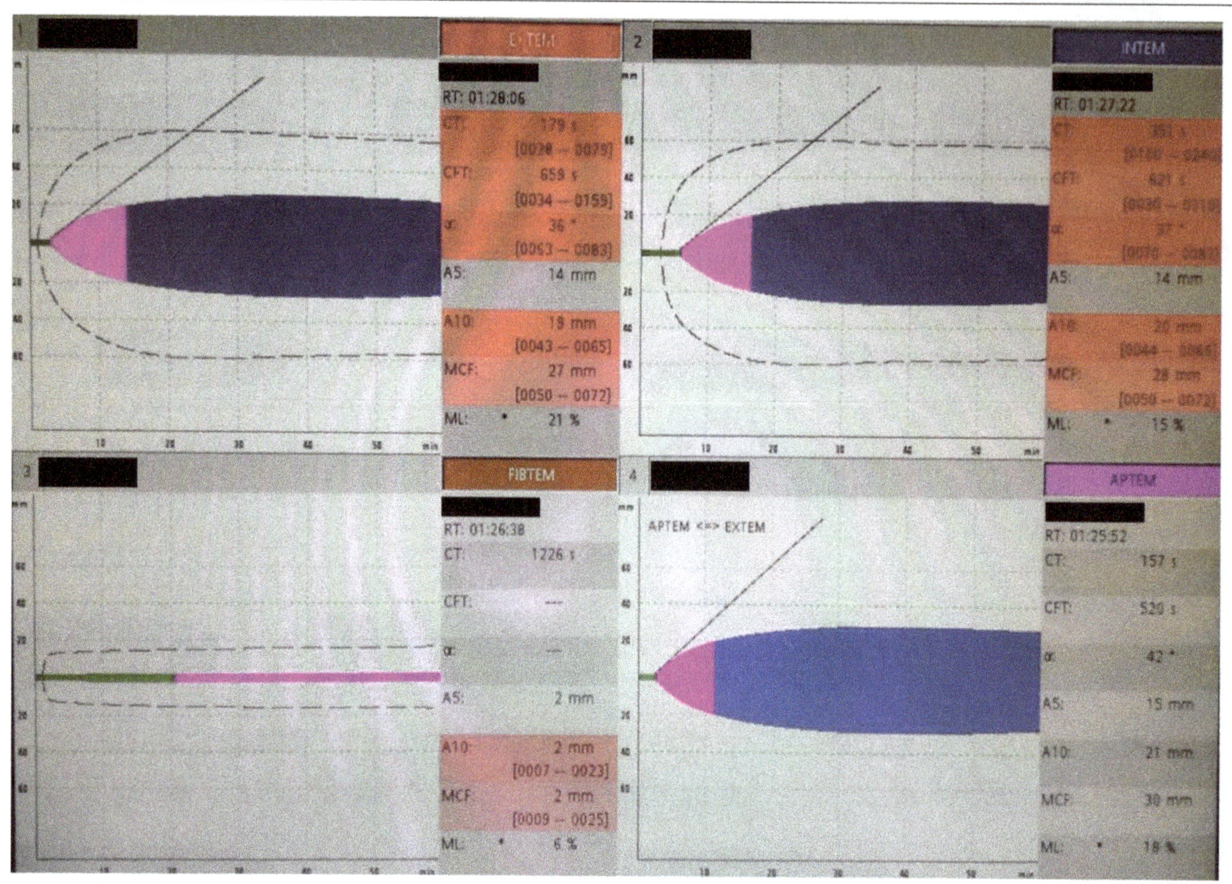

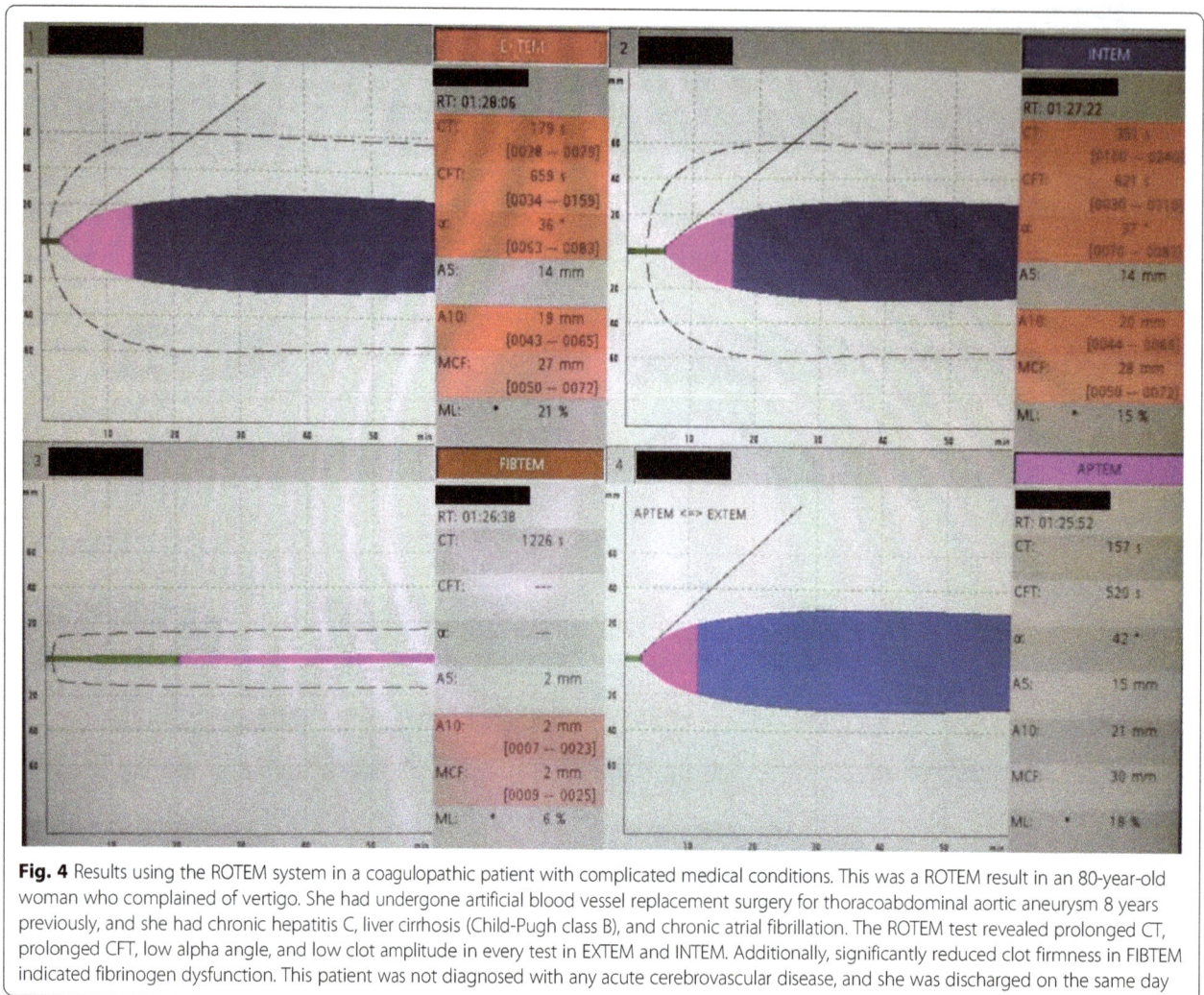

Fig. 4 Results using the ROTEM system in a coagulopathic patient with complicated medical conditions. This was a ROTEM result in an 80-year-old woman who complained of vertigo. She had undergone artificial blood vessel replacement surgery for thoracoabdominal aortic aneurysm 8 years previously, and she had chronic hepatitis C, liver cirrhosis (Child-Pugh class B), and chronic atrial fibrillation. The ROTEM test revealed prolonged CT, prolonged CFT, low alpha angle, and low clot amplitude in every test in EXTEM and INTEM. Additionally, significantly reduced clot firmness in FIBTEM indicated fibrinogen dysfunction. This patient was not diagnosed with any acute cerebrovascular disease, and she was discharged on the same day

Platelets bind to collagen on the inner surface of the simulated blood vessel via von Willebrand factor (VWF) to generate shear stress. Platelets activated by shear stress aggregate and trigger thrombus formation in cooperation with fibrinogen and VWF. Figure 6 shows the actual monitor during measurement with a PL-chip. Figure 7 shows the actual monitor during measurement with an AR-chip. The built-in software for analyzing thrombus formation, T-TAS® Zia (Fig. 8), allows us to observe thrombus formation in a simulated vessel of the AR-chip in detail.

In other tests using POC devices and routine coagulation tests in clinical laboratories such as PT and APTT, a coagulation accelerant is directly added and mixed with the whole blood or plasma sample. On the other hand, in the T-TAS® system, collagen or tissue factor that had been coated on the inner surface of a simulated blood vessel activates platelets or the coagulation system in a part of the whole blood sample and then triggers physiological thrombus formation.

We discovered the change in coagulation function of a patient before and after the patient received hyperbaric oxygen therapy (HBOT) [24]. Figure 9 shows a graph of HBOT significantly reduced the clot formation ability of whole blood.

Viscoelastic devices in the guidelines for the treatment of traumatic coagulopathy in the USA and Europe

The importance of taking into consideration traumatic coagulopathy in the treatment strategy of trauma patients in Europe can be understood from the title of the European guidelines for the treatment of trauma patients. We showed only part of monitoring with viscoelastic devices. Please check other authors' comments to help the understanding for full guideline. And a European guideline is mentioning as which use is being just recommended, but an American guideline is mentioned until an in-depth numerical analysis. The title of the guidelines published in 2007 [25] was "Management of bleeding

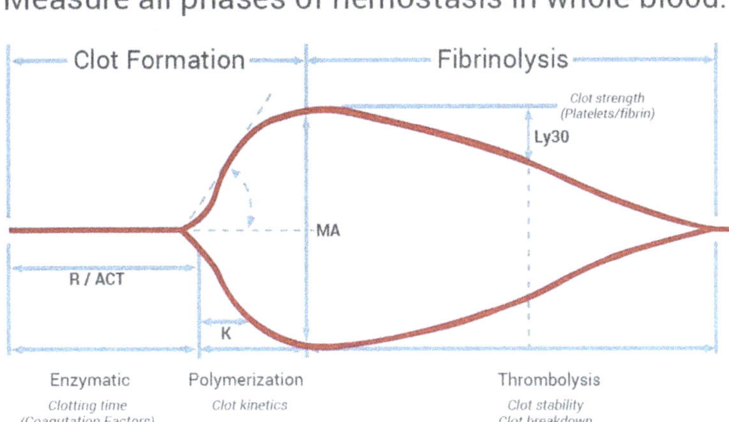

Fig. 5 Example of TEG findings. The typical presentation of measurement data obtained by TEG® is shown. The data are displayed in a graph in which the horizontal axis is time (min) and the vertical axis is clot firmness, similar to the ROTEM® system. Parameters are the duration from the start of the measurement to the beginning of clotting (*R*-time), duration from the beginning of clotting to the time when the amplitude of clot firmness reaches 20 mm (*K*-time), clot firmness (MA) and the fibrinolytic index (LY30)

following major trauma: the European guidelines," whereas that published in 2013 [26] was "Management of bleeding and coagulopathy following major trauma: updated European guidelines"; the word "coagulopathy" was added to the title of the more recent guidelines, indicating the growing importance of taking into consideration coagulopathy in the treatment strategy of trauma. The guidelines published in 2013 mentioned that viscoelastic devices were beneficial for establishing the treatment strategy and assessing the status of coagulopathy in patients with hemorrhagic shock (grade 1C). Judging from the description in the European guidelines, the importance of viscoelastic devices in understanding the disease condition of patients with traumatic coagulopathy has been widely recognized in Europe.

In the USA, the ACS TQIP Massive Transfusion in Trauma Guidelines proposed by the American College of Surgeons in 2013 presented the test results obtained by the viscoelastic devices, TEG® 5000 and ROTEM®, as the standard for transfusion or injection of blood plasma, cryoprecipitate, platelet concentrate, or anti-fibrinolytic agents in the treatment strategy for traumatic coagulopathy and hemorrhagic shock [27]. This description indicates that the clinical application of viscoelastic device is more widespread in the USA than in Japan. The guidelines proposed cutoff points using test values obtained by TEG® that indicate the need for transfusion or infusion as follows: plasma replacement if the duration from the start of measurement to the beginning of clotting (*R*-time) > 9 s; administration of plasma or cryoprecipitate (fibrinogen

Table 1 Comparisons of various parameters between TEG® and ROTEM®

TEG	ROTEM	Interpretation of the finding
R (reaction time)	CT (clotting time)	Time to initiation of clot formation
	A (amplitude)	Viscoelasticity of the blood clot. Reflecting the function and counts of platelet and fibrinogen about thrombogenicity of fibrin clot.
K (clot kinetics)	CFT (clot formation time)	Time from starting of blood clotting to the clot amplitude reaches at 20 mm. Reflecting the speed of clot polymerization.
α	*α* (alpha angle)	Rate of increase of clot amplitude. Reflecting the speed of fibrin clot.
MA (maximum amplitude)	MCF (maximum clot firmness)	Maximum of amplitude. Reflecting the clot strength.
TMA (time to maximum amplitude)		Time to maximum amplitude. Reflecting the clot formation time.
LY	LI (lysis index)	Rate of decrease of clot amplitude. Reflecting the degree of fibrinolytic activity.
CLT (clot lysis time)		Time from maximum to minimum of clot amplitude. Reflecting the degree of fibrinolysis.
	ML (maximum lysis)	Maximum rate of decrease of clot amplitude to MCF.

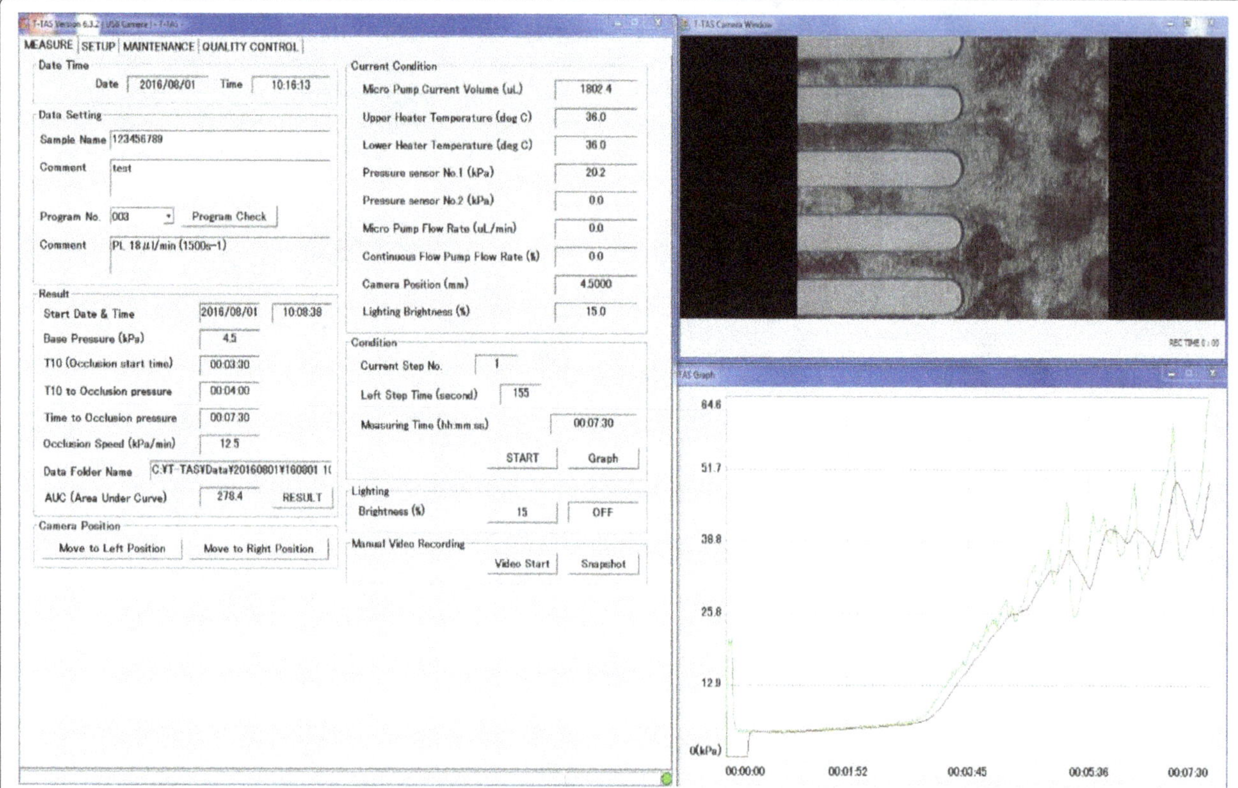

Fig. 6 Display screen during measurement with a PL-chip in the T-TAS system. The *left window* shows the measurement conditions such as flow rate of blood and temperature in the simulated vessel. The status of blood flowing can be observed in the *upper right window*. The *lower right window* shows a graph presenting the time course of thrombus formation. Blood flowing in a simulated blood vessel taken by a microcamera can be observed in real time in the *upper right window*. The *lower right window* shows a graph presenting the time course of thrombus formation in which the horizontal axis is time and the vertical axis is the measured pressure. This graph allows us to observe the process of thrombus formation visually. The *left window* shows the measured numerical data and measurement conditions. Measurement conditions are the flow rate of blood flowing in the simulated vessel and the temperature in the vessel, and these flowing conditions can be set freely. Therefore, this device allows us to simulate thrombus formation in various blood vessels in the body. Another chip, the AR-chip, has a built-in simulated blood vessel in which the inner lumen is coated with collagen and tissue factor. After adding Ca^{++} in the simulated vessel, citrated whole blood is activated by the collagen and tissue factor. Then, a very firm thrombus is formed by activated platelets and coagulation factors. Therefore, the AR-chip enables us to assess the cooperative capacity of platelets and the coagulation system in thrombus formation

preparation) if the duration from the beginning of clotting to the time when the amplitude of clot firmness reaches 20 mm (*K*-time) > 9 s; administration of cryoprecipitate (or fibrinogen preparation) or plasma if *α* angle <60°; administration of platelet concentrate if the maximum amplitude (MA) < 55 mm; and injection of anti-fibrinolytic agents such as tranexamic acid if the fibrinolytic index (LY30) is >7.5%. The cutoff points using rapid TEG® that indicate the need for transfusion or infusion are as follows: plasma replacement if ACT > 128 s; administration of plasma or cryoprecipitate (fibrinogen preparation) preparations if *K*-time > 2.5 s; administration of cryoprecipitate (or fibrinogen preparation) or plasma if *α* angle <60°; administration of platelet concentrate if MA < 55 mm; and administration of anti-fibrinolytic agents such as tranexamic acid if LY30 > 3%. On the other hand, cutoff points using test values obtained using ROTEM® that indicate the need for transfusion or infusion are as follows: plasma replacement if clotting time >100 s with EXTEM and/or if clotting time >230 s with INTEM; administration of cryoprecipitate (fibrinogen preparation) and/or plasma if MCF < 8 mm with FIBTEM; administration of platelet concentrate if MCF < 45 mm with EXTEM and MCF > 10 mm with FIBTEM; and administration of fibrinolytic agents such as tranexamic acid if ML > 15% with EXTEM.

Reports on the relationship between the use of viscoelastic devices and the outcome of trauma

Treatment outcome has been considered as an index of the usefulness of information obtained by viscoelastic devices for acute-phase treatment of trauma. There have been a number of reports on the relationship between the test results obtained by viscoelastic devices and outcome in trauma patients [28–31]. One study reported that mortality was 100% in patients manifesting fulminant hyperfibrinolysis with a mean injury severity score (ISS) of

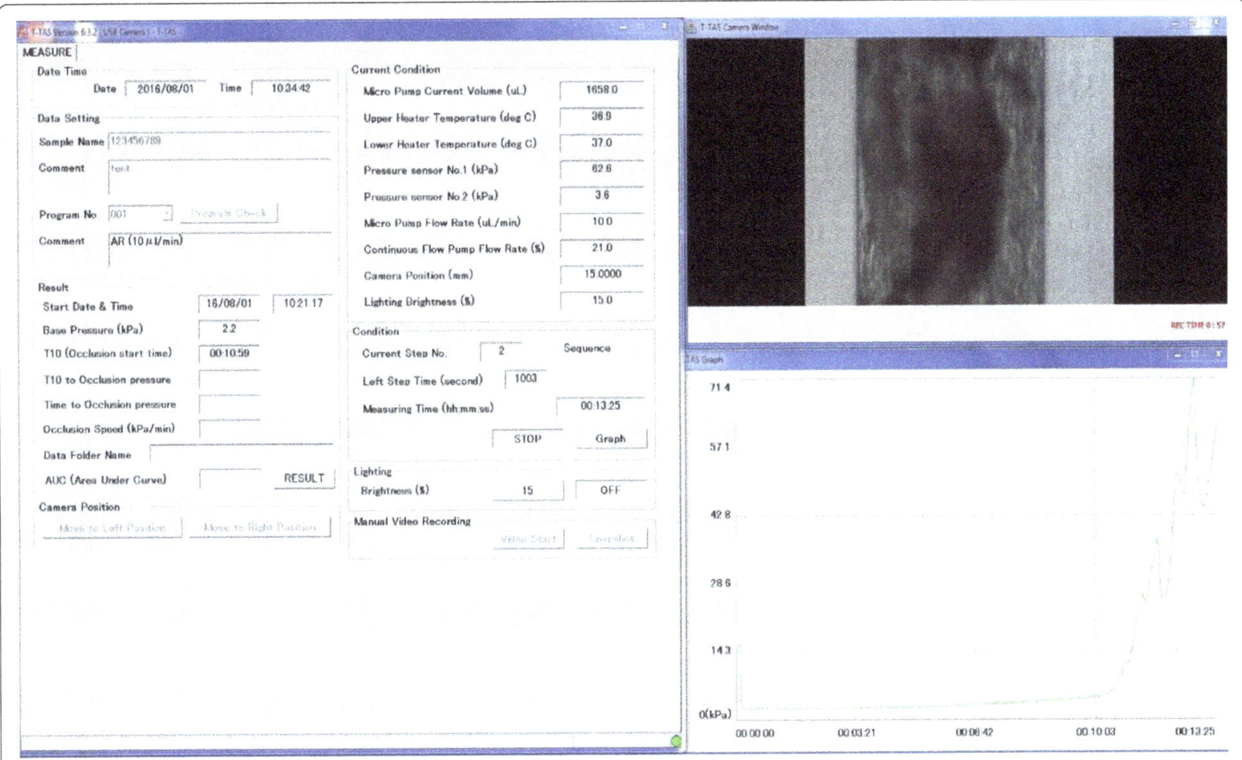

Fig. 7 Display screen during measurement with an AR-chip in the T-TAS system. The configuration of the screen is similar to that shown in Fig. 6

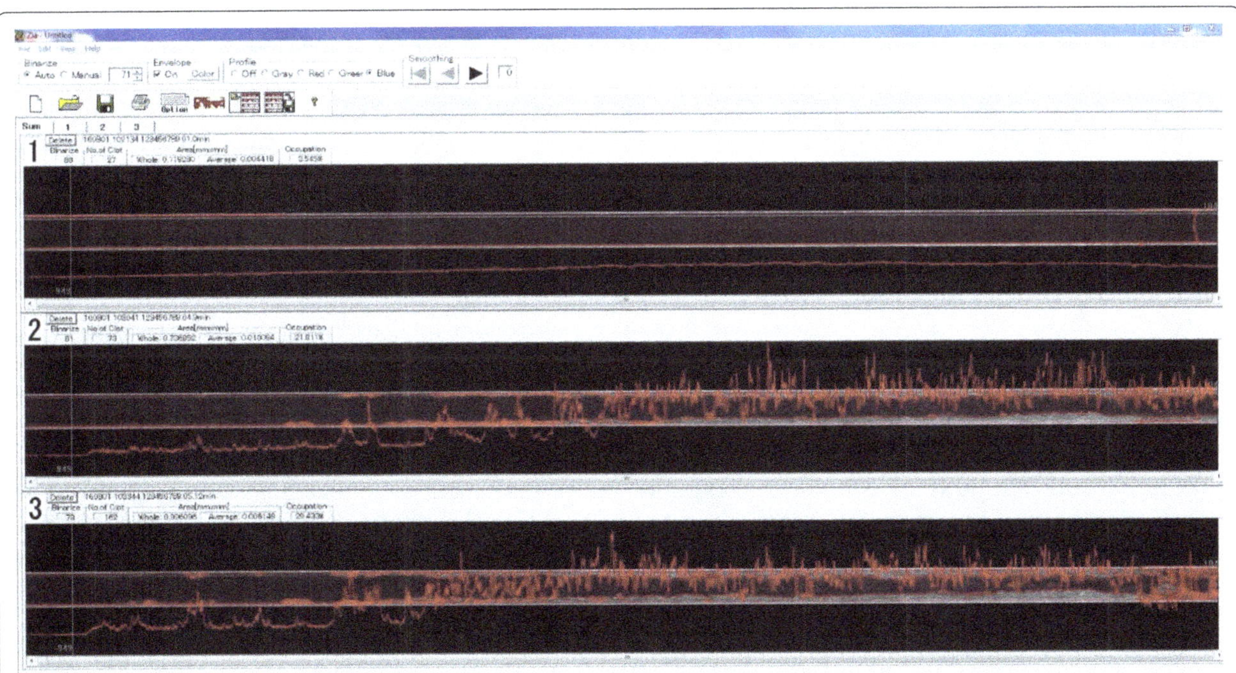

Fig. 8 Display screen of T-TAS Zia®. T-TAS Zia® is the built-in software that can analyze thrombus conditions in detail (thrombus formation in the PL-chip can also be analyzed with the software in the most recent model, T-TAS plus®)

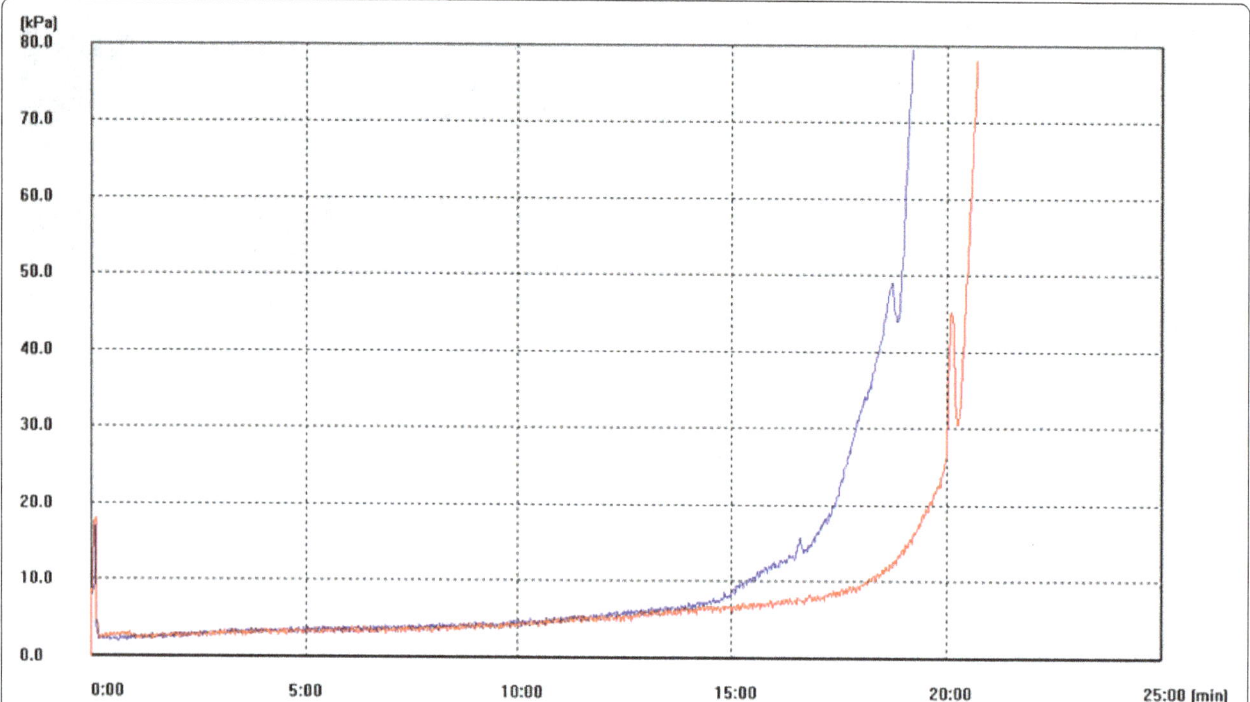

Fig. 9 T-TAS® measurement of thrombus formation in a patient who underwent HBOT. The *blue line* represents the result obtained before HBOT, and the *red line* represents the result obtained after HBOT. After HBOT, the coagulation function decreased

48 [32]. It was also reported that abnormalities of R and MA values measured by TEG® were independent predictive factors for poor outcome [33–36]. It has been demonstrated that prolongation of CFT and a decrease in MCF which indicate a decrease in platelet count measured by ROTEM® were correlated more strongly with poor outcome than with mortality calculated with the Trauma and Injury Severity Score (TRISS) equation [32, 37]. It has been reported that a decrease in fibrinogen level which is detectable in the early stage of coagulopathy was also correlated with poor outcome, suggesting the use of fibrinogen level as the standard for administration of cryoprecipitate and fibrinogen preparations [30]. The study also reported improved survival with infusion and transfusion based on the measurement of the fibrinogen level.

Abnormal findings in platelet mapping analysis with TEG® that represented reduced platelet function were frequently observed among patients who died of head injury [38]. It was also reported that the outcome was better in patients in a hypercoagulable state than in patients in a hypocoagulable state [31].

Algorithms for trauma care using viscoelastic devices

A specific algorithm for transfusion strategy in trauma patients based on test results obtained with ROTEM® was reported from Parkland Memorial Hospital in 2015, indicating the current spread of viscoelastic devices in clinical practice in the USA [39]. In this algorithm, patients were treated as follows: If ML was prolonged with EXTEM, the patient was judged to have hyperfibrinolysis and tranexamic acid was administered as antifibrinolytic treatment. If the clotting time was prolonged with EXTEM, the patient was judged to have reduced coagulability, and a plasma preparation was administered. If the amplitude was reduced with FIBTEM, the patient was judged to have fibrinogen dysfunction and cryoprecipitate or a fibrinogen preparation was administered. If the amplitude was not reduced, the patient was judged to have platelet dysfunction and platelet concentrate was transfused.

On the other hand, Yin et al. [40] reported a goal-directed transfusion protocol based on the results of TEG® in patients with abdominal trauma in Nanjing Hospital, China, in 2014. If the *R* value that represents the time to early clot formation was prolonged, fresh frozen plasma was administered and its dose was decided according to the degree of prolongation. If the α angle which is the angle of slope at 20 mm in amplitude and represents the rate of fibrin cross-linkage is depressed, the patient was considered to have fibrinogen dysfunction and cryoprecipitate was additionally administered after fresh frozen plasma infusion. If the α angle was normal but MA which represents the strength of the blood clot was reduced, the patient was considered to have platelet dysfunction or a coagulopathy, and platelet concentrate or recombinant factor VII was administered. Several studies conducted in other countries reported the use of viscoelastic devices in trauma care and demonstrated their usefulness for the assessment of traumatic coagulopathy [32, 35, 41–44].

These viscoelastic devices will become an important tool for establishing the treatment strategy in trauma care patients in Japan in the future.

However, some studies have reported limitations of these viscoelastic devices. A review in the Cochrane Library published in 2015 pointed out the presence of biases in the abovementioned reports in trauma patients and the absence of a quality study in this field thus far [45]. The review concluded that PT and INR are the most reliable parameters for monitoring traumatic coagulopathy although these parameters are not perfect. Thus, it mentioned that POC tests should be done with devices used in clinical laboratories because the way of processing was not established for hardly interpretable results obtained with POC devices. At present, the usefulness of viscoelastic devices has been demonstrated only for control of intraoperative bleeding in cardiac surgery, and there has not been favorable evidence for the usefulness of POC devices for transplantation control and improvement of outcomes in trauma patients with other pathologies [46]. To make good use of POC devices in establishing the treatment strategy for patients with traumatic coagulopathy in the future, it is necessary to compare the results obtained from POC devices with the results of PT and INR obtained by laboratory devices. In addition, it may be necessary to clarify and solve the problems of measurement using POC devices and to verify the usefulness of viscoelasticity as a supplementary test item after understanding its characteristics in clinical application.

Conclusions

Viscoelastic devices will become an important tool in establishing the treatment strategy in trauma care patients in the future. However, some studies have reported limitations of these viscoelastic devices. A quality study on the relationship between traumatic coagulopathy and the results obtained with viscoelastic devices is needed.

Abbreviations

ACT: Activated clotting time; DCS: Damage control surgery; POC: Point-of-care; PT: Prothrombin time

Funding

There was no funding for this review report.

Authors' contributions

SY, KH, and MT wrote the manuscript. All authors read and approved the final manuscript.

Competing interests

SY has received speaking fees from Asahi Kasei.

References

1. MacLeod JBA, Lynn M, McKenney MG, Cohn SM, Murtha M. Early coagulopathy predicts mortality in trauma. J Trauma. 2003;55:39–44.
2. Bolliger D, Gorlinger K, Tanaka KA. Pathophysiology and treatment of coagulopathy in massive hemorrhage and hemodilution. Anesthesiology. 2010;113:1205–19.
3. Wohlauer MV, Moore EE, Droz NM, Harr J, Gonzalez E, Fragoso MF, et al. Hemodilution is not critical in the pathogenesis of the acute coagulopathy of trauma. J Surg Res. 2012;173:26–30.
4. Winstedt D, Thomas OD, Nilsson F, Olanders K, Schott U. Correction of hypothermic and dilutional coagulopathy with concentrates of fibrinogen and factor XIII: an in vitro study with ROTEM. Scand J Trauma Resusc Emerg Med. 2014;22:73.
5. Brohi K, Cohen MJ, Davenport RA. Acute coagulopathy of trauma: mechanism, identification and effect. Curr Opin Crit Care. 2007;13:680–5.
6. Germanos S, Gourgiotis S, Villias C, Bertucci M, Dimopoulos N, Salemis N. Damage control surgery in the abdomen: an approach for the management of severe injured patients. Int J Surg. 2008;6:246–52.
7. Rotondo MF, Schwab CW, McGonigal MD, Phillips GR, Fruchterman TM, Kauder DR, et al. 'Damage control': an approach for improved survival in exsanguination penetrating abdominal injury. J Trauma. 1993;35:375–82.
8. Davenport R, Manson J, De'Ath H, Platton S, Coates A, Allard S, et al. Functional definition and characterization of acute traumatic coagulopathy. Crit Care Med. 2011;39:2652–8.
9. Brummel KE, Paradis SG, Butenas S, Mann KG. Thrombin functions during tissue factor-induced blood coagulation. Blood. 2002;100:148–52.
10. Martini WZ, Cortez DS, Dubick MA, Park MS, Holcomb JB. Thrombelastography is better than PT, aPTT, and activated clotting time in detecting clinically relevant clotting abnormalities after hypothermia, hemorrhagic shock and resuscitation in pigs. J Trauma. 2008;65:535–43.
11. Hartert H. Blutgerinnungsstudien mit der Thrombelastographie, einem neuen Untersuchungsverfahren. Klin Wochenschr. 1948;26:577–83.
12. Jeger V, Zimmermann H, Exadaktylos AK. Can RapidTEG accelerate the search for coagulopathies in the patient with multiple injuries? J Trauma. 2009;66:1253–7.
13. Kang YG, Martin DJ, Marquez J, Lewis JH, Bontempo FA, Shaw BW, et al. Intraoperative changes in blood coagulation and thrombelastographic monitoring in liver transplantation. Anesth Analg. 1985;64:888–96.
14. Whiting D, DiNardo JA. TEG and ROTEM: technology and clinical applications. Am J Hematol. 2014;89:228–32.
15. Sankarankutty A, Nascimento B, da Luz LT, Rizoli S. TEG and ROTEM in trauma: similar test but different results? World J Emerg Surg. 2012;7 Suppl 1:S3.
16. Katori N, Tanaka KA, Szlam F, Levy JH. The effects of platelet count on clot retraction and tissue plasminogen activator-induced fibrinolysis on thromboelastography. Anesth Analg. 2005;100:1781–5.
17. Koami H, Sakamoto Y, Ohta M, Goto A, Narumi S, Imahase H, et al. Can rotational thromboelastometry predict septic DIC? Blood Coagul Fibrinolysis. 2015;26:778–83.
18. Koami H, Sakamoto Y, Sakurai R, Ohta M, Imahase H, Yahata M, et al. The thromboelastometric discrepancy between septic and trauma induced disseminated intravascular coagulation diagnosed by the scoring system from the Japanese Association for Acute Medicine. Medicine. 2016;95:e4514.
19. Koami H, Sakamoto Y, Furukawa T, Imahase H, Iwamura T, Inoue S. Utility of rotational thromboelastometry (ROTEM) for the diagnosis of asymptomatic hyperfibrinolysis secondary to anaphylaxis. Blood Coagul Fibrinolysis. 2016;27:450–3.
20. Koami H, Sakamoto Y, Sakurai R, Ohta M, Goto A, Imahase H, et al. Utility of measurement of serum lactate in diagnosis of coagulopathy associated with peripheral circulatory insufficiency: retrospective evaluation using thromboelastometry from a single center in Japan. J Nippon Med Sch. 2016;83:150–7.

hyperfibrinolysis secondary to anaphylaxis. Blood Coagul Fibrinolysis. 2016;27:450–3.

20. Koami H, Sakamoto Y, Sakurai R, Ohta M, Goto A, Imahase H, et al. Utility of measurement of serum lactate in diagnosis of coagulopathy associated with peripheral circulatory insufficiency: retrospective evaluation using thromboelastometry from a single center in Japan. J Nippon Med Sch. 2016;83:150–7.
21. Yamaguchi Y, Moriki T, Igari A, Matsubara Y, Ohnishi T, Hosokawa K, et al. Studies of a microchip flow-chamber system to characterize whole blood thrombogenicity in healthy individuals. Thromb Res. 2013;132:263–70.
22. Hosokawa K, Ohnishi T, Fukasawa M, Kondo T, Sameshima H, Koide T, et al. A microchip flow-chamber system for quantitative assessment of the platelet thrombus formation process. Microvasc Res. 2012;83:154–61.
23. Hosokawa K, Ohnishi T, Kondo T, Fukasawa M, Koide T, Maruyama I. A novel automated microchip flow-chamber system to quantitatively evaluate thrombus formation and antithrombotic agents under blood flow conditions. J Thromb Haemost. 2011;9:2029–37.
24. Miike T, Sakamoto Y, Sakurai R, Ohta M, Goto A, Imahase H, et al. Effects of hyperbaric exposure on thrombus formation. Undersea Hyperb Med. 2016;43:233–8.
25. Spahn DR, Cerny V, Coats TJ, Duranteau J, Fernandez-Mondejar E, Gordini G, et al. Management of bleeding following major trauma: a European guideline. Crit Care. 2007;11:R17.
26. Spahn DR, Bouillon B, Cerny V, Coats TJ, Duranteau J, Fernandez-Mondejar E, et al. Management of bleeding and coagulopathy following major trauma: an updated European guideline. Crit Care. 2013;17:R76.
27. Camazine MN, Hemmila MR, Leonard JC, Jacobs RA, Horst JA, Kozar RA, et al. Massive transfusion policies at trauma centers participating in the American College of Surgeons Trauma Quality Improvement Program. J Trauma Acute Care Surg. 2015;78:S48–53.
28. Da Luz LT, Nascimento B, Shankarakutty AK, Rizoli S, Adhikari NKJ. Effect of thromboelastography (TEG®) and rotational thromboelastometry (ROTEM®) on diagnosis of coagulopathy, transfusion guidance and mortality in trauma: descriptive systematic review. Crit Care. 2014;18:518.
29. Schochl H, Frietsch T, Pavelka M, Jambor C. Hyperfibrinolysis after major trauma: differential diagnosis of lysis patterns and prognostic value of thrombelastometry. J Trauma. 2009;67:125–31.
30. Levy JH, Welsby I, Goodnough LT. Fibrinogen as a therapeutic target for bleeding: a review of critical levels and replacement therapy. Transfusion. 2014;54:1389–405.
31. Carroll RC, Craft RM, Langdon RJ, Clanton CR, Snider CC, Wellons DD, Dakin PA, Lawson CM, Enderson BL, Kurek SJ. Early evaluation of acute traumatic coagulopathy by thrombelastography. Transl Res. 2009;154:34–9.
32. Park MS, Salinas J, Wade CE, Wang J, Martini W, Pusateri AE, Merrill GA, Chung K, Wolf SE, Holcomb JB. Combining early coagulation and inflammatory status improves prediction of mortality in burned and nonburned trauma patients. J Trauma. 2008;64:S188–94.
33. Nystrup KB, Windeløv NA, Thomsen AB, Johansson PI. Reduced clot strength upon admission, evaluated by thrombelastography (TEG®), in trauma patients is independently associated with increased 30-day mortality. Scand J Trauma Resusc Emerg Med. 2011;19:52.
34. Kornblith LZ, Kutcher ME, Redick BJ, Calfee CS, Vilardi RF, Cohen MJ. Fibrinogen and platelet contributions to clot formation: implications for trauma resuscitation and thromboprophylaxis. J Trauma Acute Care Surg. 2014;76:255–63.
35. Schöchl H, Frietsch T, Pavelka M, Jambor C. Hyperfibrinolysis after major trauma: differential diagnosis of lysis patterns and prognostic value of thromboelastometry. J Trauma. 2009;67:125–31.
36. Tauber H, Innerhofer P, Breitkopf R, Westermann I, Beer R, El Attal R, Strasak A, Mittermayr M. Prevalence and impact of abnormal ROTEM® assays in severe blunt trauma: results of the 'Diagnosis and Treatment of Trauma-Induced Coagulopathy (DIA-TRE-TIC) study'. Br J Anaesth. 2011;107:378–87.
37. Collins PW, Solomon C, Sutor K, Crispin D, Hochleitner G, Rizoli S, et al. Theoretical modelling of fibrinogen supplementation with therapeutic plasma, cryoprecipitate, or fibrinogen concentrate. Br J Anaesth. 2014;113:585–95.
38. Davis PK, Musunuru H, Walsh M, Cassady R, Yount R, Losiniecki A, Moore EE, Wohlauer MV, Howard J, Ploplis VA, Castellino FJ, Thomas SG. Platelet dysfunction is an early marker for traumatic brain injury-induced coagulopathy. Neurocrit Care. 2013;18:201–8.
39. Abdelfattah K, Cripps MW. Thromboelastography and rotational thromboelastometry use in trauma. Int J Surg. 2016;33:196–201.
40. Yin J, Zhao Z, Li Y, Wang J, Yao D, Zhang S, et al. Goal-directed transfusion protocol via thrombelastography in patients with abdominal trauma: a retrospective study. World J Emerg Surg. 2014;9:28.
41. Jansen JO, Luke D, Davies E, Spencer P, Kirkman E, Midwinter MJ. Temporal changes in ROTEM®-measured coagulability of citrated blood samples from coagulopathic trauma patients. Injury. 2013;44:36–9.
42. Schochl H, Cotton B, Inaba K, Nienaber U, Fischer H, Voelckel W, et al. FIBTEM provides early prediction of massive transfusion in trauma. Crit Care. 2011;15:R265.
43. Scholchl H, Nienaber U, Hofer G, Voelckel W, Jambor C, Scharbert G, et al. Goal-directed coagulation management of major trauma patients using thromboelastometry (ROTEM®)-guided administration of fibrinogen concentrate and prothrombin complex concentrate. Crit Care. 2010;14:R55.
44. Tanaka KA, Bolliger D, Vadlamudi R, Nimmo A. Rotational thromboelastometry (ROTEM)-based coagulation management in cardiac surgery and major trauma. J Cardiothorac Vasc Anesth. 2012;26:1083–93.
45. Hunt H, Stanworth S, Curry N, Woolley T, Cooper C, Ukoumunne O, et al. Thromboelastography (TEG) and rotational thromboelastometry (ROTEM) for trauma induced coagulopathy in adult trauma patients with bleeding. Cochrane Database Syst Rev. 2015;2:CD010438.
46. Levi M, Hunt BJ. A critical appraisal of point-of care coagulation testing in critically ill patients. J Thromb Haemost. 2015;13:1960–7.

14

Lung ultrasound—a primary survey of the acutely dyspneic patient

Francis Chun Yue Lee[1,2]

Abstract

There has been an explosion of knowledge and application of clinical lung ultrasound (LUS) in the last decade. LUS has important applications in the ambulatory, emergency, and critical care settings and its deployability for immediate bedside assessment allows many acute lung conditions to be diagnosed and early interventional decisions made in a matter of minutes. This review detailed the scientific basis of LUS, the examination techniques, and summarises the current applications in several acute lung conditions. It is to be hoped that clinicians, after reviewing the evidence within this article, would see LUS as an important first-line modality in the primary evaluation of an acutely dyspneic patient.

Keywords: Lung ultrasound, A-lines, B-lines, Z-lines, I-lines, Curtain sign

Abbreviations: ACPE, Acute cardiogenic pulmonary edema; ARDS, Acute respiratory distress syndrome; COPD, Chronic obstructive pulmonary disease; CXR, Chest X-rays; LUS, Lung ultrasound; MHz, Megahertz; SLF, Sonographic lung field

Background

Lung ultrasound (LUS) is an effective and sensitive tool compared to the traditional chest auscultation and chest X-rays [1–3]. Its use as a primary survey tool in the acutely dyspneic or hypoxemic patient gives an immediate understanding of the state of the lung and influences therapeutic decisions. Proper LUS practise requires the following: the understanding of pathophysiology of acute lung conditions; the sonographic features they produce; and the ability to elucidate the LUS signs in the clinical context of the patient.

Lung ultrasound examination

LUS examination is best performed with a low frequency transducer (3–5 MHz), such as the commonly available curvilinear transducer, set to a study depth of about 12–18 cm (depending on body habitus). Microconvex transducers have the additional advantage of a smaller footprint for better intercostal imaging and application in younger patients. High-frequency transducers are helpful for the search of lung comets and detailed visualisation of pleural layers and small subpleural lesions. The phased-array transducer for echocardiographic applications could be used, but defining near field pathology such as consolidation or atelectasis would be a challenge.

Filters, such as compounding and harmonic imaging, cancel off artifacts and noise; is unhelpful in LUS; and should be turned off. The rest of this article will introduce LUS signs that are identifiable with the first two types of transducers mentioned above.

The transducer should be applied onto the chest wall in the longitudinal cranial-caudal plane, straddling across the intercostal space, with the marker oriented towards the head. All the images; with the exception of image B in Fig. 2, which is a transverse study; presented in this article are studies in the cranial-caudal axis with the left side of image oriented towards the head.

LUS examination is performed with the patient in the supine or reclined position, starting with right anterior chest, followed by the right lateral chest, and ends with a careful examination of the lower lung and the costophrenic recesses (in this article, the term "lung base" will be used to denote these two areas); this is repeated on the left side. The posterior lung should also be examined with the

Correspondence: Lee.francis@alexandrahealth.com.sg
[1]Acute and Emergency Care Centre, Khoo Teck Puat Hospital, Singapore, Singapore
[2]Yong Loo Lin School of Medicine, National University of Singapore, Singapore, Singapore

patient turned or in the sitting position. During LUS examination, the transducer should be held still for a few seconds observation, avoiding unnecessary movements. Care must be taken to keep the probe perpendicular to the chest wall during scanning. Excessive tilting or angulation may orientate the ultrasound beam out of the plane of the lung, producing uninterpretable images; this is especially a problem at the clavipectoral triangle and axillary area.

There are several approaches to studying, documenting and communicating LUS findings. At the author's centre, each hemithorax is divided into six sectors for study (Fig. 1 and Table 1). Other methods, dividing the chest into sectors or quadrants [4, 5]; using the anatomical lines [6] as a guide; and marking three key scanning points on the chest [7] have been proposed.

Regardless of the study convention used, thorough scanning is important. This must include the posterior lung and the lung bases, as acute disease processes commonly start in these areas.

Basic lung signs

Pleural line—the starting point

Identification of the pleural line is the first step in LUS. It is important to start with the transducer positioned in a longitudinal plane (cranio-caudal axis), straddled across the intercostal space and the ribs. The ribs will serve as a guide to the correct identification of the pleural line and avoid confusion with hyperechoic lines cast by tissue planes (Fig. 2); and for this reason, the transverse oriented study is not recommended as a start. Without visualising the pleural line, one cannot be certain that the lung is being examined. The area below the pleural line and between the acoustic shadows cast by the ribs is the sonographic lung field (SLF), the focus of LUS examination.

Lung sliding

The first question in LUS evaluation is whether there is lung sliding. In the normal lung, where the visceral and parietal pleural are closely applied and slides with respiration, an artifact known as lung sliding is generated. This appears as an actual movement, shimmering or flickering at the pleural line, depending on how the transducer beam interacts with the pleural line. Lung sliding may be subtle: at the end of the respiratory cycle; near the apex of the lung which has much less respiratory excursion; in clinical situations of hypopnea and bradypnea. The subject should be asked to take deliberate breaths to overcome this problem; otherwise, the operator should patiently observe the pleural line. The key to lung sliding observation is to train the eyes on the pleural line and not be distracted by other disturbances such as chest wall movements.

The appearance of lung air on ultrasound

Air has low acoustic impedance to ultrasound. When ultrasound traverses from tissue to air, the large acoustic impedance mismatch causes 99 % of the ultrasound to be reflected, resulting in a hyperechoic image in the SLF (Fig. 3). In the backdrop of this image, a number of LUS artifacts have been described and classified using an alphabetical system [8, 9]. Four basic artifacts of fundamental

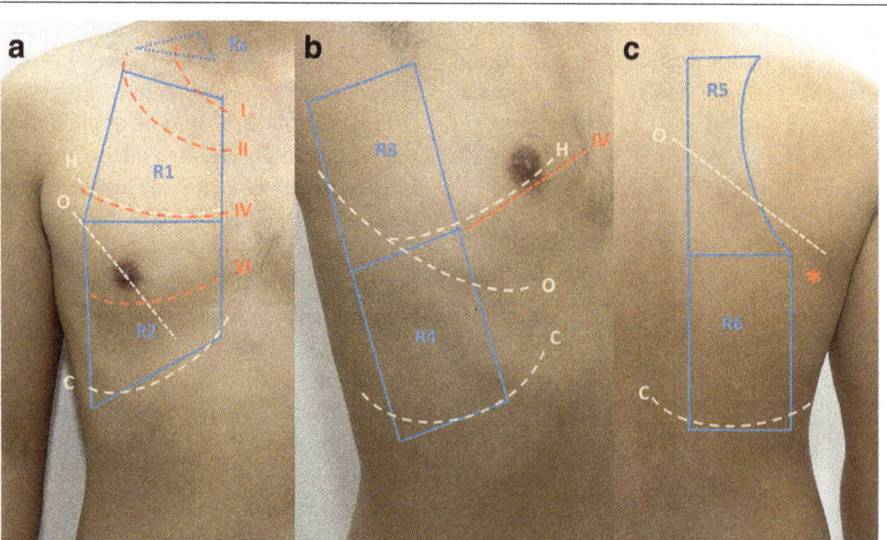

Fig. 1 Scanning sectors (as used at the author's centre). Zones on the right hemithorax. **a** *R1* right anterior upper zone, *R2* right anterior lower zone, *Rs* right supraclavicular fossa **b** *R3* right lateral axilla zone, *R4* right lateral lower zone **c** *R5* right posterior upper zone *R6* right posterior lower zone. *I, II, III, IV* first, second, third, fourth ribs, respectively, *H* horizontal fissure, *O* oblique fissure, *C* costophrenic recess, lowest limit of LUS study where curtain sign is found, *inferior angle of scapula

Table 1 Detailed descriptions of scanning sectors in LUS

Chest	Sector	Boundaries	Anatomical/study significance
Anterior	R1 or Ll (anterior upper)	Upper: clavicle; lower: 4th rib; medial: sternal edge; lateral: defined by LUS image of lung; beyond this border are contents of the axilla and clavipectoral triangle	• Horizontal fissure is in line with the 4th rib; therefore, this zone contains the upper lobe of the lung
	R2 or L2 (anterior lower)	Upper: 4th rib; lower: variable, depending on body habitus and defined by curtain sign in LUS and appearance of abdominal contents;liver on the right side, bowel and spleen on the left; medial: sternal edge; lateral: anterior axillary line	• The 6th rib approximates the inferior most part of the lung and anterior insertion of diaphragm (not seen in normal LUS with curtain sign). Beyond the 6th rib is the potential space: costophrenic recess • This sector contains mainly the middle lobe; on the left lung, lingular lobe; with a small portion of the lower lobe on the lateral side • The sector on the left hemithorax is very small due to the position of the heart; no sector in cardiomegaly states
	Rs or Ls supraclavicular fossa	Triangle formed by the clavicle, lower parts of sternomastoid and trapezius	• Optional study area for the following: first rib; apical pneumothorax; pulmonary tuberculosis
Lateral	R3 or L3 lateral axilla	Upper: axilla; lower: the axis of the 4th rib; anterior: anterior axillary line; posterior: posterior axillary line	• This sector contains primarily the upper lobe of the lung with a small portion of the lower lobe
	R4 or L4 lateral lower	Upper: the axis of the 4th rib; lower: variable, depending on body habitus. Defined by curtain sign in LUS; anterior: anterior axillary line; posterior: posterior axillary line	• This sector contains primarily the lower lobe of the lung
Posterior	R5 or L5 posterior upper	Upper: defined by LUS image of the lung; medial: thoracic spine; lateral: medial border of scapula; lower: level of the inferior angle of the scapula	• This sector contains the upper lobe and lower lobe of the lung in almost equal proportion
	R6 or L6 posterior lower	Upper: level of the inferior angle of the scapula; medial: thoracic spine Lateral: posterior axillary line; lower: defined by curtain sign in LUS and appearance of abdominal contents ; liver on the right side; bowel and spleen on the left	• This sector contains primarily the lower lobe of the lung

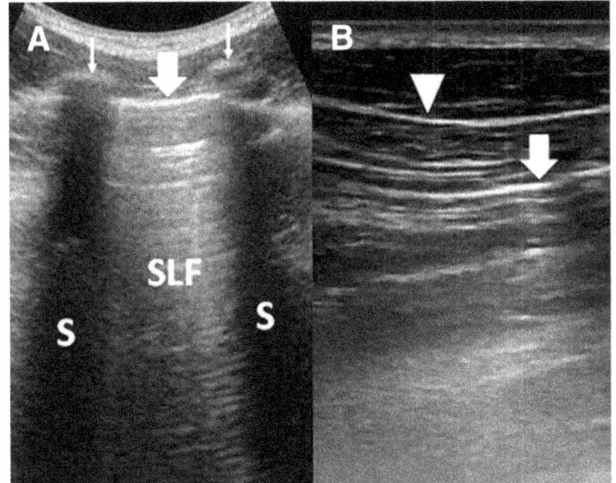

Fig. 2 Comparing two scanning planes in LUS. **a** LUS performed in the longitudinal or cranio-caudal plane showed ribs (*thin arrows*) and their acoustic shadows (*S*). Just below the level of the ribs is the pleural line (*thick arrow*) and the sonographic lung field (SLF). **b** Subcutaneous tissue lines (*arrowhead*) could be mistaken for the pleural line (*arrow*) when LUS is performed in a transverse plane, without the guidance of the rib structure

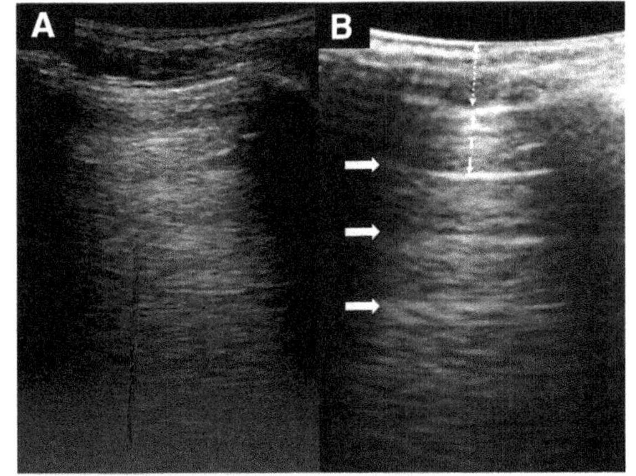

Fig. 3 Two different appearances of air in LUS. **a** A hyperehoic appearance of lung air without A-lines. **b** LUS appearance with A-lines (*solid arrows*). The distance between the A-lines (*dashed arrow*) is equal to that between the transducer and the pleural line (*dotted arrow*). A-lines, other than that indicating a strong reflector is present, have no clinical significance

importance to LUS practise, with distinct mechanism of genesis, are described below with their corresponding alphabetic nomenclature.

A-lines (repetition artifacts) When the incident ultrasound wave is perfectly perpendicular to a highly reflective surface, it will be reflected back and forth between the transducer face and the reflector (c.f. short-paths reverberations), creating repetition artifacts consisting of a series of equally spaced horizontal lines [10, 11]. The distance between each horizontal line is equal to that between the transducer and the reflector, but the strength of the images decrease with depth as energy is lost through repetitive reflections. Examples where repetition artifacts could be generated include:

- Inner layer of the trachea in airway scanning
- Needle in ultrasound guided procedures
- Trapped air bubble within a condom in transvaginal or endorectal scanning [10]

The pleural line is a strong reflector creating similar repetition artifacts. A-lines is a specific name given to these artifacts found in LUS. The significance of A-lines is simply that the ultrasound has encountered a strong reflector and in itself has no clinical meaning.

Lung comets (I-lines) In the right conditions, when ultrasound waves are trapped within small confines of tissue or structure, short-paths reverberations [10] could occur, producing short vertical artifacts that fades with increasing depth. These are the characteristics of the comet-tail artifact [12, 13] (Fig. 4). In LUS, the important type of comet-tail artifacts are the ones that start from the pleural line and move with lung sliding and this property indicates their likely origin from peripheral lung intersititia. They share similarity to B-lines (described below), albeit being short in length and weak in appearance. They are commonly referred to as lung comets or simply comet-tail artifacts (an unrefined term). The closest description of this artifact in Lichtenstein's alphabetical nomenclature is the I-lines [7, 8]. An important point to note is that lung comets (I-lines) are readily seen with high-frequency linear transducer but difficult to visualise with low frequency transducers. The presence of lung comets is a good confirmation that the two pleural layers are in contact, which is useful in excluding a pneumothorax. However, because lung comets are commonly seen in normal lung, they cannot be used in lung intersitial disease diagnosis.

Z-lines (reverberation artifacts) These artifacts could be randomly found in any part of the lungs during LUS exam and are likely to be caused by short-paths reverberations between the parietal pleural and the endothoracic fascia. Because of the extra-pulmonary location, they are often seen as static vertical artifacts which do not move with lung sliding. Z-lines do not have any clinical significance except that they could easily be misinterpreted as B-lines (Fig. 4).

B-lines (ring-down artifacts) The ring-down artifact (Fig. 4) has been shown to be generated by a bubble-

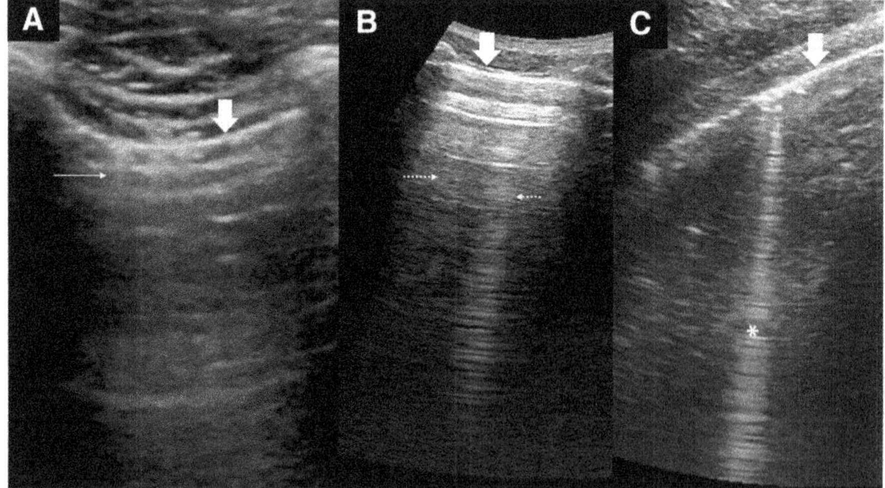

Fig. 4 Vertical artifacts in LUS. **a** Lung comet (*thin arrows*) or I-lines arising from the pleural line (*thick arrows*) as seen with a high-frequency transducer at 8.5 MHz. **b** Static reverberation artifacts or Z-lines (*dotted arrows*) within the SLF are weak images with no relationship with the pleural line (*thick arrow*) and fades with depth. **c** A strong ring-down artifact or B-line (*asterisk*) starts from the pleural line (*thick arrow*) and reaches the depths without fading. It also swings side to side with lung sliding

tetrahedron bugle mechanism [11, 14]. When a series of bubble-tetrahedron (small amount of fluid is trapped between four microbubbles) are aligned, they form a "bugle" that is able to oscillate continuously when struck by ultrasound, persistently emitting signals back to the transducer. The resulting effect is a strong vertical artifact consisting of closely spaced horizontal echoes that "ring-down" the end of the screen.

The ring-down artifact within the lungs could only arise from the subpleural interstitia, intralobular interstitia, interlobular septa, and interlobar fissures where the conditions for forming bubble-tetrahedral complexes are potentially available.

In most part of the normal lung, air predominates and the parenchyma does not provide sufficient acoustic windows to generate ring-down artifacts. In contrast, the lung bases [15] where hydrostatic pressure gives a more fluid-rich interstitia; at fissures where there is abundance of connective tissue with pulmonary vasculature, ring-down artifacts could be seen. These normal ring-down artifacts are usually thin and transient (changes with posture), and there should not be more than three within one SLF or intercostal space.

Disease processes that alter the fluid-air composition of the interstitia and alveoli provide the environment to form bubble-tetrahedron bugles and, hence, generate ring-down artifacts. Ring-down artifacts arising from the diaphragmatic pleural have also been shown to be useful in the diagnosis of pulmonary diseases [16], a sign of interstitial involvement in the lung bases as examined through the liver window. B-lines is a term used to describe ring-down artifacts found within the SLF in LUS. B-lines are technically not comet-tail artifacts contrary to popular nomenclature.

Basic LUS artifacts: a comparative summary Terms like comet-tail artifacts, lung comets, and B-lines are often used loosely and interchangeably in current LUS literature, creating some confusion and the misunderstanding. Taking reference from the mechanism of artifact generation, a comparative summary is made to help readers understand the nuances (Table 2).

Curtain sign at the lung bases—the end point

As one survey from the upper lung to the lung bases, one could appreciate that the SLF ends abruptly with a sharply demarcated edge called the curtain sign (Fig. 5). A normal curtain sign must have two characteristics. First, it must be dynamic, i.e., moves to and fro with respiration. Second, the unique anatomy of the thorax (and hence the lung) overlapping the abdomen means that the lateral diaphragm is always hidden under the curtain. Any deviation from these characteristics causes an abnormal curtain sign and should alert one that a change in the lung or pleural anatomy at the lung base has occurred. A careful review of that area is necessary to define the actual pathology.

A normal lung ultrasound study

A normal LUS study is therefore defined as

- The presence of lung sliding
- Demonstration of the typical appearance of air in the SLF of the entire lung
- The presence of the normal curtain sign at the lung bases

Lung ultrasound signs of disease

The lung can be diseased or injured in many ways but all share some common pathophysiological end points (Fig. 6). Many of these endpoints involve the alteration of air contents within the lung tissues leading to the loss of sonographic picture of air, creates new artifacts, and opens up acoustic windows for ultrasound access.

Loss of lung sliding

A loss of lung sliding occurs when there is no dynamic interaction of the parietal and visceral pleural. The possible causes are summarised in Table 3.

The M-mode is sometimes used to document the nature of lung sliding (Fig. 7). The M-mode image of the SLF is a grainy pattern of movement artifacts generated by lung sliding, in contrast to the extra-pulmonary soft tissues which presents a quiet and still linear image. This pattern is known as the "seashore sign" which indicate the presence of lung sliding. When lung sliding is absent, the M-mode does not register any disturbance at the pleural line and therefore gives a quiet trace of SLF. This pattern is called the "stratosphere" sign. In practise, lung sliding is best appreciated by careful visualisation of the pleural line rather than an M-mode study.

Conditions causing pathological B-lines

B-lines in lung diseases (Fig. 8) are caused by pathological thickening of the lung interstitia and septa. They are sensitive markers of interstitial lung involvement, appearing way before chest X-rays (CXR) changes but are non-specific as they could be seen in a myriad of acute and chronic lung conditions (Table 4). Acute interstitial syndrome [15] is a term used in the BLUE protocol [7, 17] to describe LUS findings of predominantly B-lines in the SLF.

Effusion

LUS was first used for the detection of pleural effusion [18] and is an important tool in the investigation of opacities in CXR [19]. Pleural effusion typically gives a hypoechoic zone in LUS with compressive atelectasis of

Table 2 Basic LUS artifacts: a comparative summary

	A-lines	Lung comets (I-lines)	Z-lines	B-lines
Artifact generation mechanism	Repetition: Long-paths reflections between transducer and reflector.	Reverberation: Short-paths reflections within tissue structures or materials.		Ring-down: Bubble-tetrahedron mechanism.
Characteristics	Short, repetitive equidistance horizontal lines. Fades with increasing depth.	Weak vertical artifacts comprising of irregularly spaced horizontal lines. Artifacts are often of variable length and fades with increasing depth. This is the typical description of a comet-tail artifact.		Strong narrow vertical artifact comprising of tightly spaced short horizontal lines. Artifact starts from point of origin to the end of the ultrasound screen. Does not fade with increasing depth. This is the typical description of a ring-down artifact.
Artifact generation mechanism in LUS	Ultrasound encounters the pleural line (strong reflector).	Created in the lung interstitial or in the? Interpleural layer.	Originate from an extra-pulmonary location probably between the parietal pleural and the endothoracic fascia.	Created by "thickened" lung interstitia and interlobular structures near lung surface parenchyma.
Additional characteristics in LUS	Found within SLF.	Weak vertical artifact readily found within SLF with high-frequency transducers. Similarity to B-lines: • I-lines arise from the pleural line. • Move with lung sliding/respiration. Unlike B-lines: • Short, often <2 cm.	Found within SLF • Does not appear to be related to the pleural line. • Static: does not move with lung sliding or respiration. • Blend with other background artifacts.	Found within SLF. • B-lines arise from the pleural line. • Move with lung sliding/respiration, like search lights. • Dominant over other \background artifacts (e.g., A-lines, Z-lines).
Significance	Signifies ultrasound interaction with a highly reflective surface. No diagnostic significance.	Signifies that the pleural layers are in contact. Important in pneumothorax diagnosis. As they are commonly found in the normal lung. Cannot be used for diagnosis of lung interstitial diseases.	No clinical significance. The uninitiated may mistake these for B-lines.	When more than 3 per SLF, may signify an interstitial disease process. Important in LUS diagnosis.
Mimics in LUS	Linear foreign body in subcutaneous area.	• Pockets of air in the subcutaneous tissue may give rise to reverberation artifacts, crossing the pleura lines and into the SLF. These are also called E-Lines or "emphysema lines" [8]. • Foreign body in subcutaneous area.	• Subcutaneous emphysema could generate this artifact, originating from the subcutaneous area, instead of the SLF. • Linear foreign body in subcutaneous area.	Pockets of air in the subcutaneous tissue may give rise to ring-down artifacts, crossing the pleura lines and into the SLF. These are also called E-lines in Lichtenstein's publications [7, 8].
Other common names (better terms in italics)	Reverberation artifact.	Comet-tails, *lung comets*	*Comet-tails*, lung comets	Comet-tails, lung comets

As could be seen from this matrix, many lung conditions share similar LUS signs. It is the knowledge of extent, combination, and distribution of the lung signs that will help achieve a more accurate diagnosis. Legends: bilateral—seen in both left and right lung; symmetrical—distribution pattern in left and right lungs are similar; patchy—uneven distribution within one lung where one part of the lung is involved while others spared; focal—localised to one area of the lung, one lobe or one lung; normal (for pleural line)—thin and smooth appearance; uneven—pleural line of varying thickness

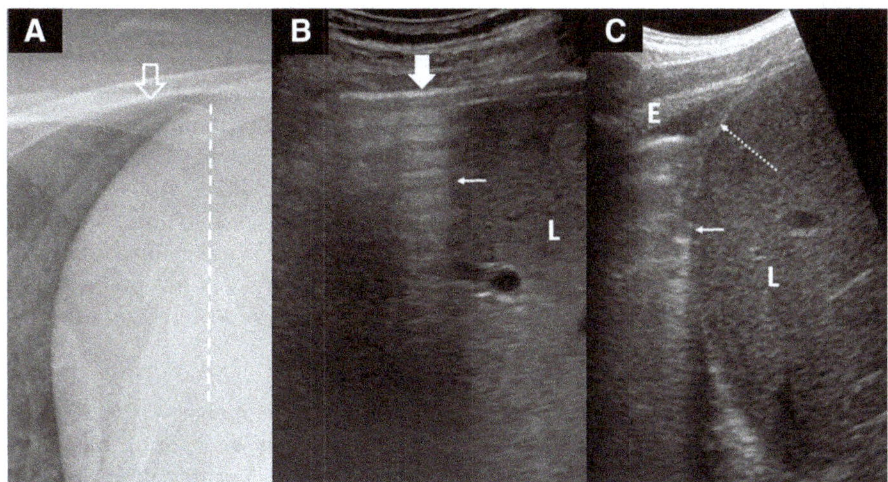

Fig. 5 Curtain sign. **a** Chest X-ray illustrates the extent (*dotted line*) to which the lower parts of the lung (*open arrow*) cover the abdomen. **b** LUS shows the pleural line (*solid arrow*) ends abruptly with an edge (*thin arrow*) forming an acoustic shadow, the "curtain sign," which slides over the liver (L) with respiration. The lateral diaphragm is always hidden by the curtain and not seen in normal LUS. **c** An example of an abnormal curtain sign: a small effusion (*E*) causing an incomplete "curtain" sign (*thin arrow*) and exposing the lateral diaphragm (*dotted arrow*)

the lung, making the visceral pleura visible (called the lung line, not pleural line). The separation of the two pleural layers also means that lung sliding is lost. The earliest LUS indication of pleural effusion is the abnormal curtain sign at the lung bases (Fig. 5). It may be possible to predict the cause of the effusion by the presence of other LUS features (Table 5), but these are non-specific signs.

LUS can ensure the safety of a thoracocentesis by defining the level of diaphragm and determining the appropriate size of effusion for safe aspiration [20]. Another

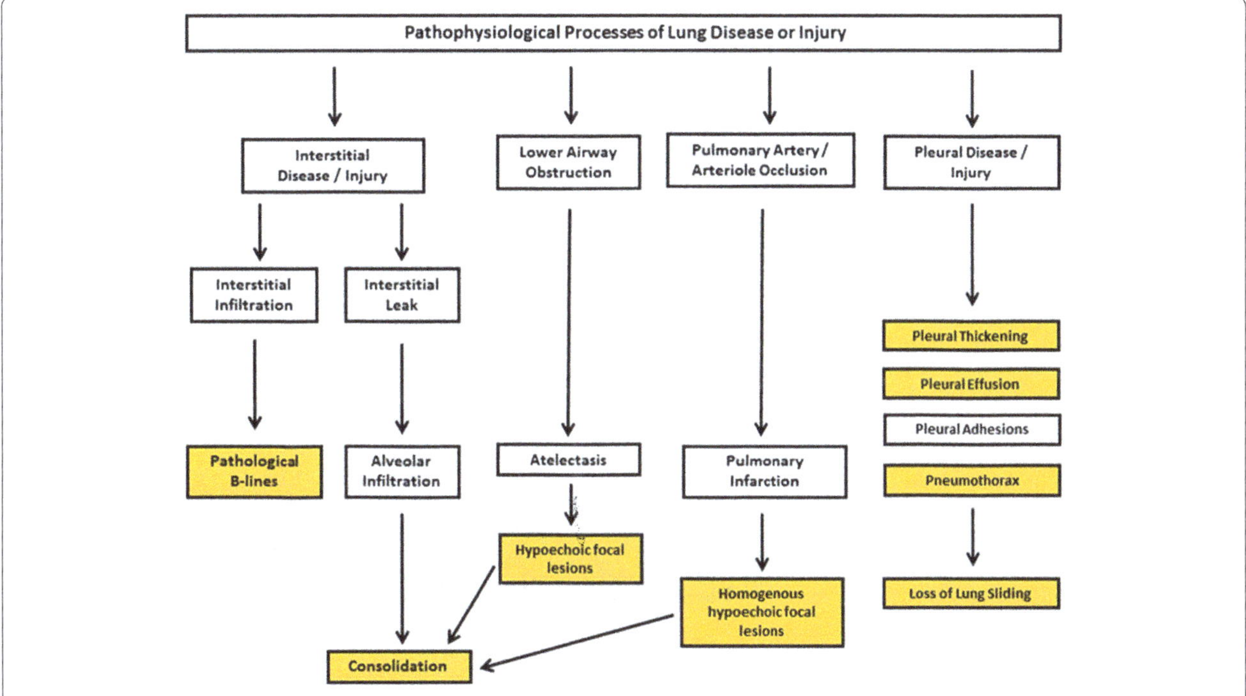

Fig. 6 Pathological processes of lung disease and injury. This summarises some of the common endpoints of the pathological processes of lung disease and injury. The endpoints result in discernible features (*yellow boxes*) in LUS

Table 3 Causes of loss of lung sliding

Pleural separation	Pleural adhesions	Non-ventilation
Pneumothorax Pleural effusion Pleural diseases *Artifact mimics* *Subcutaneous emphysema* *Tissue planes*	Inflammatory adhesions • Pneumonia • Acute lung injury Pleurodesis Pleural fibrosis • Interstitial lung disease • Fibrotic lung disease Pleural diseases	Apnea Severe hyperinflation • Asthma • Chronic obstructive pulmonary disease (COPD) Non-ventilated patient • cEndotracheal tube complications • One-lung intubation Atelectasis

important application is the investigation of the lung underlying the effusion [19].

Consolidation

In consolidation (Fig. 9), the air in the alveoli is replaced by fluid, inflammatory exudates, and cellular infiltrates. This process removes the acoustic impedance posed by air and thus allows visualisation of the affected lung parenchyma itself. Early small consolidations appear as subpleural defects and gradually enlarge to assume a wedge-shaped appearance as more lung parenchyma is involved. The interface of the consolidation with the unaffected aerated lung creates an irregular hyperechoic border called the shred sign. A fully formed consolidation appears solid, "liver-like," and very often with pockets of trapped air (air-alveologram) and highlighting air-filled bronchioles (air bronchogram) [21]. In consolidation, the bronchioles are often patent and communicate with the large airways. This gives rise to an air bronchogram sign that changes with respiration, called dynamic air bronchogram [22]. Hypoechoic tubes known as fluid bronchogram have also been observed. The discovery of hypoechoic regions within the consolidation may signify lung necrosis and the formation of an abscess. Consolidations involving the base of the lung, in addition, cause abnormal curtain sign.

Consolidation is a common endpoint of many disease processes such as pneumonia, atelectasis, infarction, and tumour infiltration; correlation with the clinical information of the patient is necessary to arrive at a diagnosis.

Atelectasis

Atelectasis or pulmonary collapse is defined as the absent of air in parts or whole of the lung. It can be divided into compressive atelectasis caused by a large effusion and obstructive atelectasis caused by lower airway obstruction. In compressive atelectasis, the underlying lung is not consolidated and therefore will change in shape with respiration, demonstrating jellyfish sign and sinusoid sign (Table 5). LUS is an accurate tool for the diagnosis of obstructive atelectasis [23]. The early appearance of atelectasis is a homogenous liver-like lesion (Fig. 10) with loss of lung sliding. Any air trapped within the atelectasis could form a static air bronchogram. The junction between atelectasis and the aerated lung may show the shred sign. Overtime, the atelectatic segment may evolve to assume the appearance of a consolidation but the dynamic air bronchogram could help distinguish the two entities [22]. Potential use of LUS in the

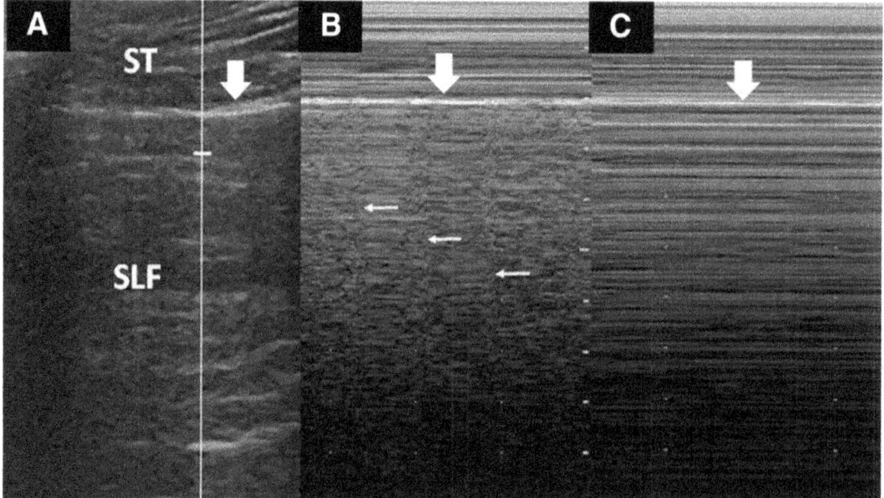

Fig. 7 M-mode studies of lung sliding. **a** A proper M-mode study begins with the cursor (*vertical line*) centred over the SLF. The pleural line (*thick arrow*) separates the extra-pulmonary soft tissues (*ST*) and the SLF. **b** The M-mode showing "seashore" sign, where the quiet ST tracing ("sea") is separated by the pleura line (*thick arrow*) from the noisy SLF tracing ("sandy shore"), caused by lung sliding. At regular intervals, the lung pulse (*thin arrows*) is seen. **c** M-mode showing "stratosphere" sign. The SLF tracing is "quiet" as there is no activity (lung sliding) at pleural line. There is also no lung pulse in this image

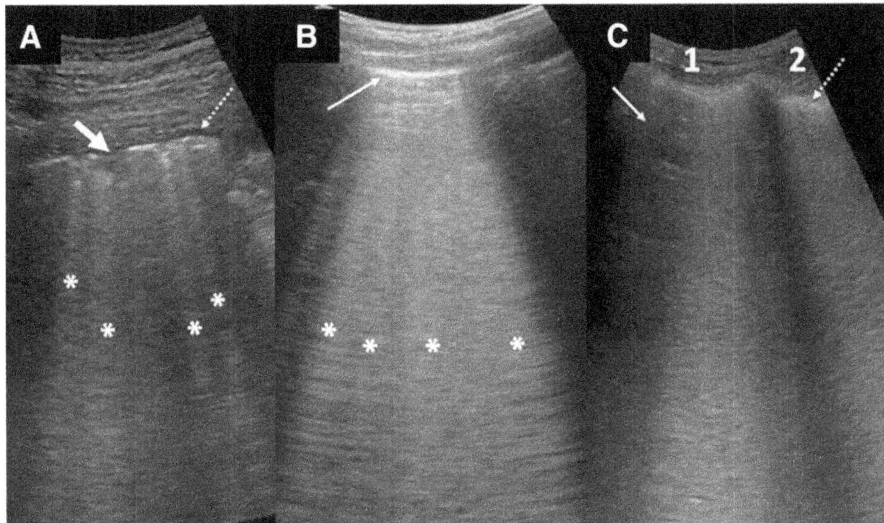

Fig. 8 Examples of conditions with B-lines. **a** Pneumonia with several LUS features: B-lines (asterisk) of uneven spacing, a small consolidation (*arrow*), and small effusion (*dotted arrow*). **b** Cardiogenic pulmonary edema with many evenly spaced B-lines (*asterisk*) banded together into a thick sheet. Note the smooth and thin pleural line (*thin arrow*). **c** ARDS with dense B-lines involving two intercostal spaces (1, 2). Note that an area in 1 (*arrow*) is spared, indicating the patchy distribution of the disease process. The pleura is thickened and uneven (*dotted arrow*)

monitoring and management of atelectasis in the intensive care unit has been demonstrated [24].

The lung ultrasound primary survey of the acutely dyspneic patient

A LUS primary survey refers to using the ultrasound as the initial assessment tool for a breathless patient in lieu of the traditional stethoscope or CXR. This approach requires a thorough study of the accessible lung surfaces to determine:

- Morphology (types of lung signs)
- Distribution of the lung signs

A good understanding of the pathophysiology and time course of pulmonary diseases will help the clinician anticipate the type of signs that could be expected during LUS. These signs must in turn be interpreted with the clinical findings and investigations such as lab tests, blood gases.

The lung signs matrix (Table 6) summarises the combination of LUS findings that could be found in various acute lung conditions.

A LUS workflow in acute lung disease diagnosis called the BLUE protocol [7, 17] could also be used. This protocol was validated in a study population with single diagnoses

Table 4 Conditions producing pathological B-lines

Fluid
Cardiogenic pulmonary edema
Fluid overload states
Inflammatory
Acute lung injury/pneumonitis
Acute respiratory distress syndrome
Pneumonia
Fibrosis
Pulmonary fibrosis
Chronic interstitial lung disease
Trauma
Pulmonary contusion
Blast lung

Table 5 Other signs described in pleural effusion [8, 37, 38]

Signs	Cause	Significance
Quad sign	Pleural effusion	Shape of effusion collection
Spine sign	Large effusion	Large effusion allowing visualisation of the spine
Plankton sign	Blood, fibrin	Hemothorax, exudate
Air-fluid level	Air	Air within effusion
Jellyfish sign	Compressive atelectasis	No consolidation of underlying lung
Sinusoid sign	Jellyfish sign in M-mode	No consolidation of underlying lung
Suspended microbubble sign	Air within lung abscess	Distinguish lung abscess from empyema

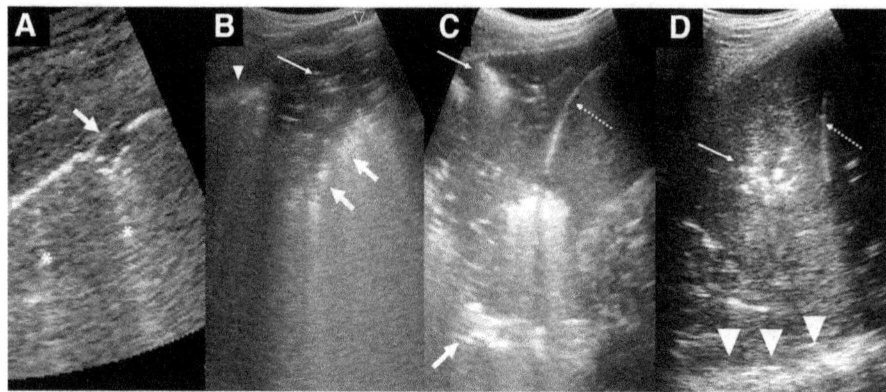

Fig. 9 Features of consolidation. **a** Small consolidations appearing as subpleural defects (*arrow*). Ring-down artifacts or B-lines are also present (*asterisks*) **b** Wedge-shaped hypoechoic consolidations with trapped air within (*thin arrow*) and shred sign (*thick arrow*). A normal looking pleural line (*open arrow head*) and a thickened uneven pleural line (*arrowhead*) are shown. **c** A larger consolidation showing shred sign (*thick arrow*) and air bronchogram (*thin arrow*). Because this occurs at the lung base, the diaphragm (*dotted arrow*) is shown and hence the curtain sign is loss. **d** A lobar consolidation at the lung base showing air bronchogram (*thin arrow*), diaphragm (*dotted arrow*), and spine sign (*arrowhead*)

with confounding cases (rare; more than one diagnoses; no diagnoses) excluded, and the authors acknowledged the limitations of the protocol in separating disease entities that share similar lung signs. The aspects not covered by the BLUE protocol were explained in detail in a subsequent publication [25].

Pneumothorax

Pneumothorax is the signature condition with loss of lung sliding. In a dyspneic patient with a previously normal lung, the loss of lung sliding is predictably due to pneumothorax and the presence of lung sliding rules out pneumothorax with a >99 % sensitivity [26, 27].

Distinguishing pneumothorax from situations involving a relatively aerated lung (such as non-ventilation, pleurodesis) is often a challenge. One scenario that illustrates the non-specificity of loss of lung sliding; in an intubated asthmatic patient with worsening hypoxemia, the finding of loss of lung sliding in one lung could be attributed to either a pneumothorax or non-ventilation of the lung (e.g., slipped endotracheal tube). Conditions such as pleural effusion, consolidation, and atelectasis are easily distinguishable from pneumothorax because there are other ultrasound features to support the respective diagnoses.

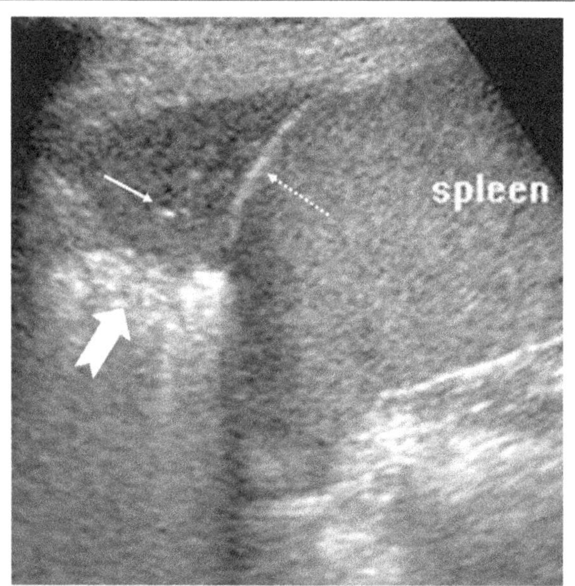

Fig. 10 Atelectasis. Hypoechoic homogenous lesion at the lung base with air bronchogram (*thin arrow*) and shred sign (*thick arrow*). The diaphragm (*dotted arrow*) is seen as the curtain sign is lost

In difficult situations, additional lung signs are needed, all with aim of determining whether the two pleural layers are in contact:

B-lines Since B-lines originate from the lung interstitia, the demonstration of B-lines signifies that the lung is fully inflated and the visceral pleura being in contact with the parietal pleura. A pneumothorax, no matter how small, will obscure any existing B-lines. The pitfalls of using B-lines as evidence are:

- They are rare in healthy lungs (without parenchymal disease), especially the upper lung, where a pneumothorax usually manifests
- There are also uncommon situations where B-lines are seen with a pneumothorax: adhesions of parts of the lung in a loculated pneumothorax [28], pneumothorax in lung fibrosis and failed pleurodesis

Lung comets (I-lines) As explained earlier, I-lines share the same origin and some characteristics as B-lines but are

Table 6 The lung signs matrix

Diagnosis	Lung signs distribution	Lung sliding	Pleural line	B-lines	Effusion	Consolidation
Acute pulmonary oedema/ fluid overload states	Bilateral/symmetrical	Present	Normal	Bilateral/symmetrical	Often present	No
Acute respiratory distress syndrome	Bilateral/asymmetrical/patchy	Present/may be absent in severe states	Thickened/uneven	Patchy distribution	May be found	Yes
Bacterial pneumonia	Usually unilateral/focal/patchy	Present/may be absent in severe states	Thickened/uneven	Focal	May be found/empyema	Yes
Viral/atypical pneumonia	Bilateral/asymmetrical/patchy	Present/may be absent in severe states	Thickened/uneven	Patchy distribution	May be found	Yes
Acute interstitial lung disease	Bilateral/asymmetrical/patchy	Present/may be absent in severe states	Thickened/uneven	Patchy distribution	May be found	Yes
Pneumothorax	Focal/starts with upper lung	Absent	Normal	No	No	No
COPD exacerbation/asthma	–	Present	Normal	No	No	No
Acute pulmonary infarction	Focal	Present/may be absent	Normal/may be thickened	No	May be found	Yes—at late stage
Atelectasis	Focal	Absent	Normal	No	May be found	Yes—at late stage

generated through a different mechanism. They are readily seen in healthy lungs (without parenchymal disease) with a high-frequency transducer and their presence means the pleural layers are in contact. The main pitfall of the search for I-lines is that they are often not visible with a low frequency transducer.

Lung pulse Lung pulse (Fig. 7) is an artifact seen in M-mode studies of the lung. It is due to cardiac pulsations conducted to the chest wall, which register a disturbance to the transducer. Logically, the lung pulse is not seen when the pleural layers are separated in a pneumothorax. Two pitfalls of lung pulse as a supporting sign are:

- The lung pulse is sometimes not seen in a normal lung because of patient factors, such as body habitus
- A very small pneumothorax may still allow the transmission of vibrations through the pleural cavity air to the transducer, registering a lung pulse

Lung point The lung point is the junction between the pneumothorax and the normal lung. In B-mode LUS, one part of the pleural line demonstrates lung sliding and the other does not. The lung point also represents the extent of the pneumothorax discoverable by ultrasound. In M-mode, there is an alternating seashore sign with stratosphere sign. However, this M-mode feature is also seen in patients with bradypnea where there are long intervals without respiratory movements; therefore, finding and visualising the lung point in B-mode is still a better approach.

Pitfalls of lung point are:

- A large pneumothorax involving the entire lung does not have a lung point
- It is difficult to find a lung point in a person with pneumothorax on top of a pre-exisiting condition of pleural adhesion (e.g., fibrotic lung disease, failed pleurodesis)

Acute respiratory distress syndrome vs acute cardiogenic pulmonary edema

Acute lung injury often goes through the stages of interstitial involvement, thus generating B-lines, to the stage of alveolar infiltration and, hence, consolidations. The severe end point is the clinical state of acute respiratory distress syndrome (ARDS). This could be distinguished from acute cardiogenic pulmonary edema (ACPE) by observing a few differing characteristics [29]. The distribution of ARDS changes are often patchy with one area of the lung more involved than another. The pleural line may be thickened and uneven as a result of inflammatory exudate and effusion often occurs.

ACPE produces bilateral symmetrical B-lines that starts in the lower parts of the lung and progressively involve the upper lung as the severity increases. When fluid floods the alveoli, an air-fluid foam mixture is created, which generates even more B-lines. In severe cases, the multiple B-lines coalesce into a thick white sheet. B-lines in ACPE is quantifiable to determine disease severity and could be used to guide therapy [30, 31]. The commonly found pleural effusion indicates the progressive development of heart failure days to weeks prior to the ACPE episode but cannot be used to determine ACPE severity. Pleural thickening and consolidations are not features of ACPE [29].

Pneumonia

LUS is a sensitive tool to pick up changes associated with pneumonia (c.f. CXR). The signs are, however, non-specific and should be interpreted in the context of the clinical findings of a patient.

Most pneumonias begin with interstitial involvement and progress to alveolar infiltration with red cells and serous infiltrates (congestion), followed by deposition of fibrin rich fluid (red hepatisation) and infiltration with inflammatory cells (grey hepatisation). The corresponding LUS signs are B-lines, hypoechoic subpleural defects, and consolidation. Parapneumonic effusions are sometimes present. Fulminant pneumonias may progress to abscess formation.

Acute interstitial pneumonias tend to present with predominantly B-lines in LUS [32], which are unevenly distributed throughout the lungs. Small consolidations and subpleural lesions are common, but there are reports of interstitial pneumonias without these, which is helpful in determining the aetiology [33].

Acutely dyspneic patient with normal lung ultrasound

Acute asthma and exacerbation of chronic obstructive pulmonary disease (COPD) are reactive airway diseases and do not produce pathophysiologic changes to the lung parenchyma and pleural per se, hence, giving a normal LUS picture. Rarely, in very severe states of air-trapping and lung hyperinflation, pulmonary excursion is severely restricted leading to loss of lung sliding. LUS in asthma and COPD is helpful to exclude other concomitant causes of breathlessness, such as pneumonia and heart failure [34].

Pulmonary embolism and pulmonary infarction

LUS has shown that pulmonary involvement is common in pulmonary embolism (PE), contrary to common beliefs. PE often produces changes that could be regarded as early infarction [35]. In the initial stage, the alveoli are infiltrated by red blood cells replacing air. Infarctions are typically wedge-shaped subpleural lesions that are homogenously hypoechoic with absent LUS features of air. There may be a linear hyperechoic region within the lesion resembling an air bronchogram. An associated pleural effusion adjacent to the infarction is often seen. An infarction at the lung base gives loss of curtain sign. Over time, the infarcted area will be infiltrated by inflammatory cells and assumes a consolidation appearance. Pulmonary infarctions are most often found in the posterior and lower half of the lung, and LUS has a high sensitivity and diagnostic accuracy for the confirmation of pulmonary infarction [36]. The further workup on these patients require risk-profiling (e.g., Well's criteria), D-Dimer test, DVT scan, or CT Pulmonary angiogram.

Conclusions

This review illustrates the fact that many acute lung conditions could be diagnosed readily with LUS. LUS offers us the precision that traditional physical examination of the lung and the chest X-ray could not provide and the ability to make important therapeutic decisions early. Practitioners of LUS should therefore be conversant with the technique and be ready to apply it in primary survey of a dyspneic patient.

Acknowledgements

Special thanks to Dr. Hong Chuen Toh, Dr. Sanjay Patel, and Dr. Michael Liu for the preparation of images used in this article.

Funding

In the course of this work, I received no funding, remuneration, or sponsorship from any company, individuals, or organisations.

Competing interests

The authors declare that they have no competing interests.

References

1. Lichtenstein D, Goldstein I, Mourgeon E, Cluzel P, Grenier P, Rouby JJ. Comparative diagnostic performances of auscultation, chest radiography and lung ultrasonography in acute respiratory distress syndrome. Anesthesiology. 2004;100:9–15.
2. Bourcier JE, Paquet J, Seinger M, Gallard E, Redonnet JP, Cheddadi F, et al. Performance comparison of lung ultrasound and chest x-ray for the diagnosis of pneumonia in the ED. Am J Emerg Med. 2014;32:115–8.
3. Pivetta E, Goffi A, Tizzani M, Porrino G, Ferreri E, Volpicelli G, et al. Lung ultrasound-implemented diagnosis of acute decompensated heart failure in the ED: A SIMEU multicentre study. Chest. 2015;148(1):202–10.
4. Vopicelli G, Mussa A, Garofalo G, Cardinale L, Casoli G, Perotto F, et al. Bedside lung ultrasound in the assessment of alveolar-interstitial syndrome. Am J Emerg Med. 2006;24:689–96.
5. Milliner BHA, Tsung JW. An evidence-based lung ultrasound scanning protocol for diagnosing pediatric pneumonia. Ann Emerg Med. 2015;66(4):S107.
6. Sonja B. Indications, technical prerequisites and investigation procedure. In: Mathis G, editor. Chest sonography. Berlin Heidelberg: Springer-Verlag; 2011.
7. Lichtenstein D, Mezière GA. The BLUE-points: three standardized points used in the BLUE-protocol for ultrasound assessment of the lung in acute respiratory failure. Crit Ultrasound J. 2011;3:109–10.
8. Lichtenstein D. Whole body ultrasonography in the critically ill. Berlin Heidelberg: Springer-Verlag; 2010.
9. Lichtenstein D. General ultrasound in the critically ill. Berlin Heidelberg: Springer-Verlag; 2005.
10. Scanlan KA. Sonographic artifacts and their origins. AJR. 1991;156:1267–72.
11. Louvet A, Bourgeois J. Lung ring-down artefact as a sign of pulmonary alveolar-interstitial disease. Vet Radiol Ultrasound. 2008;49(4):374–7.
12. Ziskin MC, Thickman DI, Goldenberg NJ, Lapayowker MS, Becker JM. The comet tail artifact. J Ultrasound Med. 1982;1(1):1–7.
13. Thickman TI, Ziskin MC, Goldenberg NJ, Linder BE. Clinical manifestations of the comet tail artifact. J Ultrasound Med. 1983;2:225–30.
14. Avruch L, Cooperberg PL. The ring-down artifact. J Ultrasound Med. 1985;4(1):21–8.
15. Lichtenstein D, Mézière G, Biderman P, Gepner A, Barré O. The comet-tail artifact. An ultrasound sign of alveolar-interstitial syndrome. Am J Respir Crit Care Med. 1997;156:1640–6.
16. Lim JH, Lee KS, Kim TS, Chung MP. Ring-down artifacts posterior to the right hemidiaphragm on abdominal sonography: sign of pulmonary parenchymal abnormalities. J Ultrasound Med. 1999;18:403–10.
17. Lichtenstein DA, Mézière G. Relevance of lung ultrasound in the diagnosis of acute respiratory failure: the BLUE Protocol. Chest. 2008;134:117–25.
18. Joyner Jr CR, Herman RJ, Reid JM. Reflected ultrasound in the detection and localisation of pleural effusion. JAMA. 1967;200(5):399–402.
19. Yu CJ, Yang PC, Wu HD, Chang DB, Kuo SH, Luh KT. Ultrasound study in unilateral hemithorax opacification. Image comparison with computed tomography. Am Rev Respir Dis. 1993;147(2):430–4.
20. Lichtenstein D, Hulot JS, Rabiller A, Tostivint I, Mézière G. Feasibility and safety of ultrasound assisted thoracentesis in mechanically ventilated patients. Intensive Care Med. 1999;25:955–8.
21. Weinberg B, Diakoumakis EE, Kass EG, Sefie B, Zvi ZB. The air bronchogram: sonographic demonstration. Am J Roentgenol. 1986;147(3):593–5.
22. Lichenstein D, Mézière G, Seitz J. The dynamic air bronchogram. Chest. 2009;135:1421–5.
23. Acosta CM, Maidana GA, Jacovitti D, Agustin B, Cerveda S, Rae E. Accuracy of transthoracic lung ultrasound for diagnosing anaesthesia-induced atelectasis in children. Anesthesiology. 2014;120:1370–9.
24. Yang JX, Zhang M, Liu ZH, Ba L, Gan JX, Xu SW. Detection of lung atelectasis/consolidation by ultrasound in multiple trauma patients with mechanism ventilation. Crit Ultrasound J. 2009;1:13–6.
25. Lichtenstein D. Lung ultrasound in the critically ill. Cham: Springer; 2016.
26. Dulchavsky SA, Schwartz KL, Kirkpatrick AW, Billica RD, Williams DR, Diebel LN, et al. Prospective evaluation of thoracic ultrasound in the detection of pneumothorax. J Trauma. 2001;50:201–5.
27. Blavais M, Lyon M, Duggard S. A prospective comparison of supine chest radiography and bedside ultrasound for the diagnosis of traumatic pneumothorax. Acad Emerg Med. 2005;12:844–9.
28. Volpicelli G, Boero E, Stefanone V, Storti E. Unusual new signs of pneumothorax at lung ultrasound. Crit Ultrasound J. 2013;5:10.
29. Copetti R, Soldati G, Copetti P. Chest sonography: a useful tool to differentiate acute cardiogenic pulmonary edema from acute respiratory distress syndrome. Cardiovasc Ultrasound. 2008;6:16.
30. Jambrik Z, Monti S, Coppola V, Agricola E, Mottola G, Miniati M, et al. Usefulness of ultrasound lung comets as a nonradiologic sign of extravascular lung water. Am J Cardiol. 2004;93:1265–70.
31. Agricola E, Bove T, Oppizzi M, Marino G, Zangrillo A, Margonato A, et al. Ultrasound comet tail images: a marker of pulmonary edema. Chest. 2005;127:1690–5.
32. Giudice VL, Bruni A, Corcioni E, Corcioni B. Ultrasound in the evaluation of interstitial pneumonia. J Ultrasound. 2008;11(1):30–8.
33. Japiassu A, Bozza F. Lung ultrasound can differentiate pneumocystis jiroveci versus other etiologies among critically ill AIDS patients with pneumonia. Crit Care. 2012;16(Supp1):86.
34. Volpicelli G, et al. Usefulness of lung ultrasound in the bedside distinction between pulmonary edema and exacerbation of COPD. Emerg Radiol. 2008;15(3):145–51.
35. Mathis G, Metzler J, Fussenegger D, Sutterlutti G, Fuerstein M, Fritzsche H. Sonographic observation of pulmonary infarction and early infarctions by pulmonary embolism. Eur Heart J. 1993;14:804–8.
36. Comert SS, Caglayan B, Arturk U, Fidan A, Kirai N, Parmaksiz E, et al. The role of thoracic ultrasonography in the diagnosis of pulmonary embolism. Ann Thorac Med. 2013;8(2):99–104.
37. Targhetta R, Bourgeois JM, Chavagneux R, et al. Ultrasound approach to diagnosing hydropneumothorax. Chest. 1992;101(4):931–4.
38. Lin FC, Chou CW, Chang SC. Differentiating pyopneumothorax and peripheral lung abscess: chest ultrasonography. Am J Med Sci. 2004;327(6):330–5.

15

Procalcitonin: a promising diagnostic marker for sepsis and antibiotic therapy

Ashitha L. Vijayan, Vanimaya, Shilpa Ravindran, R. Saikant, S. Lakshmi, R. Kartik and Manoj. G*

Abstract

Background: Sepsis is a global healthcare problem, characterized by whole body inflammation in response to microbial infection, which leads to organ dysfunction. It is becoming a frequent complication in hospitalized patients. Early and differential diagnosis of sepsis is needed critically to avoid unnecessary usage of antimicrobial agents and for proper antibiotic treatments through the screening of biomarkers that sustains with diagnostic significance.

Main body of abstract: Current targeting conventional markers (C-reactive protein, white blood cell, tumour necrosis factor-α, interleukins, etc.) are non-specific for diagnosing sepsis. Procalcitonin (PCT), a member of the calcitonin super family could be a critical tool for the diagnosis of sepsis. But to distinguish between bacterial versus viral infections, procalcitonin alone may not be effective. Rapid elevation in the concentration of procalcitonin and other newly emerging biomarkers during an infection and its correlation with severity of illness makes it an ideal biomarker for bacterial infection. Beside this, the procalcitonin levels can be used for monitoring response to antimicrobial therapy, diagnosis of secondary inflammations, diagnosis of renal involvement in paediatric urinary tract infection, etc.
The present article summarizes the relevance of procalcitonin in the diagnosis of sepsis and how it can be useful in determining the therapeutic approaches.

Conclusion: Further studies are needed to better understand the application of PCT in the diagnosis of sepsis, differentiating between microbial and non-microbial infection cases and determining the therapeutic approaches for sepsis.

Keywords: Procalcitonin, Sepsis, Antibiotic therapy, Diagnostic marker

Background

During the course of evolution, our immune system has eventually developed to deal with infectious pathogen invasions by various host defence mechanisms. Inflammatory response is one of the primary responses to a microbial invasion, [1] which leads to the systemic illness which is referred to as sepsis. Its severity correlates with mortality [2–5]. It may occur as a result of infections acquired from community, hospitals or other healthcare facilities. There is an alarming number of 18 million new sepsis cases reported each year worldwide with mortality rate ranging from 30–50% [6]. Intensive care case pattern study reported frequent prevalence of sepsis in India, with 28.3% of patients contact sepsis during ICU stay and have 34% mortality rate [7].

All types of microbes like bacteria, virus, fungi and parasites can cause sepsis, but bacteria cause the most common pathogenic invasion [8–10]. During sepsis, the microorganisms invade to the blood stream and directly proliferate locally and release various virulent factors into the bloodstream [11]. These products can stimulate the release of endogenous mediators of sepsis from endothelial cells, monocytes, macrophages neutrophils and plasma cell precursors [12]. Sepsis-related inflammatory response arise when the body attempts to neutralize pathogenic infection which in turn leads to the activation of various mechanism with the immune cells to secrete inflammatory protein which in turn damage tissues and organs of the host [13, 14]. Clinical symptoms of sepsis include tachycardia, tachypnea, fever, leucocytosis, etc. Usually severe sepsis is accompanied with hypoperfusion or dysfunction of at least one organ. Sepsis associated with multiple organ dysfunction syndrome (MODS) or hypotension is known as septic shock [15].

* Correspondence: manojg@lifecarehll.com
Diagnostic Products Division, Corporate R&D Centre, HLL Lifecare Limited, Akkulam, Sreekariyam (P.O), Trivandrum, Kerala, India

Early diagnosis and prompt antimicrobial therapy is crucial in the treatment of sepsis for saving lives. Sepsis is a systemic inflammatory response syndrome (SIRS) that affect all organs. Hence, host responses including cytokine, cell markers, receptor biomarkers, coagulations, vascular endothelial damage, vasodilation, organ failure and scientific advancement in the field of molecular biology can equip us to screen wide range of protein markers in acute phase of sepsis development that helps in identifying relevant biomarkers to diagnose sepsis [16].WBC, C-reactive protein (CRP) and interleukin-1 (IL-1) are the conventional markers used for diagnosis of sepsis. Compared to CRP, PCT has better diagnostic and prognostic value and will clearly distinguish viral and bacterial meningitis [17]. Cytokines like TNF-α, IL-1 and IL-6 are elevated during sepsis, but they do not possess sufficient sensitivity or specificity for the development of clinical markers [18]. Blood culture is considered as the gold standard for the confirmation of bacteraemia which can isolate and identify the causative agent and subsequently test the antimicrobial sensitivity, but the delayed process of bacterial culture emphasises the early diagnosis of sepsis [19]. Several studies mentioned the advantages of the precursor molecule of calcitonin, namely procalcitonin as a biomarker for sepsis. The serum PCT level rises rapidly than CRP levels and peaks within very short time; moreover, if the patient responds appropriately to the treatment, the level of PCT returns to normal range faster than CRP which makes it a better biomarker for sepsis [20]. In general, PCT alone or in combination with other biomarkers would serve as a promising tool for understanding the prediction, cause, diagnosis, progression, regression and outcome of the treatment regimes.

History of procalcitonin

In 1975, Moya F et al. suggested the existence of a precursor for calcitonin in chicken. The large biosynthetic molecule splits intracellularly to generate the hormone, and they named it as procalcitonin [21]. Allison's study (1981) in RNA isolated from human medullary carcinoma demonstrated the synthesis of calcitonin as a precursor protein molecule in human [22]. Later studies show that calcitonin is secreted after a sequential Co and post translational modification like glycosylation protiolytic cleavage, etc. [23]. In healthy individuals, PCT is produced in thyroid C cells, from a CALC-1 gene located on chromosome 11. The mRNA product is known as preprocalcitonin. It is further modified to 116 amino acid procalcitonin. Finally, it is cleaved into 3 distinct molecules; active calcitonin (32 amino acid), katacalcitonin (21 amino acid) and N-terminal procalcitonin (57 amino acid). Calcitonin hormone is involved in the homeostasis of calcium and phosphorous [24]. Normally, CALC-1 gene in thyroid C cells are induced by elevated calcium level, glucocorticoid, calcitonin gene-related peptide (CGRP), glucagon, gastrin or β-adregenic stimulations. Practically, all the PCT formed in thyroid C cells are converted to calcitonin so that no PCT is released into the circulation. Hence, the PCT level in healthy subjects is very low (0.05 ng/mL) but the inflammatory release of PCT is independent of the above regulations. During inflammation, PCT is produced mainly by two alternative mechanisms; direct pathway induced by lipopolysaccharide (LPS) or other toxic metabolite from microbes and indirect pathway induced by various inflammatory mediators like IL-6, TNF-α, etc. (Fig. 1).

In bacterial septicaemia, PCT is produced by alternate pathways, either directly or indirectly. For better understanding of the pathophysiology of calcitonin precursor in sepsis, an experiment was conducted in animal (hamsters) analogue to human sepsis [25]. During sepsis, ubiquitous and uniform expressions of calcitonin (CT) mRNA in multiple tissues were observed in hamsters. In healthy hamsters, PCT mRNA was isolated primarily from the thyroid with minute amounts of synthesis associated with lung tissue. The next set of hamsters was infected with gram-negative bacteria, and the level of PCT mRNA in various tissues and cells were observed. White blood cells (WBC), spleen, kidney, adipocytes, pancreas, colon and brain showed a significantly elevated level of PCT mRNA. Many reports are available which shows that PCT levels are elevating rapidly between 2 and 6 h which peaks within 6–24 h during bacterial infection.

Procalcitonin as diagnostic tool

An ideal biomarker should possess high diagnostic accuracy, for an early and rapid diagnosis. PCT is a recently re-discovered biomarker that fulfils many of these requirements especially in comparison to conventional and widely used other biomarkers that have demonstrated superior diagnostic accuracy for a variety of infections, including sepsis. PCT is helpful for early detection of sepsis as well as to monitor the antimicrobial treatment regimen. In fact, PCT can be a useful tool for antimicrobial stewardship and its utilization may safely lead to significant reduction of unnecessary administration of antimicrobial therapy. Laboratories and clinicians must comprehend the precincts of the present microbiological methods and the need for highly sensitive biomarker assays to facilitate accurate diagnosis and goal directed therapy in patients suspected of sepsis.

During sepsis conditions, microbes and their antigens stimulate numerous anti-inflammatory mediators, which will trigger the host immune response. Precursors, mature forms and degradation products of these mediators penetrate from the site of action into the circulation, where which can be measured theoretically. These

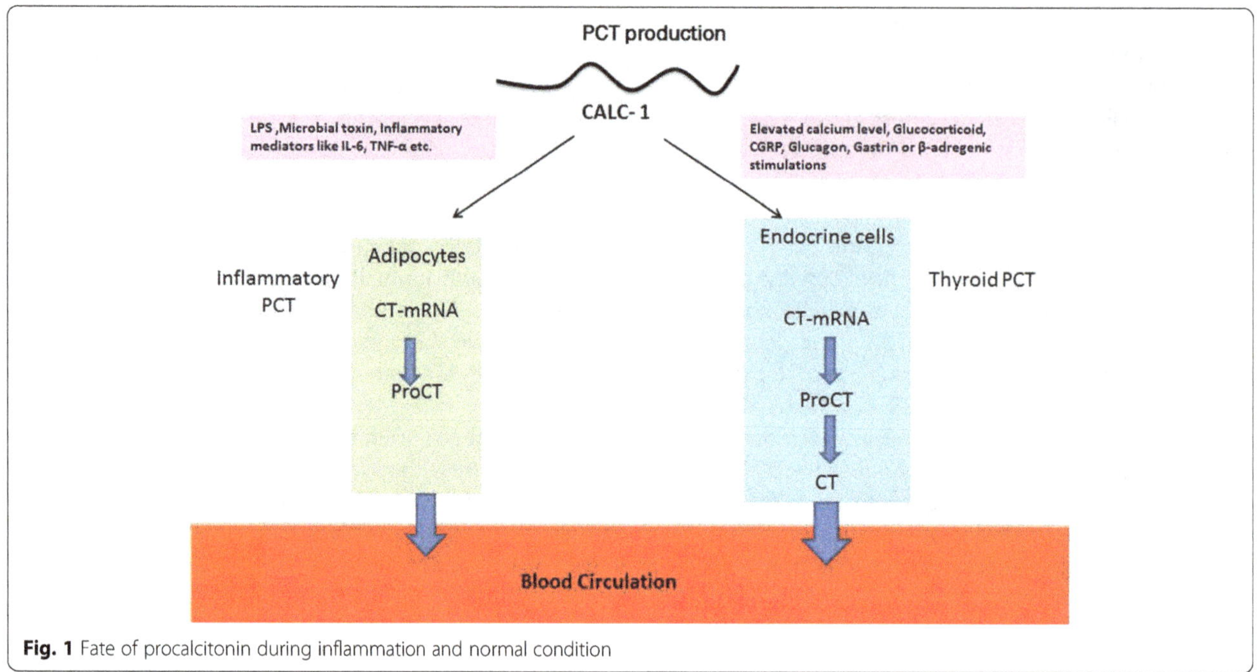

Fig. 1 Fate of procalcitonin during inflammation and normal condition

substances can be measured as surrogate markers for the diagnosis and the severity of infection. Exalted production of PCT during bacterial and its association with sepsis was first demonstrated by Asscot et al. [26]. The actual mechanism of production of PCT during infection is not known, but it assumes that bacterial lipopolysaccharides and sepsis released cytokines modulate the liver and peripheral blood mononuclear cells to produce PCT. Microbial infection induces the elevated expression of CALC 1 gene followed by the release of PCT product which is correlated with severity of disease and mortality.

The PCT as a biomarker proved successfully its clinical usefulness in determining the presence of sepsis. Moreover, it has been shown to correlate the extent and the severity of microbial invasion. It clearly showed the significance of early diagnosis of bacterial infected sepsis. PCT can be used for early detection of sepsis and prediction of outcome after major trauma. Muller et al. conducted a study in patients with community-acquired pneumonia; the serum PCT concentration could differentiate bacterial from viral causes. Out of 545 patients with pneumonia symptoms consulting at the emergency department (ED), 373 were suspected with true bacterial pneumonia, with an area under the receiver operating characteristics (AUROC) curve for the PCT to predict bacterial pneumonia of 0.88. CRP was slightly less efficient (AUROC = 0.76) than PCT. PCT 0.1 ng/ml predicted bacterial pneumonia with 90% sensitivity and 59% specificity, whereas PCT 1 ng/ml showing 43% sensitivity and 96% specificity [27]. Several meta-analysis data suggest of heterogeneity for the PCT testing; however, elevated PCT concentrations strongly associated with all-cause mortality in sepsis patients [28].

Muller and colleagues conducted a study in consecutive critically ill patients to compare the usefulness of serum concentration of calcitonin precursor, CRP, IL-6 and lactate for the diagnosis of sepsis. Blood samples were collected at variable intervals during the course of disease (systemic inflammatory response syndrome (SIRS), sepsis and severe sepsis and septic shock. Serum concentration of calcitonin precursor, CRP, IL-6 and lactate were elevated according to the severity of illness. Based on receiver operating characteristic (ROC) curve analysis, they concluded that PCT is the most reliable marker for the diagnosis of sepsis, with 89% of sensitivity and 94% of specificity [29]. Ibrahim et al. evaluated the utility of PCT as a routine biochemical tool compared to the traditional inflammatory marker CRP. They simultaneously measured PCT and CRP in 73 medico surgical ICU patients; according to the American College of Chest Physician (ACCP) criteria-based study group, 75% cases revealed SIRS in clinical representation. They observed 75% of diagnostic accuracy, 72% of specificity and sensitivity of 76% for PCT and concluded that PCT is superior to CRP in terms of accuracy in identification and assessment of severity of sepsis [30].

Study of Young et al. [31] evaluated the ability of PCT as an early detector of septic shock in patients with acute pyelonephritis secondary to ureteral calculi. They considered 49 patients and divided them into 2 groups: with and without septic shock. Platelet count, PCT, CRP, creatinine, erythrocyte sedimentation rate (ESR), albumin and white blood cells (WBC) were measured at the time of admission to the emergency department before administrating antibiotic treatment. Univariate analysis shows higher PCT and CRP level and higher positive blood culture rate during septic shock. The multivariate model reveals that lower platelet count and higher PCT level are independent risk factors of septic shock. In ROC curve, the AUC (area under curve) was wider for PCT (0.929) compared to platelet count (0.822). At the cut-off of 0.52 ng/ml, PCT shows high sensitivity (86.7%) and specificity (85.3%). The study demonstrated that elevated PCT is an early independent predictor of development of septic shock in patients with sepsis induced by acute pyelonephritis associate with ureteral calculi.

Comparison of procalcitonin and presepsin/sCD-14

In 2004, presepsin was identified as a diagnosis marker and evaluated for sepsis. It became an alternative biomarker to aid the diagnosis of sepsis [32]. Recent studies shows that soluble cluster of differentiation 14 (sCD14) plays a significant role as biomarker with respect to diagnosis of sepsis. CD14 is a surface marker constituent of glycoprotein on monocytes and macrophages (mCD14) and serves as a high-affinity receptor towards lipopolysaccharides (LPSs), which is an essential building block of outer cell wall of gram-negative bacteria, and LPS-binding proteins (LPBs). CD14 binding to toll-like receptor 4 (TLR4) lead to activation of pro-inflammatory signalling cascade in bacterial infection [33, 34].

Along with PCT, other biomarkers alone or in combination are used in the diagnosis of sepsis, including presepsin, C-reactive protein (CRP), interleukin (IL), etc. However, the clinical value of these biomarkers independently or in combination is still at investigative stages [35]. Presepsin exists in the blood and urine of humans and comprises 99% of the total amount of CD14 in the human body, with a normal concentration of 2–6 μg/ml in serum [36]. When this was compared to PCT, presepsin also showed a similar diagnostic accuracy for sepsis with respect to area under curve (AUC) (Table 1) [37–40]. Accuracy of presepsin was similar to that of PCT, although presepsin had some superiority in the management of patients but Food and Drug Administration (FDA) approved PCT as a more reliable marker for sepsis. PCT level above 2.0 ng/ml on the first day of ICU admission could be associated with a higher risk for progression to severe sepsis and/or septic shock than PCT levels below 0.5 ng/mL. This diagnostic approach is also recommended in various guidelines [41].

Procalcitonin as a tool for antibiotic therapy

The introduction of antibiotics was in mid-20th century. Misuse and overuse of antibiotics launch the next misery known as antibiotic resistance by pathogens. Judicious use of antibiotics is of vital importance in clinical therapy [42]. Scott Fridin et al. analysed the Centres for Disease Control and Prevention (CDC) which conducted Emerging Infections Program (EIP), and thus a national administrative database (Marketscn Hospital Drug Database) was prepared to assess the potential for improvement of inpatient antibiotic prescribing. According to their study, reduction of incorrect antibiotic prescription can improve the use and patient safety [43].

Implementation of antibiotic stewardship helps to control unnecessary antibiotic prescribing as well as ensure the efficiency of treatment [44]. Inappropriate usage of medicines may lead to the development of antibiotic resistance in patients [45]. It is obligatory to reduce 'blind' prescription of drugs to avoid the evolution of secondary infection to antibiotics and obstruct the occurrence of drug resistance. An ideal marker should assist early diagnosis and capabilities to track the disease and facilitate the therapeutic interventions and decisions. The PCT is a better choice, compared to other markers which satisfy these features. An algorithm based on serial measurement of PCT can reduce the antibiotic exposure in septic patients [46]. According to the level of serum PCT, therapeutic decisions in patients were taken (Fig. 2). Based on reports, in transplant recipients, to minimize delays in the diagnosis of sepsis, it is paramount to recognize the specific risk factors for infection associated with each allograft type. Hence, PCT can be a better biomarker in detecting bacterial sepsis at initial stages. But the major limitations are to identify the causative bacteria. In addition, the particular surgical techniques involved in each type of transplantation may be closely related to the clinical manifestations of the infection process. Hence, further culturing and gram staining is required to identify the type of bacteria for further accurate treatments.

Table 1 Comparison of diagnostic potential of procalcitonin and presepsin

Reports	No. of subject	Area under curve (AUC) for the diagnosis of sepsis	
		Procalcitonin	Presepsine
Dunja Mihajlovic et al. (2017) [3]	100	0.750	0.730
Christian Leli et al.(2016) [38]	0 92	0.876	0.788
Kada Klouche et al. (2016) [39]	144	0.800	0.750
Enguix-Armada A et al.(2016) [40]	388	0.989	0.948

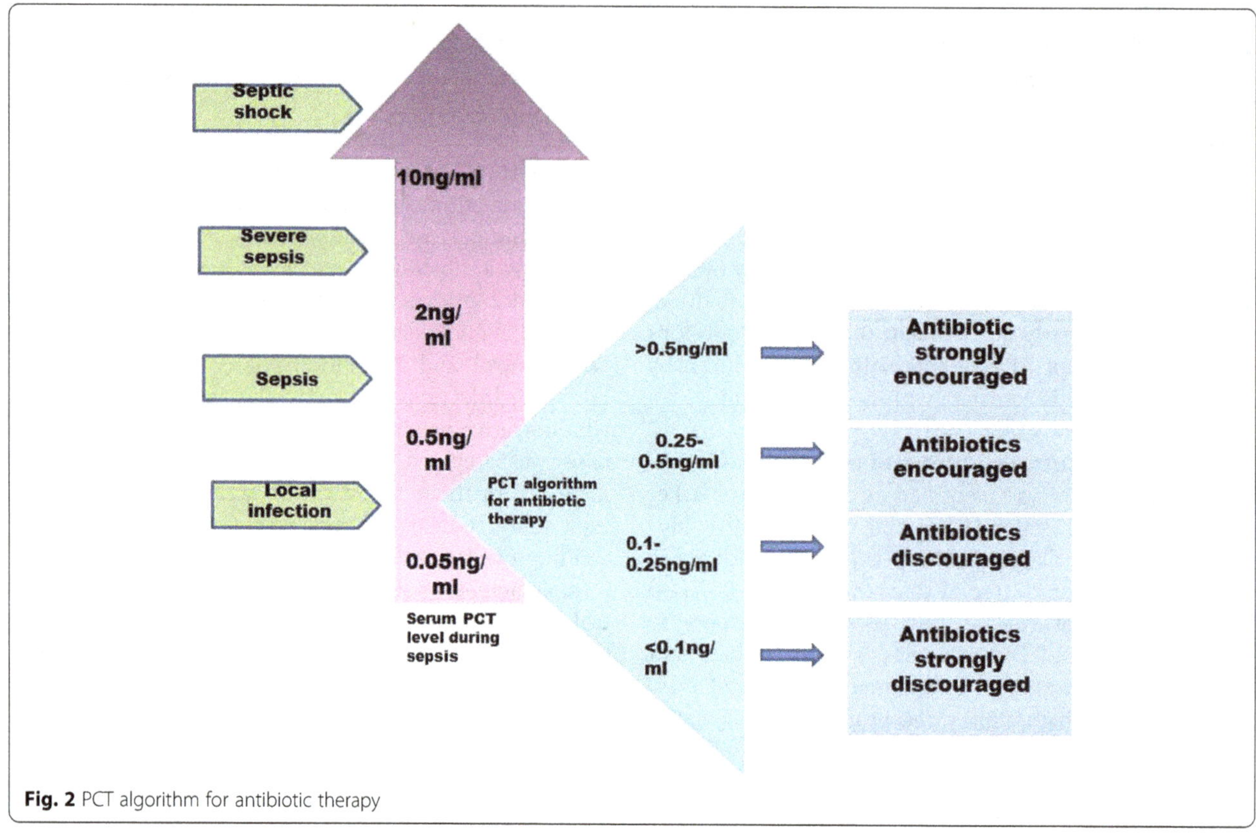

Fig. 2 PCT algorithm for antibiotic therapy

A study conducted in acutely febrile patients reveals that measurement of PCT is helpful in differentiating bacteria and non-bacterimic infectious episodes in patients. Based on the above observations, serum PCT level measurement is recommended for the guidance of antibiotic therapy [47]. Stolz D et al. evaluated the efficacy and safety of PCT guidance compared to standard therapy with antibiotic prescriptions in patients experiencing exacerbations of chronic obstructive pulmonary disease (COPD) [48]. Compared to standard therapy, PCT guidance reduce the antibiotic exposure (relative risk (RR), 0.56; 95% confidence interval (CI), 0.43 to 0.73; $p < 0.0001$) and antibiotic prescription (40 vs. 72%, respectively; $p < 0.0001$).

Schroeder et al. conducted a study in surgical intensive care patients with severe sepsis in which two classes were considered, PCT guided and control. For all patients, drug administration was based on microbiological spectrum. When the clinical signs of infection improved and PCT level decreased to <35% of the initial value, the antibiotic treatment was discontinued in PCT-guided patients. In control group, treatment was based on empirical rules. They observed that PCT-based algorithm reduces the use of antibiotic as well as the expense of treatment [49]. Lavrentieva et al. reported that PCT-guided algorithm for antibiotic therapy may contribute to the reduction of antibiotic exposure in burn intensive care unit. They enrolled 46 burn ICU patients for the study, wherein 24 patients received the therapy based on PCT guidance, which resulted in a smaller antibiotic exposure (10.1 ± 4 vs. 15.3 ± 8 days) without any negative impact on clinical outcome [50].

Kip and colleagues assessed the cost effectiveness of PCT-based algorithm. It was found to reduce the length of hospital stay, number of blood cultures and the duration of antibiotic therapy [51]. Antibiotic treatment based on PCT monitoring is a sensitive way of antibiotic usage in ICU patient with severe sepsis and septic shock [52]. Anna Prkno and co-workers reviewed various studies regarding the clinical trials and compared PCT-guided antibiotic stewardship with standard care and hospital mortality, duration of antimicrobial therapy and length of stay in the ICU. It was noticed that PCT guidance could not make better change in the mortality rate, but there was definitely a noteworthy effect on the duration of antimicrobial treatment [53, 54].

Future of PCT for the management of sepsis

Various studies are published revealing the wide application of PCT in medical field. Before selecting PCT as a biomarker, its limitations have to be studied. Further studies should be conducted to disclose even more application of PCT. The assay used for the detection must distinguish PCT levels between healthy individuals, non-bacteremia patients and progressing SIRS. More sensitive assays should be developed to take forward the studies to the clinical level [55, 56].

Conclusion

The PCT is a unique biomarker having wide range of application in the medical field, compared to other conventional markers for sepsis. However, to diagnose invasive bacterial infection and their severity assessment of PCT levels alone may not be enough. Because of the possible complication in diagnosis of sepsis and the challenge in differentiating between microbial and non-microbial infection cases, it is unlikely that a single biomarker serve as an effective diagnosis tool. A combination of biomarkers may be more functional in the case of clinical application, but this may require further investigation in various aspects as a reliable diagnostic tool [57, 58]. Measurement of combinational biomarkers may require reliable and cost effective technology development. Selection of biomarkers plays a crucial role in technology development; consequently, assessment of combination of biomarkers like procalcitonin, sCD14-ST and other new biomarkers can be made use in evaluation of sepsis in all age groups. Combination of emerging new biomarkers with PCT could be used in terms of good clinical judgement based on which antimicrobial therapy may suggested, thus reducing the prescription and duration of antibiotic treatment. Combinational biomarker with PCT-guided antibiotic stewardship could be properly fabricated to develop a safer and affordable strategy for diagnosis of sepsis and its prognosis.

Acknowledgements

The authors would like to thank the management team of HLL for the extended support and guidance. The authors are thankful to Dr. Rajmohan G (Scientist E3) for the valuable comments during scripting of this article. We are also thankful to Ms. Jeslin Varghese (Senior Project Fellow) for the technical support in completing the study.

Funding

Not applicable.

Authors' contributions

AV, VM, SR, SK, LS, KR and MG participated in drafting and revising the manuscript. All authors have read and approved the final manuscript.

Authors' information

Ms. Ashitha Vijayan, M. Sc Microbiology, working as Research Intern in Diagnostic Products lab of CRDC, HLL and involved in diagnostic kit developments.
Ms. Vani Maya, M. Sc Biochemistry, working as Junior Project Fellow in Diagnostic Products lab of CRDC, HLL and involved in diagnostic kit developments.
Ms. Shilpa Ravindran, M. Sc Biochemistry, Working as Senior Project Fellow in Diagnostic Products lab of CRDC, HLL and involved in diagnostic kit developments.
Mr. Saikant R, M. Sc Biotechnology, working as Junior Scientist in Diagnostic Products lab of CRDC, HLL and involved in diagnostic kit developments.
Dr. Lakshmi S, Ph.D Biotechnology, working as Junior Scientist in Diagnostic Products lab of CRDC, HLL and involved in drug developments.
Dr. Kartik Ramaswami, Ph.D Biotechnology, working as Junior Scientist in Diagnostic Products lab of CRDC, HLL and involved in clinical research.
Dr. Manoj G, Ph. D Biotechnology, working as Scientist E2 in Diagnostic Products lab of CRDC, HLL and involved in diagnostic kit developments.

Competing interests

The authors declare that they have no competing interests.

References

1. Markus B, Peter AW. The inflammatory response in sepsis. Trends Immunol. 2013;34(3):129–36.
2. Lever A, Mackenzie I. Sepsis: definition, epidemiology, and diagnosis. Br Med J. 2007;335:879–83.
3. Dunja M, Snezana B, Arsen U, Biljana D, Vladimir V. Use of presepsin and procalcitonin for prediction of SeptiFast results in critically ill patients. J Crit Care. 2017;40:197–201.
4. Angus DC, Van der Poll T. Severe sepsis and septic shock. N Engl J Med. 2013;369:840–51.
5. Moore LJ, McKinley BA, Turner K. The epidemiology of sepsis in general surgery patients. J Trauma. 2011;70(3):672–80.
6. Slade E, Tamber PS, Vincent JL. The surviving sepsis, campaign, raising awareness to reduce mortality. Crit Care. 2003;7(1):1–2.
7. Divatia JV, Amin PR, Ramakrishnan N, Kapadia FN, Todi S, Sahu S, Govil D, Chawla R, Kulkarni AP, Samavedam S, Jani CK, Rungta N, Samaddar DP, Mehta S, Venkataraman R, Hegde A, Bande BD, Dhanuka S, Singh V, Tewari R, Zirpe K, Sathe P, INDICAPS Study Investigators. Intensive care in India: the Indian intensive care case mix and practice patterns study. Indian J Crit Care Med. 2016;20(4):216–25.
8. Feldmann H, Geistbert TW. Ebola, hemorrhagic, fever. Lancet. 2011; 377(97768):849–62.
9. Calrk IA, Alleva LM, Mills AC, Cowden WB. Pathogen of malaria and clinically similar conditions. Clin Microbio Rev. 2004;17(3):509–39.
10. Paessler S, Walker DH. Pathogenesis of the viral hemorrhagic fever. Annu Rev Pathol. 2013;8:411–40.
11. Livorsi DJ, Stenehjem E, Stephens DS. Virulence factors of gram-negative bacteria in sepsis with a focus on Neisseria meningitidis. Contrib Microbiol. 2011;17:31–47.
12. Willey J, Sherwood L, Christopher JW. Prescotts's Microbiol, International edition. 8th ed; 2011. p. 97.
13. Rimmelé T, Leli C, Payen D, Cantaluppi V, Marshall J, Gomez H, Gomez A, Murray P, Kellum JA. Immune cell phenotype and function in sepsis. Shock. 2016;45(3):282–91.
14. Chen X-h, Yin Y-j, Zhang J-x. Sepsis and immune response. World J Emerg Med. 2011;2(2):88–92.
15. Reinhart K, Bauer M, Reideman NC, Hartog CS. New approaches to sepsis: molecular diagnostics and biomarkers. J Cln Microbiol. 2010;25:609–34.
16. Sakr Y, Brgett U, Nacul FE, Reinhart K, Brunkhorst F. Lipopolysaccharide binding protein in a surgical intensive care unit: a marker of sepsis? Crit Care Med. 2008;36:2014–22.
17. Usama M, Nermin A, Ayman A, Sultan MH. Serum procalcitonin in viral and bacterial meningitis. J Glob Infect Dis. 2011;3:14–8.
18. Hina C, Juhua Z, Yin Z, Mir MA, Franklin M, Prakash SN, Mitzi N. Role of Cytokines as a Double-edged Sword in Sepsis. In Vivo. 2013;27(6):669–84.
19. Angus DC, Linde-Zwirble WT, Lidicker J, Clermont G, Carcillo J, Pinsky MR. Epidemology of severe sepsis in the United States. Analysis of incidence, outcome and associated cost of care. Crit Care Med. 2001;29:1303–10.
20. Standage SW, Wong HR. Biomarkers for paediatric sepsis and septic shock. Expert Rev Anti-Infect Ther. 2011;9(1):71–9.
21. Moya F, Nieto A, Jose LR. Calcitonin biosynthesis: evidence for a precursor. Eur J Biochem. 1975;55:407–13.
22. Allison J, Hall L, MacIntyre I, Craig RK. The construction and partial characterisation of plasmid containing complimentary DNA sequences to human calcitonin precursor poly protein. Biochem J. 1981;199:725–31.
23. Jacobs JW, Lund PK, Potts JT, Bell NH, Habener JF. Procalcitonin is a glycoprotein. J Biol Chem. 1981;25(256):2803–7.
24. Katherine S, Roma LH. Proclacitonin: an emerging biomarker of bacterial sepsis. Clin Microbiol Newsletter. 2001;3:171–8.

25. Müller B, White JC, Nylén ES, Snider RH, Becker KL, Habener JF. Ubiquitous expression of the calcitonin-1 gene in multiple tissues in response to sepsis. J Clin Endocrinol Metab. 2001;86:396–404.
26. Assicot M, Gendrel D, Carsin H, Raymond J, Guilbaud J, Bohuon C. High serum procalcitonin concentrations in patients with sepsis and infection. Lancet. 1993;341:515–8.
27. Müller B, Harbarth S, Stolz D, Bingisser R, Mueller C, Leuppi J, Nusbaumer C, Tamm M, Christ-Crain M. Diagnostic and prognostic accuracy of clinical and laboratory parameters in community-acquired pneumonia. BMC Infect Dis. 2007;7:10.
28. Dan L, Longxiang S, Gencheng H, Peng Y, Lixin X. Prognostic value of Procalcitonin in adult patients with sepsis: a systematic review and meta-analysis. PLoS One. 2015;10(6):e0129450.
29. Müller B, Becker KL, Schächinger H, Rickenbacher PR, Huber PR, Zimmerli W, Ritz R. Calcitonin precursors are reliable markers of sepsis in a medical intensive care unit. Crit Care Med. 2000;28:977–83.
30. Nargis W, Ibrahim MD, Ahamed BU. Procalcitonin versus C-reactive protein: usefulness as biomarker of sepsis in ICU patient. Int J CritIlln Inj Sci. 2014;4:195–9.
31. Young HK, Yoon SJ, Sin-Youl P, Kim SJ, Song PH. Procalcitonin determined at emergency department as an early indicator of progression to septic shock in patient with sepsis associated with ureteral calculi. Int Braz J Urol. 2016;42(2):270–6.
32. Yaegashi Y, Shirakawa K, Sato N, Suzuki Y, Kojika M, Imai S, et al. Evaluation of a newly identified soluble CD14 subtype as a marker for sepsis. J Infect Chemother. 2005;11:234–8.
33. Romualdo LG, Torrella PE, González MV, Sánchez RJ, Holgado AH, Freire AO. Diagnostic accuracy of presepsin (soluble CD14 subtype) for prediction of bacteremia in patients with systemic inflammatory response syndrome in the emergency department. Clin Biochem. 2014;47:505–8.
34. Camussi G, Mariano F, Biancone L, De Martino A, Bussolati B, Montrucchio G, et al. Lipopolysaccharide binding protein and CD14 modulate the synthesis of platelet-activating factor by human monocytes and mesangial and endothelial cells stimulated with lipopolysaccharide. J Immunol. 1995;155:316–24.
35. Jiayuan W, Liren H, Gaohua Z, Fenping W, Taiping H. Accuracy of presepsin in sepsis diagnosis: a systematic review and meta-analysis. PLoS One. 2015;10(7):e0133057.
36. Wacker C, Prkno A, Brunkhorst FM. Procalcitonin as a diagnostic marker for sepsis: a systematic review and meta-analysis. Lancet Infect Dis. 2013;13: 426–35.
37. Cargnin S, Jommi C, Canonico PL, Genazzani AA, Terrazzino S. Diagnostic accuracy of HLAB*57:01 screening for the prediction of abacavir hypersensitivity and clinical utility of the test: a meta-analysis review. Pharmacogenonics. 2014;15:963–76.
38. Christian L, Marta F, Umberto M, Zainab SD, Silvia B, Elio C, Antonella M. Diagnostic accuracy of presepsin (sCD14-ST) and procalcitonin for prediction of bacteremia and bacterial DNAaemia in patients with suspected sepsis. J Med Microbiol. 2016;65:713–9.
39. Kada K, Jean PC, Julie D, Vincent G, Nils K, Romaric L, Laurent A, Philippe C, Olivier J, Anne MD. Diagnostic and prognostic value of soluble CD14 subtype (presepsin) for sepsis and community-acquired pneumonia in ICU patients. Ann Intensive Care. 2016;6:59.
40. Enguix-Armada A, Escobar-Conesa R, García-De La Torre A, De La Torre-Prados MV. Usefulness of several biomarkers in the management of septic patients: C-reactive protein, procalcitonin, presepsin and mid-regional pro-adrenomedullin. Clin Chem Lab Med. 2016;54(1):163–8.
41. Michael M. Update on procalcitonin measurements. Ann Lab Med. 2014;34:263–73.
42. Lieberman JM. Appropriate antibiotic use and why it is important: the challenges of bacterial resistance. Pediatr Infect Dis J. 2003;22(12):1143–51.
43. Scott F, James B, Ryan F, Shelley M, Lori AP, Paul M, Rachel S, Karim K, Michael AR, Makoto J, Matthew HS, Dumyati G, Elizabeth DA, James M, Kimberly YH, Jernigan J, Shehab N, Herrera R, LC MD, Schneider A, Arjun S. Vital signs: improving antibiotic use among hospitalized patients. Mob Mort Wkly Rep. 2014;63(09):194–200.
44. Liew YX, Chlebicki MP, Lee W, Hsu LY, Kwa AL. Use of procalcitonin (PCT) to guide discontinuation of antibiotic use in an unspecified sepsis is an antimicrobial stewardship program (ASP). Eur J Clin Microbiol Infect Dis. 2011;30:853–5.
45. Larson E. Community factors in the development of antibiotic resistance. Annu Rev Public Health. 2007;28:435–47.
46. Simon P, Milbrandt EB, Emlet LL. PCT-guided antibiotics in severe sepsis. Crit Care. 2008;12:309.
47. Chirouze C, Schuhmacher H, Rabaud C, Gil H, Khayat N, Estavoyer JM, May T, Hoen B. Low-serum procalcitonin level accuracy predicts the absence of bacteraemia in adult patients with acute fever. Clin Infect Dis. 2002;35:156–61.
48. Stolz D, Christ-Crain M, Bingisser R, Leuppi J, Miedinger D, Müller C, Huber P, Müller B, Tamm M. Antibiotic treatment of exacerbations of COPD: a randomized, controlled trial comparing procalcitonin-guidance with standard therapy. Chest. 2007;131:9–19.
49. Schroeder S, Hochreiter M, Koehler T, Schweiger AM, Bein B, Keck FS, von Spiegel T. Procalcitonin (PCT)-guided algorithm reduces length of antibiotic treatment in surgical intensive care patients with severe sepsis: results of a prospective randomized study. Langenbeck's Arch Surg. 2009;394(2):221–6.
50. Lavrentieva A, Kontou P, Soulountsi V, Kioumis J, Chrysou O, Bitzani M. Implementation of a procalcitonin-guided algorithm for antibiotic therapy in the burn intensive care unit. Ann Burns Fire Disasters. 2015;28(3):163–70.
51. Kip MM, Kusters R, IJzerman J, Steuten MA. PCT algorithm for discontinuation of antibiotic therapy is a cost-effective way to reduce antibiotic exposure in adult intensive care patients with sepsis. J Med Econ. 2015;18(11):944–53.
52. Nobre V, Harbarth S, Graf JD, Rohner P, Jerome P. Use of procalcitonin to shorten antibiotic treatment duration in septic patients. Am J Resp Crit Care Med. 2008;177:498–505.
53. Prkno A, Wacker C, Brunkhorstand FM, Schlattmann P. Procalcitonin-guided therapy in intensive care unit patients with severe sepsis and septic shock—a systematic review and meta-analysis. Crit Care. 2013;17:R291.
54. Nylen E, Muller B, Becker KL, Snider R. The future diagnostic role of procalcitonin levels: the need for improved sensitivity. Clin Infect Dis. 2003;36:823–4.
55. Pradeep M, Xu J, Karen DHM. Biomarkers for neonatal sepsis: recent developments. Dovepress. 2014;4:157–68.
56. Taylor R, Jones A, Kelly S, Simpson M, Mabey J. A review of the value of procalcitonin as a marker of infection. Cureus. 2017;9(4):e1148.
57. Cakır Madenci O, Yakupoglu S, Benzonana N, Yucel N, Akbaba D, Orçun KA. Evaluation of soluble CD14 subtype (presepsin) in burn sepsis. Burns. 2013;40:664–9.
58. Elisa P, Marco U, Claudia G, Manuela L, Tilde M, Enrico L, Giulio M, Stefania B. Role of presepsin for the evaluation of sepsis in the emergency department. Clin Chem Lab Med. 2014;52(10):1395–400.

Fluid responsiveness prediction using Vigileo FloTrac measured cardiac output changes during passive leg raise test

Anton Krige[1*], Martin Bland[1] and Thomas Fanshawe[2]

Abstract

Background: Passive leg raising (PLR) is a so called self-volume challenge used to test for fluid responsiveness. Changes in cardiac output (CO) or stroke volume (SV) measured during PLR are used to predict the need for subsequent fluid loading. This requires a device that can measure CO changes rapidly. The Vigileo™ monitor, using third-generation software, allows continuous CO monitoring. The aim of this study was to compare changes in CO (measured with the Vigileo device) during a PLR manoeuvre to calculate the accuracy for predicting fluid responsiveness.

Methods: This is a prospective study in a 20-bedded mixed general critical care unit in a large non-university regional referral hospital. Fluid responders were defined as having an increase in CO of greater than 15 % following a fluid challenge. Patients meeting the criteria for circulatory shock with a Vigileo™ monitor (Vigileo™; FloTrac; Edwards™; Lifesciences, Irvine, CA, USA) already in situ, and assessed as requiring volume expansion by the clinical team based on clinical criteria, were included. All patients underwent a PLR manoeuvre followed by a fluid challenge.

Results: Data was collected and analysed on stroke volume variation (SVV) at baseline and CO and SVV changes during the PLR manoeuvre and following a subsequent fluid challenge in 33 patients. The majority had septic shock. Patient characteristics, baseline haemodynamic variables and baseline vasoactive infusion requirements were similar between fluid responders (10 patients) and non-responders (23 patients). Peak increase in CO occurred within 120 s during the PLR in all cases. Using an optimal cut point of 9 % increase in CO during the PLR produced an area under the receiver operating characteristic curve of 0.85 (95 % CI 0.63 to 1.00) with a sensitivity of 80 % (95 % CI 44 to 96 %) and a specificity of 91 % (95 % CI 70 to 98 %).

Conclusions: CO changes measured by the Vigileo™ monitor using third-generation software during a PLR test predict fluid responsiveness in mixed medical and surgical patients with *vasopressor-dependent circulatory* shock.

Keywords: Passive leg raising, Edwards Vigileo FloTrac monitoring, Fluid responsiveness, Cardiac output monitoring, Vasoplegic shock, Septic shock,

Background

Circulatory insufficiency is common in critically ill patients and may lead to organ dysfunction. Increasing cardiac preload may increase stroke volume (SV) and consequently cardiac output (CO) and thus tissue perfusion [1]. However, it has been shown that only half of critically ill patients thought to be preload responsive, based on static predictors of preload, actually show an increase in SV, and therefore CO, following volume expansion (VE) [2, 3]. The administration of fluid in the group that is not preload responsive not only delays the appropriate management of their circulatory insufficiency but is also an independent predictor of delayed respiratory weaning and survival [4–11].

Functional haemodynamic monitoring has been shown to accurately predict fluid responsiveness but unfortunately several caveats, which include constant tidal volumes of adequate size and sinus rhythm, must be

* Correspondence: anton.krige@elht.nhs.uk
[1]Department of Anaesthesia and Critical Care, Royal Blackburn Hospital, Haslingden Road, Blackburn, UK
Full list of author information is available at the end of the article

present [12–17]. Unfortunately, this precludes a large proportion of critically ill patients.

Passive leg raising (PLR), whereby the patients legs are transiently raised by 45°, and the torso flattened, results in a reversible flow of 150–300 ml of blood from the venous capacitance vessels of the lower body, to the thoracic compartment, a so called self-volume challenge [18–20]. Boulain et al. [21] first demonstrated the potential of this phenomenon to predict fluid responsiveness by measuring blood pressure changes during a PLR.

Subsequent studies have shown even greater accuracy, without the limitations of functional haemodynamic monitoring, using a variety of minimally invasive devices capable of rapid measurement of changes in flow or stroke volume during PLR. Examples include esophageal Doppler [22, 23], transthoracic Doppler ultrasound [24], transthoracic echocardiography (TTE) [25–29], pulse contour techniques [28, 30–33], bioreactance [34–36], end tidal carbon dioxide change [37] and bio-impedance cardiography [38]. These studies have been summarised in three recent systematic reviews [39–41], and all reported a high sensitivity regarding prediction of fluid responsiveness (all three reported the same pooled area under the receiver operating characteristic curve (AUC) of 0.95, with similar confidence intervals).

Only one of these [28] studies used the Vigileo™ monitor but with second-generation software.

The aim of this study was to assess the accuracy of the Vigileo™ monitor (Vigileo™; FloTrac; Edwards™; Lifesciences, Irvine, CA, USA) using third-generation software (version 3.02), in predicting preload responsiveness by measuring changes in CO during a PLR manoeuvre, in a mixture of medical and surgical critically ill patients with circulatory shock, with or without spontaneous breathing efforts or arrhythmias. In addition, we included an assessment of the accuracy of stroke volume variation (SVV) measured by the same device to predict responsiveness. We evaluated a cut point of 9.6 % at baseline (derived by Li et al. [42]), and the change in SVV during PLR were both evaluated as predictors of fluid responsiveness.

Methods

Patients

This prospective study was conducted on a mixed medical and surgical general critical care unit in a large non-university regional referral hospital. The study received research ethics committee approval and patients were enrolled following written informed consent.

Inclusion criteria

Critical care patients, over 18 years of age, requiring a fluid challenge as decided by the attending critical care physician, were included. The research team had no influence over this decision, and patients were only approached for enrolment following the decision to administer a fluid challenge.

This decision was based on the presence of at least one clinical sign of inadequate tissue perfusion, i.e. (a) systolic blood pressure <90 mmHg (or a decrease of >50 mmHg in previously hypertensive patients) or the need for vasoconstrictor drugs (vasopressin or norepinephrine); (b) urine output <0.5 ml/kg/h for ≥2 h; (c) tachycardia (heart rate >100/min); or (d) presence of skin mottling.

The Vigileo system (Edwards Lifescience, Irvine, CA) with arterial pressure waveform analysis device via special blood flow sensor (FloTrac Sensor, Edwards Lifesciences, Irvine, CA) using third-generation software must already be in situ.

Exclusion criteria

Any patients that were unable to perform PLR and who had any contraindications to fluid challenge, defined as life-threatening hypoxaemia, and evidence of blood volume overload and/or hydrostatic pulmonary oedema, were excluded.

Measurements

All haemodynamic data was continuously recorded on a Draeger monitoring system and a Vigileo system (Edwards Lifesciences, Irvine, CA) using third-generation software (version 3.02).

VigileoTM monitor measurements

The FloTrac transducer (FloTracTM, Edwards Lifesciences, Irvine, CA, USA) connected the indwelling arterial line to the VigileoTM System (Edwards Lifesciences, Irvine, CA, USA). This non-calibrated continuous CO monitor software analyses the arterial waveform with a frequency of a 100 Hz over 20 s. SV is calculated as $k \times$ pulsatility, where pulsatility is the standard deviation of arterial pressure over the preceding 20 s, and k is a factor which describes vascular compliance and resistance over the preceding 1 to 5 min, depending on the setting. This factor (so called proprietary Dynamic Tone Technology) is derived from a multivariate regression model taking into account Langewouter's aortic compliance [43], mean arterial pressure (MAP), along with variance, skewness, and kurtosis of the arterial pressure wave [43, 44]. A greater number of hyperdynamic and vasodilated patients were incorporated into the algorithm database, and additional physiologically based variables were added to the algorithm's vascular tone k factor in order to adjust automatically for hyperdynamic and vasodilated patients in the third-generation software update. This has increased the accuracy of SV measurement in vasodilated patients [45–47].

Other measurements

The presence of any arrhythmias was recorded. Respiratory data was collated regarding the mode of ventilation, presence of spontaneous respiratory efforts, peak inspiratory pressures, plateau pressures, PEEP value and tidal volume. Dosages of any vasoactive drugs were recorded.

Study design

The study design is illustrated in Fig. 1. The following peak haemodynamic parameters were all recorded at each of the four stages in the protocol: heart rate (HR), mean arterial pressure (MAP), central venous pressure (CVP), cardiac index (CI), CO, SV, stroke volume index (SVI) and stroke volume variation (SVV). At the first baseline stage, measurements were taken while the patient was 45° semi-recumbent. During the next stage (PLR), the remote control of the bed was used to tilt the trunk to a horizontal position, and the legs were tilted 45° upwards. The patient was then returned to the 45° semi-recumbent position until the haemodynamic parameters stabilised to similar values as the original baseline. These values were recorded as representing the second baseline stage. Following this, a VE of 250 ml of Gelofusine[R] was administered at the maximum rate allowed by the volumetric pump (within 15 min). The final stage, denoted as post volume expansion (PVE), occurred immediately following the fluid challenge, when all haemodynamic parameters were recorded once again.

Statistical analysis

Continuous data are reported as mean and standard deviation or median and inter-quartile range. A change in CO from baseline of >15 and <15 % following the volume challenge was used to classify the patients as 'responders' and 'non-responders', respectively [3]. Measured variables were then compared between responders and non-responders using *t* tests, chi-squared tests or Fisher's exact test for low counts, as appropriate for the data type, and reported as *p* values. The positively skewed variables of time to admission, tidal volume and norepinephrine dose were analysed after log-transforming the original data values. A receiver operating characteristic (ROC) curve was used to measure the sensitivity and specificity of the PLR test to predict responders to the fluid challenge.

p values of less than 0.05 were considered to be statistically significant. Statistical analysis was performed using R version 2.15.2 [48].

Results

Patient characteristics

Thirty-seven patients with CO monitoring in situ and meeting clinical criteria for a fluid challenge were initially included and four were subsequently excluded. Three had different diagnoses (cardiogenic shock with blood volume overload which was an exclusion criteria), and one had missing baseline and PLR CO data. The data from the remaining 33 patients who received a fluid challenge were analysed. Patient characteristics are summarised in Table 1 and were similar between groups. The majority (80 %), overall and in each group, were on a controlled mode of ventilation, with similar tidal volumes between groups. Cardiac arrhythmias were present in 9 % of all patients and balanced between the groups. The aetiology of circulatory insufficiency was septic shock in the majority (82 %) and severe systemic inflammatory response syndrome (SIRS) in the remainder.

Baseline haemodynamic variables and vasoactive infusions

There were no statistically significant differences in baseline haemodynamic variables (Table 2). Vasoactive drug infusions (Table 3) were similar between groups, and only two patients did not receive any vasoactive infusions at the time of the PLR test. Thirty (91 %) patients received a norepinephrine infusion with a mean dose of 0.30 (0.17) mcg/kg/min. Seven patients received Dobutamine, and this was split between responders and non-responders. Vasopressin infusions were used in two patients. It was combined with norepinephrine in one patient and used as sole vasopressor in the other.

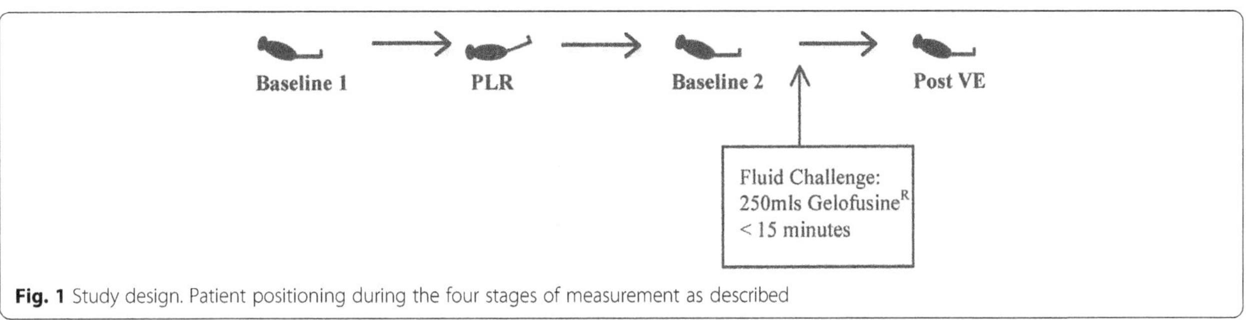

Fig. 1 Study design. Patient positioning during the four stages of measurement as described

Table 1 Patient characteristics

	All *n* = 33	Responders *n* = 10	Non-responders *n* = 23	*p*
Age	60.0 (13.6)	58.4 (16.2)	60.7 (12.7)	0.70
Sex				
Male	15 (45 %)	4 (40 %)	11 (48 %)	0.97
Female	18 (55 %)	6 (60 %)	12 (52 %)	
Weight (kg)	72.1 (12.9)	75.0 (14.1)	70.9 (12.4)	0.44
APACHE II score	19.9 (6.9)	19.0 (5.8)	20.4 (7.5)	0.58
Died in hospital				
Yes	16 (48 %)	7 (70 %)	9 (39 %)	0.21
No	17 (52 %)	3 (30 %)	14 (61 %)	
Admission to PLR (h)	26 [18, 52]	38 [21,102]	26 [16, 42]	0.25
Arrhythmia				
Present	3/32 (9 %)	1/9 (11 %)	2/23 (9 %)	1.00
Absent	29/32 (91 %)	8/9 (89 %)	21/23 (91 %)	
Tidal volume (ml)	510 [463, 563]	540 [473, 660]	491 [460, 549]	0.39
Plateau pressure (cmH_2O)	26.6 (7.1)	26.4 (5.5)	26.7 (7.7)	0.90
PEEP (cmH_2O)	8.5 (2.5)	8.9 (2.8)	8.4 (2.4)	0.60
Respiratory rate (/min)	16.8 (4.2)	15.5 (2.4)	17.3 (4.7)	0.15
Spontaneous breathing				
Yes	6/30 (20 %)	2/9 (22 %)	4/21 (19 %)	1.00
No	24/30 (80 %)	7/9 (78 %)	17/21 (81 %)	
Arterial line site:				
Femoral	4 (12 %)	1 (10 %)	3 (13 %)	1.00
Other (radial and brachial)	29 (88 %)	9 (90 %)	20 (87 %)	
Diagnostic groups:				
Septic shock	27 (82 %)	7 (70 %)	20 (87 %)	0.34
- Endocarditis	1 (3 %)	0 (0 %)	1 (4 %)	-
- Occult	7 (21 %)	2 (20 %)	5 (22 %)	-
- Peritonitis	8 (24 %)	2 (20 %)	6 (26 %)	-
- Pneumonia	11 (33 %)	3 (30 %)	8 (35 %)	-
SIRS	6 (18 %)	3 (30 %)	3 (13 %)	-
- Ischaemic bowel	2 (6 %)	1 (10 %)	1 (4 %)	-
- Occult	1 (3 %)	0	1 (4 %)	-
- Pancreatico-duodenectomy	1 (3 %)	0	1 (4 %)	-
- Pancreatitis	2 (6 %)	2 (20 %)	0	-

Data are shown as mean (standard deviation), median (inter-quartile range), or number (percentage) with *p* value comparing responders to non-responders for certain characteristics. Sample sizes are as in column headings unless stated (some variables had small numbers of missing values)

Effects of PLR and VE on CO and other haemodynamic variables

The peak increase in CO occurred within 120 s in all cases. CO change during PLR was positively related to subsequent VE (correlation = 0.65) (Fig. 2). Spontaneous breathing and/or arrhythmia was only present in a few patients in each group thus not allowing any meaningful analysis of the influence of these two factors on the association (Table 1).

Effects of PLR and VE on changes in CO

The changes in CO induced by PLR were significantly greater in responders than in non-responders ($p = 0.02$). In fluid responders, CO increased by an average of 1.43 l/min (95 % CI 0.53 to 2.33) from baseline (average 5.98) to during PLR (average 7.41), corresponding to a 24 % increase from baseline (95 % CI 8 to 39 %), and by an average of 1.94 l/min (95 % CI 0.99 to 2.89) from

Table 2 Haemodynamic variables at baseline

	All	Responders	Non-responders	p
	n = 33	n = 10	n = 23	
HR (/min)	100 (19.5)	106 (19.9)	98 (19.2)	0.29
CVP (mmHg)	10.6 (5.7)	9.9 (6.1)	10.9 (5.7)	0.66
MAP (mmHg)	69.5 (10.7)	65.1 (8.8)	71.5 (11.0)	0.09
PP (mmHg)	52.6 (13.1)	51.6 (17.8)	52.9 (11.2)	0.85
SV (ml/beat)	60.8 (14.5)	56.7 (16.3)	62.7 (13.7)	0.33
SVI (ml/m^2/beat)	33.4 (7.8)	30.9 (8.8)	34.4 (7.4)	0.28
CO (L/min)	6.1 (1.5)	6.0 (1.6)	6.1 (1.5)	0.84
CI (L/min/m^2)	3.3 (0.8)	3.3 (1.0)	3.4 (0.8)	0.81
SVV (%)	14.2 (11.0)	18.4 (10.5)	12.3 (11.0)	0.15
SVR (dynes s/cm^5)	842 (347)	917 (504)	810 (259)	0.54

Data are shown as mean (standard deviation) or number (percentage) with p value comparing responders to non-responders.
HR heart rate, *CVP* central venous pressure, *MAP* mean arterial pressure, *PP* pulse pressure, *SV* stroke volume, *SVI* stroke volume index, *CO* cardiac output, *CI* cardiac index, *SVV* stroke volume variation, *SVR* systemic vascular resistance

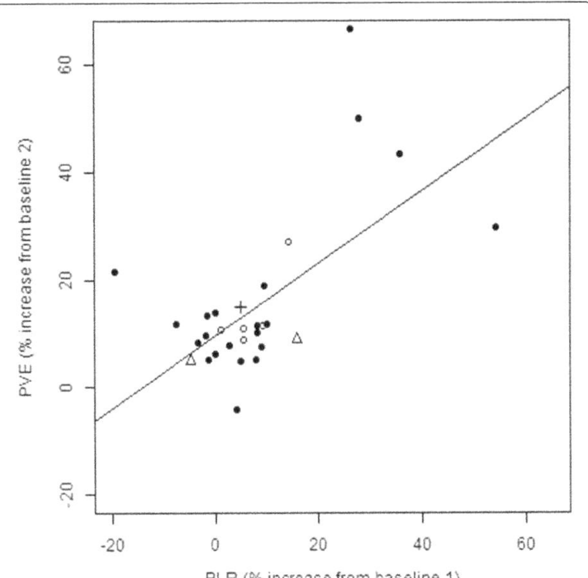

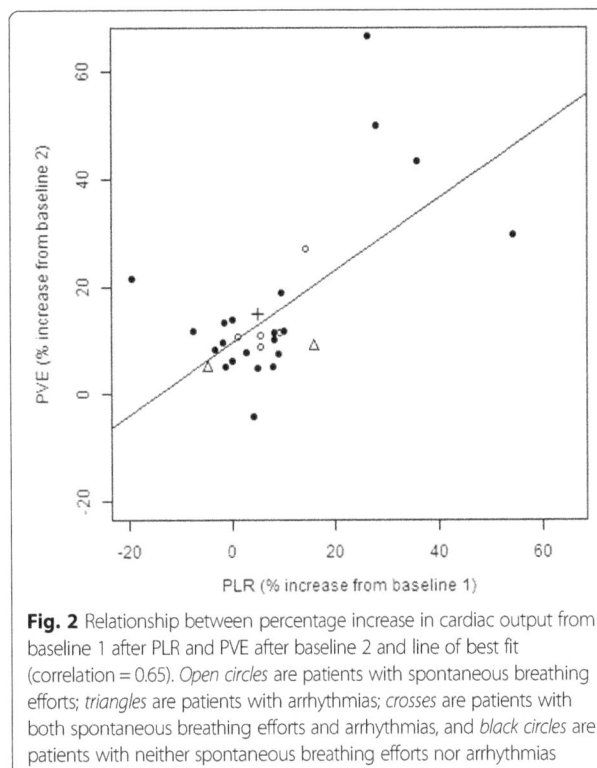

Fig. 2 Relationship between percentage increase in cardiac output from baseline 1 after PLR and PVE after baseline 2 and line of best fit (correlation = 0.65). *Open circles* are patients with spontaneous breathing efforts; *triangles* are patients with arrhythmias; *crosses* are patients with both spontaneous breathing efforts and arrhythmias, and *black circles* are patients with neither spontaneous breathing efforts nor arrhythmias

before VE (average 5.39) to after VE (average 7.33), corresponding to a 35 % increase from baseline (95 % CI 24 to 47 %).

In fluid non-responders, CO increased by an average of 0.24 l/min (95 % CI 0.09 to 0.39) from baseline (average 6.10) to during PLR (average 6.34), corresponding to a 3 % increase from baseline (95 % CI 1 to 6 %), and by an average of 0.45 l/min (95 % CI 0.31 to 0.59) from before VE (average 5.94) to after VE (average 6.39), corresponding to a 7 % increase from baseline (95 % CI 5 to 10 %).

Seven patients had an insignificant reduction in their CO during PLR (Fig. 2).

Prediction of fluid responsiveness

The ROC curve (Fig. 3) shows the varying predictive performance of the PLR test as the cut point changes. The optimal cut point on the ROC curve for this dataset was approximately 9 %, i.e. an increase in CO of 9 % or greater during PLR predicts fluid responsiveness with the greatest accuracy generating a sensitivity of 80 % (95 % CI 44 to 96 %) and a specificity of 91 % (95 % CI 70 to 98 %).

Although there was little distinction between a range of 10 to 15 % (for a 15 % cut point the sensitivity and specificity was 60 % (95 % CI 27 to 86 %) and 96 (95 % CI 76 to 99.8 %), the positive and negative predictive values were 86 % (695 % CI 42 to 99 %) and 85 % (95 % CI 64 to 95 %), respectively).

The area under the empirical ROC curve was 0.85 (95 % CI 0.63 to 1.00).

Using the increase in SVV during the PLR test as the predictor provides no better predictive performance than would be expected by chance with an area under the ROC curve of 0.56 (95 % CI 0.34 to 0.77).

An SVV cut point of 9.6 % at baseline, rather than change during PLR, as the predictor of fluid responsiveness, gives an area under the ROC curve of 0.74 (95 % CI 0.53 to 0.91), with 70 % sensitivity and 57 % specificity.

Discussion

Our study shows that changes in CO measured using the Vigileo™ monitor during a PLR manoeuvre is a useful

Table 3 Vasoactive drug infusions

	All	Responders	Non-responders	p
Norepinephrine (mcg/kg/min)	0.28 (0.20, 0.36) (n = 30)	0.31 (0.16, 0.37) (n = 10)	0.28 (0.21, 0.34) (n = 20)	0.92
Vasopressin (mcg/min)	–	4.5 (n = 1)	3.0 (n = 1)[a]	–
Dobutamine (mcg/kg/min)	4.6 (1.2) (n = 7)	4.4 (1.3) (n = 4)	4.8 (1.2) (n = 3)	–

Data are shown as mean (standard deviation) or median (inter-quartile range), and number of patients (n) (p value compares dose between responders and non-responders in the case of norepinephrine). In the case of vasopressin, the only dose is given, as there was one patient only in each group
[a]The only patient requiring vasopressor support that did not include norepinephrine

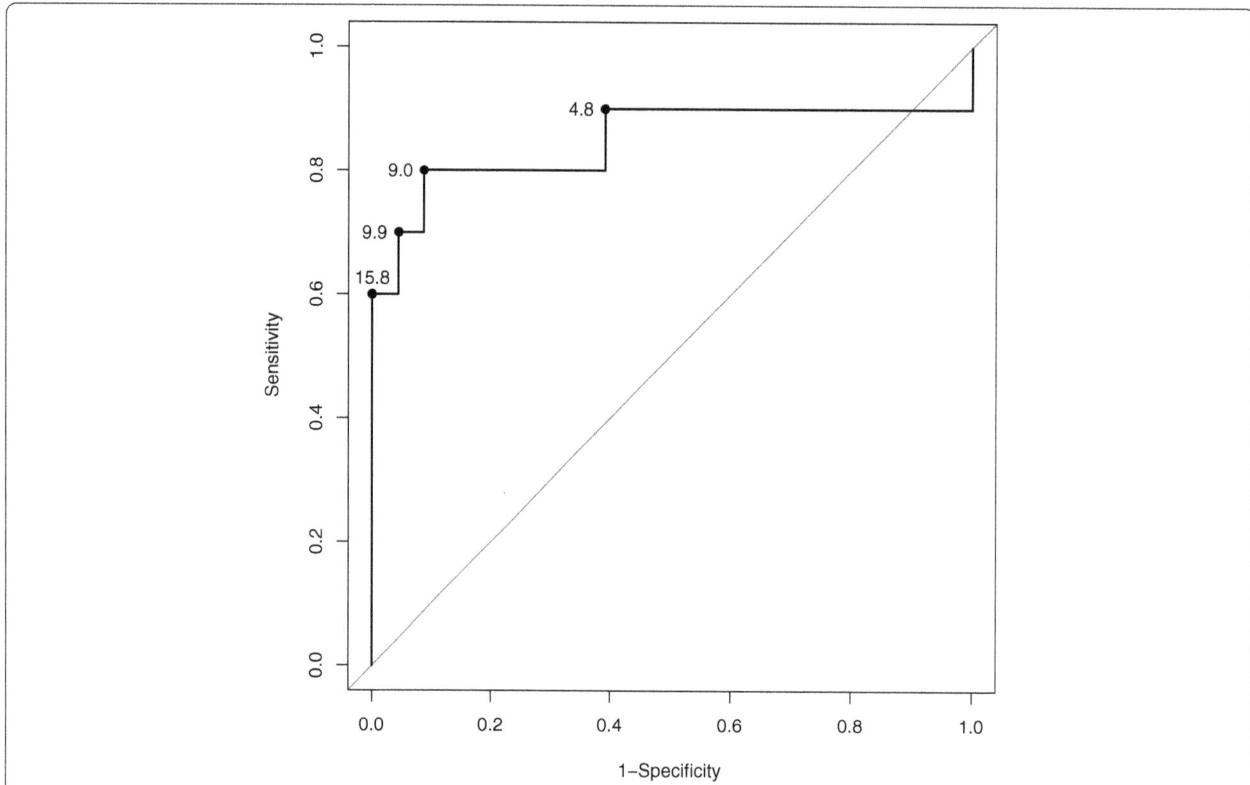

Fig. 3 ROC curve demonstrating predictive performance after PLR on cardiac output response to PVE (AUC 0.85). Figures on the curve indicate the relevant cut point of cardiac output response (% change from baseline)

predictor of fluid responsiveness in mixed critically ill patients with vasopressor-dependent circulatory shock. An increase in CO of ≥ 9 % during the PLR predicted an increase in CO of ≥15 % following subsequent volume expansion with good sensitivity (80 %) and specificity (91 %) resulting in an AUC of 0.85 (95 % CI 0.63 to 1.00). The high specificity has the potential to avoid the deleterious effects of unnecessary volume expansion in this patient group [4, 6, 7, 11].

Our results were consistent with previous validation studies of the PLR manoeuvre [21–38, 49] which are encapsulated in three recent systematic reviews [39–41]. These included nine, 21 and 23 studies assessing a total of 353, 991 and 1013, patients respectively. Our results were similar to the only other study using the Vigileo FloTrac device conducted by Biais et al. [14]. They reported a sensitivity of 85 % and a specificity of 90 % with a sample size of 34 patients and a peak change in flow within 120 s. Their study differed from our study in the following respects. They used second-generation FloTrac software whereas we used third-generation FloTrac software. Almost all the patients in the Biais study were surgical as opposed to an even split between medical and surgical in our study. The patients in our sample were much sicker, i.e. only 65 % were invasively ventilated in their study and all were breathing spontaneously with none receiving vasoactive drugs. That is in contrast with our study where all the patients were invasively ventilated and receiving vasoactive drugs (mean norepinephrine dosage was 0.3 ± 0.17mcg/kg/min). We reported a high APACHE2 score and hospital mortality.

Our study had the following limitations. Firstly, we identified less than one third of our sample as fluid responders (ten out of 33 subjects), whereas 50 % of patients were identified as responders in the systematic review by Michard et al. [3] and similarly in the PLR systematic reviews [39–41]. This may have weakened our calculated sensitivity and specificity. Responders were defined using a cut off of 15 %, as this definition was used consistently throughout the other published PLR studies [21–41, 49, 50], and we used the recommended PLR manoeuvre, i.e. patients started from a semi-recumbent position. This has been indentified as essential to ensure that splanchnic blood redistribution occurs thereby ensuring an adequate self-volume challenge [49].The small sample size and the volume chosen for our fluid challenges may have contributed to this lower rate of fluid responders. However, the sample size was still larger than half of all other PLR studies published [21–38, 49]. We chose 250 ml of Gelofusine for our fluid challenges as this was a pragmatic study which followed the local clinical practice at that time. Although most of the studies in the systematic reviews [39–41] used volumes of 500 ml, the study by Kang et al. [31] used

250 ml, and the study by Boulain et al. [21] used 300 ml of Gelatin. Both of these studies reported the usual rate of fluid responders and the Kang et al. study reported very high sensitivity and specificity. Boulain et al. discussed the rationale for choosing that volume, i.e. it is roughly equal to the volume of blood redistributed by the PLR manoeuvre. The volume and type of fluid we used were also consistent with the 2008 Surviving Sepsis Campaign Guidelines [51], a review by Vincent et al. [52] on circulatory shock and Trof et al. showed a more rapid change in SV with colloid boluses [53]. We delivered our volume challenge within fifteen minutes which is in keeping with the other studies.

Secondly, we measured CO using a single non-calibrated device and did not include a second calibrated device. However, the study by Biais et al. [28] had simultaneously measured haemodynamic changes during PLR with the Vigileo™ monitor and transthoracic echocardiography and found that the changes induced by volume expansion correlated well between these two devices ($r^2 = 0.77$, $p < 0.0001$). This was despite Biais et al. using the less accurate second-generation Vigileo software (version 1.14). In addition, several studies have validated the Vigileo third-generation software in the patient population we recruited. Meng et al. [46] assessed the trending ability of the Vigileo third-generation software using directly measured Oesophageal Doppler blood flow as the comparison device and found that the two devices showed 96 % concordance when measuring a change in preload induced by whole body tilting. De Backer et al. [45] reported acceptable accuracy using the third-generation software in patients with vasoplegia (septic shock and liver failure) as did Slagt et al. [47] in a systematic review comparing the different generations of Vigileo software. Despite the absence of a second calibrated device in our study, we derived a similar optimal cut point as the other published PLR studies [21–41, 49, 50] and specifically in the subgroups that also used pulse contour methods [28, 30–33].

Thirdly, in the majority of our patients (88 %), measurement was via a peripheral artery which may be less accurate than via a central artery in vasodilated patients [54]. The number receiving a central (femoral) arterial catheter was too few to analyse for this effect.

Finally, 39 % of the patients included in our study were surgical and therefore had the potential for intra-abdominal hypertension which has been shown by Mahjoub et al. [50] to reduce the accuracy of PLR for predicting fluid responsiveness. We did not have sufficient data on intra-abdominal pressures to analyse for this effect.

Conclusions

We have demonstrated that changes in cardiac output measured using the Vigileo™ monitor with third-generation software during a PLR test were predictive of fluid responsiveness in both medical and surgical patients with vasopressor-dependent circulatory shock. As the EV1000™ monitoring system, which has replaced the Vigileo™ monitor, continues to use the third-generation software for the FloTrac device these findings remain valid.

Abbreviations

AUC: Area under the receiving operating characteristic curve; CO: Cardiac output; PLR: Passive leg raise; PVE: Post volume expansion; SV: Stroke volume; TTE: Transthoracic echocardiography; VE: Volume expansion

Acknowledgements

Lynne Bullock and Donna Harrison-Briggs participated in the data collection. This study received no financial support. The Vigileo™ monitor (Vigileo™; FloTrac; Edwards™; Lifesciences, Irvine, CA, USA) was part of our routine flow monitoring on our critical care unit for 3 years prior to this study.

Funding

This study was undertaken by the authors and the acknowledged members of the clinical team without any external funding.

Authors' contributions

AK conceived and designed the study, participated in the data collection and drafted the manuscript. MB participated in the data collection and contributed to drafting the manuscript. TF provided the statistical analysis and contributed to drafting the manuscript. AK has full access to all the study data and takes responsibility for data integrity and accuracy of data analysis. All authors read and approved the final manuscript.

Competing interests

The authors declare that they have no competing interests.

Author details

[1]Department of Anaesthesia and Critical Care, Royal Blackburn Hospital, Haslingden Road, Blackburn, UK. [2]Nuffield Department of Primary Care Health Sciences, University of Oxford, Oxford, UK.

References

1. Rivers E, Nguyen B, Havstad S, Ressler J, Muzzin A, Knoblich B, Peterson E, Tomlanovich M. Early goal-directed therapy in the treatment of severe sepsis and septic shock. N Engl J Med. 2001;345:1368–77.
2. Kumar A, Anel R, Bunnell E, Habet K, Zanotti S, Marshall S, Neumann A, Ali A, Cheang M, Kavinsky C, Parillo J. Pulmonary artery occlusion pressure and central venous pressure fail to predict ventricular filling volume, cardiac performance, or the response to volume infusion in normal subjects. Crit Care Med. 2004;32(3):691–9.
3. Michard F, Teboul JL. Predicting fluid responsiveness in ICU patients: a critical analysis of the evidence. Chest. 2002;121:2000–8.

4. Alsous F, Khamiees M, DeGirolamo A, Amoateng-Adjepong Y, Manthous CA. Negative fluid balance predicts survival in patients with septic shock. Chest. 2002;117:1749–54.
5. Holte K, Kehlet H. Fluid therapy and surgical outcomes in elective surgery: a need for reassessment in fast-track surgery. J Am Coll Surg. 2006;202:971–89.
6. Wiedemann HP, Wheeler AP, Bernard GR, et al. Comparison of two fluid-management strategies in acute lung injury. N Engl J Med. 2006;354:2564–75.
7. Boyd JH, Forbes J, Nakada TA, et al. Fluid resuscitation in septic shock: a positive fluid balance and elevated central venous pressure are associated with increased mortality. Crit Care Med. 2011;39:259–65.
8. Nisanevich V, Felsenstein I, Almogy G, et al. Effect of intraoperative fluid management on outcome after intra-abdominal surgery. Anesthesiology. 2005;103:25–32.
9. Bundgaard-Nielsen M, Secher NH, Kehlet H. 'Liberal' vs. 'restrictive' perioperative fluid therapy—a critical assessment of the evidence. Acta Anaesthesiol Scand. 2009;53:843–51.
10. Holte K, Klarskov B, Christensen DS, et al. Liberal versus restrictive fluid administration to improve recovery after laparoscopic cholecystectomy: a randomized, double-blind study. Ann Surg. 2004;240:892–9.
11. Weidemann HP, Wheeler AP, Bernard GR, Thompson BT, Hayden D, deBoisblanc B, Connors Jr AF, Hite RD, Harabin AL. Comparison of two fluid management strategies in acute lung injury. N Engl J Med. 2006;354:2564–75.
12. Cavallaro F, Sandroni C, Antonelli M. Functional hemodynamic monitoring and dynamic indices of fluid responsiveness. Minerva Anestesiol. 2008;74:137–43.
13. Marik PE, Cavallazzi R, Vasu T, Hirani A. Dynamic changes in arterial waveform derived variables and fluid responsiveness in mechanically ventilated patients: a systematic review of the literature. Crit Care Med. 2009;37:2642–7.
14. Michard F, Teboul JL. Using heart-lung interactions to assess fluid responsiveness during mechanical ventilation. Crit Care. 2000;4:282–9.
15. Perner A, Faber T. Stroke volume variation does not predict fluid responsiveness in patients with septic shock on pressure support ventilation. Acta Anaesthesiol Scand. 2006;50:1068–73.
16. Hofer CK, Senn A, Weibel L, Zollinger A. Assessment of stroke volume variation for prediction of fluid responsiveness using the modified FloTrac and PiCCOplus system. Crit Care. 2008;12:R82.
17. Soubrier S, Saulnier F, Hubert H, Delour P, Lenci H, Onimus T, Nseir S, Durocher A. Can dynamic indicators help the prediction of fluid responsiveness in spontaneously breathing critically ill patients? Intensive Care Med. 2007;33: 1117–24.
18. Rutlen DL, Wackers FJ, Zaret BL. Radionuclide assessment of peripheral intravascular capacity: a technique to measure intravascular volume changes in the capacitance circulation in man. Circulation. 1981;64:146–52.
19. Gaffney FA, Bastian BC, Thal ER, et al. Passive leg raising does not produce a significant or sustained autotransfusion effect. J Trauma. 1982;22:190–3.
20. Wong DH, O'Connor D, Tremper KK, et al. Changes in cardiac output after acute blood loss and position change in man. Crit Care Med. 1989;17:979–83.
21. Boulain T, Achard JM, Teboul JL, Richard C, Perrotin D, Ginies G. Changes in BP induced by passive leg raising predict response to fluid loading in critically ill patients. Chest. 2002;121:1245–52.
22. Lafaneche're A, P'ene F, Goulenok C, Delahaye A, Mallet V, Choukroun G, Chiche JD, Mira JP, Cariou A. Changes in aortic blood flow induced by passive leg raising predicts fluid responsiveness in critically ill patients. Crit Care. 2006;10:R132–40.
23. Monnet X, Rienzo M, Osman D, Anguel N, Richard C, Pinsky MR, Teboul JL. Passive leg raising predicts fluid responsiveness in the critically ill. Crit Care Med. 2006;34:1402–7.
24. Thiel SW, Kollef MH, Isakow W. Non-invasive stroke volume measurement and passive leg raising predicts volume responsiveness in medical ICU patients: an observational cohort study. Crit Care. 2009;13:R111–20.
25. Lamia B, Ochagavia A, Monnet X, Chemla D, Richard C, Teboul JL. Echocardiographic prediction of volume responsiveness in critically ill patients with spontaneous breathing activity. Intensive Care Med. 2007; 33:1133–8.
26. Maizel J, Airapetian N, Lorne E, Tribouilloy C, Massy Z, Slama M. Diagnosis of central hypovolemia by using passive leg raising. Intensive Care Med. 2007;33:1133–8.
27. Caille V, Jabot J, Belliard G, Charron C, Jardin F, Vieillard-Baron A. Hemodynamic effects of passive leg raising: an echocardiographic study in patients with shock. Intensive Care Med. 2008;34:1239–45.
28. Biais M, Vidil L, Sarrabay P, Cottenceau V, Revel P, Sztark F. Changes in stroke volume induced by passive leg raising in spontaneously breathing patients: comparison between echocardiography and Vigileo TM/FloTracTM device. Crit Care. 2009;13:R195.
29. Pr'eau S, Saulnier F, Dewavrin F, Durocher A, Chagnon JL. Passive leg raising is predictive of fluid responsiveness in spontaneous breathing patients with severe sepsis or acute pancreatitis. Crit Care Med. 2010;38:819–25.
30. Lakhal K, Ehrmann S, Runge I, et al. Central venous pressure measurements improve the accuracy of leg raising-induced change in pulse pressure to predict fluid responsiveness. Intensive Care Med. 2010;36:940–8.
31. Kang WS, Kim SH, Kim SY, Oh CS, Lee SA, Kim JS. The influence of positive end-expiratory pressure on stroke volume variation in patients undergoing cardiac surgery: an observational study. J Thorac Cardiovasc Surg. 2014;148:3139–45.
32. Geerts B, de Wilde R, Aarts L, et al. Pulse contour analysis to assess hemodynamic response to passive leg raising. J Cardiothorac Vasc Anesth. 2011;25:48–52.
33. Dong ZZ, Fang Q, Zheng X, et al. Passive leg raising as an indicator of fluid responsiveness in patients with severe sepsis. World J Emerg Med. 2012;3:191–6.
34. Benomar B, Ouattara A, Estagnasie P, et al. Fluid responsiveness predicted by noninvasive bioreactance-based passive leg raise test. Intensive Care Med. 2010;36:1875–81.
35. Marik PE, Levitov A, Young A, et al. The use of bioreactance and carotid Doppler to determine volume responsiveness and blood flow redistribution following passive leg raising in hemodynamically unstable patients. Chest. 2013;143:364–70.
36. Duus N, Shogilev DJ, Skibsted S, et al. The reliability and validity of passive leg raise and fluid bolus to assess fluid responsiveness in spontaneously breathing emergency department patients. J Crit Care. 2015;30:217.e1–5.
37. Monge García MI, Gil Cano A, Gracia Romero M, et al. Non-invasive assessment of fluid responsiveness by changes in partial end-tidal CO_2 pressure during a passive leg-raising maneuver. Ann Intensive Care. 2012;2:9.
38. Fellahi JL, Fischer MO, Dalbera A, et al. Can endotracheal bioimpedance cardiography assess hemodynamic response to passive leg raising following cardiac surgery? Ann Intensive Care. 2012;2:26.
39. Cavallaro F, Sandroni C, Marano C, La Torre G, Chiara A, De Waure C, Bello G, Maviglia R, Antonelli M. Diagnostic accuracy of passive leg raising for prediction of fluid responsiveness in adults: systematic review and meta-analysis of clinical studies. Intensive Care Med. 2010;36:1475–83.
40. Monnet X, Marik P, Teboul J-L: Passive leg raising for predicting fluid responsiveness: a systematic review and meta-analysis. Intensive Care Med. published online 20th Jan 2016
41. Chernapath TGV, Hirsch A, Geerts BF, et al. Predicting fluid responsiveness by passive Leg raising: a systematic review and meta-analysis of 23 clinical trials. Crit Care Med. 2016;44(5):981–91.
42. Cheng L, Lin F-q, Shu-kun F, et al. Stroke volume variation for prediction of fluid responsiveness in patients undergoing gastrointestinal surgery. Int J Med Sci. 2013;10(2):148–55.
43. Langewouters GJ, Wesseling KH, Goedhard WJ. The pressure dependent dynamic elasticity of 35 thoracic and 16 abdominal human aortas in vitro described by a five component model. J Biomech. 1985;18:613–20.
44. Pratt B, Roteliuk L, Hatib F, Frazier J, Wallen RD. Calculating arterial pressure-based cardiac output using a novel measurement and analysis method. Biomed Instrum Technol. 2007;41:403–11.
45. De Backer D, Marx G, Tan A, et al. Arterial pressure-based cardiac output monitoring: a multicenter validation of the third-generation software in septic patients. Intensive Care Med. 2011;37:233–40.
46. Meng L, Tran PS, Brenton AS, Lanning K, et al. The impact of phenyephrine, ephedrine and increased preload on the third-generation Vigileo-Flotrac and esophageal Doppler cardiac output measurements. Anesth Analg. 2011;113:751–7.
47. Slagt C, Malagon I, Groeneveld ABG. Systematic review of uncalibrated arterial pressure waveform analysis to determine cardiac output and stroke volume variation. Br J Anaesth. 2014;112(4):626–37.
48. R Development Core Team (2008). R: a language and environment for statistical computing. R Foundation for Statistical Computing. *Vienna, Austria. ISBN 3-900051-07-0, URL* http://www.R-project.org.
49. Jabot J, Teboul JL, Richard C, Monnet X. Passive leg raising for predicting fluid responsiveness: importance of the postural change. Intensive Care Med. 2009;35:85–90.
50. Mahjoub Y, Touzeau J, Airapetian N, Lorne E, Hijazi M, Zogheb E, Tinturier F, Slama M, Dupont H. The passive leg-raising maneuver cannot accurately predict fluid responsiveness in patients with intra-abdominal hypertension. Crit Care Med. 2010;38(9):1824–9.

51. Dellinger RP, Levy MM, Carlet JM, et al. Surviving sepsis campaign: international guidelines for management of severe sepsis and septic shock. Crit Care Med. 2008;36:296–327.
52. Vincent JL, Weil MH. Fluid challenge revisited. Crit Care Med. 2006;34:1333–7.
53. Trof RJ, Sukul SP, Twisk JW, et al. Greater cardiac response of colloid than saline fluid loading in septic and non-septic critically ill patients with clinical hypovolaemia. Intensive Care Med. 2010;36:697–701.
54. Dorman T, Breslow MJ, Lipsett PA, Rosenberg JM, Balser JR, Almog Y, Rosenfeld BA. Radial artery pressure monitoring underestimates central arterial pressure during vasopressor therapy in critically ill surgical patients. Crit Care Med. 1998;26:1646–9.

17

Achieving the earliest possible reperfusion in patients with acute coronary syndrome

Takahiro Nakashima and Yoshio Tahara*

Abstract

Acute coronary syndrome (ACS) remains one of the leading causes of mortality worldwide. Appropriate management of ACS will lead to a lower incidence of cardiac arrest. Percutaneous coronary intervention (PCI) is the first-line treatment for patients with ACS. PCI techniques have become established. Thus, the establishment of a system of health care in the prehospital and emergency department settings is needed to reduce mortality in patients with ACS. In this review, evidence on how to achieve earlier diagnosis, therapeutic intervention, and decision to reperfuse with a focus on the prehospital and emergency department settings is systematically summarized.

The purpose of this review is to generate current, evidence-based consensus on scientific and treatment recommendations for health care providers who are the initial points of contact for patients with signs and symptoms suggestive of ACS.

Keywords: ACS, STEMI, NSTEMI, PCI

Background

Acute coronary syndrome (ACS) remains one of the leading causes of mortality worldwide. Appropriate management of this disease will lead to a reduced incidence of cardiac arrest. One major focus of research worldwide is improving outcomes in patients with ACS. In 2015, the Japan Resuscitation Council (JRC) guidelines were updated based on the 2015 International Consensus on Cardiopulmonary Resuscitation and Cardiovascular Care Science with Treatment Recommendations (CoSTR). CoSTR is a systematic and explicit approach to making judgments about the quality of evidence and strength of recommendations. The purpose of this review is to generate current, evidence-based consensus on scientific and treatment recommendations for health care providers who are the initial point of contact for patients with signs and symptoms suggestive of ACS based on the 2015 JRC guidelines.

* Correspondence: tahara@ncvc.go.jp
Department of Cardiovascular Medicine, National Cerebral and Cardiovascular Center, 5-7-1 Fujishirodai, Suita 565-8565, Japan

Review

Primary health care algorithm for ACS

Figure 1 shows the primary algorithm for ACS. In patients presenting to the emergency department (ED) with chest pain of suspected cardiac etiology, prompt diagnosis and treatment of ACS are the key concepts. The urgency and severity of ACS are evaluated using the history and physical examination in the ED. Twelve-lead electrocardiogram (ECG) plays a central role in the triage process. For patients with ST-elevation myocardial infarction (STEMI), the physician cooperates with the cardiologist to prioritize revascularization. On the other hand, for patients with no ST elevation but non-STEMI (NSTEMI) or high-risk unstable angina is suspected, the emergency physician and cardiologist should work together on cardiac care unit admission. These patients have a high rate of adverse cardiac events (death, nonfatal myocardial infarction, and urgent revascularization). Thus, an invasive strategy such as percutaneous coronary intervention (PCI) is often selected in addition to medical therapy. In patients with suspected ACS, normal initial biomarkers and nonischemic ECG, 0 h/1 h or 0 h/3 h rule-out algorithm of NSTEMI using high-sensitivity cardiac troponin (hs-cTn) may be recommended as a safe and effective strategy in the

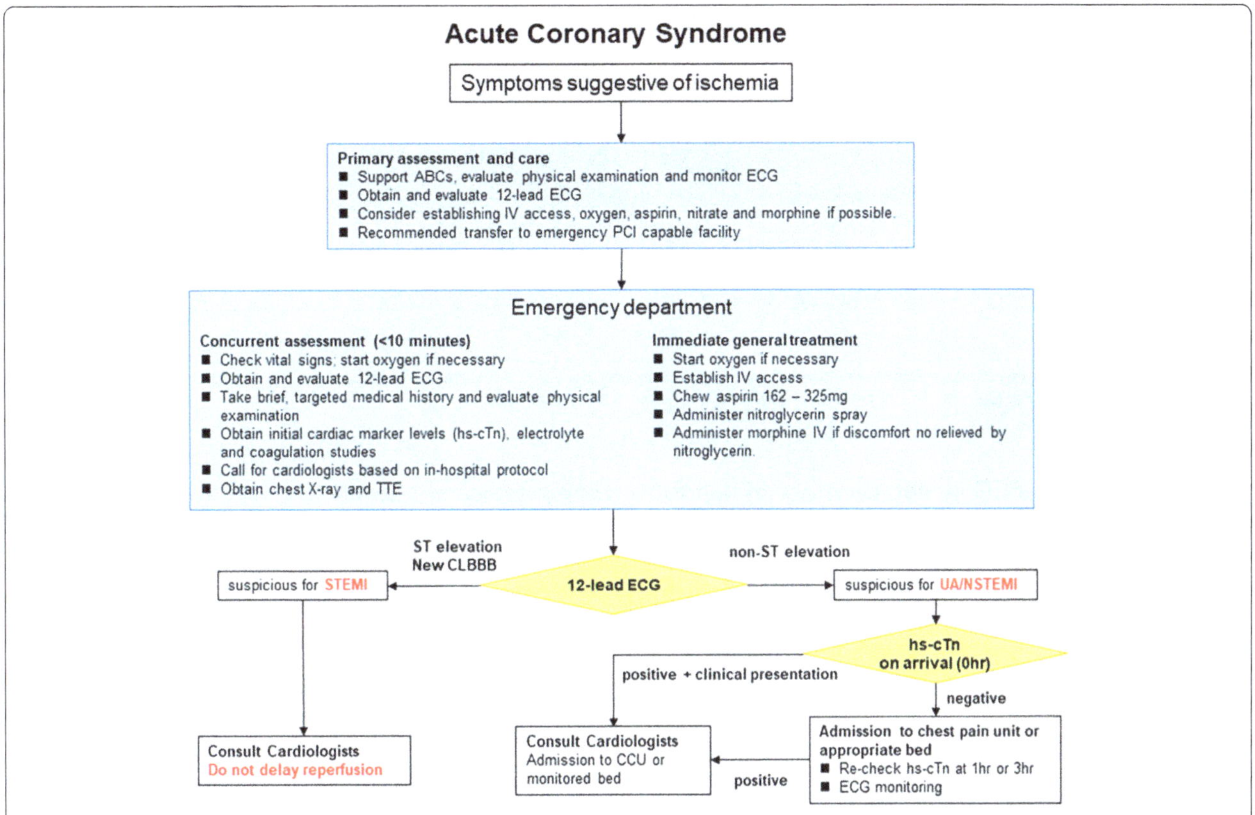

Fig. 1 Primary health care algorithm for acute coronary syndrome. *ABC* airway, breathing, and circulation; *CCU* cardiac care unit; *CLBBB* complete left bundle block; *ECG* electrocardiogram; *EMS* emergency medical services; *hs-cTn* high-sensitivity cardiac troponin; *IV* intravenous; *MI* myocardial infarction; *PCI* percutaneous coronary intervention; TTE transthoracic echocardiography; *UA* unstable angina

ED (see the "Biomarkers in ACS" section). Transthoracic echocardiography is helpful not only in the evaluation of wall motion abnormality, left ventricular function, and mechanical complications such as ventricular free wall rupture, ventricular septal perforation, and papillary muscle rupture, but also in the diagnosis of conditions such as acute aortic dissection, acute pulmonary embolism, and acute pericarditis. Chest X-ray is helpful in diagnosing and assessing the severity of ACS, but is not always necessary if ACS is strongly suspected and obtaining a chest X-ray will delay revascularization. Furthermore, waiting for the results of laboratory data to diagnose ACS should not cause delay in revascularization. Time from hospital arrival to transport to facilities capable of performing emergency PCI capable should be within 30 min.

Diagnostic interventions in ACS

Risk stratification in ACS

Various patient demographic factors might impede seeking medical help rapidly and add to further in-hospital treatment delay. Many reports have suggested that older age, female gender, racial or ethnic minority status, low socioeconomic status, and residing alone are independent factors associated with in-hospital treatment delay [1, 2]. Providers should be trained to expeditiously identify patients with ACS irrespective of age, gender, socioeconomic status, or living arrangement. On the other hand, signs and symptoms may be useful in combination with other important information such as biomarkers, risk factors, ECG, and other diagnostic test results, in triaging and making some treatment and investigational decisions for ACS in the out-of-hospital and ED settings. The Global Registry of Acute Coronary Events (GRACE) score provides accurate stratification of risk on admission and discharge (Table 1) [3, 4].

ECG

The ECG is essential for the initial triage and initiation of management in patients with possible ACS, especially in the ED and out-of-hospital settings. Many observational studies have shown the benefit of prehospital 12-lead ECG in reducing 30-day mortality, first-medical contact-to-reperfusion time, door-to-balloon time, and door-to-needle time compared with no ECG in patients with STEMI [5–13]. The 2015 JRC guidelines recommend prehospital 12-lead ECG acquisition with hospital notification for adult patients with suspected STEMI (strong recommendation, low-quality evidence). However,

Table 1 The Global Registry of Acute Coronary Events (GRACE) score

Age (year)	Score	Heart rate (bpm)	Score	Systolic BP (mmHg)	Score	Killip class	Score	Creatinine (mg/dL)	Score		Score
< 40	0	< 70	0	< 80	63	Class I	0	0.0–0.39	2	Cardiac arrest at admission	43
40–49	18	70–89	7	80–99	58	Class II	21	0.4–0.79	5		
50–59	36	90–109	13	100–119	47	Class III	43	0.8–1.19	8	Elevated cardiac markers	15
60–69	55	110–149	23	120–139	37	Class IV	64	1.2–1.59	11		
70–79	73	150–199	36	140–159	26			1.6–1.99	14	ST-segment deviation	30
80 <	91	200 <	46	160–199	11			2.0–3.99	23		
				200 <	0			4.0 <	31		

In-hospital mortality: low risk (≤ 10), intermediate risk (109–140), and high risk (> 140) are < 1%, 1–3%, and > 3%, respectively. Post-discharge to 6 months death: low risk (≤ 88), intermediate risk (89–118), and high risk (> 8) are < 3%, 3–8%, and > 8%, respectively
BP blood pressure

prehospital 12-lead ECG is not currently widespread in Japan. Thus, we should consider the use of prehospital 12-lead ECG in order to start specific therapy for STEMI more quickly. At the same time, we need to develop a computer-assisted ECG interpretation system for STEMI and an educational program for nurses and paramedics in ECG interpretation for STEMI [14–18].

Biomarkers in ACS

Some observational studies have shown that hs-cTn is helpful for excluding the diagnosis of ACS [19–26]. The 2015 JRC guidelines recommend against using only hs-cTnT and hs-cTnI measured at 0 and 2 h to rule out ACS (strong recommendation, very low-quality evidence). However, in low-risk patients (as defined by the Vancouver rule or a Thrombolysis in Myocardial Infarction Trial [TIMI] score of 0 or 1), the guidelines suggest that negative hs-cTnI at 0 and 2 h and negative hs-cTnI or hs-cTnT at 0 and 3–6 h may be used to rule out ACS (weak recommendation, low-quality evidence). Further studies are needed to evaluate the combination of troponins and clinical risk scores to determine which patients with chest pain may be safely discharged from the ED.

Imaging techniques

Noninvasive tests such as cardiac computed tomography (CT), cardiac magnetic resonance (MR), myocardial perfusion imaging, and echocardiography may be considered in selected patients who present to the ED with chest pain and an initial nondiagnostic conventional work-up that included 12-lead ECG or cardiac biomarkers. It is reasonable to consider both radiation and iodinated contrast exposure when using cardiac CT and myocardial perfusion imaging. Moreover, in some low-risk patients, these noninvasive tests may decrease cost, length of stay, and time to diagnosis [27–29]. They might provide valuable short-term and long-term prognostic information on future major cardiac events. However, there are insufficient data to assess the impact of imaging techniques on mortality. A combination of these techniques and chest pain observation units may be useful, and the spread of chest pain observation units is expected in Japan.

Therapeutic interventions for ACS

Oxygen therapy

Some randomized controlled trials (RCTs) have shown no difference between no oxygen and supplementary oxygen administration with regards to mortality (odds ratio [OR], 0.91; 95% confidence interval [CI], 0.25–3.34) [30–34]. The 2015 JRC guidelines suggest withholding routine high-concentration oxygen supplementation (8 L/min) in normoxic ($SpO_2 > 93\%$) patients with ACS (weak recommendation, very low-quality evidence), except for patients with previous myocardial infarction, severe chronic obstructive pulmonary disease, respiratory failure, cardiogenic shock, central cyanosis, $SpO_2 < 85\%$, or dyspnea from any other cause. Moreover, two recent RCTs show that routine supplementary oxygen administration is not beneficial [33, 35]. However, there is lack of evidence regarding low-concentration oxygen supplementation.

Nitroglycerin

Although it is reasonable to consider early administration of nitroglycerin in selected patients without contraindications, insufficient evidence exists to support or refute the routine administration of nitroglycerin in the ED or prehospital setting in patients with suspected ACS. There may be some benefit if nitroglycerin results in pain relief. When non-cardiologist physicians administer nitroglycerin, they give one sublingual nitroglycerin tablet or spray every 3 to 5 min, which may be repeated a total of 3 times if the patient remains hemodynamically stable. If right ventricular (RV) infarction is suspected, vasodilators, including nitroglycerin, are contraindicated because hemodynamic status with RV infarction depends on RV filling pressure. Relief of chest discomfort with nitroglycerin is neither sensitive nor specific for ACS; gastrointestinal etiologies as well as other causes of chest discomfort can respond to nitroglycerin administration.

Analgesics and sedation

Morphine can relieve chest pain, alleviate the work of breathing, reduce anxiety, and favorably affect ventricular loading conditions [36]. Despite limited direct evidence to support or refute the practice, morphine should be administered intravenously and titrated to pain relief in patients with STEMI. Morphine may be considered for pain relief in patients with suspected NSTEMI. Physicians give patients morphine 2 to 4 mg via intravenous injection, which may be increased to 8 mg every 5 to 15 min if it is not effective [37]. Other forms of analgesia (e.g., buprenorphine 0.1 to 0.2 mg) should be considered for patients with active chest discomfort. While anxiolytics may be administered to patients with ACS to alleviate anxiety, there is no evidence that anxiolytics facilitate ECG resolution, reduce infarct size, or decrease mortality in patients with suspected ACS. Non-steroidal anti-inflammatory drugs (NSAIDs) should not be administered because they may be harmful in patients with suspected ACS. Some studies have shown that NSAIDs are associated with an increased risk of mortality, reinfarction, hypertension, heart failure, and myocardial rupture in patients with STEMI [38, 39]. Patients with suspected ACS who are taking NSAIDs should have them discontinued when feasible.

Aspirin (acetylsalicylic acid) and adenine diphosphate (ADP) receptor antagonists

Despite limited direct evidence to support or refute the practice [40], the 2015 CoSTR guidelines mentioned that it may be reasonable to consider aspirin as soon as possible, without a history to exclude a true allergy or bleeding disorder. Moreover, some RCTs have shown that compared with in-hospital administration, there is no additional benefit with prehospital administration of an ADP receptor antagonist in terms of 30-day mortality (OR, 1.58; 95% CI, 0.90–2.78) and major bleeding (OR, 1.12; 95% CI, 0.72–1.74) [41–43]. These studies suggest that ADP receptor antagonists can be given to patients with suspected STEMI and planned primary PCI in either the prehospital or the in-hospital setting (very low-quality evidence, weak recommendation). However, in Japan, administration of aspirin for suspected STEMI outside of the hospital by emergency medical service (EMS) personnel is prohibited by law. When a primary PCI approach is being planned, physicians can give patients aspirin (162 to 325 mg) and ADP receptor antagonists (clopidogrel 300 mg or prasugrel 20 mg). Further investigation is needed to confirm the benefit of prehospital aspirin and ADP receptor antagonist administration in the doctor car or medical helicopter.

Anticoagulants

In patients with suspected out-of-hospital STEMI, a non-RCT showed no benefit of prehospital unfractionated heparin (UFH) on 30-day mortality compared with in-hospital UFH (OR, 1.07; 95% CI, 0.595–1.924) [44]. The 2015 CoSTR guidelines suggest that UFH administration can occur in either the prehospital or in-hospital setting in patients with suspected STEMI and a planned primary PCI approach. There is insufficient evidence to change existing practice (weak recommendation, very low-quality evidence). However, in Japan, EMS personnel cannot administer anticoagulants in the prehospital setting. Further investigation is needed to confirm the benefit of prehospital fibrinolysis in the doctor car or medical helicopter. Physicians administer UFH as a single intravenous injection with a target activated clotting time (ACT) of > 250 s. We note that most evidence about UFH in patients ACS were from the pre-primary PCI era. Further investigation is needed to approve prehospital anticoagulant administration by EMS personnel and the use of enoxaparin for STEMI in Japan.

Reperfusion decisions in patients with STEMI

The 2015 JRC guidelines address the question of which reperfusion strategy is best under specific circumstances. The options available for reperfusion will depend on the local prehospital system and availability of PCI centers. They consider reperfusion decisions in relation to regional availability (e.g., prehospital fibrinolysis versus ED or prehospital fibrinolysis versus direct transport to PCI). Table 2 shows the most appropriate reperfusion strategy by time from symptom onset and anticipated treatment delay.

Table 2 Most appropriate reperfusion strategy by time from symptom onset and anticipated treatment delays

Treatment delay	Time from symptom onset		
	< 2 h	2–3 h	3–6 h*
< 60 min	Primary PCI	Primary PCI or fibrinolysis†	Primary PCI
60–120 min	Fibrinolysis†	Primary PCI or fibrinolysis†	Primary PCI
> 120 min	Fibrinolysis†	Fibrinolysis†	Fibrinolysis†

Patients with higher risk, including those with Killip class > 1, may benefit from primary PCI even when there are treatment delays up to 120 min

PCI percutaneous coronary intervention

*If time from symptom onset is greater than 6 h, primary PCI is appropriate regardless of treatment delay

†In case of fibrinolytic therapy, immediate transfer to a PCI center after fibrinolysis should be considered for cardiac angiography within 3 to 24 h

Prehospital fibrinolysis versus ED fibrinolysis

Some RCTs have shown that prehospital fibrinolysis reduced in-hospital mortality without increasing intracranial hemorrhage and bleeding compared with in-hospital fibrinolysis (OR, 0.46; 95% CI, 0.23–0.93) [44–47]. When fibrinolysis is the planned treatment strategy, the 2015 JRC guidelines recommend prehospital fibrinolysis over in-hospital fibrinolysis for STEMI in health systems where typical transport time is greater than 30 min and prehospital fibrinolysis can be accomplished by a physician in the ambulance or medical helicopter with well-established protocols, comprehensive training programs, and quality assurance programs in place (strong recommendation, moderate-quality evidence).

Prehospital triage to a PCI center versus prehospital fibrinolysis

There is moderate-quality evidence that mortality is not reduced and low-quality evidence of harm from fibrinolysis [48, 49]. The 2015 JRC guidelines suggest that direct triage and transport for PCI is preferred in geographic regions where PCI facilities are not available (weak recommendation, low-quality evidence). On the other hand, the 2015 CoSTR suggest that prehospital fibrinolysis is a reasonable alternative to triage and direct transport to a PCI center in geographic regions where PCI facilities are not available. In Japan, prehospital fibrinolysis is preferred but a physician must be present because only physicians can perform fibrinolysis. Further investigation is needed to confirm the benefit of prehospital fibrinolysis in the doctor car or medical helicopter.

Delayed PCI versus fibrinolysis stratified by time since symptom onset

Some RCTs have shown that compared with fibrinolysis, delayed PCI is associated with higher 30-day mortality (OR, 2.6; 95% CI, 1.2–5.64) and 5-year mortality (OR, 2.03; 95% CI, 1.1–5.64) [50, 51]. In patients with STEMI presenting less than 2 h after symptom onset for whom primary PCI will result in a delay of greater than 60 min, the 2015 JRC guidelines suggest fibrinolysis over primary PCI (weak recommendation, low-quality evidence) [49, 52, 53]. Further investigation on delayed PCI versus fibrinolysis is needed.

ED fibrinolysis, transport only for rescue PCI, routine early angiography, transport for PCI or only rescue PCI

In adult patients with STEMI in the ED of a hospital without PCI capabilities, some RCTs have shown that transfer without fibrinolysis to a PCI center for angiography is associated with lower 30-day mortality compared with immediate in-hospital fibrinolysis and only transfer for ischemia-driven PCI in the first 24 h (OR, 0.66; 95% CI, 0.50–0.86) [54, 55]. For adult patients presenting with STEMI in the ED of a hospital not capable of performing PCI, the 2015 JRC guidelines recommend emergency transfer without fibrinolysis to a PCI center as opposed to immediate in-hospital fibrinolysis and transfer only for rescue PCI (strong recommendation, moderate-quality evidence). On the other hand, some RCTs have shown no difference in 30-day mortality between immediate in-hospital fibrinolysis and routine transfer for angiography compared with transfer to a PCI center (OR, 0.84; 95% CI, 0.24–2.98) [49, 56]. They suggest fibrinolytic therapy with routine transfer for angiography as an alternative to immediate transfer to PCI (weak recommendation, very low-quality evidence). Some RCTs have shown no difference in 30-day and 1-year mortality between either immediate in-hospital fibrinolysis and routine transfer for angiography at 3 to 6 h (or up to 24 h) and immediate in-hospital fibrinolysis and only transfer for ischemia-driven PCI (rescue PCI) (OR, 0.96; 95% CI, 0.64–1.44, OR 0.54; 95% CI, 0.16–1.89, respectively) [49, 57, 58]. Thus, for patients with STEMI who underwent ED fibrinolysis when primary PCI was not available on-site, the 2015 JRC guidelines suggest transport for early routine angiography in the first 3 to 6 h (or up to 24 h) rather than only transport for ischemia-guided angiography (weak recommendation, moderate-quality evidence).

The current evidence indicates that PCI from 3 to 24 h after fibrinolysis reduces reinfarction. The optimal timing within this time window has not been established. Similarly, the optimal management is unclear for patients after fibrinolysis in remote areas where transport to PCI is difficult or prolonged [54, 58–64].

Medications for ACS

To reduce the incidence of major adverse cardiac event and improve long-term survival, some additional medical therapies have been proposed. However, most of the data supporting the use of these therapies were gathered from patients after admission. To date, there is no evidence on which additional medical therapies in the prehospital or ED setting are important for patients with ACS.

Antiarrhythmics

Avoiding preventive administration of antiarrhythmics is reasonable in patients with ACS.

β-blockers

Avoiding routine intravenous administration of β-blockers during the initial prehospital or ED evaluation is reasonable for patients with ACS. For patients with ACS, there is no evidence to support routine intravenous administration of β-blockers during the initial prehospital or ED evaluation. Intravenous administration of β-blockers may be reasonable for selected patients with severe hypertension and tachycardia [65, 66]. On the other hand, contraindications to β-blockers include moderate to severe left ventricular failure, pulmonary edema, bradycardia, and hypotension. The effect of early β-blocker administration has not been fully studied in the primary PCI era.

After the patient is stabilized, starting an oral agent of β-blocker at a low dose before discharge is reasonable [67]. A recent multicenter registry of AMI in the PCI era has shown that β-blockers are associated with reduced mortality during long-term follow-up [68].

Angiotensin-converting enzyme inhibitors (ACE-Is) and angiotensin II receptor blockers (ARBs)

ACE-I and ARB administration after admission is known to reduce mortality in patients with acute myocardial infarction [69, 70]. However, there is insufficient evidence to support the routine administration of ACE-Is and ARBs in the prehospital and ED settings.

HMG-CoA reductase inhibitors (statins)

Statin therapy for patients with ACS soon after admission is reasonable in patients without contraindications [71]. Statins should be continued for patients with ACS who are already being treated with statins [72].

Hospital reperfusion decisions after return of spontaneous circulation (ROSC)

PCI after ROSC with or without ST elevation

After ROSC, some observational studies have shown that emergency cardiac catheterization in patients with ST elevation is associated with increased in-hospital survival (OR, 0.35; 95% CI, 0.31–0.41) and favorable neurological survival (OR 2.54; 95% CI, 2.17–2.99) compared with catheterization laboratory evaluation later in the hospital stay or no catheterization [73–76]. On the other hand, after ROSC in patients without ST elevation, two observational studies have shown the benefit of emergency cardiac catheterization on in-hospital mortality (OR, 0.51; 95% CI, 0.35–0.73) and favorable neurological survival (OR 1.96; 95% CI, 1.35–2.85) compared with catheterization laboratory evaluation later in the hospital stay or no catheterization [73, 76]. Thus, the 2015 JRC guidelines recommend emergency cardiac catheterization laboratory evaluation rather than cardiac catheterization later in the hospital stay or no catheterization in selected adult patients with ROSC after out-of-hospital cardiac arrest of suspected cardiac origin with ST elevation (strong recommendation, low-quality evidence) or without ST elevation on ECG (weak recommendation, very low-quality evidence). In patients with ST elevation, a variety of factors were more likely to be associated with cardiac catheterization: male gender, younger age, ventricular fibrillation as the presenting cardiac arrest rhythm, witnessed arrest, bystander cardiopulmonary resuscitation (CPR), and being supported with vasopressors or left ventricular assist devices. Patient characteristics that were less likely to be associated with angiography were diabetes mellitus, renal failure, and heart failure. On the other hand, in patients without ST elevation, a variety of factors such as patient age, CPR duration, hemodynamic instability, presenting cardiac rhythm, neurologic status upon hospital arrival, and perceived likelihood of cardiac etiology influenced the decision for intervention. Further investigation is needed to confirm the benefit seen in the first two observational studies. Ideally, randomized studies would help identify if there are certain subgroups of patients that would benefit more from angiography after ROSC.

Mechanical support for ACS with cardiogenic shock or cardiac arrest

ACS patients are often hemodynamically unstable. Management of these patients can be challenging. The use of mechanical support is taken into consideration for ACS patients with cardiogenic shock, defined as systolic blood pressure of less than 90 mmHg, use of catecholamines to maintain a systolic pressure of at least 90 mmHg, clinical signs of pulmonary congestion, or signs of impaired organ perfusion. In ACS patients with shock, use of an intra-aortic balloon pump (IABP), percutaneous left ventricular support device (Impella®, Abiomed, Danvers, Massachusetts), or veno-arterial extracorporeal membrane oxygenation (VA-ECMO) can be considered. Although the American Heart Association and European Society of Cardiology guidelines have downgraded the use of IABP [36, 77], the Japanese Cardiology Society guidelines give the use of IABP for cardiogenic shock a class I recommendation because percutaneous left ventricular support device (Impella®) was not yet approved in Japan at the time. Percutaneous left ventricular support device (Impella®) has been approved in Japan since 2017. Further accumulation of

Table 3 Ways to improve systems of care for acute coronary syndrome

- Emergency physician calls for the catheterization team
- Single call to a central operator
- Real-time data feedback
- Institutional commitment
- Team-based approach
- Catheterization team arrival within 20 min of being called
- Having an interventional cardiologist immediately available at the hospital

It is reasonable for hospitals to consider these measures to improve systems of care for acute coronary syndrome

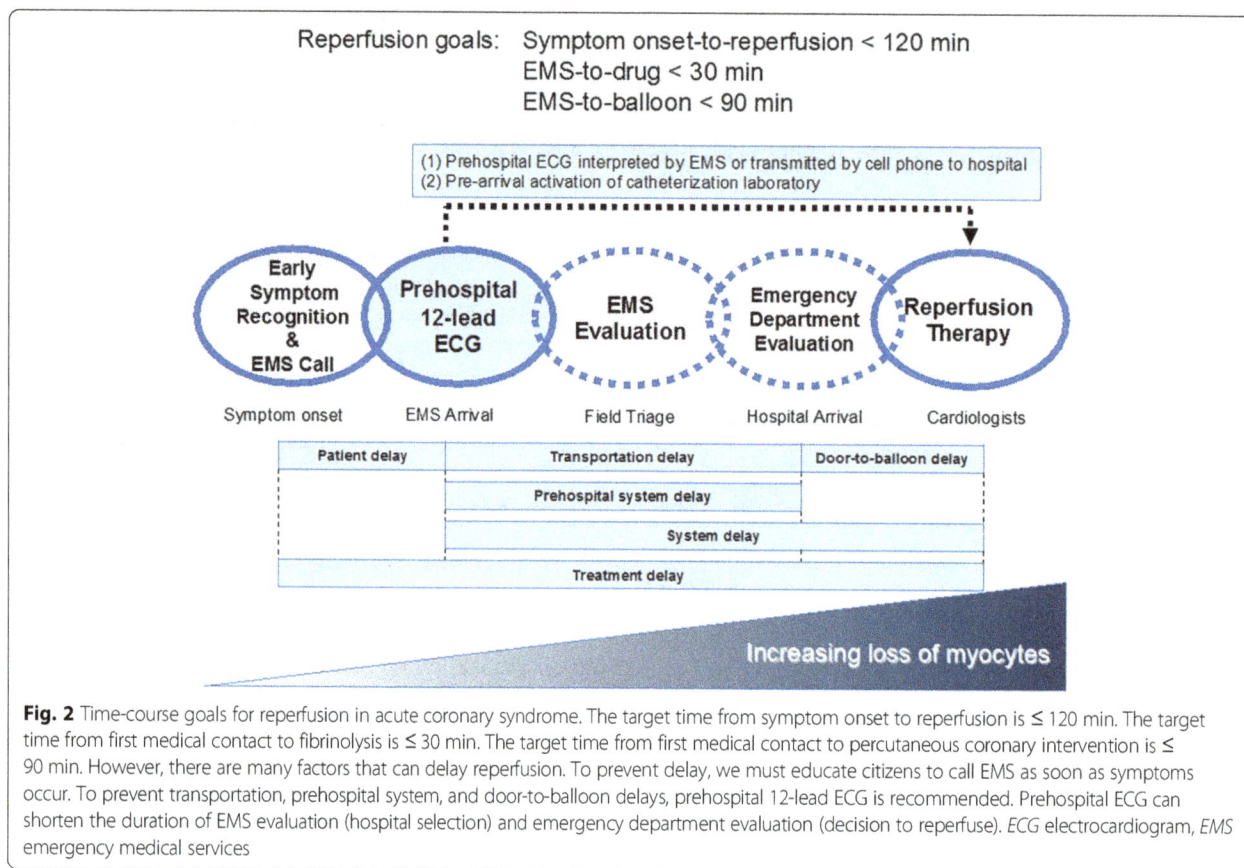

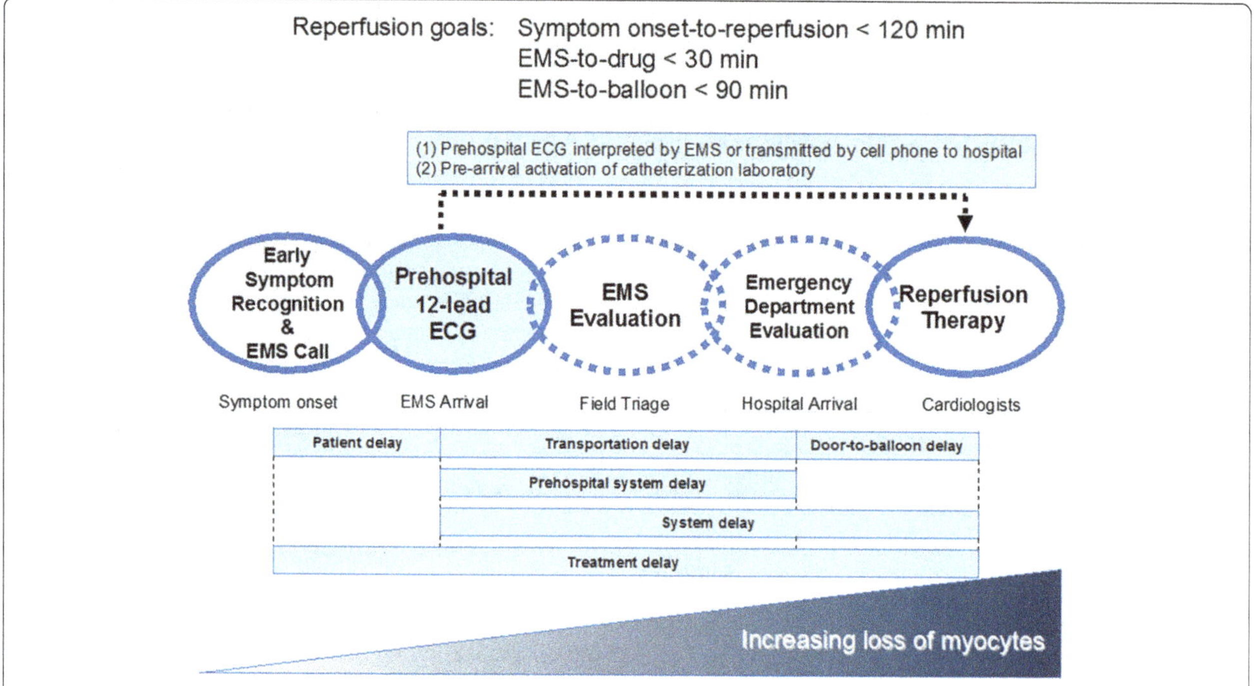

Fig. 2 Time-course goals for reperfusion in acute coronary syndrome. The target time from symptom onset to reperfusion is ≤ 120 min. The target time from first medical contact to fibrinolysis is ≤ 30 min. The target time from first medical contact to percutaneous coronary intervention is ≤ 90 min. However, there are many factors that can delay reperfusion. To prevent delay, we must educate citizens to call EMS as soon as symptoms occur. To prevent transportation, prehospital system, and door-to-balloon delays, prehospital 12-lead ECG is recommended. Prehospital ECG can shorten the duration of EMS evaluation (hospital selection) and emergency department evaluation (decision to reperfuse). *ECG* electrocardiogram, *EMS* emergency medical services

clinical data in Japan is needed. On the other hand, the 2015 JRC guidelines suggest that VA-ECMO is a reasonable rescue therapy for selected patients with cardiac arrest refractory to conventional CPR (weak recommendation, very low-quality evidence) [78, 79]. In patients with cardiac arrest due to ACS, VA-ECMO may allow providers additional time to treat acute coronary artery occlusion [80]. However, these techniques require adequate vascular access and specialized equipment.

Health care system interventions for ACS

Prehospital notification for activation of the cardiac catheterization laboratory and calling for the catheterization team

To prepare for primary PCI, the 2015 JRC guidelines recommend prehospital notification to activate the cardiac catheterization laboratory and calling for the catheterization team (strong recommendation, very low-quality evidence). Some observational studies have shown that prehospital activation of the catheterization team reduces 30-day mortality (OR, 0.41; 95% CI, 0.30–0.56) [7, 10, 81]. Establishment of a health care system in the prehospital and ED settings is needed (Table 3).

Conclusion

Several systems-related strategies have been developed to improve quality of care for patients with ACS and reduce reperfusion delays for patients with STEMI. Some strategies that focus on patients identified as having ACS in the prehospital and ED settings (Fig. 2) include the use of prehospital 12-lead ECG and time-saving strategies to facilitate early diagnosis and rapid treatment for patients with STEMI. Recently, PCI technique has become established. Thus, we must construct a system of health care to achieve early reperfusion in the prehospital and ED settings to reduce mortality in patients with ACS.

Abbreviations

ACE-Is: Angiotensin-converting enzyme inhibitors; ACS: Acute coronary syndrome; ACT: Activated clotting time; ARBs: Angiotensin II receptor blockers; CoSTR: Consensus on Cardiopulmonary Resuscitation and Cardiovascular Care Science with Treatment Recommendations; CPR: Cardiopulmonary resuscitation; CT: Computed tomography; ECG: Electrocardiogram; ED: Emergency department; EMS: Emergency medical service; GRACE: Global Registry of Acute Coronary Events; hs-cTn: High-sensitivity cardiac troponin; IABP: Intra-aortic balloon pump; JRC: Japan Resuscitation Council; MR: Magnetic resonance; NSAID: Non-steroidal anti-inflammatory drug; NSTEMI: Non-ST-elevation myocardial infarction; PCI: Percutaneous coronary intervention; ROSC: Return of spontaneous circulation; RV: Right ventricular; STEMI: ST-elevation myocardial infarction; TIMI: Thrombolysis in Myocardial Infarction Trial;

UFH: Unfractionated heparin; VA-ECMO: Veno-arterial extracorporeal membrane oxygenation

Acknowledgements
We thank the members of the 2015 JRC resuscitation guidelines working group.

Funding
None

Authors' contributions
TN wrote the main manuscript. YT critically reviewed and revised the manuscript for intellectual content. Both authors read and approved the final manuscript.

Competing interests
The authors declare that they have no competing interests.

References
1. Lefler LL, Bondy KN. Women's delay in seeking treatment with myocardial infarction: a meta-synthesis. J Cardiovasc Nurs. 2004;19:251–68.
2. Moser DK, Kimble LP, Alberts MJ, et al. Reducing delay in seeking treatment by patients with acute coronary syndrome and stroke: a scientific statement from the American Heart Association Council on cardiovascular nursing and stroke council. Circulation. 2006;114:168–82.
3. Aragam KG, Tamhane UU, Kline-Rogers E, et al. Does simplicity compromise accuracy in ACS risk prediction? A retrospective analysis of the TIMI and GRACE risk scores. PLoS One. 2009;4:e7947.
4. de Araujo GP, Ferreira J, Aguiar C, Seabra-Gomes R. TIMI, PURSUIT, and GRACE risk scores: sustained prognostic value and interaction with revascularization in NSTE-ACS. Eur Heart J. 2005;26:865–72.
5. Canto JG, Rogers WJ, Bowlby LJ, French WJ, Pearce DJ, Weaver WD. The prehospital electrocardiogram in acute myocardial infarction: is its full potential being realized? National Registry of Myocardial Infarction 2 Investigators. J Am Coll Cardiol. 1997;29:498–505.
6. Terkelsen CJ, Lassen JF, Norgaard BL, et al. Reduction of treatment delay in patients with ST-elevation myocardial infarction: impact of pre-hospital diagnosis and direct referral to primary percutanous coronary intervention. Eur Heart J. 2005;26:770–7.
7. Carstensen S, Nelson GC, Hansen PS, et al. Field triage to primary angioplasty combined with emergency department bypass reduces treatment delays and is associated with improved outcome. Eur Heart J. 2007;28:2313–9.
8. Brown DW, Gauvreau K, Powell AJ, et al. Cardiac magnetic resonance versus routine cardiac catheterization before bidirectional Glenn anastomosis in infants with functional single ventricle: a prospective randomized trial. Circulation. 2007;116:2718–25.
9. Martinoni A, De Servi S, Boschetti E, et al. Importance and limits of pre-hospital electrocardiogram in patients with ST elevation myocardial infarction undergoing percutaneous coronary angioplasty. Eur J Cardiovasc Prev Rehabil. 2011;18:526–32.
10. Sorensen JT, Terkelsen CJ, Norgaard BL, et al. Urban and rural implementation of pre-hospital diagnosis and direct referral for primary percutaneous coronary intervention in patients with acute ST-elevation myocardial infarction. Eur Heart J. 2011;32:430–6.
11. Chan AW, Kornder J, Elliott H, et al. Improved survival associated with pre-hospital triage strategy in a large regional ST-segment elevation myocardial infarction program. JACC Cardiovasc Interv. 2012;5:1239–46.
12. Ong ME, Wong AS, Seet CM, et al. Nationwide improvement of door-to-balloon times in patients with acute ST-segment elevation myocardial infarction requiring primary percutaneous coronary intervention with out-of-hospital 12-lead ECG recording and transmission. Ann Emerg Med. 2013;61:339–47.
13. Quinn T, Johnsen S, Gale CP, et al. Effects of prehospital 12-lead ECG on processes of care and mortality in acute coronary syndrome: a linked cohort study from the Myocardial Ischaemia National Audit Project. Heart. 2014;100: 944–50.
14. Ducas RA, Wassef AW, Jassal DS, et al. To transmit or not to transmit: how good are emergency medical personnel in detecting STEMI in patients with chest pain? Can J Cardiol. 2012;28:432–7.
15. Trivedi K, Schuur JD, Cone DC. Can paramedics read ST-segment elevation myocardial infarction on prehospital 12-lead electrocardiograms? Prehosp Emerg Care. 2009;13:207–14.
16. Lee CH, Van Gelder CM, Cone DC. Early cardiac catheterization laboratory activation by paramedics for patients with ST-segment elevation myocardial infarction on prehospital 12-lead electrocardiograms. Prehosp Emerg Care. 2010;14:153–8.
17. Young DR, Murinson M, Wilson C, et al. Paramedics as decision makers on the activation of the catheterization laboratory in the presence of acute ST-elevation myocardial infarction. J Electrocardiol. 2011;44:18–22.
18. Dorsch MF, Greenwood JP, Priestley C, et al. Direct ambulance admission to the cardiac catheterization laboratory significantly reduces door-to-balloon times in primary percutaneous coronary intervention. Am Heart J. 2008;155: 1054–8.
19. Aldous SJ, Richards AM, Cullen L, Than MP. Early dynamic change in high-sensitivity cardiac troponin T in the investigation of acute myocardial infarction. Clin Chem. 2011;57:1154–60.
20. Parsonage WA, Greenslade JH, Hammett CJ, et al. Validation of an accelerated high-sensitivity troponin T assay protocol in an Australian cohort with chest pain. Med J Aust. 2014;200:161–5.
21. Cullen L, Greenslade JH, Than M, et al. The new Vancouver Chest Pain Rule using troponin as the only biomarker: an external validation study. Am J Emerg Med. 2014;32:129–34.
22. Cullen L, Mueller C, Parsonage WA, et al. Validation of high-sensitivity troponin I in a 2-hour diagnostic strategy to assess 30-day outcomes in emergency department patients with possible acute coronary syndrome. J Am Coll Cardiol. 2013;62:1242–9.
23. Scheuermeyer FX, Wong H, Yu E, et al. Development and validation of a prediction rule for early discharge of low-risk emergency department patients with potential ischemic chest pain. CJEM. 2014;16:106–19.
24. Kelly AM, Klim S. Prospective external validation of an accelerated (2-h) acute coronary syndrome rule-out process using a contemporary troponin assay. Int J Emerg Med. 2014;7:42.
25. Mahler SA, Miller CD, Hollander JE, et al. Identifying patients for early discharge: performance of decision rules among patients with acute chest pain. Int J Cardiol. 2013;168:795–802.
26. Hess EP, Brison RJ, Perry JJ et al. Development of a clinical prediction rule for 30-day cardiac events in emergency department patients with chest pain and possible acute coronary syndrome. Ann Emerg Med 2012;59:115–125 e1.
27. Hoffmann U, Truong QA, Schoenfeld DA, et al. Coronary CT angiography versus standard evaluation in acute chest pain. N Engl J Med. 2012;367:299–308.
28. Miller CD, Hwang W, Case D, et al. Stress CMR imaging observation unit in the emergency department reduces 1-year medical care costs in patients with acute chest pain: a randomized study for comparison with inpatient care. JACC Cardiovasc Imaging. 2011;4:862–70.
29. Miller CD, Hwang W, Hoekstra JW, et al. Stress cardiac magnetic resonance imaging with observation unit care reduces cost for patients with emergent chest pain: a randomized trial. Ann Emerg Med. 2010;56:209–19. e2
30. Rawles JM, Kenmure AC. Controlled trial of oxygen in uncomplicated myocardial infarction. Br Med J. 1976;1:1121–3.
31. Ukholkina GB, Kostianov I, Kuchkina NV, Grendo EP, Gofman Ia B. Effect of oxygenotherapy used in combination with reperfusion in patients with acute myocardial infarction. Kardiologiia. 2005;45:59.
32. Ranchord AM, Argyle R, Beynon R, et al. High-concentration versus titrated oxygen therapy in ST-elevation myocardial infarction: a pilot randomized controlled trial. Am Heart J. 2012;163:168–75.

33. Stub D, Smith K, Bernard S, et al. Air versus oxygen in ST-segment-elevation myocardial infarction. Circulation. 2015;131:2143–50.
34. Wilson AT, Channer KS. Hypoxaemia and supplemental oxygen therapy in the first 24 hours after myocardial infarction: the role of pulse oximetry. J R Coll Physicians Lond. 1997;31:657–61.
35. Hofmann R, James SK, Jernberg T, et al. Oxygen therapy in suspected acute myocardial infarction. N Engl J Med. 2017;377:1240–9.
36. O'Gara PT, Kushner FG, Ascheim DD, et al. 2013 ACCF/AHA guideline for the management of ST-elevation myocardial infarction: a report of the American College of Cardiology Foundation/American Heart Association Task Force on Practice Guidelines. Circulation. 2013;127:e362–425.
37. Meine TJ, Roe MT, Chen AY, et al. Association of intravenous morphine use and outcomes in acute coronary syndromes: results from the CRUSADE quality improvement initiative. Am Heart J. 2005;149:1043–9.
38. McGettigan P, Henry D. Cardiovascular risk and inhibition of cyclooxygenase: a systematic review of the observational studies of selective and nonselective inhibitors of cyclooxygenase 2. JAMA. 2006;296:1633–44.
39. Kearney PM, Baigent C, Godwin J, Halls H, Emberson JR, Patrono C. Do selective cyclo-oxygenase-2 inhibitors and traditional non-steroidal anti-inflammatory drugs increase the risk of atherothrombosis? Meta-analysis of randomised trials. BMJ. 2006;332:1302–8.
40. Every NR, Parsons LS, Hlatky M, Martin JS, Weaver WD. A comparison of thrombolytic therapy with primary coronary angioplasty for acute myocardial infarction. Myocardial Infarction Triage and Intervention Investigators. N Engl J Med 1996;335:1253–1260.
41. Zeymer U, Arntz HR, Mark B, et al. Efficacy and safety of a high loading dose of clopidogrel administered prehospitally to improve primary percutaneous coronary intervention in acute myocardial infarction: the randomized CIPAMI trial. Clin Res Cardiol. 2012;101:305–12.
42. Ducci K, Grotti S, Falsini G, et al. Comparison of pre-hospital 600 mg or 900 mg vs. peri-interventional 300 mg clopidogrel in patients with ST-elevation myocardial infarction undergoing primary coronary angioplasty. The Load&Go randomized trial. Int J Cardiol. 2013;168:4814–6.
43. Montalescot G, van 't Hof AW, Lapostolle F, et al. Prehospital ticagrelor in ST-segment elevation myocardial infarction. N Engl J Med. 2014;371:1016–27.
44. Zijlstra F, Ernst N, de Boer MJ, et al. Influence of prehospital administration of aspirin and heparin on initial patency of the infarct-related artery in patients with acute ST elevation myocardial infarction. J Am Coll Cardiol. 2002;39:1733–7.
45. Steg PG, Van 't Hof A, Hamm CW, et al. Bivalirudin started during emergency transport for primary PCI. N Engl J Med. 2013;369:2207–17.
46. Sejersten M, Nielsen SL, Engstrom T, Jorgensen E, Clemmensen P. Feasibility and safety of prehospital administration of bivalirudin in patients with ST-elevation myocardial infarction. Am J Cardiol. 2009;103:1635–40.
47. Hirschl MM, Mayr H, Erhart F, et al. Prehospital treatment of patients with acute myocardial infarction with bivalirudin. Am J Emerg Med. 2012;30:12–7.
48. Bonnefoy E, Lapostolle F, Leizorovicz A, et al. Primary angioplasty versus prehospital fibrinolysis in acute myocardial infarction: a randomised study. Lancet. 2002;360:825–9.
49. Armstrong PW, Committee WS. A comparison of pharmacologic therapy with/without timely coronary intervention vs. primary percutaneous intervention early after ST-elevation myocardial infarction: the WEST (Which Early ST-elevation myocardial infarction Therapy) study. Eur Heart J. 2006;27: 1530–8.
50. Westerhout CM, Bonnefoy E, Welsh RC, Steg PG, Boutitie F, Armstrong PW. The influence of time from symptom onset and reperfusion strategy on 1-year survival in ST-elevation myocardial infarction: a pooled analysis of an early fibrinolytic strategy versus primary percutaneous coronary intervention from CAPTIM and WEST. Am Heart J. 2011;161:283–90.
51. Bonnefoy E, Steg PG, Boutitie F, et al. Comparison of primary angioplasty and pre-hospital fibrinolysis in acute myocardial infarction (CAPTIM) trial: a 5-year follow-up. Eur Heart J. 2009;30:1598–606.
52. Thiele H, Eitel I, Meinberg C, et al. Randomized comparison of pre-hospital-initiated facilitated percutaneous coronary intervention versus primary percutaneous coronary intervention in acute myocardial infarction very early after symptom onset: the LIPSIA-STEMI trial (Leipzig immediate prehospital facilitated angioplasty in ST-segment myocardial infarction). JACC Cardiovasc Interv. 2011;4:605–14.
53. Armstrong PW, Gershlick AH, Goldstein P, et al. Fibrinolysis or primary PCI in ST-segment elevation myocardial infarction. N Engl J Med. 2013; 368:1379–87.
54. Andersen HR, Nielsen TT, Rasmussen K, et al. A comparison of coronary angioplasty with fibrinolytic therapy in acute myocardial infarction. N Engl J Med. 2003;349:733–42.
55. Perez de Arenaza D, Taneja AK, Flather M. Long distance transport for primary angioplasty vs immediate thrombolysis in acute myocardial infarction (PRAGUE-2 trial). Eur Heart J. 2003;24:1798.
56. Fernandez-Aviles F, Alonso JJ, Pena G, et al. Primary angioplasty vs. early routine post-fibrinolysis angioplasty for acute myocardial infarction with ST-segment elevation: the GRACIA-2 non-inferiority, randomized, controlled trial. Eur Heart J. 2007;28:949–60.
57. Scheller B, Hennen B, Hammer B, et al. Beneficial effects of immediate stenting after thrombolysis in acute myocardial infarction. J Am Coll Cardiol. 2003;42:634–41.
58. Widimsky P, Groch L, Zelizko M, Aschermann M, Bednar F, Suryapranata H. Multicentre randomized trial comparing transport to primary angioplasty vs immediate thrombolysis vs combined strategy for patients with acute myocardial infarction presenting to a community hospital without a catheterization laboratory. The PRAGUE study Eur Heart J. 2000;21:823–31.
59. Widimsky P, Budesinsky T, Vorac D, et al. Long distance transport for primary angioplasty vs immediate thrombolysis in acute myocardial infarction: final results of the randomized national multicentre trial—PRAGUE-2. Eur Heart J. 2003;24:94–104.
60. Dieker HJ, van Horssen EV, Hersbach FM, et al. Transport for abciximab facilitated primary angioplasty versus on-site thrombolysis with a liberal rescue policy: the randomised Holland Infarction Study (HIS). J Thromb Thrombolysis. 2006;22:39–45.
61. Dobrzycki S, Kralisz P, Nowak K, et al. Transfer with GP IIb/IIIa inhibitor tirofiban for primary percutaneous coronary intervention vs. on-site thrombolysis in patients with ST-elevation myocardial infarction (STEMI): a randomized open-label study for patients admitted to community hospitals. Eur Heart J. 2007;28:2438–48.
62. Grines CL, Westerhausen DR Jr, Grines LL, et al. A randomized trial of transfer for primary angioplasty versus on-site thrombolysis in patients with high-risk myocardial infarction: the Air Primary Angioplasty in Myocardial Infarction study. J Am Coll Cardiol. 2002;39:1713–9.
63. Svensson L, Aasa M, Dellborg M, et al. Comparison of very early treatment with either fibrinolysis or percutaneous coronary intervention facilitated with abciximab with respect to ST recovery and infarct-related artery epicardial flow in patients with acute ST-segment elevation myocardial infarction: the Swedish Early Decision (SWEDES) reperfusion trial. Am Heart J. 2006;151:798 e1–7.
64. Vermeer F, Oude Ophuis AJ, vd Berg EJ, et al. Prospective randomised comparison between thrombolysis, rescue PTCA, and primary PTCA in patients with extensive myocardial infarction admitted to a hospital without PTCA facilities: a safety and feasibility study. Heart. 1999;82:426–31.
65. Chen ZM, Pan HC, Chen YP, et al. Early intravenous then oral metoprolol in 45,852 patients with acute myocardial infarction: randomised placebo-controlled trial. Lancet. 2005;366:1622–32.
66. Herlitz J, Edvardsson N, Holmberg S, et al. Goteborg Metoprolol Trial: effects on arrhythmias. Am J Cardiol. 1984;53:27D–31D.
67. Freemantle N, Cleland J, Young P, Mason J, Harrison J. Beta blockade after myocardial infarction: systematic review and meta regression analysis. BMJ. 1999;318:1730–7.
68. Goldberger JJ, Bonow RO, Cuffe M, et al. Effect of beta-blocker dose on survival after acute myocardial infarction. J Am Coll Cardiol. 2015;66:1431–41.
69. ISIS-4: a randomised factorial trial assessing early oral captopril, oral mononitrate, and intravenous magnesium sulphate in 58,050 patients with suspected acute myocardial infarction. ISIS-4 (fourth international study of infarct survival) collaborative group. Lancet 1995;345:669–685.
70. GISSI-3: effects of lisinopril and transdermal glyceryl trinitrate singly and together on 6-week mortality and ventricular function after acute myocardial infarction. Gruppo Italiano per lo studio della Sopravvivenza nell'infarto Miocardico. Lancet. 1994;343:1115–22.
71. Kayikcioglu M, Can L, Kultursay H, Payzin S, Turkoglu C. Early use of pravastatin in patients with acute myocardial infarction undergoing coronary angioplasty. Acta Cardiol. 2002;57:295–302.
72. Heeschen C, Hamm CW, Laufs U, et al. Withdrawal of statins increases event rates in patients with acute coronary syndromes. Circulation. 2002;105:1446–52.
73. Hollenbeck RD, McPherson JA, Mooney MR, et al. Early cardiac catheterization is associated with improved survival in comatose survivors of cardiac arrest without STEMI. Resuscitation. 2014;85:88–95.

74. Mooney MR, Unger BT, Boland LL, et al. Therapeutic hypothermia after out-of-hospital cardiac arrest: evaluation of a regional system to increase access to cooling. Circulation. 2011;124:206–14.
75. Grasner JT, Meybohm P, Lefering R, et al. ROSC after cardiac arrest–the RACA score to predict outcome after out-of-hospital cardiac arrest. Eur Heart J. 2011;32:1649–56.
76. Bro-Jeppesen J, Kjaergaard J, Wanscher M, et al. Emergency coronary angiography in comatose cardiac arrest patients: do real-life experiences support the guidelines? Eur Heart J Acute Cardiovasc Care. 2012;1:291–301.
77. Ibanez B, James S, Agewall S, et al. ESC guidelines for the management of acute myocardial infarction in patients presenting with ST-segment elevation: the task force for the management of acute myocardial infarction in patients presenting with ST-segment elevation of the European Society of Cardiology (ESC). Eur Heart J. 2017;2017
78. Maekawa K, Tanno K, Hase M, Mori K, Asai Y. Extracorporeal cardiopulmonary resuscitation for patients with out-of-hospital cardiac arrest of cardiac origin: a propensity-matched study and predictor analysis. Crit Care Med. 2013;41:1186–96.
79. Sakamoto T, Morimura N, Nagao K, et al. Extracorporeal cardiopulmonary resuscitation versus conventional cardiopulmonary resuscitation in adults with out-of-hospital cardiac arrest: a prospective observational study. Resuscitation. 2014;85:762–8.
80. Yannopoulos D, Bartos JA, Raveendran G, et al. Coronary artery disease in patients with out-of-hospital refractory ventricular fibrillation cardiac arrest. J Am Coll Cardiol. 2017;70:1109–17.
81. Brown JP, Mahmud E, Dunford JV, Ben-Yehuda O. Effect of prehospital 12-lead electrocardiogram on activation of the cardiac catheterization laboratory and door-to-balloon time in ST-segment elevation acute myocardial infarction. Am J Cardiol. 2008;101:158–61.

18

Evaluating the discriminating capacity of cell death (apoptotic) biomarkers in sepsis

Christopher Duplessis[1*], Michael Gregory[1], Kenneth Frey[1], Matthew Bell[1], Luu Truong[1], Kevin Schully[1], James Lawler[1], Raymond J. Langley[2], Stephen F. Kingsmore[3], Christopher W. Woods[4,5,6], Emanuel P. Rivers[7], Anja K. Jaehne[7], Eugenia B. Quackenbush[8], Vance G. Fowler[4], Ephraim L. Tsalik[4,5,9] and Danielle Clark[1]

Abstract

Background: Sepsis biomarker panels that provide diagnostic and prognostic discrimination in sepsis patients would be transformative to patient care. We assessed the mortality prediction and diagnostic discriminatory accuracy of two biomarkers reflective of cell death (apoptosis), circulating cell-free DNA (cfDNA), and nucleosomes.

Methods: The cfDNA and nucleosome levels were assayed in plasma samples acquired in patients admitted from four emergency departments with suspected sepsis. Subjects with non-infectious systemic inflammatory response syndrome (SIRS) served as controls. Samples were acquired at enrollment (T0) and 24 h later (T24). We assessed diagnostic (differentiating SIRS from sepsis) and prognostic (28-day mortality) predictive power. Models incorporating procalcitonin (diagnostic prediction) and APACHE II scores (mortality prediction) were generated.

Results: Two hundred three subjects were included (107 provided procalcitonin measurements). Four subjects exhibited uncomplicated sepsis, 127 severe sepsis, 35 septic shock, and 24 had non-infectious SIRS. There were 190-survivors and 13 non-survivors. Mortality prediction models using cfDNA, nucleosomes, or APACHEII yielded AUC values of 0.61, 0.75, and 0.81, respectively. A model combining nucleosomes with the APACHE II score improved the AUC to 0.84. Diagnostic models distinguishing sepsis from SIRS using procalcitonin, cfDNA(T0), or nucleosomes(T0) yielded AUC values of 0.64, 0.65, and 0.63, respectively. The three parameter model yielded an AUC of 0.74.

Conclusions: To our knowledge, this is the first head-to-head comparison of cfDNA and nucleosomes in diagnosing sepsis and predicting sepsis-related mortality. Both cfDNA and nucleosome concentrations demonstrated a modest ability to distinguish sepsis survivors and non-survivors and provided additive diagnostic predictive accuracy in differentiating sepsis from non-infectious SIRS when integrated into a diagnostic prediction model including PCT and APACHE II. A sepsis biomarker strategy incorporating measures of the apoptotic pathway may serve as an important component of a sepsis diagnostic and mortality prediction tool.

Keywords: Cell-free DNA, Nucleosomes, Severe Sepsis, Procalcitonin, Sepsis prognostication, Sepsis diagnosis

Background

Sepsis remains a leading cause of mortality globally. Despite concerted research into improving treatment and survival, few novel efficacious therapies have been identified. Sepsis contributes up to 750,000 hospitalizations annually in the USA, is the most common etiology of ICU-associated mortality, and incurs 50% mortality rates in severe cases [1–7]. The pathophysiology of sepsis is complex, multifactorial, and heterogeneous involving multiple interdependent pathways (proinflammatory, anti-inflammatory, regulatory, and coagulation/fibrinolysis) which become dysregulated and uncoordinated [8].

Given the heterogeneity of sepsis, accurate diagnosis, stratification, and prognosis will require biomarker panels to capture the evolving and dynamic information provided by multiple unique and interdependent cascades [9, 10]. Sepsis biomarker panel candidates may require representation of (1) multiple non-collinear

* Correspondence: Christopher.a.duplessis.mil@mail.mil
[1]Biological Defense Research Directorate, Naval Medical Research Center, 503 Robert Grant Avenue, Silver Spring, MD 20910, USA
Full list of author information is available at the end of the article

pathways (from a potentially infinite orthogonal space), (2) counter-regulatory biomarkers (capturing uncoordinated and dysregulated activity), and (3) temporal trends ("kinetics") [11]. For example, procalcitonin (PCT) dynamics are superior in sepsis prognostication than isolated measurements [12]. Apoptosis is a process in which intracellular death programs are activated (programmed cell death). Apoptotic cells shrink and condense with a collapse of the cytoskeleton accompanied by dissemblance of the nuclear envelope and leakage of intact and degraded DNA fragments [3, 13].

The apoptosis pathway is increasingly recognized as integral to sepsis pathophysiology, and therefore, representative biomarkers may provide additive discriminatory power in sepsis biomarker panels [3, 13]. Apoptotic pathway activation increases with sepsis severity often leading to marked lymphopenia within the initial 24 h [14, 15]. Apoptotic depletion of immune cells can undermine host immunity by engendering anergy, latent infection reactivation, and susceptibility to secondary infections [4, 14, 15]. Apoptosis-induced cellular debris increases immunogenic cellular by-products (including damage-associated molecular patterns (DAMPs)) contributing to immune tolerance and deleterious immune activation and dysregulation [3, 4, 14–17]. As apoptotic biomarkers represent the integrated cumulative organ injury and systemic inflammation portending future tissue damage [13], they may provide independent, non-collinear (additive) discriminatory predictive power when combined with traditional biomarkers or the APACHEII score [3, 13, 15, 18]. Extracellular cell-free DNA (cfDNA) and nucleosome levels both reflect cellular apoptosis activity and may serve as representative biomarkers of this pathway [3, 19, 20].

Circulating cfDNA (encompassing nuclear and mitochondrial-DNA) derives from cellular necrosis, lysis, apoptosis, and secretion (i.e., neutrophil extracellular traps (NETs)) [3, 13, 21–23]. Although bacteria may contribute, it appears to be a minor contributor in infectious syndromes [3]. Nucleosomes are basic units of DNA packaging stemming from chromatin degradation by endonucleases during apoptosis or necrosis [24, 25]. Nucleosomes are the basic unit of DNA packaging whereby DNA is wound around histone core proteins. Histones represent a class of DAMP molecules, are cytotoxic to endothelial and epithelial cells, and contribute to NETosis, which also directly participates in inflammation and the response to infection (activating TLR2, TLR4, and NF-κβ signaling) [1, 26]. In healthy individuals, circulating cfDNA and nucleosome levels are low, exhibiting short half-lives (15 min) given efficient clearance (in the liver) [1, 22]. In illness, levels rise from excessive cellular injury/death, insufficient clearance, or decrements in endogenous DNase [1, 15, 24]. Improvement in detection has fostered studies in many clinical arenas (cancer, trauma, stroke, myocardial infarction, rheumatoid arthritis, and sepsis) to assess their utility as discriminative diagnostic and prognostic biomarkers [3, 15, 17, 20–22, 27]. Furthermore, pilot studies suggest cfDNA and nucleosome concentrations correlate with sepsis severity [15, 22]. The origins of both cfDNA and nucleosomes depend on the particular clinical syndrome. For example, extracellular nucleic acids are plausibly released from the direct injurious insult sustained in trauma, or the rapidly dividing tumor cells in cancer. In sepsis, it is thought these extracellular nucleic acids derive from hematologic cells (neutrophils and lymphocytes) participating in the immune response to infection, with contributions from tissue injury sustained in organ damage [3, 17, 23]. We are unaware of associations between cfDNA and nucleosome concentrations with preceding neutrophil and lymphocyte levels (i.e., immune-suppressed patients), nor attributable contributions from the hematological cells vice tissue injury across sepsis severity all warranting future study.

We measured cfDNA and nucleosome levels in archived plasma samples acquired from the Community Acquired Pneumonia and Sepsis Outcome Diagnostic (CAPSOD) study. Our primary objectives were to assess the diagnostic (differentiating SIRS and sepsis) and prognostic (28-day mortality) performance of both biomarkers. In this preliminary biomarker discovery effort, we included PCT and APACHE II score to determine if apoptotic biomarkers offered independent classification utility. Specifically, models incorporating procalcitonin (for diagnostic prediction) and APACHE II scores (for mortality prediction) were also generated.

Methods

Archived samples from the CAPSOD investigation

In the CAPSOD study (ClinicalTrials.gov NCT00258869), 1152 individuals with suspected community-acquired sepsis [≥ 2 Systemic Inflammatory Response Syndrome (SIRS) criteria presumed due to an infection] were enrolled prospectively in the emergency departments at three urban, tertiary-care hospitals in the USA (Duke University, Durham VA Medical Center, and Henry Ford Hospital) from 2005 to 2009 (Fig. 1). Later, a fourth emergency department was added (UNC Medical Center) where enrollment occurred in 2010. Some were later adjudicated as having non-infectious SIRS. Medical history, physical examination, and acute illness scores (APACHE II) were recorded at enrollment (T0) and 24 h later (T24). Blood specimens were acquired at the corresponding time-points [6].

The primary outcome was survival at day-28, which along with infectious status was adjudicated by board-certified clinicians. Definitions that were standard

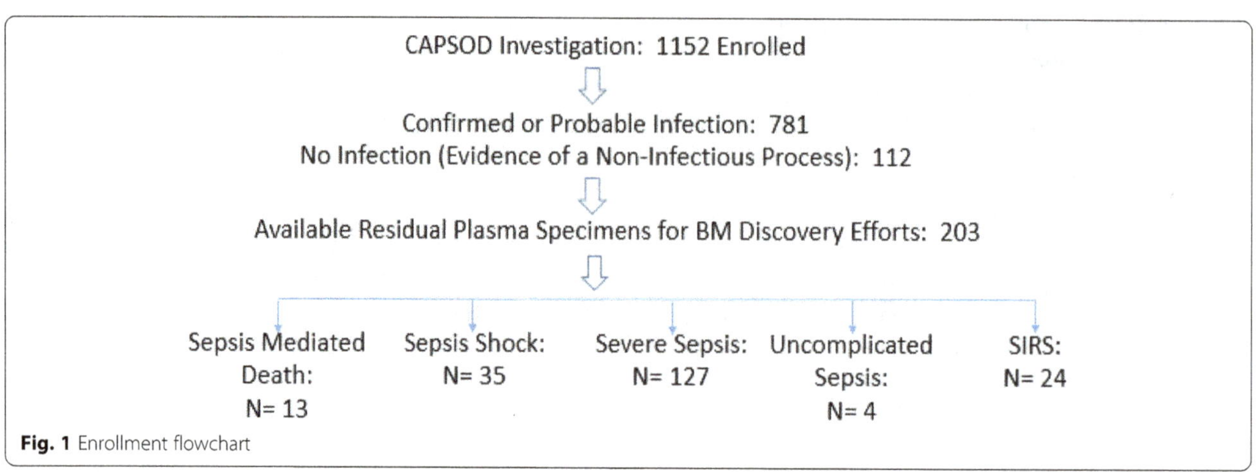

Fig. 1 Enrollment flowchart

at that time were employed for organ dysfunction and shock [6]. The definitions used for the adjudication process were based on the 2001 Consensus definition for sepsis [28]. The investigators pursued proteomics and metabolomics on patient samples to identify novel signatures predicting sepsis-associated mortality and have published a parsimonious set of metabolites exhibiting excellent prognostication for sepsis-associated mortality [6].

We accessed a sub-sample ($n = 203$) of the enrolled patients in this effort. Subject selection from the pool of 1152 subjects was first constrained by removing indeterminate adjudications where individual subjects could not be definitively assigned as having sepsis or SIRS. Sample selection was further constrained by those subjects for whom an adequate volume of residual plasma remained. This resulted in 203 evaluable subjects. We did not identify an introduction of any significant systematic bias imposed by the two constraints in this subcohort analyzed in terms of demographics (age, gender), source of infection, infectious pathogen, or representation across the various sepsis categories save for uncomplicated sepsis. Sample processing was harmonized at all participating sites with immediate separation of plasma subsequently frozen at − 20 °C and underwent one freeze-thaw cycle prior to assaying. This retrospective analysis of previously acquired specimens was approved by the Naval Medical Research Center (NMRC) institutional review board (IRB) as exempt (non-human subjects research) under protocol NRMC.2014.0008.

Assays

cfDNA

The cfDNA was assayed using SYBR® Gold Nucleic Acid Gel Stain, (Invitrogen, Paisley, UK) via the fluorometric method [3]. This assay yields similar cfDNA levels employing serum or plasma, correlates significantly with conventional β-globin gene DNA quantification [R^2 = 0.9987 ($p < 0.0001$)], and remains immune to organic molecular interference when samples are diluted to < 30% [3]. We executed the assay with slight modification (improving assay resolution). Specifically, SYBR® Gold was diluted at 1:1000 in dimethyl sulphoxide (DMSO, Sigma-Aldrich) and then at 1:8 in phosphate-buffered saline. An eight-point standard curve was created employing ultrapure salmon sperm DNA (Life Technologies, Carlsbad, CA, USA) diluted in 2% BSA/100 mM HEPES from 4 to 0.13 μg/ml [yielding a robust linear curve ($R^2 > 0.99$) between 0.25 and 4 μg/ml] (corresponding to a sample range: 20 to 1.25 μg/ml upon 1:5 dilution in the assay) aligning with 1:5 dilutions (in 2% BSA/100 mM HEPES) applied to samples and controls [10 μg/ml and 5 μg/ml (2 μg/ml and 1 μg/ml upon 1:5 dilutions)]. A common plasma control was applied to all plates to control for plate-to-plate variability. Twenty microliters of standards, controls, and samples were applied to black 96-well plates (Greiner Bio-One, Frickenhausen, Germany). Diluted SYBR® Gold was added (80 μl) to each well (final dilution 1:10,000), and fluorescence measured with a 96-well fluorometer (Ultra Evolution; Tecan, Durham, NC, USA) at an emission wavelength of 535-nm and an excitation wavelength of 485-nm. The low end of our linear curve overlaps the anticipated upper end of the normal range of healthy patients (1 μg/ml) which is known to exhibit significant intra- and inter-individual variability [3]. The intra-day CV is 16%, 7.9%, and 4.8% and inter-day CV is 31%, 6.7%, and 8% in the low (383 ng/ml), elevated (1152 ng/ml), and high DNA range (2735 ng/mL), respectively [3].

Nucleosomes The nucleosomes were quantified using the Cell Death Detection ELISAPlus kit (Roche Life Science, Indianpolis, IN, USA) according to the manufacturer's instructions. This assay employs two murine antibodies directed at DNA (detection) and histones (capture). An eight-point standard curve was generated by twofold standard dilution of purified human nucleosomes (Human native nucleosomes; EMD Millipore, Billerica, MA, USA) in the incubation buffer from the enzyme-linked immunosorbent assay (ELISA) kit. Samples (18 uL) were assayed in duplicate. Standards and samples were applied followed by 80 uL of immunoreagent. Plates were incubated at (21 °C) for 2 h while shaking gently (300 rpm). Plates were decanted and washed thrice using 250 uL of incubation buffer/well. ABTS (100 uL) solution was added per well and incubated at room temperature with gentle shaking (250 rpm) for 15 min. The detection reaction was stopped with 100 uL of stop solution/well. The optical density of the wells at 405 nm were read on an Epoch microplate spectrophotometer (BioTek; Winooski, VT, USA). Standard curves were fitted to a five-parameter logistic curve using the GEN5 Data Analysis Software version 2.01 (BioTek) allowing interpolation for sample concentrations.

Procalcitonin Procalcitonin (PCT) was measured from serum samples on a Roche Elecsys 2010 analyzer (Roche Diagnostics) by electrochemiluminescence or on the miniVIDAS immunoassay (bioMerieux). When serum was unavailable, measurements were made by the Phadia Immunology Reference Laboratory in plasma-EDTA by immunofluorescence using the BRAHMS PCT sensitive KRYPTOR (Thermo Fisher Scientific). Replicates were performed for some paired serum and plasma samples, revealing equivalence in concentrations. Therefore, all PCT measurements (ng/ml) were treated equivalently, regardless of testing platforms.

Statistical analyses

Demographic and clinical data were compared with chi-squared, Student's t test, or Wilcoxon rank sum test. Non-normal data were log-transformed. Spearman's rank-order correlation coefficients were calculated to evaluate correlations between biomarkers and APACHE II scores. Statistical significance was defined as $p < 0.05$. Prediction of 28-day mortality and discrimination between SIRS and sepsis were performed using logistic regression models. Performance was evaluated using area under the curve (AUC). All analyses were done with Stata (version-14).

Results

Study population

This was a nested case-control study focusing on subjects within the CAPSOD cohort. After identifying individuals with residual plasma, we identified 203 subjects with clinically adjudicated sepsis ($n = 179$) or non-infectious SIRS ($n = 24$) (Table 2). The sepsis group was further stratified by sepsis severity using definitions available during the enrollment period (i.e., before Sepsis-3) and as previously defined [6]. The cohort was further stratified by 28-day survival. Overall mortality was low (6.4% mirroring the 4.9% in the full CAPSOD cohort) resulting in 190 survivors and 13 non-survivors. All the mortality events were in subjects with sepsis. Although the original investigation enrolled from four sites, most of our samples were derived from a single site (Duke). There were no significant differences in age, gender, or race between survivors and non-survivors. We did observe a significant difference in comorbidities. Non-survivors had a higher prevalence of cirrhosis, chronic kidney disease, and chronic pulmonary disease. Bacterial pathogens were recovered from 28% of subjects. *Staphylococcus aureus* was most common ($n = 16$) followed by *Escherichia coli* ($n = 10$), *Klebsiella pneumoniae* ($n = 9$), and *Streptococcus pneumoniae* ($n = 7$). Influenza A was identified from two patients: one survivor and one non-survivor (Table 1).

Assessment of significance across sepsis stratifications in biomarkers (cfDNA, nucleosome, and procalcitonin concentrations) and APACHE II score (Table 2)

Under the hypothesis that apoptosis is a prominent host pathway in response to infection, we systematically compared cfDNA and nucleosome concentrations (seeking significant differences) among patients exhibiting various categories of sepsis (Table 2). Saliently, the sepsis severity categories delineated in Table 2 are based on the maximum severity achieved. Our subsequent analyses included comparing sepsis as compared to non-infectious SIRS, sepsis severities (i.e., uncomplicated sepsis, severe sepsis, and septic shock), and sepsis survival outcomes. Moreover, we compared concentrations at the time of enrollment (T0) and 24 h later (T24). Our reporting framework will assess cfDNA, followed by nucleosomes, PCT, and the APACHE II score.

For the cfDNA evaluation, as expected, we observed a trend toward higher cfDNA concentrations as sepsis severity increased. Specifically, we noted significant differences (increases) in the mean cfDNA concentrations between SIRS patients (3.0 μg/ml) when compared to patients experiencing severe sepsis (3.9 μg/ml; $p = 0.02$), septic shock (4.8 μg/ml; $p = 0.01$), and death (3.9 μg/ml; $p = 0.04$). There was a significant difference in the cfDNA concentrations between subjects experiencing sepsis vice SIRS ($p = 0.009$). We did not identify a significant difference in the cfDNA levels between survivors and non-survivors.

With respect to nucleosomes, there were significant differences observed in the mean nucleosome concentrations between SIRS patients (1.1 μg/ml) when compared to patients experiencing septic shock (5.5 μg/ml; $p = 0.012$) and those who died (5.0 μg/ml; $p = 0.001$). We

Table 1 Demographic table

Characteristic	Died ($N = 13$)	Survived ($N = 190$)
Age [median (IQR)]	64 (53–76)	54 (40–67)
Male [*n* (%)]	8 (62)	107 (56)
Caucasian [*n* (%)]	11 (85)	116 (61)
Comorbidities [*n* (%)] +	9 (69)*	67 (35)*
CAP [*n* (%)]	7 (54)*	29 (15)*
Pathogen [*n* (%)]		
Unidentified	7 (54)	139 (73)
Staphylococcus aureus	1 (8)	15 (8)
Escherichia coli	1 (8)	9 (5)
Klebsiella pneumoniae	0 (0)	9 (5)
Streptococcus pneumoniae	1 (8)	6 (3)
Other	3 (23)	12 (6)

*Significant difference between survivors and non-survivors ($p < 0.05$)
+Comorbidities include liver failure, heart failure, renal failure, neoplasm, chronic lung disease, immunosuppression, neutropenia, HIV, hemodialysis, corticosteroid use, or chemotherapy
CAP community-acquired pneumonia

also noted significant differences between patients experiencing severe sepsis (3.0 μg/ml) and death ($p = 0.003$). There was a significant difference in the nucleosome concentrations between subjects experiencing sepsis vice SIRS ($p = 0.036$). We noted a significant difference in nucleosome concentrations between survivors and non-survivors ($p = 0.007$).

With respect to PCT, there were significant differences observed in the mean PCT concentration between patients experiencing SIRS (7.5 μg/ml) and septic shock (20.7 μg/ml; $p = 0.002$). We did observe a significant decrement in PCT levels from SIRS to severe sepsis (6.5 μg/ml; $p < 0.002$). There was no significant difference in PCT concentrations in subjects experiencing sepsis vice SIRS. There were too few mortality cases with PCT measurements for meaningful interpretation in mortality prediction models nor to assert differences between survivors and non-survivors.

The average APACHE II score was significantly lower in SIRS patients (8.3) when compared to patients experiencing septic shock (15.5; $p < 0.001$) or those who died (17.5; $p < 0.001$). APACHE II was also lower in patients experiencing severe sepsis (9.0) compared to septic shock and death ($p < 0.001$ for both comparisons). The APACHE II score was significantly elevated in subjects experiencing sepsis vice SIRS ($p = 0.044$). The APACHE II score was significantly higher in non-survivors vice survivors ($p < 0.001$).

Finally, we identified no significant difference in the cfDNA biomarker concentrations measured at T0 and T24. Unlike the cfDNA levels, we did identify significant elevations in the nucleosome levels from T0 to T24, accompanied by increased variability at T24 relative to cfDNA in all groups (SIRS, death, and all severities of sepsis). Given the increased variability and the fact that there was no difference in the predictive accuracy when exploiting nucleosomes at T0 vice T24, we present the concentrations for nucleosomes (and all biomarkers) at T0 in Table 2 and all analyses assessing predictive accuracy utilizes values at T0 (see Figs. 2 and 3).

Table 2 Mean biomarker concentrations and APACHE II scores at enrollment (T0) stratified by sepsis categories (maximum sepsis severity achieved)

	cfDNA (μg/ml) Mean (SD)[6]	Nucleosome (μg/ml) Mean (SD)[7]	APACHE II Mean (SD)[9]	[5,8]PCT (ng/ml) Mean (SD)
Non-infectious SIRS[1] ($N = 24$)	3.0 (1.5)	1.1 (1.7)	8.3 (4.7)	7.5 (24.8)
Uncomplicated sepsis[2] ($N = 4$)	3.6 (1.0)	1.7 (1.9)	11.5 (3.8)	0.4 (0.4)
Severe sepsis[3] ($N = 127$)	3.9 (4.3)	3.0 (9.4)	9.0 (5.3)	6.5 (15.6)
Shock[4] ($N = 35$)	4.8 (5.8)	5.5 (10.9)	15.5 (6.3)	20.7 (34.4)
Survivors ($N = 190$)	3.9 (4.3)	3.2 (9.1)	10.1 (5.9)	9.1 (21.9)
Non-survivors ($N = 13$)	3.9 (1.4)	5.0 (4.9)	17.5 (5.9)	–

[1]SIRS (no infection with two or more of the following): 1 temp > 38.3 or < 36 °C, 2 heart rate > 90 bpm, 3 tachypnea resp. > 20 bpm or pCO2 < 32 mmHg, 4 WBC < 4000mm^3 or > 12,000mm^3 or 10% bands
[2]Sepsis (infection with two or more of the aforementioned SIRS criteria)
[3]Severe sepsis: sepsis accompanied by organ dysfunction: 1 arterial hypotension (SAP < 90 mmHg, MAP < 70 mmHg), 2 reduced urine output (< 0.5 mL/kg/h for > 2 h); 3 acute lung injury (PaO_2/FIO_2 < 250 if without pneumonia or < 200 if afflicted with pneumonia) based on the ACCP/SCCM consensus document. The following organ systems surveillance was available: cardiovascular, pulmonary, renal, and hematologic
[4]Septic shock: sepsis-induced hypotension persisting despite adequate fluid resuscitation
[5]There were only three subjects available in the non-survivor group in which the PCT level was available
[6]Significance between SIRS and sepsis ($p = 0.009$), SIRS and severe sepsis ($p = 0.02$), SIRS and septic shock ($p = 0.01$), and SIRS and death ($p = 0.04$)
No significance between survivors and non-survivors
[7]Significance between SIRS and septic shock ($p = 0.012$); between SIRS and death ($p = 0.001$); between severe sepsis and death ($p = 0.003$); between sepsis vice SIRS ($p = 0.036$); between survivors and non-survivors ($p = 0.007$)
[8]Significance between SIRS and septic shock ($p = 0.002$); SIRS and severe sepsis ($p < 0.002$)
[9]Significance between SIRS and septic shock ($p < 0.001$); between SIRS and death ($p < 0.001$); between severe sepsis and septic shock and death ($p < 0.001$); between SIRS and sepsis ($p = 0.044$); between survivors and non-survivors ($p < 0.001$)

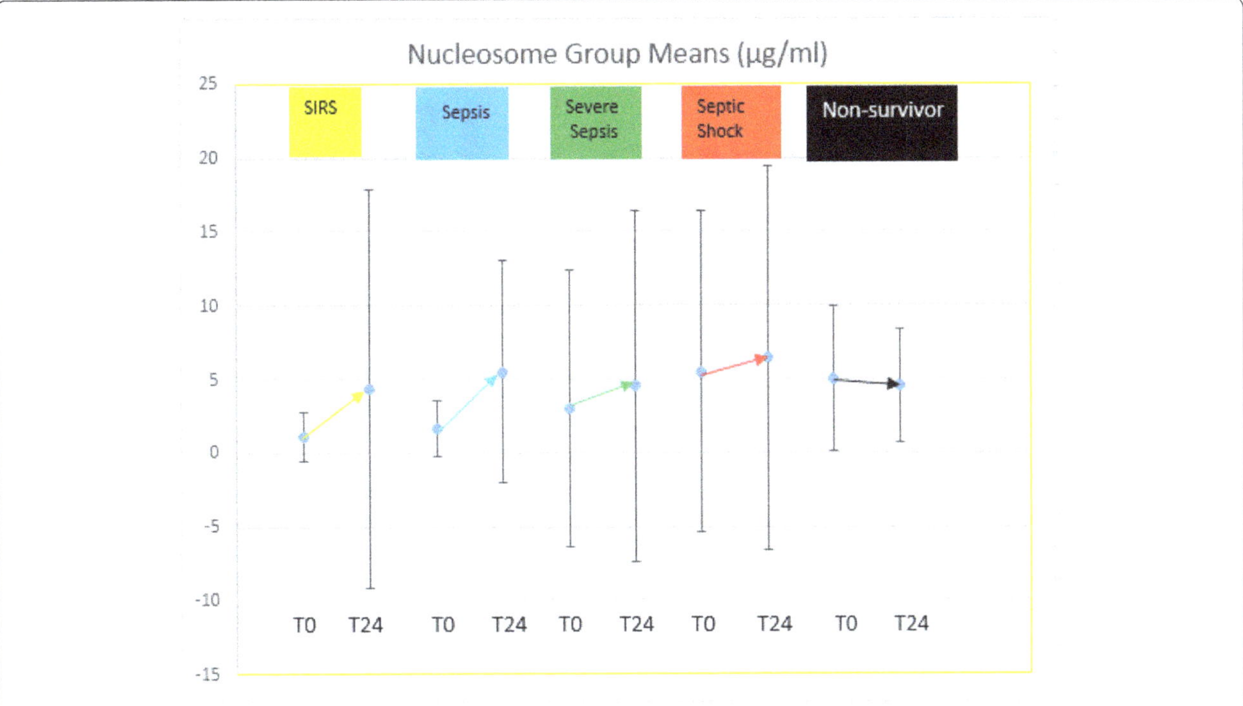

Fig. 2 Nucleosome group means and standard deviations at T0 and T24. Gold (SIRS); blue (sepsis); green (severe sepsis); red (septic shock); black (non-survivors)

Biomarker correlations

Even though cfDNA and nucleosomes are both apoptotic biomarkers, they may reflect different aspects of that process. We therefore correlated concentrations of these two biomarkers with each other. Furthermore, these two apoptotic biomarkers may be co-linear or complementary with other prognostic biomarkers, specifically PCT and APACHE II score. We therefore also assessed correlations between cfDNA, nucleosomes, PCT, and APACHE II (Table 3). While there was a modest correlation between cfDNA and nucleosomes (0.41), there was a smaller correlation between cfDNA and PCT and APACHE II (0.29 and 0.21, respectively). The nucleosome levels exhibited a similarly low correlation with PCT and APACHE II (0.07 and 0.24, respectively).

Predicting 28-day mortality

Mortality prediction models using cfDNA (at T0), nucleosomes (at T0), or APACHE II (at T0) yielded AUC values of 0.61, 0.75, and 0.81, respectively (Table 4). As asserted in Table 2, there were too few subjects in our cohort possessing PCT levels to provide meaningful interpretation. Permutations of a mortality prediction tool that used various combinations of cfDNA, nucleosomes, and APACHE II revealed that only nucleosome concentrations added to the predictive accuracy of APACHE II alone (0.84).

Discriminating SIRS from sepsis

Procalcitonin has been widely used as a sepsis diagnostic biomarker. We therefore determined whether measuring cfDNA or nucleosome improved the ability of procalcitonin to discriminate sepsis from SIRS. When used alone, we observed similarly modest AUCs for both cfDNA (0.62) and nucleosomes (0.63). When restricting to the subset of subjects who had available PCT results ($n = 107$), the AUC values for sepsis vs. SIRS discrimination were 0.64 for procalcitonin, 0.65 for cfDNA (at T0), and 0.63 for nucleosomes (at T0). There was no significant difference in the AUC for cfDNA and nucleosomes in the entire data set relative to the subset providing procalcitonin. A model incorporating all three biomarkers had an improved AUC of 0.74 (Table 5).

Discussion

Apoptosis is a well-recognized biological pathway in the host's response to infection [3, 13]. It is therefore plausible that cfDNA and nucleosomes, both by-products of the apoptosis pathway exhibiting biological roles (primarily originating from lymphocytes and neutrophils), could serve as useful sepsis biomarkers [29]. These biomarkers are inextricably linked within the interdependent innate and adaptive immunity (including NETosis), modulating endothelial homeostasis, and biasing the delicate balance within several pathways and their counter-regulatory cascades (including inflammatory, coagulation,

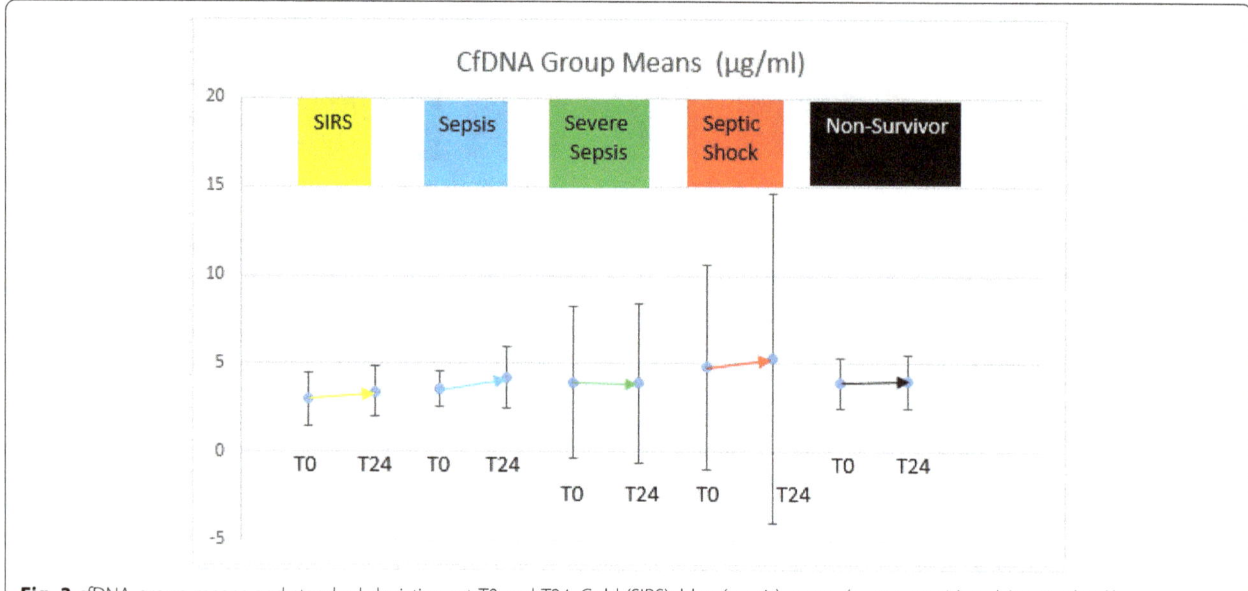

Fig. 3 cfDNA group means and standard deviations at T0 and T24. Gold (SIRS); blue (sepsis); green (severe sepsis); red (septic shock); black (non-survivors)

and fibrinolytic) [1, 26, 30]. It is not yet known if altering cfDNA or nucleosome levels or their dynamics could influence the evolution and outcomes in sepsis. In this study, we sought to answer a more proximal question, which is whether cfDNA or nucleosomes correlated with various aspects of sepsis such as diagnosis, severity, and prognosis. Furthermore, we wished to assess how these biomarkers compared with each other and what importance might they serve when combined with other sepsis-related biomarkers and predictive scores. As prior studies suggested that the cfDNA level in sepsis patients are primarily host derived (nuclear) in origin (not secondary to prokaryotic origins), we did not pursue a rigorous delineation of the source of nucleic acid in this effort as the major impetus was to seek a clinically relevant and reliable predictive diagnostic and prognostic biomarker panel [3, 13].

The prognostic accuracy of cfDNA to predict sepsis-mediated mortality was modest in this study (AUC of 0.61) but is comparable to that reported in the literature for non-ICU admitted subjects exhibiting AUCs (0.61 to 0.84) [3, 17, 22]. Notably, hitherto enrollment has been restricted to severely septic patients admitted to the ICU wherein the cfDNA exhibited superior prognostic accuracy (AUC of 0.7–0.97) [3, 13, 15, 17, 22, 27]. The lower accuracy observed in our investigation may be attributed to the (1) small sample size (and most saliently few subjects experiencing mortality), (2) inclusion of less ill sepsis patients irrespective of ICU admission, (3) possible sample degradation from long-term storage (although speculative should have been minimized exploiting our chosen assay), (4) the pronounced intra and inter-individual variability in cfDNA levels, (5) differential renal clearance, and (6) differential comorbidities that likely contribute to poorer predictive accuracy in patients experiencing less severe sepsis (and non-infectious SIRS). Of note, we had too few cases of specific clinical syndromes (comorbidities) and most specifically renal insufficiency to control for and evaluate their independent influence upon mortality and certainly warrants attention in future investigations. *Thus,*

Table 3 Correlation table

	cfDNA	Nucleosome	PCT[2]	APACHE II
cfDNA	1	0.41	0.29	0.21
Nucleosome		1	0.07	0.24
PCT[1]			1	0.41
APACHE II				1

Spearman's correlation coefficient
[1]PCT concentrations available for 107 patients

Table 4 AUC for predicting mortality

AUC for predicting mortality	
Biomarker or APACHE II Scoring System	AUC ($N = 203$) predicting mortality
cfDNA (T0)	0.61 (0.46–0.75)
cfDNA (T24)	0.62 (0.47–0.76)
Nucleosome (T0)	0.75 (0.62–0.87)
Nucleosome (T24)	0.67 (0.52–0.81)
APACHE II (T0)	0.81 (0.69–0.93)
APACHE II (T0) + cfDNA (T0)	0.81 (0.70–0.93)
APACHE II (T0) + nucleosome (T0)	0.84 (0.72–0.96)

Table 5 AUC for diagnosis (differentiating SIRS from sepsis)

	AUC ($N = 203$) Predicting sepsis
cfDNA (T0)	0.62 (0.50–0.74)
Nucleosome (T0)	0.63 (0.52–0.73)
Subset of patients ($N = 107$) possessing PCT values	
	AUC ($N = 107$) Predicting sepsis
Nucleosome (T0)	0.63 (0.46–0.79)
CfDNA (T0)	0.65 (0.44–0.85)
PCT (T0)	0.64 (0.49–0.79)
PCT (T0) + nucleosome (T0) + cfDNA (T0)	0.74 (0.60–0.88)

cfDNA levels may be best exploited in severe sepsis patients admitted to the ICU. Finally, of note, there have been no significant differences in cfDNA levels observed relative to the type of infecting organism [31].

The prognostic accuracy of nucleosomes for predicting sepsis-associated mortality was higher than that predicted by cfDNA and more consistent with published literature [14, 19]. We observed a modest correlation between these two biomarkers, which was less than expected given their shared biology. We speculate this may attributed to (1) differential nucleosome and cfDNA levels generated via variable apoptosis/necrosis ratios and NETosis, (2) cfDNA encompassing non-nuclear (mtDNA), (3) differential half-lives and clearance kinetics of their components, and (4) variability introduced by the assay method (ELISA) [1]. These observations suggest that in addition to concerted attention to consider potential representation in predictive biomarker panels, multiple apoptotic biomarkers (cfDNA, mucleosomes, histones) may be considered.

Both cfDNA and nucleosome (the latter significantly) were higher in non-survivors, but neither biomarker discriminated sepsis severity among survivors consistent with published data [3, 17, 18, 21, 22, 27, 32–35]. Increased levels among non-survivors may stem from a discrete increase in immune cell destruction, and bias to necrosis relative to caspase-dependent apoptosis in non-survivors [1, 32]. This suggests a reproducible dichotomy in host molecular responses highlighting allostasis (pathway normalization or compensation) in survivors and maladaption (pathway dysregulation and funneling to conserved death pathways) in non-survivors.

PCT is a host response biomarker that is secreted primarily in the context of bacterial infection but can also be elevated in certain non-infectious conditions. However, it is frequently used to help discriminate sepsis from non-infectious conditions. Moreover, it is part of the host's inflammatory pathway and presumably represents biology that is largely orthogonal to apoptosis. The subjects from which PCT was acquired may have experienced clinical endpoints deviating systematically from the entire cohort. However, we did not identify any systematic differences in demographics or salient clinical parameters between these cohorts, as delineated in Table 1. APACHE II is a commonly used clinical score that incorporates a variety of host factors such as age, comorbidity, and organ function assessments to create a sepsis severity score which correlates with mortality. Regrettably, as intimated earlier, the CAPSOD investigation experienced a lower percentage of non-survivors than historical or contemporary reported sepsis-associated mortality rates. Thus, we had too few non-survivors possessing PCT levels to pursue a mortality prediction model. Given the poor correlation of these apoptotic biomarkers with both PCT and the APACHE II, and the known biology of apoptosis, we conjecture that apoptotic biomarkers reflect an important septic pathway non-collinear or not otherwise reflected in the APACHE II or other biomarkers (PCT) and thus would be complimentary to them, thus adding accuracy to the mortality prediction model [3, 13]. We observed a modest increase in the AUC (from 0.81 to 0.84) appending nucleosomes to the APACHE II which although unlikely to add clinically significant predictive prognostic discrimination, we suspect that the additive predictive accuracy of the apoptotic biomarkers was muted by the unusually high predictive value of the APACHE II score in this cohort secondary to the low numbers of non-survivors.

The rates of non-infectious etiologies misdiagnosed as sepsis are estimated to be 14–18% in the emergency department population [36]. Most biomarkers studied to date are insensitive in differentiating SIRS stemming from infectious or non-infectious etiologies [21]. Improvements in predictive diagnostic accuracy would expedite accurate diagnoses, promoting prompt and appropriate therapeutic intervention and circumventing unnecessary antibiotic exposure. Both apoptotic biomarkers exhibited poor diagnostic accuracy to differentiate SIRS from sepsis (we speculate due to dilution with non-ICU admitted patients), yet was consistent with prior literature (nucleosomes exhibited a diagnostic AUC for discriminating sepsis in ICU patients of 0.7 [4]). However, we did observe a significant increase in AUC (0.74) exploiting our three-parameter model demonstrating independent and additive diagnostic predictive power from the apoptosis pathways.

Serial testing of sepsis biomarkers (e.g., procalcitonin, caspase, cleaved cytokeratin18, and protein C) may provide superior discriminatory power [3, 37]. However, cfDNA may not be useful for serial monitoring since concentrations remain stable for several days following sepsis presentation suggesting a fixed burden of cumulative tissue injury dictated by sepsis severity [3, 13, 17,

37]. We corroborated these observations identifying nonsignificant differences in the cfDNA levels in our investigation at T0 and T24. We acknowledge that the "stationary" kinetics encompasses a dynamic of fluctuating nucleic acid derived from NETosis, apoptosis, necrosis, and endogenous DNase activity. Unlike the cfDNA levels, we did identify significant elevation in the nucleosome levels from T0 to T24 (accompanied by increased variability). However, we did not identify differential predictive value for diagnosis or prognosis at T24 from T0 (likely attributed to the wide variability). We are not aware of any literature describing nucleosome kinetics; thus, this is the first report revealing the increasing nucleosome concentrations in septic patients in the first 24 h, which deviates from the stationary kinetics exhibited by cfDNA. Given the relative dearth of research specific to nucleosomes in sepsis, further research is necessary to define its kinetics and variability as a function of clinical state. Whereas biomarker dynamics provide useful information about a patient's state of illness and response to treatment, stable biomarkers can be useful clinically as they may provide a reliable inference as to the severity of sepsis at presentation (regardless of its heterogeneity), although not informing changing clinical states or treatment response.

Technology will need to be developed potentiating real-time measurement of cfDNA or nucleosomes so their relevance to clinical practice may be realized. Future research may attempt partitioning the source of cfDNA (mitochondrial, nuclear) and clarifying the predictive accuracy of the constituents of nucleosomes (histones) which may provide further insight into differentiating their relative propensity to promoting inflammation, coagulation, anti-fibrinolysis, antibacterial activity, and predictive (diagnostic and prognostication) power [2]. Alternative apoptotic biomarkers may be superior in their discriminatory potential and targeted for future research [31, 38]. Finally, all apoptotic biomarkers would ideally be developed as a real-time point of care testing platform.

Limitations

We employed a convenience sampling constrained by subjects with definitive adjudicated diagnoses and who had sufficient banked plasma for biomarker measurements (although did not observe any significant systematic bias from the full cohort in terms of demographics (age, gender), source of infection, infectious pathogen, or representation across the various sepsis categories save for uncomplicated sepsis). The low mortality in this cohort may have resulted in a lower sensitivity of these biomarkers for severe disease. However, this did represent a more realistic cohort of patients with sepsis, not all of whom are managed in the ICU. Long-term storage may have led to differential cfDNA and nucleosome degradation which is uncontrolled with the retrospective analyses employed herein (however, we acknowledge the cfDNA fluorometric assay employed circumvents concerns in DNA fragmentation) [3]. Finally, samples underwent one freeze-thaw cycle, however, again the fluorometric assay circumvents concerns in DNA fragmentation, while nucleosome concentrations were shown to remain stable through several freeze-thaw cycles [25].

Conclusions

To our knowledge, this is the first head-to-head comparison of cfDNA and nucleosomes in diagnosing sepsis and predicting sepsis-related mortality. Both cfDNA and nucleosome concentrations demonstrated a modest ability to distinguish sepsis survivors and non-survivors and provided additive diagnostic predictive accuracy in differentiating sepsis from non-infectious SIRS when integrated into a diagnostic prediction model including PCT and APACHE II. A sepsis biomarker strategy incorporating measures of the apoptotic pathway may serve as an important component of a sepsis diagnostic and mortality prediction tool.

Abbreviations

AUC: Area under the curve; BSA: Bovine serum A; CAP: Community-acquired pneumonia; CAPSOD: Community Acquired Pneumonia and Sepsis Outcome Diagnostic; cfDNA: Cell-free DNA; DAMP: Damage-associated molecular pattern; ELISA: Enzyme-linked immunosorbent assay; NMRC: Naval Medical Research Center; PCT: Procalcitonin; SIRS: Systemic Inflammatory Response Syndrome; T0: Lab acquisition upon initial enrollment; T24: Lab acquisition at 24 h later

Acknowledgements

None.

Funding

This study was funded by JSTO (Joint Science and Technology Office) and is supported by grants from the NIH (U01AI066569, P20RR016480, HHSN266200400064C).

Disclaimer

The views expressed in this article are those of the author and do not necessarily reflect the official policy or position of the Department of the Navy, Department of Defense, Department of Veterans Affairs, nor the U.S. Government. This is a US Government work. There are no restrictions on its use. There were no financial conflicts of interests among any of the authors.

Authors' contributions

CD, MG, KF, KS, and JL contributed to the study design, assay execution, and manuscript preparation. MB and LT are responsible for the assay execution. RL, SK, CW, ER, AJ, EQ, and VF took part in the study design, sample acquisition (clinical trial investigator = CAPSOD). ET contributed to the study design, sample acquisition (clinical trial investigator = CAPSOD), and manuscript preparation. DC contributed to the study design, statistical analysis, and manuscript preparation. All authors read and approved the final manuscript.

Author information
N/A

Competing interests
The authors declare that they have no competing interests.

Author details
[1]Biological Defense Research Directorate, Naval Medical Research Center, 503 Robert Grant Avenue, Silver Spring, MD 20910, USA. [2]Department of Pharmacology and Center for Lung Biology, University of South Alabama College of Medicine, Mobile, USA. [3]Rady Pediatric Genomic and Systems Medicine Institute, Rady Children's Hospital, Encinitas, USA. [4]Division of Infectious Diseases and International Health, Department of Medicine, Duke University School of Medicine, Durham, USA. [5]Center for Applied Genomics and Precision Medicine, Department of Medicine, Duke University School of Medicine, Durham, USA. [6]Section on Infectious Diseases, Durham Veteran's Affairs Medical Center, Durham, USA. [7]Department of Emergency Medicine, Henry Ford Hospital, Wayne State University, Detroit, USA. [8]Department of Emergency Medicine, University of North Carolina Health Care, Chapel Hill, USA. [9]Emergency Medicine Service, Durham Veteran's Affairs Medical Center, Durham, USA.

References

1. Gould TJ, Vu TT, Stafford AR, Dwivedi DJ, Kim PY, Fox-Robichaud AE, et al. Cell-free DNA modulates clot structure and impairs fibrinolysis in sepsis. Arterioscler Thromb Vasc Biol. 2015;35(12):2544–53. https://doi.org/10.1161/ATVBAHA.115.306035 Epub 2015/10/22, PubMed PMID: 26494232.
2. Bhagirath VC, Dwivedi DJ, Liaw PC. Comparison of the proinflammatory and procoagulant properties of nuclear, mitochondrial, and bacterial DNA. Shock. 2015;44(3):265–71. https://doi.org/10.1097/SHK.0000000000000397 PubMed PMID: 25944792.
3. Dwivedi DJ, Toltl LJ, Swystun LL, Pogue J, Liaw KL, Weitz JI, et al. Prognostic utility and characterization of cell-free DNA in patients with severe sepsis. Crit Care. 2012;16(4):R151. https://doi.org/10.1186/cc11466 Epub 2012/08/13 PubMed PMID: 22889177; PubMed Central PMCID: PMCPMC3580740.
4. Chen Q, Ye L, Jin Y, Zhang N, Lou T, Qiu Z, et al. Circulating nucleosomes as a predictor of sepsis and organ dysfunction in critically ill patients. Int J Infect Dis. 2012;16(7):e558–64. https://doi.org/10.1016/j.ijid.2012.03.007 Epub 2012/05/18. PubMed PMID: 22609014.
5. Heron M. Deaths: leading causes for 2014. Natl Vital Stat Rep. 2016;65(5):1–96 PubMed PMID: 27376998.
6. Langley RJ, Tsalik EL, van Velkinburgh JC, Glickman SW, Rice BJ, Wang C, et al. An integrated clinico-metabolomic model improves prediction of death in sepsis. Sci Transl Med. 2013;5(195):195ra95. https://doi.org/10.1126/scitranslmed.3005893 PubMed PMID: 23884467; PubMed Central PMCID: PMCPMC3924586.
7. Rivers EP, Jaehne AK, Nguyen HB, Papamatheakis DG, Singer D, Yang JJ, et al. Early biomarker activity in severe sepsis and septic shock and a contemporary review of immunotherapy trials: not a time to give up, but to give it earlier. Shock. 2013;39(2):127–37. https://doi.org/10.1097/SHK.0b013e31827dafa7 PubMed PMID: 23324881.
8. Stearns-Kurosawa DJ, Osuchowski MF, Valentine C, et al. The pathogenesis of sepsis. Annu Rev Pathol. 2011;6:19–48.
9. Sandquist M, Wong HR. Biomarkers of sepsis and their potential value in diagnosis, prognosis and treatment. Expert Rev Clin Immunol. 2014;10(10):1349–56. https://doi.org/10.1586/1744666X.2014.949675 Epub 2014/08/21. PubMed PMID: 25142036; PubMed Central PMCID: PMCPMC4654927.
10. Faix JD. Biomarkers of sepsis. Crit Rev Clin Lab Sci. 2013;50((1):23–36. https://doi.org/10.3109/10408363.2013.764490 PubMed PMID: 23480440; PubMed Central PMCID: PMCPMC3613962.
11. Llewelyn MJ, Berger M, Gregory M, Ramaiah R, Taylor AL, Curdt I, et al. Sepsis biomarkers in unselected patients on admission to intensive or high-dependency care. Crit Care. 2013;17(2):R60. https://doi.org/10.1186/cc12588 Epub 2013/03/26 PubMed PMID: 23531337; PubMed Central PMCID: PMCPMC3672658.
12. Schuetz P, Maurer P, Punjabi V, Desai A, Amin DN, Gluck E. Procalcitonin decrease over 72 hours in US critical care units predicts fatal outcome in sepsis patients. Crit Care. 2013;17(3):R115. https://doi.org/10.1186/cc12787 Epub 2013/06/20 PubMed PMID: 23787145; PubMed Central PMCID: PMCPMC4057444.
13. Avriel A, Paryente Wiessman M, Almog Y, Perl Y, Novack V, Galante O, et al. Admission cell free DNA levels predict 28-day mortality in patients with severe sepsis in intensive care. PLoS One. 2014;9(6):e100514. https://doi.org/10.1371/journal.pone.0100514 Epub 2014/06/23 PubMed PMID: 24955978; PubMed Central PMCID: PMCPMC4067333.
14. Zeerleder S, Zwart B, Wuillemin WA, Aarden LA, Groeneveld AB, Caliezi C, et al. Elevated nucleosome levels in systemic inflammation and sepsis. Crit Care Med. 2003;31(7):1947–51. https://doi.org/10.1097/01.CCM.0000074719.40109.95 PubMed PMID: 12847387.
15. Huttunen R, Kuparinen T, Jylhävä J, Aittoniemi J, Vuento R, Huhtala H, et al. Fatal outcome in bacteremia is characterized by high plasma cell free DNA concentration and apoptotic DNA fragmentation: a prospective cohort study. PLoS One. 2011;6(7):e21700. Epub 2011/07/01. doi: https://doi.org/10.1371/journal.pone.0021700. PubMed PMID: 21747948; PubMed Central PMCID: PMCPMC3128600.
16. Condotta SA, Cabrera-Perez J, Badovinac VP, Griffith TS. T-cell-mediated immunity and the role of TRAIL in sepsis-induced immunosuppression. Crit Rev Immunol. 2013;33(1):23–40 PubMed PMID: 23510024; PubMed Central PMCID: PMCPMC3625932.
17. Saukkonen K, Lakkisto P, Pettilä V, Varpula M, Karlsson S, Ruokonen E, et al. Cell-free plasma DNA as a predictor of outcome in severe sepsis and septic shock. Clin Chem. 2008;54(6):1000–7. Epub 2008/04/17. doi: https://doi.org/10.1373/clinchem.2007.101030. PubMed PMID: 18420731.
18. Clementi A, Virzì GM, Brocca A, Pastori S, de Cal M, Marcante S, et al. The role of cell-free plasma DNA in critically ill patients with sepsis. Blood Purif. 2016;41(1–3):34–40. Epub 2015/10/20. doi: https://doi.org/10.1159/000440975. PubMed PMID: 26960212.
19. Zeerleder S, Stephan F, Emonts M, de Kleijn ED, Esmon CT, Varadi K, et al. Circulating nucleosomes and severity of illness in children suffering from meningococcal sepsis treated with protein C. Crit Care Med. 2012;40(12):3224–9. https://doi.org/10.1097/CCM.0b013e318265695f PubMed PMID: 22932399.
20. Moreira VG, Prieto B, Rodríguez JS, Alvarez FV. Usefulness of cell-free plasma DNA, procalcitonin and C-reactive protein as markers of infection in febrile patients. Ann Clin Biochem. 2010;47(Pt 3):253–8. Epub 2010/04/26. doi: https://doi.org/10.1258/acb.2010.009173. PubMed PMID: 20421309.
21. Hou YQ, Liang DY, Lou XL, Zhang M, Zhang ZH, Zhang LR. Branched DNA-based Alu quantitative assay for cell-free plasma DNA levels in patients with sepsis or systemic inflammatory response syndrome. J Crit Care. 2016;31(1):90–5. Epub 2015/11/10. doi: https://doi.org/10.1016/j.jcrc.2015.10.013. PubMed PMID: 26589770.
22. Forsblom E, Aittoniemi J, Ruotsalainen E, Helmijoki V, Huttunen R, Jylhävä J, et al. High cell-free DNA predicts fatal outcome among *Staphylococcus aureus* bacteraemia patients with intensive care unit treatment. PLoS One. 2014;9(2):e87741. Epub 2014/02/10. doi: https://doi.org/10.1371/journal.pone.0087741. PubMed PMID: 24520336; PubMed Central PMCID: PMCPMC3919733.
23. Rhodes A, Cecconi M. Cell-free DNA and outcome in sepsis. Crit Care. 2012;16(6):170. Epub 2012/11/08. doi: https://doi.org/10.1186/cc11508. PubMed PMID: 23140420; PubMed Central PMCID: PMCPMC3672553.
24. Holdenrieder S, Stieber P. Clinical use of circulating nucleosomes. Crit Rev Clin Lab Sci. 2009;46(1):1–24. https://doi.org/10.1080/10408360802485875 PubMed PMID: 19107649.
25. Holdenrieder S, Mueller S, Stieber P. Stability of nucleosomal DNA fragments in serum. Clin Chem. 2005;51(6):1026–9. https://doi.org/10.1373/clinchem.2005.048454 PubMed PMID: 15914786.
26. Hampson P, Dinsdale RJ, Wearn CM, Bamford AL, Bishop JRB, Hazeldine J, et al. Neutrophil dysfunction, immature granulocytes, and cell-free DNA are early biomarkers of sepsis in burn-injured patients: a prospective observational cohort study. Ann Surg. 2017;265(6):1241–9. https://doi.org/10.1097/SLA.0000000000001807 PubMed PMID: 27232244.
27. Wijeratne S, Butt A, Burns S, Sherwood K, Boyd O, Swaminathan R. Cell-free plasma DNA as a prognostic marker in intensive treatment unit patients. Ann N Y Acad Sci. 2004;1022:232–8. https://doi.org/10.1196/annals.1318.036 PubMed PMID: 15251966.
28. Gould TJ, Lysov Z, Liaw PC. Extracellular DNA and histones: double-edged swords in immunothrombosis. J Thromb Haemost. 2015;13(Suppl 1):S82–91.
29. Levy MM, et al. 2001 SCCM/ ESICM/ ACCP/ ATS/ SIS International Sepsis Definitions Conference. Intensive Care Med. 2003;29(4):530–8.
30. Schneck E, Samara O, Koch C, Hecker A, Padberg W, Lichtenstern C, Weigand MA, Uhle F. Plasma DNA and RNA differentially impact coagulation during abdominal sepsis-an explorative study. J Surg Res. 2017;210:231–43.

31. Clementi A, Virzi GM, Brocca A, Pastori S, de Cal M, Marcante S, Granata A, Ronco C. The role of cell-free plasma DNA in critically ill patients with sepsis. Blood Purif. 2016;41(1–3):34–40.
32. Raffray L, Douchet I, Augusto JF, Youssef J, Contin-Bordes C, Richez C, et al. Septic shock sera containing circulating histones induce dendritic cell-regulated necrosis in fatal septic shock patients. Crit Care Med. 2015;43(4): e107–16. https://doi.org/10.1097/CCM.0000000000000879 PubMed PMID: 25654179.
33. Moore DJ, Greystoke A, Butt F, Wurthner J, Growcott J, Hughes A, et al. A pilot study assessing the prognostic value of CK18 and nDNA biomarkers in severe sepsis patients. Clin Drug Investig. 2012;32(3):179–87. https://doi.org/10.2165/11598610-000000000-00000 PubMed PMID: 22217154.
34. Wildhagen KC, Wiewel MA, Schultz MJ, Horn J, Schrijver R, Reutelingsperger CP, et al. Extracellular histone H3 levels are inversely correlated with antithrombin levels and platelet counts and are associated with mortality in sepsis patients. Thromb Res. 2015;136(3):542–7. Epub 2015/07/23. doi: https://doi.org/10.1016/j.thromres.2015.06.035. PubMed PMID: 26232351.
35. Ekaney ML, Otto GP, Sossdorf M, Sponholz C, Boehringer M, Loesche W, et al. Impact of plasma histones in human sepsis and their contribution to cellular injury and inflammation. Crit Care. 2014;18(5):543. Epub 2014/09/24. doi: https://doi.org/10.1186/s13054-014-0543-8. PubMed PMID: 25260379; PubMed Central PMCID: PMCPMC4201918.
36. Tsalik EL, Jaggers LB, Glickman SW, Langley RJ, van Velkinburgh JC, Park LP, et al. Discriminative value of inflammatory biomarkers for suspected sepsis. J Emerg Med. 2012;43(1):97–106. Epub 2011/11/06. doi: https://doi.org/10.1016/j.jemermed.2011.05.072. PubMed PMID: 22056545; PubMed Central PMCID: PMCPMC3740117.
37. Garnacho-Montero J, Huici-Moreno MJ, Gutiérrez-Pizarraya A, López I, Márquez-Vácaro JA, Macher H, et al. Prognostic and diagnostic value of eosinopenia, C-reactive protein, procalcitonin, and circulating cell-free DNA in critically ill patients admitted with suspicion of sepsis. Crit Care. 2014; 18(3):R116. Epub 2014/06/05. doi: https://doi.org/10.1186/cc13908. PubMed PMID: 24903083; PubMed Central PMCID: PMCPMC4229882.
38. Huttunen R, Syrianen J, Vuento R, Laine J, Hurme M, Aittoniemi J. Apoptosis markers soluble Fas (sFas), Fas ligand (FasL) and sFas/FasL ratio in patients with bacteremia: a prospective cohort study. J Inf Secur. 2012;64(3):276–81.

19

Daily use of extracorporeal CO_2 removal in a critical care unit: indications and results

Hadrien Winiszewski[1,2*], François Aptel[1], François Belon[1], Nicolas Belin[1], Claire Chaignat[1], Cyrille Patry[1], Cecilia Clermont[1], Elise David[1], Jean-Christophe Navellou[1], Guylaine Labro[1], Gaël Piton[1,4] and Gilles Capellier[1,3,4]

Abstract

Background: While outcome improvement with extracorporeal CO_2 removal ($ECCO_2R$) is not demonstrated, a strong pathophysiological rational supports its use in the setting of acute respiratory distress syndrome (ARDS) and COPD exacerbation. We aimed to describe our single-center experience of $ECCO_2R$ indications and outcome.

Methods: Patients treated with $ECCO_2R$ in our medial ICU, from March 2014 to November 2017, were retrospectively enrolled. Primary end point was evolution of ventilator settings during the two first days following $ECCO_2R$ start.

Results: Thirty-three patients received $ECCO_2R$. Seventeen were managed with Hemolung®, 10 with Prismalung®, 4 with ILA®, and 2 with Cardiohelp®. Indications for $ECCO_2R$ were mild or moderate ARDS ($n = 16$), COPD exacerbation ($n = 11$), or uncontrolled hypercapnia due to other causes ($n = 6$). Four patients were not intubated at the time of $ECCO_2R$ start. Median duration of $ECCO_2R$ treatment was 7 days [5–10]. In ARDS patients, between baseline and day 2, median tidal volume and driving pressure decreased from 5.3 [4.4–5.9] mL/kg and 10 [8–15] to 3.8 [3.3–4.1] mL/kg and 9 [8–11], respectively. Prone positioning was performed in 10 of the 16 patients, without serious adverse event. In COPD patients, between baseline and day 2, median ventilation minute and PaCO2 decreased significantly from respectively 7.6 [6.6–8.7] L/min and 9.4 [8.4–10.1] kPa to 5.8 [4.9–6.2] L/min and 6 [5.3–6.8] kPa. Four out of 11 COPD patients were extubated while on $ECCO_2R$. Device thrombosis occurred in 5 patients (15%). Hemolysis was documented in 16 patients (48%). One patient died of intracranial hemorrhage, while on $ECCO_2R$. Twenty-four patients were discharged from ICU alive. Twenty-eight day mortality was 31% in ARDS, 9% in COPD patients, and 50% in other causes of refractory hypercapnic respiratory failure.

Conclusion: $ECCO_2R$ was useful to apply ultra-protective ventilation among ARDS patients and improved $PaCO_2$, pH, and minute ventilation in COPD patients.

Keywords: Extracorporeal CO2 removal, Acute respiratory distress syndrome, Chronic obstructive pulmonary disease exacerbation

Background

There is not yet enough data to make strong recommendation about extracorporeal CO_2 removal ($ECCO_2R$) devices, as the benefits-risks ratio is not established. Because of its low flow, this technology is unable to provide adequate extracorporeal oxygenation. However, 350 to 500 mL/min is sufficient to remove half of CO_2 production, making $ECCO_2R$ an interesting tool in several situations.

First, in the setting of acute respiratory distress syndrome (ADRS), it is well established that low tidal volume and limited plateau pressure are associated with better survival [1]. Recent guidelines recommend to aim for tidal volume of 4–8 mL/kg of predicted body weight (PBW) and plateau pressure less than 30 cmH_2O [2]. However, ventilator-induced lung injury (VILI) due to hyperinflation has been documented even with low tidal volume [3]. Because some data suggest that decreasing plateau pressure, even if it is < 30 cmH_2O, might be associated with reduced mortality [4], using tidal volume lower than 6 mL/kg has been proposed [5]. Three studies have showed the feasibility and safety of ultra-protective ventilation, with 4 mL/kg

* Correspondence: hadrien51@hotmail.com
[1]Medical Intensive Care Unit, Besançon, France
[2]Service de Réanimation Médicale, CHU de Besançon, 25030 Besançon, France
Full list of author information is available at the end of the article

tidal volume and plateau pressure < 25 cmH_2O [6–8]. However, at this time, no prospective trial has demonstrated an impact on outcome.

Second, in the setting of chronic obstructive pulmonary disease (COPD) exacerbation, noninvasive ventilation is the first option [9]. Indeed, the need for invasive mechanical ventilation is associated with higher mortality [10]. By providing extracorporeal CO_2 clearance, $ECCO_2R$ might decrease respiratory rate and limit auto-PEEP, resulting in reduced respiratory work. Three case-control studies have suggested that $ECCO_2R$ decrease the intubation rate of severe COPD exacerbation [11–13]. It might also allow an earlier extubation and rehabilitation.

Finally, $ECCO_2R$ might also be useful in the setting of refractory respiratory acidosis with pH < 7.20 despite usual care. For example, successful treatment of near-fatal asthma using $ECCO_2R$ has been reported [14].

In this monocentric retrospective cohort study, we aimed to describe indications, ventilatory settings, gas exchanges, and outcome of patients receiving $ECCO_2R$ in our ICU.

Methods

Patients

We performed a retrospective chart review of all patients admitted to our tertiary regional intensive care unit (ICU) and started on $ECCO_2R$ from March 2014 to November 2017. Cases were identified through a prospectively maintained electronic database.

Ethical issues

$ECCO_2R$ therapy was started while all patients were on high-intensity treatment. Families were informed of the rescue treatment and the benefits-risks ratio. As a rule, all COPD patients required either to be intubated or to fail noninvasive ventilation (NIV) or refuse intubation to be started on $ECCO_2R$. Four ARDS patients were involved in ongoing studies related to $ECCO_2R$.

$ECCO_2R$ system

Four veno-venous $ECCO_2R$ systems were used, including ILA® (Novalung, Germany), Hemolung® (ALung Technologies, Inc., Pittsburgh, PA, USA), Prismalung® (Baxter Healthcare/Gambro Lund, Sweden), and CardioHelp® (Maquet, Germany). CardioHelp® was the only system using two venous cannulas. Others were associated to dual-lumen catheters, usually inserted by jugular access. There was no protocol guiding the choice of $ECCO_2R$ device, which was let to the clinician in charge. When renal replacement therapy was required, Prismalung® was preferentially used. $ECCO_2R$ weaning strategy was let to clinician's discretion.

Data recording

Demographic data collected included age, gender, primary admission diagnosis, cause of respiratory failure, and any known comorbidities. Physiologic data collected included vasopressor therapy and renal replacement therapy. Ventilatory data included ventilator mode, respiratory rate, tidal volume, plateau pressure when available, minute ventilation, and results of daily arterial blood gases (Additional file 1). $ECCO_2R$-related data included indication of extracorporeal support, type of device, blood flow, sweep gas flow, and anticoagulation level evaluated by anti-Xa activity. Ventilation settings were gathered just before starting $ECCO_2R$, at 4 hourly intervals for the first 24 h, and at day 2. Arterial blood gases were recorded once a day for 48 h.

$ECCO_2R$-related or potentially linked complications included bleeding, catheter or pump thrombosis, hemolysis, thrombocytopenia, obvious local infection, and bacteremia. Bleeding at catheter insertion site was considered if associated with at least one red blood cell transfusion. Because plasma-free hemoglobin assessment was not available in our center, hemolysis was defined as anemia associated to haptoglobin less than 0,1 g/L. Thrombocytopenia was defined as a platelet count inferior to 150 G/L or a decrease of more than 50% since $ECCO_2R$ start.

Statistical analysis

Qualitative variables were expressed as number percentage. Quantitative variables were expressed as median and interquartile range. Comparisons between two qualitative variables were performed using the Fischer exact test. Comparisons between two quantitative variables were performed using the Wilcoxon test. For the study of the evolution of quantitative variables over time among patients, the Wilcoxon rank sum test was performed. All analyses were performed using SAS 9.4.

Results

Description of the overall population

Over 4 years, 33 patients received $ECCO_2R$ therapy, including 16 mild or moderate ARDS patients, and 11 COPD patients with severe exacerbation. The remaining six patients had refractory hypercapnic acidosis secondary to severe acute asthma ($n = 2$), nosocomial pneumonia, bronchiolitis obliterans, exacerbation of pulmonary fibrosis, and bilateral bronchial compression by germinal tumor. Among ARDS patients who received $ECCO_2R$, three were enrolled in SUPERNOVA study (NCT02282657), and one in PRISMA-LUNG study [15]. All COPD patients except one were intubated. Among COPD patients, 7 (63%) benefited from long-term oxygen therapy and 4 (36%) from noninvasive home ventilation. Baseline characteristics of the study population are shown in Table 1.

Table 1 Baseline characteristics

Variables	Patients ($n = 33$)
Age (years)	63 [59–68]
Gender (male/female)	20/13
Body mass index (kg/m^2)	26 [23–30]
IGS2 score	49 [36–65]
SOFA score	
At ICU admission	7 [5–10]
At the time of ECCO$_2$R start	10 [7–12]
Indication	
Mild or moderate ARDS	16 (48)
COPD exacerbation	11 (33)
Other	6 (19)
Associated organ dysfunction	
Maximum noradrenaline dose (μg/kg/min)	0.16 [0.00–0.25]
Need for renal replacement therapy	7 (21)
Comorbidities	
Chronic obstructive pulmonary disease	16 (48)
Arterial hypertension	22 (66)
Coronary artery disease	7 (21)
Cardiac insufficiency	6 (18)
Chronic renal impairment	2 (6)
Stroke	2 (6)
Obesity	9 (27)
Ongoing treatments	
Antiplatelet therapy	10 (30)
Anticoagulation	4 (12)
Home oxygen therapy	11 (33)
Home noninvasive ventilation	4 (12)

Numbers are *n* (%) and median [interquartile range]

Outcome

For the 29 invasively ventilated patients, ECCO$_2$R therapy was started after a median time of 1 [1–5] day of invasive mechanical ventilation. In the overall population, median duration of ECCO$_2$R therapy was 7 [5–10] days, with no obvious difference between ARDS and COPD patients. Twenty-one patients were weaned from ECCO$_2$R while still intubated. Median duration of invasive mechanical ventilation after ECCO$_2$R weaning was 2 [0–6] days. Four COPD patients were extubated while on ECCO$_2$R therapy. Only 2 ARDS patient have benefited from a tracheostomy for respiratory support weaning. Mortality at day 28 was 27% in the whole cohort and seemed to be higher in ARDS patients than in COPD patients (31 vs 9%). Three of the 6 patients with refractory respiratory acidosis died. Median length of stay in ICU was 16 [10–22] days (Table 2).

Description of ECCO$_2$R therapy in ARDS patients

Results of ECCO2R therapy in ARDS patients are shown in Table 3. Median baseline tidal volume, plateau pressure, driving pressure, and respiratory rate were 5.3 [4.4–5.9] mL/kg, 26 [24–27] cmH$_2$O, 10 [8–15] cmH$_2$O, and 26 [22–28] respectively. Twenty-four hours after ECCO$_2$R start, tidal volume significantly decreased to 3.9 [3.5–4.2] mL/kg, without increase of PaCO$_2$. Although there was no difference for plateau pressure, driving pressure significantly decreased to 7 [6–10] cmH$_2$O. The decrease of respiratory rate was not significant. However, minute ventilation significantly decreased to 4.6 [3.9–5.8] L/min. Neuromuscular blockers were respectively used in 94, 81, and 56% of patients at baseline, day 1, and day 2. Among the 16 ARDS patients, 10 were proned while on ECCO$_2$R support. Among those 10 patients, two supported by ILA®, one by Hemolung®, and one by Prismalung® had three sessions of prone positioning or more.

Considering ultra-protective ventilation when tidal volume was ≤ 4 mL/kg of PBW and plateau pressure $\leq$ 25 cmH$_2$O, ECCO$_2$R did not allow a complete target attainment. Indeed, at baseline, 3/16 patients (19%) were ventilated with tidal volume ≤ 4 mL/kg of PBW. Plateau pressures at baseline was known for only 12/16 patients (75%) and was ≤ 25 cmH$_2$O in 6/12 (50%). At baseline, only 1/12 patient (8%) has both tidal volume ≤ 4 mL/kg of PBW and plateau pressures ≤ 25 cmH$_2$O (Additional file 1). Twenty-four hours after ECCO$_2$R beginning, 8/16 patients (50%) were ventilated with tidal volume ≤ 4 mL/kg of PBW, 5/12 (42%) with plateau pressures ≤ 25 cmH$_2$O, and 2/12 (17%) with both tidal volume ≤ 4 mL/kg of PBW and plateau pressures ≤ 25 cmH$_2$O.

Description of ECCO$_2$R therapy in COPD patients

Results of ECCO$_2$R therapy in COPD patients are shown in Table 4. Median baseline tidal volume, respiratory rate, minute ventilation, and PaCO$_2$ were 5.5 [5.5–5.9] mL/kg; 22 [20–23]; 7.6 [6.6–8.7] L/min; and 9.4 [8.4–10.1] kPa respectively. Forty-eight hours after ECCO$_2$R start, minute ventilation significantly decreased to 5.8 [4.9–6.2] L/min, while PaCO$_2$ significantly decreased to 6 [5.3–6.8] kPa. Sedation was used in 72, 54, and 45% of patients at baseline, day 1, and day 2 respectively.

Description of ECCO$_2$R therapy in non-intubated patients

Only four patients were not intubated at the beginning of ECCO$_2$R therapy. Patient no. 1 was a 61-year-old man who had a history of kidney transplantation. He had refractory hypercapnic COPD exacerbation with NIV failure. He received 2 days of ECCO$_2$R by Hemolung® device until successful weaning without need for intubation. Patient no. 2 was a 90-year-old woman with refractory hypercapnic pneumonia without hypoxemia. She was weaned from Prismalung® device after 5 days, but she died 48 h later in

Table 2 Outcomes of the 33 patients receiving $ECCO_2R$

Outcome	Total ($n = 33$)	ARDS ($n = 16$)	COPD ($n = 11$)	Others ($n = 6$)
28-day mortality	9 (27)	5 (31)	1 (9)	3 (50)
Length of stay in ICU, days	16 [10–22]	18 [11–26]	14 [11–19]	11 [8–18]
Duration of invasive ventilation before ECCO2R, days	1 [1–5]	3 [1–5]	1 [1–3]	0 [0–0]
Duration of ECCO2R therapy	7 [5–10]	6 [5–9]	7 [5–11]	6 [5–15]
Prone positioning, number of patients	15 (45)	10 (62)	3 (27)	2 (33)
Duration of invasive ventilation after ECCO2R weaning	2 [0–6]	4 [2–10]	2 [0–4]	1 [0–2]
Extubated while on ECCO2R, number of patients	4 (12)	0 (0)	4 (36)	0 (0)

Numbers are *n* (%) and median (interquartile range)

a context of withdrawal of active treatments. Patient no. 3 was a 59-year-old man with a history of lung transplantation and chronic graft rejection. He was assisted by Hemolung®. As he was not eligible for re-transplantation, he died at day 19 while still on $ECCO_2R$, in a context of withdrawal of active treatments. Patient no. 4 was a 29-year-old man with microscopic polyangeitis with end-stage renal failure associated to lung fibrosis. He benefited from Prismalung® at day 0. He was intubated at day 6 and died at day 17 of septic shock.

$ECCO_2R$ devices

Among the 33 enrolled patients, 17 were treated with Hemolung®, 10 with Prismalung®, 4 with ILA, and 2 with Cardiohelp®. Hemolung® was used in 9 of 11 COPD patients, whereas Prismalung® was used in 6 of 16 ARDS patients. ILA® and Cardiohelp® were used only in ARDS patients. Evolution of anti-Xa activity and platelet levels are reported in Table 5.

Complications

No decannulation was reported during the studied period. Thrombocytopenia was the most frequently reported adverse event (72%). Since day 2 of $ECCO_2R$ treatment, at least half of treated patients have less than 150 G/L of platelets and at least 25% have less than 90 G/L of platelets. However, only four patients (12%) received platelet transfusion. Half of the treated patients received at least one red blood cell transfusion during $ECCO_2R$ therapy. One patient treated with Hemolung® died of intracranial hemorrhage, while on $ECCO_2R$. At the diagnosis, he had 189 G/L of platelets, and 0,44 UI/mL of antiXa. Hemolysis was reported in 16 patients (48%) but did not lead to $ECCO_2R$ withdrawal. Device thrombosis occurred in 5 patients (15%). Among them, one ARDS patient treated with CardioHelp® has necessitated urgent circuit change for complete pump thrombosis. Interruption of CO_2 removal for $ECCO_2R$ change or withdrawal was well tolerated in all cases.

Discussion

In this retrospective chart review, we aimed to describe our experience of $ECCO_2R$ devices and to help clinician volunteers to use those devices beyond the scope of experimental studies. We have found that $ECCO_2R$ system allowed ultra-protective ventilation in ARDS patients by decreasing tidal volume. We also found that $ECCO_2R$ was effective to reduce minute ventilation and improve blood pH in ventilated COPD patient. Furthermore, it

Table 3 Evolution of ventilatory settings and gas exchanges in 16 ARDS patients

Ventilatory parameters	Baseline	4 h	8 h	12 h	24 h	48 h
Ventilatory mode (VC/PSV), number	16/0	16/0	16/0	16/0	15/1	14/2
TV (mL kg^{-1})	5.3 [4.4–5.9]	3.8 [3.5–4.1]*	3.7 [3.5–4.1]*	3.7 [3.6–4.1]*	3.9 [3.5–4.2]*	3.8 [3.3–4.1]*
RR (min^{-1})	26 [22–28]	23 [20–25]	22 [19–25]*	22 [20–25]*	21 [18–23]*	23 [17–26]
Minute ventilation (L min^{-1})	8.5 [6.0–9.5]	5.2 [4.0–6.1]*	4.5 [3.9–6.3]*	4.3 [3.9–6.3]*	4.6 [3.9–5.8]*	5.3 [4.0–6.9]*
PEEP (cmH_2O)	13 [10–15]	14 [10–15]	14 [10–18]	14 [10–18]	14 [12–18]	14 [11–17]
Plateau pressure (cmH_2O)	26 [24–27]	–			26 [22–29]	25 [22–27]
Driving pressure (cmH_20)	10 [8–15]	–			7 [6–10]*	9 [8–10]*
$PaCO_2$ (kPa)	6.7 [6.1–7.5]	5.7 [5.1–7.0]*			5.6 [4.8–7.6]	5.4 [4.8–8.2]
pH	7.31 [7.25–7.41]	7.39 [7.30–7.42]			7.40 [7.33–7.45]	7.41 [7.35–7.43]
PaO_2/FiO_2	145 [116–161]	207 [127–226]*			182 [149–211]	201 [168–263]*
Neuromuscular blockers use, number	15 (94%)	–			13 (81%)	9 (56%)

*$p < 0.05$ vs baseline; *V* volume control, *PSV* pressure support ventilation; numbers are *n* (%) and median (interquartile range)

Table 4 Evolution of ventilatory settings and gas exchanges in 11 COPD patients

Ventilatory parameters	Baseline	4 h	8 h	12 h	24 h	48 h
Ventilatory mode (VC/PSV/NIV), number	8/2/1	7/3/1	7/3/1	7/3/1	5/5/1	5/5/1
TV (mL kg^{-1})	5.5 [5.5–5.9]	5 [4.4–6.1]	4.6 [4.4–4.8]*	4.5 [4.2–5]*	5.6 [4.4–5.8]	5.2 [4.1–5.8]
RR (min^{-1})	22 [20–23]	18 [17–22]	18 [15–24]	18 [15–21]	20 [17–20]	20 [16–24]
Minute ventilation (L min^{-1})	7.6 [6.6–8.7]	5.9 [5–7.2]	4.7 [3.8–5.2]*	4.9 [3.8–5.9]*	6.2 [4.1–6.8]	5.8 [4.9–6.2]*
PEEP (cmH_2O)	6 [4–8]	6 [5–8]	6 [5–8]	6 [5–8]	8 [5–10]	8 [7–10]
$PaCO_2$ (kPa)	9.4 [8.4–10.1]	6.6 [5.7–7.1]*			6 [5.1–7.1]*	6 [5.3–6.8]*
pH	7.32 [7.26–7.34]	7.43 [7.41–7.45]*			7.45 [7.41–7.47]*	7.44 [7.42–7.46]*
PaO_2/FiO_2	174 [158–207]	192 [177–254]			225 [186–262]	210 [181–254]
Sedative use, number	8 (72%)	–			6 (54%)	5 (45%)
Neuromuscular blockers use, number	6 (54%)	–			4 (36%)	3 (27%)

*$p < 0.05$ vs baseline; *VC* volume control *PSV* pressure support ventilation, *NIV* noninvasive ventilation; [1]when VC is used; numbers are *n* (%) and median (interquartile range)

allowed extubation in some patients while on extracorporeal support.

In the setting of ARDS patients, our results are in line with those of the three main studies assessing veno-venous low-flow $ECCO_2R$. Indeed, in a recent pilot study in 15 mild to moderate ARDS patients, the use of Hemolung® allowed ultra-protective ventilation with tidal volume of 4 mL/kg [8]. Some similar results have been observed with Polystan SAFE® (Maquet, Rastatt, Germany), a membrane lung connected to a veno-venous hemofiltration system [6]. Interestingly, in our ARDS cohort, 6 of the 16 patients have benefited from Prismalung® device, connected to a renal replacement machine. In a recently published proof-of-concept study, Prismalung® allowed ultra-protective ventilation in 20 mild-to-moderate ARDS patients. However, mean duration treatment was only 31 h (± 22), limiting conclusion about longer use and safety [15]. Although significant, the reduction of driving pressure secondary to tidal volume decrease was quite small in our study. This could be due to a relatively low tidal volume at baseline. Indeed, in our practice, we usually target low plateau pressure, with tidal volume lower than 6 mL/kg as reported by other authors [16]. After $ECCO_2R$ start, we have noted a trend to decrease of respiratory rate. This is another potential aspect of the ultra-protective strategy, as some authors have suggested that respiratory rate could be a determinant of VILI [17]. Because median baseline PaO_2/FiO_2 ratio was 145 [116–161] mmHg, patients were a priori susceptible to have an indication for prone positioning. It is noteworthy that 10 have benefited from this therapy without any adverse event. Because prone positioning has been found to decrease mortality in ADRS with PaO_2/FiO_2 ratio less than 150 mmHg, it is mandatory that novel therapy do not limit its use [18]. While neuromuscular blockers use in moderate to severe ARDS is recommended for 48 h [19], we have noted a trend towards early interruption. This might be explained by the early improvement of oxygenation and the control of hypercapnia. In this situation, our clinicians favored decrease sedations and awakeness.

In the three largest studies enrolling COPD patients, the primary end point was the avoidance of intubation [11–13]. In our cohort, only one COPD patient has benefited from such pre-intubation strategy. However, whether $ECCO_2R$ should be started before or after intubation is still a matter of debate. Indeed, because NIV failure is hard to predict, and $ECCO_2R$ is associated with additional septic and hemorrhagic risks, appropriate selection of patients which might benefit from $ECCO_2R$ is difficult. Considering this, our policy is to start $ECCO_2R$ early after intubation. Moreover, such strategy may facilitate insertion of the $ECCO_2R$ catheter, allowing safe conditions, as no complication was reported during catheter insertion in our patients. In our cohort, 50% of the patients were started on day 1 and 75% before day 3 of mechanical ventilation. While the global effect of $ECCO_2R$ was the lowering of minute ventilation and $PaCO_2$, in our cohort, it was more marked during the 24 first hours. This might be potentially explained by the decrease of sedative use, resulting in more patients with spontaneous ventilation, with uncontrolled tidal volume and respiratory rate.

Considering safety, our data point out that $ECCO_2R$ use cannot be dissociated from the potential risks of anticoagulation in critically ill patients. Indeed, as it occurred during $ECCO_2R$ therapy, the fatal case of intracranial hemorrhage has to be underlined. Even if no heparin overdosing has been reported, there is an obvious link between anticoagulation and this complication. Even if the hemorrhagic risk was not obvious, as there was no other indication for anticoagulation, responsibility of $ECCO_2R$ therapy is here plausible. Otherwise, although frequent, thrombocytopenia was moderate, and hemolysis did not result in need for $ECCO_2R$ withdrawal. Finally, because interruption of CO_2 removal was well tolerated, $ECCO_2R$ circuit thrombosis

Table 5 Hemostatic parameters during $ECCO_2R$ therapy

Devices	Duration of therapy (days)	Platelets count (G/L)						Anti-Xa activity (UI/mL)						Hemolysis	RBC transfusion during $ECCO_2R$
		J0	J1	J2	J3	J4	J5	J0	J1	J2	J3	J4	J5		
All patients (*n* = 33)	7 [5–10]	202 [137–286]	167 [95–243]	143 [88–199]	130 [79–192]	128 [89–156]	124 [86–153]	0.22 [0.14–0.47]	0.26 [0.16–0.40]	0.33 [0.24–0.44]	0.33 [0.25–0.41]	0.30 [0.20–0.39]	0.35 [0.21–0.47]	16 (48)	16 (48)
Hemolung® (*n* = 17)	7 [5–10]	210 [163–264]	184 [108–243]	136 [88–208]	121 [79–174]	128 [89–153]	130 [88–151]	0.24 [0.15–0.50]	0.26 [0.20–0.36]	0.41 [0.30–0.53]	0.31 [0.25–0.42]	0.30 [0.20–0.38]	0.35 [0.30–0.49]	13 (76)	9 (53)
Prismalung® (*n* = 10)	5 [3–6]	153 [104–272]	126 [65–241]	124 [72–195]	105 [57–183]	82 [57–98]	77 [55–87]	0.13 [0.10–0.43]	0.17 [0.10–0.24]	0.25 [0.10–0.41]	0.37 [0.14–0.40]	0.23 [0.12–0.35]	0.20 [0.11–0.36]	1 (10)	4 (40)
ILA® (*n* = 4)	10 (5–19)*	226 [150–288]	181 [155–225]	172 [142–206]	186 [167–208]	151 [134–184]	173 [146–199]	0.19 [0.16–0.28]	0.36 [0.29–0.39]	0.26 [0.25–0.29]	0.37 [0.32–0.42]	0.31 [0.24–0.34]	0.26 [0.22–0.31]	1 (25)	3 (75)
Maquet® (*n* = 2)	6.5 (6–7)*	258 [205–311]	179 [163–195]	151 [141–162]	142 [130–153]	142 [130–153]	153 [153–153]	0.27 [0.25–0.30]	0.49 [0.44–0.53]	0.47 [0.46–0.47]	0.45 [0.42–0.47]	0.58 [0.55–0.61]	0.47 [0.46–0.47]	1 (50)	0 (0)

Numbers are *n* (%) and median (interquartile range), except for * which corresponds to min and max. *RBC* red blood cells

only resulted in loss of 250 mL of blood, corresponding to the circuit volume of purge.

Because, no trial demonstrating its clinical benefit has been published, $ECCO_2R$ systems are not widely used. Indeed, in a recent survey, among 239 French ICUs, only 15% declared having used at least once $ECCO_2R$ between 2010 and 2015 [20]. However, $ECCO_2R$ technology has improved, and because of a strong rational, several randomized trials enrolling ARDS and COPD patients are ongoing [21]. The mortality rate in our ARDS and COPD patients is in the lower range [16, 22], and early use of ECCO2R might contribute to our results. If well-designed studies bring proof of the $ECCO_2R$ benefit, a very large number of patients would be concerned, asking the question of where to perform $ECCO_2R$. Indeed, in the setting of ECMO, a large retrospective cohort analysis has suggested a negative link between ECMO cases volume and hospital mortality [23]. As well as the concept of "ECMO center," the need for "$ECCO_2R$ center" has to be assessed.

Our study has several limitations. First, because of the retrospective design, some data are lacking. Whereas tidal volume, respiratory rate, and positive end expiratory pressure are monitored hourly by the nurses in our unit, plateau pressure is usually monitored by the clinicians and not systematically reported in the medical record. It explains why complete data on plateau pressure and driving pressure were available for only 8 on 16 ARDS patients. Second, heterogeneity and small sample size limit internal validity. However, $ECCO_2R$ is not widely used, and previous studies in the setting of $ECCO_2R$ have included no more than 40 ARDS patients [7] and 25 COPD patients [12, 13]. Third, we reported a single-center experience limits the generalization of our conclusions. For example, our paramedical team is widely used to prone positioning and extracorporeal circulations. Even if prone positioning in patients receiving $ECCO_2R$ has only concerned a few patients, team practice might have decreased the risk of severe adverse events such as accidental decannulation. Our patients represent 256 $ECCO_2R$ days. Fourth, except in the setting of SUPERNOVA or PRISMALUNG studies, we did not have preset criteria for $ECCO_2R$ implantation, which was left to the clinician's judgment. Fifth, we reported only initial $ECCO_2R$ settings. However, because of maximal CO_2 is targeted, sweep gas was usually kept at his maximal value. $ECCO_2R$ rotation per minute (RPM) was set to reach a blood flow of at least 300, 450, 700 and 1000 mL/min, with Prismalung®, Hemolung®, ILA®, and CardioHelp® respectively. $ECCO_2R$ RPM were decreased only when significant hemolysis was documented. Finally, plasma-free hemoglobin assessment was not available in our center, resulting in a more difficult diagnosis of hemolysis.

Conclusion

In ARDS patients, $ECCO_2R$ use was associated with a significant decrease of tidal volume and driving pressure during the first 48 h of therapy. Prone positioning was performed in 10 (62%) patients without adverse event. In COPD patients, $ECCO_2R$ use was associated with a significant decrease of minute ventilation, normalization of pH, and decrease of $PaCO_2$. Although $ECCO_2R$ therapy was globally well tolerated, a case of fatal intracranial hemorrhage points out that this procedure cannot be dissociated from the potential risks of anticoagulation in critically ill patients.

Authors' contributions

HW helped analyze the data, write the manuscript, and perform the literature search.

FA, FB, NB, CCh, CP, CCl, ED, JCN, GL, GP, and GC helped analyze the data and write the manuscript. All authors read and approved the final manuscript.

Competing interests

Pr Capellier has received lecture fees from Baxter and Alung. Prismalung® devices were provided by Baxter. The other authors declare that they have no competing interests.

Author details

[1]Medical Intensive Care Unit, Besançon, France. [2]Service de Réanimation Médicale, CHU de Besançon, 25030 Besançon, France. [3]Department of Epidemiology and Preventive Medicine, School of Public Health and Preventive Medicine, Faculty of Medicine, Nursing and Health Sciences, Clayton, Australia. [4]Research Unit EA 3920 and SFR FED 4234, University of Franche Comté, Besançon, France.

References

1. Acute Respiratory Distress Syndrome Network, Brower RG, Matthay MA, et al. Ventilation with lower tidal volumes as compared with traditional tidal volumes for acute lung injury and the acute respiratory distress syndrome. N Engl J Med. 2000;342:1301–8.
2. Fan E, Del Sorbo L, Goligher EC, et al. An official American Thoracic Society/European Society of Intensive Care Medicine/Society of Critical Care Medicine clinical practice guideline: mechanical ventilation in adult patients with acute respiratory distress syndrome. Am J Respir Crit Care Med. 2017;195:1253–63.
3. Terragni PP, Rosboch G, Tealdi A, et al. Tidal hyperinflation during low tidal volume ventilation in acute respiratory distress syndrome. Am J Respir Crit Care Med. 2007;175:160–6.
4. Hager DN, Krishnan JA, Hayden DL, et al. Tidal volume reduction in patients with acute lung injury when plateau pressures are not high. Am J Respir Crit Care Med. 2005;172:1241–5.
5. Slutsky AS, Ranieri VM. Ventilator-induced lung injury. N Engl J Med. 2013;369:2126–36.
6. Terragni PP, Del Sorbo L, Mascia L, et al. Tidal volume lower than 6 ml/kg enhances lung protection: role of extracorporeal carbon dioxide removal. Anesthesiology. 2009;111:826–35.
7. Bein T, Weber-Carstens S, Goldmann A, et al. Lower tidal volume strategy (≈3 ml/kg) combined with extracorporeal CO2 removal versus "conventional" protective ventilation (6 ml/kg) in severe ARDS: the prospective randomized Xtravent-study. Intensive Care Med. 2013;39:847–56.
8. Fanelli V, Ranieri MV, Mancebo J, et al. Feasibility and safety of low-flow extracorporeal carbon dioxide removal to facilitate ultra-protective ventilation in patients with moderate acute respiratory distress syndrome. Crit Care Lond Engl. 2016;20:36.
9. Lindenauer PK, Stefan MS, Shieh M-S, et al. Outcomes associated with invasive and noninvasive ventilation among patients hospitalized with exacerbations of chronic obstructive pulmonary disease. JAMA Intern Med. 2014;174:1982–93.

10. Stefan MS, Nathanson BH, Higgins TL, et al. Comparative effectiveness of noninvasive and invasive ventilation in critically ill patients with acute exacerbation of chronic obstructive pulmonary disease. Crit Care Med. 2015;43:1386–94.
11. Kluge S, Braune SA, Engel M, et al. Avoiding invasive mechanical ventilation by extracorporeal carbon dioxide removal in patients failing noninvasive ventilation. Intensive Care Med. 2012;38:1632–9.
12. Del Sorbo L, Pisani L, Filippini C, et al. Extracorporeal Co2 removal in hypercapnic patients at risk of noninvasive ventilation failure: a matched cohort study with historical control. Crit Care Med. 2015;43:120–7.
13. Braune S, Sieweke A, Brettner F, et al. The feasibility and safety of extracorporeal carbon dioxide removal to avoid intubation in patients with COPD unresponsive to noninvasive ventilation for acute hypercapnic respiratory failure (ECLAIR study): multicentre case-control study. Intensive Care Med. 2016;42:1437–44.
14. Pavot A, Mallat J, Vangrunderbeeck N, et al. Rescue therapeutic strategy combining ultra-protective mechanical ventilation with extracorporeal CO2 removal membrane in near-fatal asthma with severe pulmonary barotraumas: a case report. Medicine (Baltimore). 2017;96:e8248.
15. Schmidt M, Jaber S, Zogheib E, et al. Feasibility and safety of low-flow extracorporeal CO2 removal managed with a renal replacement platform to enhance lung-protective ventilation of patients with mild-to-moderate ARDS. Crit Care Lond Engl. 2018;22:122.
16. Bellani G, Laffey JG, Pham T, et al. Epidemiology, patterns of care, and mortality for patients with acute respiratory distress syndrome in intensive care units in 50 countries. JAMA. 2016;315:788–800.
17. Gattinoni L, Tonetti T, Cressoni M, et al. Ventilator-related causes of lung injury: the mechanical power. Intensive Care Med. 2016;42:1567–75.
18. Guérin C, Reignier J, Richard J-C, et al. Prone positioning in severe acute respiratory distress syndrome. N Engl J Med. 2013;368:2159–68.
19. Papazian L, Forel J-M, Gacouin A, et al. Neuromuscular blockers in early acute respiratory distress syndrome. N Engl J Med. 2010;363:1107–16.
20. Deniau B, Ricard JD, Messika J, et al. Use of extracorporeal carbon dioxide removal (ECCO2R) in 239 intensive care units: results from a French national survey. Intensive Care Med. 2016;42:624–5.
21. Taccone FS, Malfertheiner MV, Ferrari F, et al. Extracorporeal CO2 removal in critically ill patients: a systematic review. Minerva Anestesiol. 2017;83:762–72.
22. Chandra D, Stamm JA, Taylor B, et al. Outcomes of noninvasive ventilation for acute exacerbations of chronic obstructive pulmonary disease in the United States, 1998-2008. Am J Respir Crit Care Med. 2012;185:152–9.
23. Barbaro RP, Odetola FO, Kidwell KM, et al. Association of hospital-level volume of extracorporeal membrane oxygenation cases and mortality. Analysis of the extracorporeal life support organization registry. Am J Respir Crit Care Med. 2015;191:894–901.

20

Treatment of patients with sepsis in a closed intensive care unit is associated with improved survival

Takayuki Ogura[1*], Yoshihiko Nakamura[2], Kunihiko Takahashi[3], Kazuki Nishida[3], Daisuke Kobashi[1] and Shigeyuki Matsui[3]

Abstract

Background: The aim of this study is to investigate the association between treatment in a closed ICU and survival at discharge in patients with sepsis.

Methods: This is a post hoc analysis utilizing data from the Japan Septic Disseminated Intravascular Coagulation study, including data from patients with sepsis from 2011 to 2013. Multiple logistic regression analysis was used to estimate the association between ICU policy and survival at discharge, and propensity score matching analysis was performed including the same covariates as a sensitivity analysis. Multiple linear regression analysis for the length of ICU stay in surviving patients was also performed with adjustments for the same covariates.

Results: Two thousand four hundred ninety-five patients were analyzed. The median Acute Physiology and Chronic Health Evaluation (APACHE) II score was 22 [17–29], the median Sequential Organ Failure Assessment (SOFA) score was 9 [7–12], and the overall mortality was 33%. There were 979 patients treated in 17 open ICUs and 1516 patients in 18 closed ICUs. In comparison, the APACHE II score and SOFA scores were significantly higher in patients in closed ICUs (closed vs open = 23 [18–29] vs 21 [16–28]; $p < .001$, 9 [7–13] vs 9 [6–12]; $p = 0.004$). There was no difference in the unadjusted mortality (closed vs open; 33.1% vs 33.2%), but in multiple logistic regression analysis, treatment in a closed ICU is significantly associated with survival at discharge (odds ratio = 1.59, 95% CI [1.276–1.827], $p = .001$). The sensitivity analysis (702 pairs of the matching) showed a significantly higher survival rate in the closed ICU (71.8% vs 65.2%, $p = 0.011$). The length of ICU stay of patients in closed ICUs was significantly shorter (20% less).

Conclusion: This Japanese nationwide analysis of patients with sepsis shows a significant association between treatment in a closed ICU and survival at discharge, and a 20% decrease in ICU stay.

Keywords: Intensive care unit, Sepsis, Intensivist, Mortality

Background

Sepsis is life-threatening organ dysfunction caused by dysregulated host responses to infection, and septic shock is a subset of sepsis in which underlying circulatory and cellular/metabolic abnormalities are sufficiently profound to substantially increase mortality [1]. According to one study, there are more than 750,000 patients annually in the USA with sepsis [2] and the incidence is rising [3]. Septic shock remains lethal even with aggressive management, with a mortality of 20 to 30% [4].

Patients with sepsis are usually treated in the intensive care unit (ICU). Sepsis results from infection, and these patients often develop multiple organ-system failure. Aggressive management, including control of the infection source and support of failing organ-systems, is needed for optimal outcomes. In recent years, guidelines for the treatment of patients with sepsis have been published [5,

* Correspondence: alongthelongestway2003@yahoo.co.jp
[1]Department of Emergency Medicine and Critical Care Medicine, Japan Red Cross Maebashi Hospital, Asahi-cho 3-21-36, Maebashi, Gunma 371-0014, Japan
Full list of author information is available at the end of the article

6], and intensivists play an important role in the care of these patients.

Intensivists improve patient outcome in the ICU [7], and the ICU organization model influences patient outcomes [8–10]. There are generally two staffing models for ICU treatment, including an "open organization model" and a "closed organization model." In the open model, there is no intensivist consultation or elective intensivist consultation. Mandatory intensivist consultation is conducted in closed model ICUs [8], in which intensivist directs patient care [11] regardless of the time of day.

However, focusing on sepsis, to the best of our knowledge, the effect of the ICU organization model (open/closed) or directing of care by an intensivist on the mortality of patients is unknown and there are no studies to answer this important clinical question. We hypothesize that a closed ICU improves the outcome of patients with sepsis and septic shock, since a closed ICU is the highest-intensity physician staffing ICU model and intensivists direct care regardless of the time of day in the ICU. The aim of this study is to investigate the association between management in a closed ICU and survival at discharge of patients with sepsis. This is a nationwide study in Japan, including an analysis of clinical data regarding the severity of sepsis, pre-existing co-morbidities, the need for mechanical organ system support, and treatments given.

Methods

Patient selection

>This is a post hoc analysis utilizing the database from the Japan Septic Disseminated Intravascular Coagulation study (JSEPTIC DIC study) (University Hospital Medical Information Network Individual Case Data Repository, UMIN000012543, http://www.umin.ac.jp/icdr/index-j.html), which was a nationwide study in Japan [12]. The JSEPTIC DIC study retrospectively collected data from patients admitted to the ICU for the treatment of sepsis [13] from January 2011 to December 2013, excluding patients younger than 16 years or who developed sepsis after admission to the ICU (the JSEPTIC DIC study used the definitions of sepsis, severe sepsis, and septic shock from [13] as it was performed before publication of the 2016 definitions [1]). The JSEPTIC DIC study was approved by the Institutional Review Boards of all participating hospitals. The requirement for informed consent was waived because of the retrospective nature of the study. Since this database was already anonymized for individual patient data and institutions, the Institutional Review Board waived the need for review of this post hoc study.

Patients were divided into two groups, the closed ICU group (treated in a closed ICU) and the open ICU group (treated in an open ICU). The JSEPTIC DIC study did not demonstrate a clear definition of open ICU or closed ICUs. Each ICU had reported subjective information about their ICU organization model (open/closed/unclassified) at the initiation of the JSEPTIC DIC study. In Japan, the closed ICU is conventionally defined as a unit that transfers all patient care to an intensive care team that directs patient care with primary responsibility for all care and the open ICU is conventionally defined as an ICU where the intensive care team provides expertise via elective or mandatory consultation without assuming primary responsibility for patient care [14]. Patients treated in an ICU which could not clearly be classified as the closed or open were excluded from the final study population.

Exposure and outcome variables

The present study used all variables collected in the JSEPTIC DIC study. Variables for which the proportion of missing data was above 10% (fibrinogen, fibrin/fibrinogen degradation products, D-dimer, antithrombin, and lactate) and primary infection site are not included. The main exposure variable was set as the closed ICU or open ICU. The primary outcome measure was survival at discharge. Due to the healthcare system in Japan, no patients were discharged to hospice care.

Covariates for patient characteristics included age, gender, weight, pre-existing organ dysfunction and hemostatic disorders (comorbidity), Acute Physiology and Chronic Health Evaluation (APACHE) II score [15] (day 1), Sequential Organ Failure Assessment (SOFA) score [16] (day 1), systemic inflammatory response syndrome score [17] (days 1), the identification of microorganisms responsible for sepsis, blood culture results, and results of laboratory tests on day 1 including white blood cell count, platelet count, hemoglobin level, and prothrombin time-international normalized ratio (PT-INR). Treatment variables reviewed included administration of medications, including anti-disseminated intravascular coagulation (DIC) or anti-thrombotic drugs, immunoglobulins, low-dose steroids, and transfusion of blood products during the first week after ICU admission. Other therapeutic interventions reviewed included renal replacement therapy, renal replacement therapy for non-renal indications, plasma exchange, polymyxin B direct hemoperfusion (PMX-DHP), extracorporeal membrane oxygenation (ECMO), and use of the intra-aortic balloon pump during the first week after ICU admission.

Statistical analysis

Baseline characteristics were compared before and after the follow-up period for patients in both the closed and open ICU groups. Distributed continuous variables without a normal distribution are presented as median with interquartile range (IQR). Categorical data are summarized using numbers or percentages. The Mann-Whitney *U* test was used for comparing continuous variables, and the Fisher's exact test was used for categorical data. As for the main result, multiple logistic regression analysis was performed to estimate the association between the closed/open ICU and survival at discharge from the hospital, adjusted by baseline patient characteristics and treatment variables. As a sensitivity analysis, propensity score matching analysis including the same covariate was performed. For propensity score matching analysis, we use calipers of width equal to 0.1 of the standard deviation. As for sub-analysis, multiple linear regression analysis for the log-transformed values of the length of ICU stay and hospital stay in survived patients was performed with adjustments for the same covariates, and estimated the ratio of the length of stay between the closed ICU and open ICU. The level of significance was set at $p < 0.05$. All statistical analyses were performed with SAS (Version 9.4, SAS Institute Inc., Cary, North Carolina, USA).

Results

A total of 3195 patients were included in the JSEPTIC DIC study, and 2700 patients were enrolled in this study after excluding patients treated in ICUs not clearly classified as closed or open. There were data deficits in 205 patients, and data for the remaining 2495 patients were analyzed (Fig. 1). The mean age was 72 years, 59.7% male, the median APACHE II score was 23 [17–29], and the median SOFA score (day 1) was 9 [7–12]. The rate of survival at discharge was 66.8% (Table 1). Participating ICUs included 17 (49%) closed and 18 (51%) open.

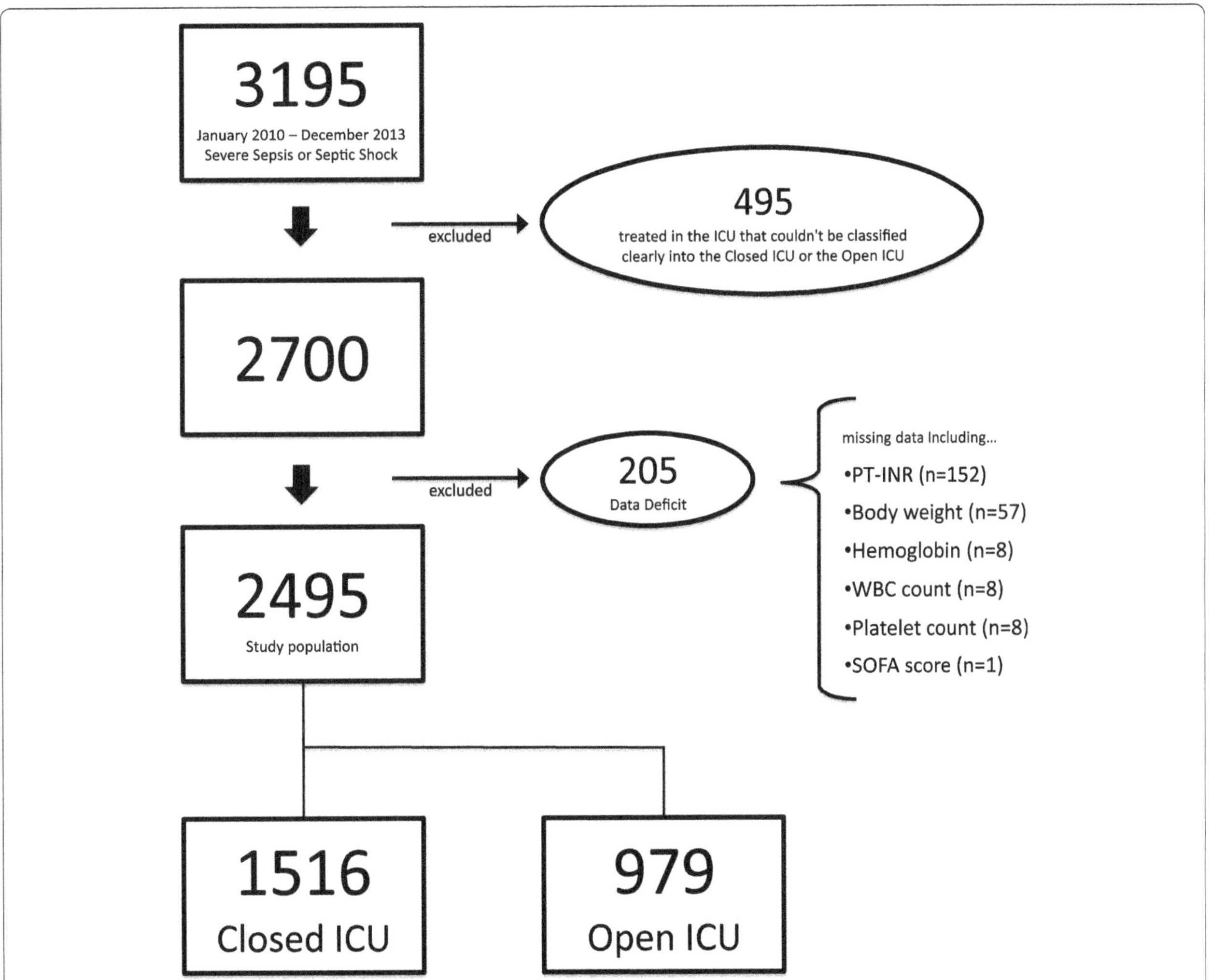

Fig. 1 Patient inclusion flow chart. Data for 3195 patients were reviewed and 495 patients did not meet inclusion criteria. There were data deficits for 205 patients, leaving a final study group of 2495 patients. The number of patients with missing data is not considered regarding duplication. PT-INR: prothrombin time international normalized ratio; WBC: white blood cell; SOFA score: Sequential Organ Failure Assessment score

Table 1 Comparison for patient characteristics and treatments ($n = 2495$)

	All patients ($n = 2495$)	Closed ICU ($n = 1516$)	Open ICU ($n = 979$)	p value
In-hospital surgical ICU	50 (2.0%)	50 (3.3%)	0 (0.0%)	< 0.001*
In-hospital general ICU	1168 (46.8%)	644 (42.5%)	5234 (53.5%)	< 0.001*
Emergency ICU	1277 (51.2%)	822 (54.2%)	455 (46.5%)	< 0.001*
Number of beds (IQR†)	12 [8–18]	10 [6–18]	12 [10–20]	< 0.001*
SOFA score (IQR†)	9 [7–12]	9 [7–13]	9 [6–12]	0.004*
APACHE II score (IQR†)	22 [17–29]	23 [18–29]	21 [16–28]	< 0.001*
SIRS score (IQR†)	3 [2–4]	3 [2–4]	3 [2–4]	0.058
Age (IQR†, year old)	72 [62–80]	72 [62–80]	73 [63–81]	0.007*
Sex (male, %)	1490 (59.7%)	916 (60.4%)	574 (58.6%)	0.373
Body weight (IQR†, kg)	54.5 [46.3–64]	54.7 [46.5–65]	54.0 [46.0–63]	0.208
White blood cell count (IQR†, $\times 10^3$)	11.2 [4.5–17.8]	11.00 [4.40–17.76]	11.66 [4.85–17.80]	0.199
Hemoglobin (IQR†, g/dl)	10.6 [9–12.4]	10.5 [8.9–12.4]	10.6 [9.1–12.5]	0.055
Platelet count (IQR†, $\times 10^3$)	120 [64–191]	121 [64–194]	118 [64–186]	0.498
Prothrombin time international normalize ratio (IQR†)	1.34 [1.17–1.61]	1.35 [1.18–1.63]	1.32 [1.16–1.56]	0.057
Co-morbidities				
Liver failure (yes, %)	104 (4.2%)	68 (4.5%)	36 (3.7%)	0.324
Respiratory failure (yes, %)	98 (3.9%)	64 (4.2%)	34 (3.5%)	0.347
Cardiac failure (yes, %)	134 (5.4%)	82 (5.4%)	52 (5.3%)	0.916
Renal failure (yes, %)	217 (8.7%)	114 (7.5%)	103 (10.5%)	0.009*
Immunological disorder (yes, %)	381 (15.3%)	263 (17.3%)	118 (12.1%)	< 0.001*
Hematologic disorder				
Cirrhosis (yes, %)	97 (3.9%)	63 (4.2%)	34 (3.5%)	0.389
Hematologic malignancy (yes, %)	84 (3.4%)	58 (3.8%)	26 (2.7%)	0.113
Chemotherapy (yes, %)	114 (4.6%)	79 (5.2%)	35 (3.6%)	0.056
Warfarin intake (yes, %)	113 (4.5%)	73 (4.8%)	40 (4.1%)	0.392
Others (yes, %)	48 (1.9%)	33 (2.2%)	15 (1.5%)	0.252
Positive blood culture	1111 (44.5%)	679 (44.8%)	432 (44.1%)	0.745
Negative blood culture	1240 (49.7%)	778 (51.3%)	462 (47.2%)	0.044*
No blood culture	144 (5.8%)	59 (3.9%)	85 (8.7%)	< 0.001*
Viral infection	22 (0.9%)	18 (1.2%)	4 (0.4%)	0.042*
GNR infection	912 (36.6%)	528 (34.8%)	384 (39.2%)	0.026*
GPC infection	586 (23.5%)	344 (22.7%)	242 (24.7%)	0.243
Fungal infection	38 (1.5%)	27 (1.8%)	11 (1.1%)	0.190
Mixed infection	339 (13.6%)	246 (16.2%)	93 (9.5%)	< 0.001*
Other infection	45 (1.8%)	33 (2.2%)	12 (1.2%)	0.081
Unknown infection	553 (22.2%)	320 (21.1%)	233 (23.8%)	0.114
Red blood cell transfusion (IQR†, units)	0 [0–4]	0 [0–4]	0 [0–4]	< 0.001*
Fresh frozen plasma transfusion (IQR†, units)	0 [0–4]	0 [0–5]	0 [0–4]	0.002*
Platelet concentration transfusion (IQR†, units)	0 [0–0]	0 [0–10]	0 [0–0]	< 0.001*
Treatment for DIC (yes, %)	1074 (43.0%)	656 (43.3%)	418 (42.7%)	0.777
Antithrombin III (yes, %)	726 (29.1%)	447 (29.5%)	279 (28.5%)	0.596
rhsTM (yes, %)	636 (25.5%)	420 (27.7%)	216 (22.1%)	0.002*
Nafamostat (yes, %)	880 (35.3%)	533 (35.2%)	347 (35.5%)	0.884
Heparin (yes, %)	453 (18.2%)	247 (16.3%)	206 (21.0%)	0.003*

Table 1 Comparison for patient characteristics and treatments ($n = 2495$) *(Continued)*

	All patients ($n = 2495$)	Closed ICU ($n = 1516$)	Open ICU ($n = 979$)	p value
Warfarin (yes, %)	39 (1.6%)	15 (1.0%)	24 (2.5%)	0.004*
Antiplatelet (yes, %)	56 (2.2%)	37 (2.4%)	19 (1.9%)	0.411
Others (yes, %)	15 (0.6%)	7 (0.5%)	8 (0.8%)	0.262
Specific treatment				
Immunoglobulin (yes, %)	743 (29.8%)	447 (29.5%)	296 (30.2%)	0.689
Low dose steroid (yes, %)	600 (24.0%)	413 (27.2%)	187 (19.1%)	< 0.001*
Renal replacement therapy (yes, %)	664 (26.6%)	452 (29.8%)	212 (21.7%)	< 0.001*
Renal replacement therapy not for renal indication (yes, %)	165 (6.6%)	58 (3.8%)	107 (10.9%)	< 0.001*
Polymyxin B direct hemoperfusion (yes, %)	547 (21.9%)	316 (20.8%)	231 (23.6%)	0.105
Plasma exchange (yes, %)	20 (0.8%)	9 (0.6%)	11 (1.1%)	0.147
Veno-arterial ECMO (yes, %)	23 (0.9%)	20 (1.3%)	3 (0.3%)	0.010*
Veno-venus ECMO (yes, %)	27 (1.1%)	26 (1.7%)	1 (0.1%)	< 0.001*
Intra-aortic balloon pumping (yes, %)	11 (0.4%)	7 (0.5%)	4 (0.4%)	0.845
Mechanical ventilation support (yes, %)	1799 (72.1%)	1184 (78.1%)	615 (62.8%)	< 0.001*
Survival discharge (yes, %)	1668 (66.9%)	1014 (66.9%)	654 (66.8%)	0.965

IQR† median [25%, 75%] for continuous variables, *ICU* intensive care unit, *SOFA score* Sequential Organ Failure Assessment score, *APACHE II score* Acute Physiology and Chronic Health Evaluation II score, *SIRS score* systemic inflammatory response syndrome score, *GNR* gram-negative rods, *GPC* gram-positive coccus, *DIC* disseminated intravascular coagulation, *rhsTM* recombinant human soluble thrombomodulin, *ECMO* extracorporeal membrane oxygenation
*$p < 0.05$

There were 979 patients treated in open ICUs and 1516 patients in closed ICUs. A comparison of the characteristics of these two groups is shown in Table 1. The closed ICU group included fewer patients with renal failure than the open ICU group (closed vs open = 7.5% vs 10.5%, $p = 0.009$), and the closed ICU group included significantly more patients with immunological disorders (closed vs open = 17.4% vs 12.1%, $p < .001$). The APACHE II and SOFA scores (day 1) of patients in the closed ICU group is significantly higher than that in the open ICU (APACHE II score: closed vs open = 23 [18–29] vs 21 [16–28], $p < 0.001$, SOFA score: closed vs open = 9 [7–13] vs 9 [6–12], $p = 0.004$). Patients in the closed ICU group were more severely ill than patients in the open ICU group, based on these scores.

The value of variables examined was different comparing treatments used during follow-up in the closed and open groups. Recombinant human soluble thrombomodulin (rhsTM) is used more frequently in the closed ICU group (closed vs open = 27.7% vs 22.1%, $p = 0.002$), but heparin and warfarin are used more often in the open ICU group (heparin; closed vs open = 16% vs 21%, $p =$ 0.003), (warfarin; closed vs open = 1.0% vs 2.5%, $p =$ 0.004). The use of low-dose steroids in patients with sepsis (closed vs open = 27.2% vs 19.1%, $p < 0.001$) and renal replacement therapy was more frequent in the closed ICU group (closed vs open = 29.8% vs 21.7%, $p < 0.001$), but renal replacement therapy for non-renal indications was more often performed in the open ICU group (closed vs open = 3.8% vs 10.9%, $p < 0.001$). Mechanical ventilation was more frequently used in the closed ICU group (closed vs open = 78.1% vs 62.8%, $p < 0.001$).

In the main analysis, the crude, the unadjusted analysis did not show a significant difference in survival at discharge between the closed and open ICU models (closed vs open = 66.9% vs 66.8%, $p = 0.97$). However, in multiple logistic regression analysis adjusted by baseline, patient characteristics and treatment variables had a significant association between treatment in a closed ICU and survival at discharge (odds ratio = 1.59, 95% CI [1.276–1.827], $p = 0.001$) (Table 2). In sensitivity analysis (702 pairs after propensity score matching), the closed ICU group showed a significantly higher survival rate, compared to the open ICU (71.8% vs 65.2%, odds ratio = 1.41 (95% CI [1.12–1.77]), $p = 0.011$) (Table 3, Additional file 1: Table S1).

In sub-analysis, multiple linear regression analysis using the data about the length of ICU stay and hospital stay as an objective variable showed that the length of ICU stay of patients treated in closed ICUs was significantly shorter (20% less) than patients in open ICUs, but this significance was not seen in the length of hospital stay (Table 4).

Discussion

In this analysis of a large nationwide Japanese cohort of patients with sepsis and septic shock, patient management in a closed ICU is significantly associated with improved rate of survival at discharge and a decrease in the length of ICU stay.

Table 2 Multiple logistic regression analysis adjusted for baseline patient characteristics and treatment ($n = 2495$)

		Coefficient	Adj OR	95% CI			p value
Closed ICU	(Ref: open ICU)	0.463	1.589	1.276	–	1.827	0.001*
Type of ICU	(Ref: in-hospital general ICU)						
In-hospital surgical ICU		– 0.525	0.592	0.286	–	1.223	0.157
Emergency ICU		0.101	1.106	0.9	–	1.36	0.338
Number of beds	(Continuous)	– 0.002	0.998	0.981	–	1.016	0.846
Blood culture	(Ref: no blood culture)						
Positive		– 0.785	0.456	0.279	–	0.746	0.002*
Negative		– 0.407	0.666	0.419	–	1.059	0.086
Infection type	(Ref: unknown infection)						
Viral infection		0.447	1.563	0.48	–	5.085	0.458
GNR infection		0.606	1.833	1.349	–	2.492	< 0.001*
GPC infection		0.224	1.251	0.898	–	1.743	0.185
Fungal infection		– 0.490	0.613	0.284	–	1.321	0.211
Mixed infection		0.015	1.015	0.715	–	1.442	0.933
Other infection		0.656	1.926	0.908	–	4.086	0.088
SOFA score	(Continuous)	– 0.133	0.876	0.845	–	0.908	< 0.001*
APACHE II score	(Continuous)	– 0.018	0.982	0.969	–	0.996	0.010*
SIRS score	(Continuous)	– 0.115	0.892	0.796	–	0.999	0.048*
Sex, female	(Ref: male)	0.373	1.451	1.171	–	1.799	< 0.001*
Age	(Continuous)	– 0.0238	0.976	0.969	–	0.985	< 0.001*
Body weight	(Continuous)	0.0193	1.020	1.011	–	1.028	< 0.001*
White blood cell count (× 103)	(Ref: 3.5~9)						
0~3.5		0.267	1.306	0.741	–	2.302	0.355
9~		– 1.407	0.245	0.019	–	3.107	0.278
Hemoglobin	(Continuous)	0.049	1.05	1.006	–	1.097	0.026*
Platelet count (per 104)	(Continuous)	0.003	1.003	0.991	–	1.015	0.624
PT-INR	(Continuous)	– 0.0614	0.94	0.868	–	1.019	0.135
Co-morbidities	(Ref: no)						
Liver failure		– 0.724	0.485	0.288	–	0.817	0.007*
Respiratory failure		– 0.434	0.648	0.404	–	1.038	0.071
Cardiac failure		– 0.486	0.615	0.403	–	0.938	0.024*
Renal failure		– 0.640	0.527	0.368	–	0.756	< 0.001*
Immunological disorder		– 0.547	0.579	0.43	–	0.779	< 0.001*
Hematologic disorder	(Ref: no)	– 0.355	0.701	0.516	–	0.952	0.023*
Red blood cell transfusion	(Continuous)	– 0.022	0.978	0.956	–	1.001	0.061
Fresh frozen plasma transfusion	(Continuous)	– 0.010	0.99	0.98	–	1.001	0.083
Platelet concentration transfusion	(Continuous)	0.002	1.002	0.996	–	1.008	0.529
Treatment for DIC	(Ref: no)						
Antithrombin III		0.185	1.203	0.938	–	1.544	0.145
rhTM		0.294	1.341	1.043	–	1.725	0.022*
Nafamostat		0.152	1.165	0.869	–	1.561	0.308
Heparin		0.334	1.396	1.06	–	1.839	0.018*
Warfarin		– 0.148	0.862	0.400	–	1.861	0.706
Antiplatelet		0.318	1.374	0.679	–	2.778	0.377

Table 2 Multiple logistic regression analysis adjusted for baseline patient characteristics and treatment ($n = 2495$) *(Continued)*

		Coefficient	Adj OR	95% CI			*p* value
Others		0.303	1.354	0.318	-	5.768	0.682
Specific treatment	(Ref: no)						
Immunoglobulin		0.147	1.158	0.909	-	1.476	0.236
Low-dose steroid		− 0.534	0.586	0.462	-	0.744	< 0.001*
Renal replacement therapy		− 0.390	0.677	0.495	-	0.926	0.015*
Renal replacement therapy not for renal indication		− 0.279	0.756	0.496	-	1.153	0.195
Polymyxin B direct hemoperfusion		0.365	1.44	1.095	-	1.894	0.009*
Plasma exchange		− 0.457	0.633	0.189	-	2.118	0.459
Veno-arterial ECMO		− 2.475	0.084	0.021	-	0.341	< 0.001*
Veno-venus ECMO		− 1.169	0.311	0.111	-	0.865	0.025*
Ventilation support		− 0.815	0.443	0.339		0.578	< 0.001*
Intra-aortic balloon pumping		0.993	2.699	0.467	-	15.608	0.268

White blood cell count (× 103)
adj OR adjusted odds ratio, *CI* confidence intervals, *ICU* intensive care unit, *GNR* gram-negative rods, *GPC* gram-positive coccus, *SOFA score* Sequential Organ Failure Assessment score, *APACHE II score* Acute Physiology and Chronic Health Evaluation II score, *SIRS score* systemic inflammatory response syndrome score, *PT-INR* prothrombin time-international normalized ratio, *DIC* disseminated intravascular coagulation, *rhsTM* recombinant human soluble thrombomodulin, *ECMO* extracorporeal
*$p < 0.05$

Efficacy of the treatment of sepsis in a closed ICU

According to multiple logistic regression analysis adjusted for baseline characteristics and treatment variables, treatment in a closed ICU had a significant association with improved survival at discharge (odds ratio = 1.59, 95% CI [1.276–1.827], $p = 0.001$) (Table 2). This result suggests that the efficacy of care in a closed ICU may depend on the management of sepsis conducted in a closed ICU. However, according to the crude comparison (Table 1), the patient cohorts were different in the closed and open ICUs. We additionally performed propensity score matching analysis as a sensitivity analysis, and the closed ICU group has a significantly higher survival rate, compared to open ICU (Table 3, Additional file 1: Table S1). The result of the main analysis is fully supported by the sensitivity analysis. There is a significant association between treatment in a closed ICU and improved survival at discharge.

A significant difference in the rate of using various treatment modalities in closed and open ICUs is identified in this study (Table 1). Although these treatments are adjuvant therapies for sepsis and their efficacy is controversial, the difference in the rate of using these treatments performed in each ICU may be partly responsible for the observed significant association between treatment in a closed ICU and survival at discharge. The present study demonstrates a significant association between prognosis and each specific treatment for sepsis including use of recombinant human soluble thrombomodulin (rhsTM), low-dose steroid therapy, or PMX-DHP.

Some DIC treatment guidelines recommend the use of rhsTM rather than heparin for patients with DIC due to sepsis [18], and both positive and negative evidence regarding the survival benefit of rhsTM have been reported [19, 20]. The result of a phase 3 trial of rhsTM [21] is awaited. The JSEPTIC DIC study using propensity score analysis reported a survival benefit with the use of rhsTM [12]. The present study, which uses the same data as the JSEPTIC DIC study, also shows a significant association between survival at discharge and rhsTM, using a different statistical analysis, and the use of rhsTM was more frequent in closed ICUs and the use of heparin was more frequent in open ICUs. This

Table 3 Cross table after propensity score matching

	Open ICU	Closed ICU	
Death	244	198	442
Survive	458	504	962
	702	702	1404

$P = 0.011$ (chi-squared test). OR = 1.41 (95% CI 1.12–1.77)
OR odds ratio, *CI* confidence intervals

Table 4 The multiple liner regression analysis for the log-transformed values of the length of ICU stay and hospital stay in survived patients

	Ratio	95% confidence interval		*p* value
Sub-analysis 1: multiple linear regression in survived patients for the length of ICU stay				
(Closed ICU/open ICU) *	0.80	0.75	0.87	< 0.001
Sub-analysis 2: multiple linear regression in survived patients for the length of hospital stay				
(Closed ICU/open ICU) *	0.98	0.90	1.07	0.642

*Adjusted by both patient backgrounds and treatment variables (exactly the same covariates in main analysis)

difference may be partly responsible for the association between improved survival at discharge and treatment in a closed ICU.

The efficacy of steroid therapy to reduce mortality in patients with sepsis has been controversial [22, 23]. In the present study, the use of low-dose steroids (which is more frequent in a closed ICU) was significantly associated with in-hospital mortality, but the route of administration, timing, and presence of side effects were not reviewed. A significant association between the use of PMX-DHP and survival at discharge was also shown, but there was no significant difference of the using rate of PMX-DHP between the closed and open ICUs. Some trials showed a survival benefit with the use of PMX-DHP [24], but others have not [25]. The effect of PMX-DHP remains controversial, and the results of another prospective multicenter randomized controlled trial is awaited, including a phase 3 trial of PMX-DHP [26].

We consider that a significant association between treatment in a closed ICU and survival at discharge can be related to the high-quality care provided in a closed ICU. A high rate of compliance with guidelines is one element of "high quality" intensive care. This element affects the patients' prognosis, and compliance is different in open and closed ICUs. Some reports show that patients with acute respiratory distress syndrome (ARDS) cared for in a closed ICU had lower hospital mortality due to the increased rate of compliance with guideline-recommended lung-protective ventilation [27] (a safety management was given for the patients with ARDS in the closed ICU). Considering the present study, a significantly lower rate of obtaining blood cultures (blood cultures are strongly recommended in the sepsis guideline [5, 6]) in the open ICU (Table 1) suggests that compliance with the guidelines in an open ICU may be lower than that in closed ICUs and the lower compliance may contribute to the higher mortality in open ICUs. Patient with sepsis commonly need ICU care, and in this decade, guidelines for the treatment of sepsis have been published from international societies [5]. The management of patients with sepsis has been qualified and standardized throughout the world, and the closed ICU can provide standardized intensive care for patients with sepsis based on the guidelines, which can improve the outcomes [28].

The safety management, prevention, or rapid and optimal response to complications is an element of "high quality" intensive care. Another report from the Leapfrog Group reported that applying ICU physician safety staffing standards could save more than 54,000 lives in the USA each year [29]. Intensivists can be an expert in safety management and complication management (prevention or appropriate response) in the ICU. Although the present study did *not* investigate the differences in incidence of complications or other safety management issues between closed and open ICUs, this potential difference may contribute to the significant association between treatment in a closed ICU and a higher survival rate at discharge. Future study should be focused on the differences in these factors.

Study limitations

This is a sub-analysis of the JSEPTIC DIC study, which used retrospective data. The 205 patients excluded because of data insufficiency may have an impact on the results although these excluded patients represent less than 10% of the study population. The J-SEPTIC DIC study did not clearly define open and closed ICUs, and each ICU had reported subjective information about their ICU model (open/closed/unclassified). This study comparing the outcomes of patients with sepsis in open and closed ICUs was conducted based on a definition that was subjectively reported from each institution. Although the present study demonstrates the potential of improved efficacy of the treatment of sepsis in a closed ICU, this result may be unreliable because of an unclear definition of the types of ICUs. Further study should clearly define open and closed ICUs to investigate the association between the outcome of patients with sepsis and ICU organization models.

This study focuses only on the association between outcomes and the type of ICU model. Details of differences in ICU treatment and quality of care in each institution have not been analyzed. Although many kinds of ICU staffing components influence ICU outcomes, the information such as hospital characteristics, general/university; the staffing numbers for open or closed ICU's in this study, nursing/junior doctors/fellows/certificated specialist intensivists/non-certificated intensivist; or nighttime coverage by certificated specialist intensivists was not available in this *post hoc* analysis. These staffing patterns must influence the outcomes of patients in the ICU, but this information was unavailable in this study. This is a severe limitation of the present study. Future studies should include staffing information to investigate a relationship between the outcomes of patients with sepsis and treatment using each ICU model (open/closed).

Although many kinds of guidelines or safety management protocols in the ICU such as hand hygiene protocols, ventilation-associated pneumonia bundles, and catheter-related blood stream infection management impact outcomes in the care of patients with sepsis, compliance with these care bundles was not evaluated in this study. Future studies should focus on compliance with sepsis and other care guidelines, treatment differences, and quality of care in the ICU. To further define the benefit of a closed ICU, additional prospective multicenter studies are warranted.

Conclusions

This nationwide retrospective *post hoc* analysis of patients with sepsis in Japan shows a significant association between treatment in a closed ICU and improved survival at discharge, although there are acknowledged study limitations. Future prospective trials are indispensable to evaluate the efficacy of treatment in a closed ICU for the treatment of patients with sepsis. These studies should define the ICU models (closed/open) clearly and focus on staffing patterns, compliance with care guidelines, treatment differences, and quality of care in ICUs with both closed and open ICU models.

Abbreviations

APACHE II score: Acute Physiology and Chronic Health Evaluation II score; ARDS: Acute respiratory distress syndrome; DIC: Disseminated intravascular coagulation; ECMO: Extracorporeal membrane oxygenation; ICU: Intensive care unit; JSEPTIC DIC study: Japan Septic Disseminated Intravascular Coagulation study; PMX-DHP: Polymyxin B direct hemoperfusion; PT-INR: Prothrombin time-international normalized ratio; SOFA score: Sequential Organ Failure Assessment score

Acknowledgements

We wish to express our gratitude to all of the J-Septic DIC study contributors: Mineji Hayakawa, Kazuma Yamakawa, Shinjiro Saito, Shigehiko Uchino, Daisuke Kudo, Yusuke Iizuka, Masamitsu Sanui, Kohei Takimoto, Toshihiko Mayumi, Kota Ono, Takeo Azuhata, Fumihito Ito, Shodai Yoshihiro, Katsura Hayakawa, Tsuyoshi Nakashima, Eiichiro Noda, Ryosuke Sekine, Yoshiaki Yoshikawa, Motohiro Sekino, Keiko Ueno, Yuko Okuda, Masayuki Watanabe, Akihito Tampo, Nobuyuki Saito, Yuya Kitai, Hiroki Takahashi, Iwao Kobayashi, Yutaka Kondo, Wataru Matsunaga, Sho Nachi, Toru Miike, Hiroshi Takahashi, Shuhei Takauji, Kensuke Umakoshi, Takafumi Todaka, Hiroshi Kodaira, Kohkichi Andoh, Takehiko Kasai, Yoshiaki Iwashita, Hideaki Arai, Masato Murata, Masahiro Yamane, Kazuhiro Shiga, and Naoto Hori.

Authors' contributions

TO conceived and designed this study, contributed to acquisition, analysis, and interpretation of the data, and was responsible for the drafting, editing, and submission of the manuscript. YN and DK contributed to interpretation of the data and drafting of the manuscript. SM, KT, and KN played a significant role in the analysis of the data and helped to draft the manuscript. All authors read and approved the final manuscript.

Competing interests

The authors declare that they have no competing interests.

Author details

[1]Department of Emergency Medicine and Critical Care Medicine, Japan Red Cross Maebashi Hospital, Asahi-cho 3-21-36, Maebashi, Gunma 371-0014, Japan. [2]Department of Emergency and Critical Care Medicine, Faculty of Medicine, Fukuoka University, Fukuoka, Japan. [3]Department of Biostatistics, Nagoya University Graduate School of Medicine, Nagoya, Japan.

References

1. Singer M, Deutschman CS, Seymour CW, Shankar-Hari M, Annane D, Bauer M, et al. The third international consensus definitions for sepsis and septic shock (Sepsis-3). JAMA. 2016;315:801–10.
2. Angus DC, Linde-Zwirble WT, Lidicker J, Clermont G, Carcillo J, Pinsky MR. Epidemiology of severe sepsis in the United States: analysis of incidence, outcome, and associated costs of care. Crit Care Med. 2001;29:1303–10.
3. Lagu T, Rothberg MB, Shieh MS, Pe-kow PS, Steingrub JS, Lindenauer PK. Hospitalizations, costs, and outcomes of severe sepsis in the United States 2003 to 2007. Crit Care Med. 2012;40:754–61.
4. Kumar G, Kumar N, Taneja A, Kaleekal T, Tarima S, McGinley E, et al. Nationwide trends of severe sepsis in the 21st century (2000-2007). Chest. 2011;140:1223–31.
5. Rhodes A, Evans LE, Alhazzani W, Levy MM, Antonelli M, Ferrer R, et al. Surviving sepsis campaign: international guidelines for management of sepsis and septic shock: 2016. Crit Care Med. 2017;45:486–552.
6. Oda S, Aibiki M, Ikeda T, Imaizumi H, Endo S, Ochiai R, Sepsis Registry Committee of The Japanese Society of Intensive Care Medicine, et al. The Japanese guidelines for the management of sepsis. J Intensive Care. 2014;2:55.
7. Vincent JL. Need for intensivists in intensive-care units. Lancet. 2000;356:695–6.
8. Pronovost PJ, Angus DC, Dorman T, Robinson KA, Dremsizov TT, Young TL. Physician staffing patterns and clinical outcomes in critically ill patients: a systematic review. JAMA. 2002;288:2151–62.
9. Wallace DJ, Angus DC, Barnato AM, Kramer AA, Khan JM. Nighttime intensivist staffing and mortality among critically ill patients. N Engl J Med. 2012;366:2093–101.
10. Wilcox ME, Chong CA, Niven DJ, Rubenfeld GD, Rowan KM, Wunsch H, et al. Do intensivist staffing patterns influence hospital mortality following ICU admission? A systematic review and meta-analyses. Crit Care Med. 2013;41:2253–74.
11. Carson SS, Stocking C, Podsadecki T, Christenson J, Pohlman A, MacRae S, et al. Effects of organizational change in the medical intensive care unit of a teaching hospital: a comparison of 'open' and 'closed' formats. JAMA. 1996;276:322–8.
12. Hayakawa M, Yamakawa K, Saito S, Uchino S, Kudo D, Iizuka Y, Japan Septic Disseminated Intravascular Coagulation (JSEPTIC DIC) study group, et al. Recombinant human soluble thrombomodulin and mortality in sepsis-induced disseminated intravascular coagulation. A multicentre retrospective study. Thromb Haemost. 2016;115:1157–66.
13. Levy MM, Fink MP, Marshall JC, Abraham E, Angus D, Cook D, et al. SCCM/ESICM/ACCP/ATS/SIS. 2001 SCCM/ESICM/ACCP/ATS/SIS international sepsis definitions conference. Crit Care Med. 2003;31:1250–6.
14. Ono Y, Tanigawa K, Shinohara K, Yano T, Sorimachi K, Sato L, et al. Difficult airway management resources and capnography use in Japanese intensive care units: a nationwide cross-sectional study. J Anesth. 2016;30:644–52.
15. Knaus WA, Draper EA, Wagner DP, Zimmerman JE. APACHE II: a severity of disease classification system. Crit Care Med. 1985;13:818–29.
16. Vincent JL, de Mendonça A, Cantraine F, Moreno R, Takala J, Suter PM, et al. Use of the SOFA score to assess the incidence of organ dysfunction/failure in intensive care units: results of a multicenter, prospective study. Working group on "sepsis-related problems" of the European Society of Intensive Care Medicine. Crit Care Med 1998;26:1793–1800.
17. Bone RC, Balk RA, Cerra FB, Dellinger RP, Fein AM, Knaus WA, et al. Definitions for sepsis and organ failure and guidelines for the use of innovative therapies in sepsis. The ACCP/SCCM Consensus Conference Committee. American College of Chest Physicians/Society of Critical Care Medicine. Chest. 1992;101:1644–55.
18. Wada H, Thachil J, Di Nisio M, Mathew P, Kurosawa S, Gando S, et al. Guidance for diagnosis and treatment of DIC from harmonization of the recommendations from three guidelines. J Thromb Haemost. 2013; https://doi.org/10.1111/jth.12155. [Epub ahead of print]
19. Yamakawa K, Ogura H, Fujimi S, Morikawa M, Ogawa Y, Mohri T, et al. Recombinant human soluble thrombomodulin in sepsis-induced disseminated intravascular coagulation: a multicenter propensity score analysis. Intensive Care Med. 2013;39:644–52.
20. Tagami T, Matsui H, Horiguchi H, Fushimi K, Yasunaga H. Recombinant human soluble thrombomodulin and mortality in severe pneumonia patients with sepsis-associated disseminated intravascular coagulation: an observational nationwide study. J Thromb Haemost. 2015;13:31–40.
21. Phase 3 safety and efficacy study of ART-123 in subjects with severe sepsis and coagulopathy. http://clinicaltrials.gov/ct2/show/NCT01598831?term=ART-123&rank=2 of subordinate document. Accessed 1st July 2015.

22. Sprung CL, Annane D, Keh D, Moreno R, Singer M, Freivogel K, et al: CORTICUS Study Group. Hydrocortisone therapy for patients with septic shock. N Engl J Med 2008;358:111–124.
23. Moran JL, Graham PL, Rockliff S, Bersten AD. Updating the evidence for the role of corticosteroids in severe sepsis and septic shock: a Bayesian meta-analytic perspective. Crit Care. 2010;14:R134.
24. Cruz DN, Antonelli M, Fumagalli R, Foltran F, Brienza N, Donati A, et al. Early use of polymyxin B hemoperfusion in abdominal septic shock: the EUPHAS randomized controlled trial. JAMA. 2009;301:2445–52.
25. Payen DM, Guilhot J, Launey Y, Lukaszewicz AC, Kaaki M, Veber B, ABDOMIX group, et al. Early use of polymyxin B hemoperfusion in patients with septic shock due to peritonitis: a multicenter randomized control trial. Intensive Care Med. 2015;41:975–84.
26. Klein DJ, Foster D, Schorr CA, Kazempour K, Walker PM, Dellinger RP. The EUPHRATES trial (Evaluating the Use of Polymyxin B Hemoperfusion in a Randomized controlled trial of Adults Treated for Endotoxemia and Septic shock): study protocol for a randomized controlled trial. Trials. 2014;15:218.
27. Treggiari MM, Martin DP, Yanez ND, Caldwell E, Hudson LD, Rubenfeld GD. Effect of intensive care unit organizational model and structure on outcomes in patients with acute lung injury. Am J Respir Crit Care Med. 2007;176:685–90.
28. Levy MM, Rhodes A, Phillips GS, Townsend SR, Schorr CA, Beale R, et al. Surviving Sepsis Campaign: association between performance metrics and outcomes in a 7.5-year study. Intensive Care Med. 2014;40:1623–33.
29. LEAPFROG PATIENT SAFETY STANDARDS. The Potential Benefits of Universal Adoption. 2000. http://www.safetyleaders.org/SafePracticeArticles/leapfrog_patient_safety_standards.pdf. Accessed 1st Apr 2018.

Cefepime dosing regimens in critically ill patients receiving continuous renal replacement therapy: a Monte Carlo simulation study

Weerachai Chaijamorn[1*], Taniya Charoensareerat[1], Nattachai Srisawat[2], Sutthiporn Pattharachayakul[3] and Apinya Boonpeng[4]

Abstract

Background: Cefepime can be removed by continuous renal replacement therapy (CRRT) due to its pharmacokinetics. The purpose of this study is to define the optimal cefepime dosing regimens for critically ill patients receiving CRRT using Monte Carlo simulations (MCS).

Methods: The CRRT models of cefepime disposition during 48 h with different effluent rates were developed using published pharmacokinetic parameters, patient demographic data, and CRRT settings. Pharmacodynamic target was the cumulative percentage of a 48-h period of at least 70% that free cefepime concentration exceeds the four times susceptible breakpoint of *Pseudomonas aeruginosa* (minimum inhibitory concentration, MIC of 8). All recommended dosing regimens from available clinical resources were evaluated for the probability of target attainment (PTA) using MCS to generate drug disposition in a group of 5000 virtual patients for each dose. The optimal doses were defined as achieving the PTA at least 90% of virtual patients with lowest daily doses and the acceptable risk of neurotoxicity.

Results: Optimal cefepime doses in critically ill patients receiving CRRT with Kidney Disease: Improving Global Outcomes (KDIGO) recommended effluent rates were a regimen of 2 g loading dose followed by 1.5–1.75 g every 8 h for Gram-negative infections with a neurotoxicity risk of < 17%. Cefepime dosing regimens from this study were considerably higher than the recommended doses from clinical resources.

Conclusion: All recommended dosing regimens for patients receiving CRRT from available clinical resources failed to achieve the PTA target. The optimal dosing regimens were suggested based on CRRT modalities, MIC values, and different effluent rates. Clinical validation is warranted.

Keywords: Cefepime, Dosing, Pharmacokinetics, Pharmacodynamics, Continuous renal replacement therapy, Critically ill patients

Background

Continuous renal replacement therapy (CRRT) is generally performed in hemodynamic unstable patients with acute kidney injury (AKI) [1]. Cefepime is an antimicrobial agent that is commonly used in critically ill patients. The low protein binding affinity (16–20%) and small volume of distribution (14–20 L) make cefepime susceptible to be removed by CRRT [2–4].

Pharmacokinetic changes in critically ill patients, such as increasing of volume of distribution and hypoalbuminemia, considerably reduce hydrophilic antimicrobial agent concentrations [5]. Consequently, we might have prescribed inadequate doses of antimicrobial agents in patients with CRRT [5] and unintentionally increase the morbidity and mortality associated with sepsis [6]. The primary aim of drug dosing in this population is to use the loading dose (LD) and adequate maintenance doses

* Correspondence: weerachai.cha@siam.edu
[1]Faculty of Pharmacy, Siam University, 38 Petkasem Road, Bangwa, Pasicharoen, Bangkok 10160, Thailand
Full list of author information is available at the end of the article

to attain pharmacokinetic and pharmacodynamic targets for maximizing antibacterial killing effect and therapeutic outcome [7].

Cefepime dosing recommendations in critically ill patients are based on previously published pharmacokinetic studies [2, 5, 8, 9]. Interestingly, Li and colleagues gathered and analyzed 64 published pharmacokinetic studies in patients receiving CRRT. They revealed that those studies did not completely report key pharmacokinetic parameters to calculate extracorporeal clearance and design drug dosing in patient with CRRT such as type of CRRT modalities, effluent rate, blood flow rate, and extraction coefficient [10]. Some studies used old CRRT techniques or hemofilters and low effluent rates [10]. Neurotoxicity from high cefepime concentrations in patients with reduced renal function has been reported [11–15].

Our study aimed to use the Monte Carlo simulation (MCS) technique to define the proper dosing of cefepime in AKI patients who require CRRT support.

Methods

Mathematical pharmacokinetic models

A literature search was performed using the following medical subject heading (MeSH) terms: (1) 'cefepime', (2) 'continuous renal replacement therapy' or 'continuous venovenous hemofiltration' or 'continuous venovenous hemodialysis', and (3) 'pharmacokinetics' and synonymous words in PubMed. EMBASE and EBSCO were searched with slightly different search terms due to differences of each database. All publications that entered the databases by 31 December 1990 were included. Two investigators (WC and TC) independently identified and evaluated studies for potential inclusion. We restricted our search to articles conducted in adult human subjects and critically ill subjects receiving CRRT. All publications focused on drug pharmacokinetics were gathered. We included only publications that reported all necessary pharmacokinetic parameters for calculation of cefepime dosing regimens. Any disagreement on inclusion was resolved by discussion between the two reviewers. We identified 50 publications, of which 6 were considered relevant and were evaluated [8, 9, 16–19]. All previously published pharmacokinetic studies of cefepime reported only basic pharmacokinetic parameters such as volume of distribution, total drug clearance, non-renal clearance, extraction coefficient, and elimination rate constant [8, 9, 16–19]. In addition, Carlier and colleagues revealed that a one-compartment pharmacokinetic model best fits to describe cefepime characteristics [19]. Consequently, a one-compartment mathematical pharmacokinetic model with first-order elimination of acute kidney disease patients receiving CRRT was developed to predict cefepime disposition in 48 h of the initial therapy. Assuming the patients were anuric, renal clearance applied in the model was 0 mL/min. Previously published cefepime pharmacokinetic parameters in critically ill patients [8, 9, 16–19] and related variability from critically ill patients receiving CRRT were gathered to create models of virtual patients with three modalities. Two thirds of patients in previously published studies were diagnosed as sepsis and septic shock and needed CRRT treatment. Different CRRT settings affect drug dosing [20], and no specific technique of CRRT modality for AKI management is recommended [1]. The commonly used modalities consisted of continuous venovenous hemofiltration (CVVH) with pre-hemofilter dilution techniques, in which replacement fluid is added in blood before going through hemofilter and continuous venovenous hemodialysis (CVVHD) [20]. To construct realistic virtual patients, we added population-specific correlation (r^2) between patient's body weight, non-renal clearance, and volume of distribution into the models. The lower limit of body weight was set at 40 kg assuming that the virtual patients are adult. In addition, body weights used in the models of virtual patients were obtained from an international database of the International Society of Nephrology (ISN)-funded prospective multicenter observational ongoing study of AKI epidemiology in Southeast Asia entitled The Epidemiology and Prognostic Factors for Mortality in Intensive Care Unit Patients with Acute Kidney Injury in Southeast Asia (SEA-AKI) [21]. It enrolled 6644 critically ill patients from Thailand, Laos, and the Philippines. All described pharmacokinetic parameters are defined in Table 1.

Transmembrane drug clearance was calculated as multiplying effluent flow rate, dialysate (Q_d) and/or ultrafiltrate (Q_{uf}) flow rate, by extraction coefficient that are sieving coefficient (SC) for hemofiltration and saturation coefficient (SA) for hemodialysis [20]. Total drug clearance was calculated from the summation of non-renal clearance and CRRT clearance. To calculate drug concentration profile in 48 h of initial therapy for evaluation of the probability of target attainment (PTA), elimination rate constant (k) was determined by total

Table 1 Parameters used in these models of virtual AKI patients receiving CRRT [14–18]

Pharmacokinetic parameters Mean ± SD (range limits)		
	Hemofiltration (HF)	Hemodialysis (HD)
Weight (kg)	60.72 ± 14.5 (40–230)	
V_d (L/kg)	0.5 ± 0.23 (0.21–1.11)	
CL_{NR} (mL/min)	24.33 ± 11.25 (13–44)	
Free fraction	0.79 ± 0.09 (0.72–0.85)	
SC or SA	0.79 ± 0.15 (0.47–0.92)	0.77 ± 0.09 (0.65–0.97)

drug clearance divided by volume of distribution. The k value was required to calculate drug concentration at a time. Blood flow rate (Q_{blood}) for all settings was prescribed as 200 mL/min. The equations used in the models were defined as follows [20]:

CL_{HD} $(L/h) = SA \times Q_d$

$CL_{HF(pre)}$ $(L/h) = SC \times Q_{uf} \times [Q_{plasma}/(Q_{plasma} + Q_{replacement})]$

$k = (CL_{NR} + CL_{HD})/V_d$

$k = (CL_{NR} + CL_{HF})/V_d$

where CL_{HF} is the transmembrane clearance in hemofiltration, Q_{plasma} is the plasma flow rate ($Q_{plasma} = Q_{blood} \times (1 - \text{hematocrit})$), hematocrit is 30%, $Q_{replacement}$ is the replacement fluid flow rate ($Q_{replacement} = Q_{uf}$), CL_{HD} is the transmembrane clearance in hemodialysis, Q_d is the dialysate flow rate, k is the elimination rate constant, CL_{NR} is the non-renal clearance, and V_d is the volume of distribution.

Effluent rates were prescribed as Kidney Disease: Improving Global Outcomes (KDIGO) recommendation of 20–25 mL/kg/h [1]. A higher effluent rate of 35 mL/kg/h was included in the models to reflect an average common effluent rate used in real-life practice or when high-volume CRRT is needed [22]. Moreover, lower effluent rates of 10–15 mL/kg/h were performed to aid cefepime dosing when low-volume CRRT was prescribed in some situations.

Cefepime dosing recommendations

Cefepime dosing regimens from available drug dosing recommendations were evaluated in the models. The dosing regimens varied from 1 to 2 g every 12 h to 2 g loading dose followed by 1 g every 8 h or 2 g every 12 h [23–25].

Monte Carlo simulation and probability of target attainment

Following a previously published method [26, 27], Monte Carlo simulation (Crystal Ball Classroom edition, Oracle) generates drug concentration-time profiles of a group of 5000 virtual patients for each dose to evaluate the PTA. PTA was predicted using pharmacodynamic target of the cumulative percentage of a 48-h period that free cefepime concentration exceeds the minimum inhibitory concentration (MIC) of *Pseudomonas aeruginosa* [28]. Given that microbiological success (eradication or presumed eradication) was significantly associated with the proportion of the dosing interval in which cefepime concentration exceeded four times MIC [29] and the cumulative percentage of free cefepime concentration needed to exceed the MIC, 70% coverage is required to achieve the maximal bactericidal effect [17, 18, 30]. In this study, at least 70% of the cumulative percentage of a 48-h period with four times MIC (70% $fT_{>4MIC}$) and susceptible breakpoint recommended by the Clinical Laboratory Standards Institute (CLSI) [31] for *P. aeruginosa* (8 mg/L) were applied in the models for the first 48 h of initial cefepime therapy. Owing to the differences of the MIC in various health care settings, we also used the MICs of 1, 2, and 4 mg/L in the models to define the optimal dosing regimens for each MIC in the study. The optimal doses were defined as achieving the PTA target of at least 90% of 5000 virtual patients with the lowest daily dose to emphasize cefepime efficacy and consider the risk of toxicity especially neurotoxicity as described below. Different cefepime dosing regimens including recommendations for critically ill patients were evaluated to define the optimal doses.

Cefepime neurotoxicity

Neurotoxicity of cefepime, defined as confusion, hallucination, convulsion, seizure, and encephalopathy, has been noted in various studies. Most studies in patients with reduced renal function reported cefepime trough concentrations associated with neurotoxicity as an average of 76 (9–224) mg/L [11–15]. We used the concentration of 70 mg/L to be a threshold for expected neurotoxicity that could occur from cefepime in AKI patients receiving CRRT. All cefepime dosing regimens were evaluated for the possibility to develop neurotoxicity at 48-h trough concentration. The optimal doses were required to achieve a previously described target and had the lowest risk of occurring ≥ 70 mg/L of cefepime concentrations in drug concentration-time profiles of 5000 virtual patients for each regimen.

Results

Characteristics of selected virtual patients who achieve the pharmacodynamic target with the optimal dosing regimens as described in the "Methods" section were compared with input parameters from previously published studies and are shown in Table 2.

Table 3 summarizes the PTA results of selected cefepime dosing regimens for treating *P. aeruginosa* using MICs of 1, 2, 4, and 8 on the first 48 h of therapy. The probability of developing neurotoxicity of each regimen of two CRRT modalities and five different effluent rates was presented in Table 4. Applying the aggressive target as CLSI recommended MIC breakpoint of 8 mg/L into the models, all recommended dosing regimens from clinical resources could not attain the targets with two different modalities. Considering efficacy from the PTA target and the probability of developing neurotoxicity, the regimen of 2 g loading dose followed by 1.5–1.75 g every 8 h achieved the aforementioned targets of > 90% for all CRRT settings with KDIGO recommended effluent rates in a range of 20–25 mL/kg/h (Table 5). In addition, the probability of neurotoxicity occurred when cefepime concentrations > 70 mg/L at 48 h was approximately 0.06–17% (Table 4). The PTA of cefepime

Table 2 Virtual patient characteristics compared with input pharmacokinetic parameters from published cefepime studies

Pharmacokinetic parameters	Literature-based values (mean ± SD (range limits)) ($N = 37$)	Simulation-based values (mean ± SD (range limits)) ($N = 5000$)
Weight (kg)	60.72 ± 14.5 (40–230)	61.88 ± 13.77 (40.01–142.22)
V_d (L/kg)	0.5 ± 0.23 (0.21–1.11)	0.49 ± 0.19 (0.21–1.11)
CL_{NR} (mL/min)	24.33 ± 11.25 (13–44)	24.21 ± 7.63 (13.00–43.99)
Free fraction	0.79 ± 0.09 (0.72–0.85)	0.78 ± 0.04 (0.72–0.85)
SC	0.79 ± 0.15 (0.47–0.92)	0.74 ± 0.10 (0.47–0.92)
SA	0.77 ± 0.09 (0.65–0.97)	0.78 ± 0.07 (0.65–0.97)

regimens according to various MICs, effluent rates, and CRRT modalities is presented in Table 3. The recommendations of cefepime regimens for critically ill patients receiving three different CRRT modalities, effluent rates, and various MICs are shown in Table 5.

If greater effluent rates such as 35 mL/kg/h are required, the cefepime dosing regimen for *P. aeruginosa* infection (MIC of 8 mg/L) using the aggressive pharmacodynamic target was 2 g LD followed by 1.75–2 g every 8 h with a higher risk of cefepime-induced neurotoxicity (≤ 33%) (Tables 4 and 5). When CRRT with lower effluent rates of 10–15 mL/kg/h was prescribed, the cefepime dosing regimen of 1.75 g loading dose followed by 1.5 g every 8 h was needed to achieve the aggressive target for *P. aeruginosa* infection (MIC of 8 mg/L) (Table 4). Figure 1 illustrates the PTA at 70% $fT_{>4MIC}$ (MIC of 8 mg/L) for selected cefepime dosing regimens of CVVHD with an effluent rate of 25 mL/kg/h.

Discussion

This is the first simulation study applying MCS technique to evaluate cefepime dosing regimens for management of *P. aeruginosa* infection in critically ill patients. Pharmacokinetic parameters collected from previously published studies [8, 9, 16–19], body weights as described in the "Methods" section, and CRRT settings with five different effluent rates (10, 15, 20, 25, and 35 mL/kg/h) [1, 22] were incorporated into the models to predict cefepime disposition in critically ill patients receiving CRRT for 48 h. Moreover, correlations between used pharmacokinetic parameters were applied in the models to create population-specific virtual patients. As shown in Table 2, this study showed that MCS technique created virtual patient pharmacokinetics that were similar to which parameters gathered from previous studies. This technique therefore could be an effective tool to build realistic patients and guide drug dosing regimens in various groups of patients, especially this population.

The pharmacodynamic target of 70% $fT_{>4MIC}$ was associated with maximum bactericidal effects [17, 18, 30]. Given the results from Tam and colleagues, bactericidal activity of cefepime is optimized at concentrations approximately four times MIC [29]. We decided to apply aggressive target as 70% $fT_{>4MIC}$ in the models as aforementioned in the "Methods" section. However, using the aggressive target could lead to excessive drug dosages with the risk of cefepime-induced neurotoxicity. Clinical monitoring of cefepime adverse reactions should be concerned.

This study revealed that the regimen of 2 g loading dose followed by 1.5–1.75 g every 8 h achieved the PTA target for *P. aeruginosa* (MIC of 8 mg/L) with two different modalities in ≥ 90% of virtual patients receiving CRRT with KDIGO recommended effluent rate of 20–25 mL/kg/h. The expected neurotoxicity risk occurred with the suggested regimen from our simulations were in a range of 0.06–17% according to the effluent rates and CRRT modalities (Table 4). Clinical monitoring of cefepime-induced neurotoxicity is needed when the recommended cefepime dosing regimen is prescribed. Notably, no clinical recommended regimens exceeded the PTA target of *P. aeruginosa*. It was aligned with the results from Seyler et al. that they used the pharmacodynamic target of 70% $fT_{>4MIC}$ (8 mg/L) which was 32 mg/L as we applied in this study for *P. aeruginosa*. They revealed that the recommended doses of cefepime could not achieve the target for critically ill patients with CRRT for the first 48 h (0% PTA) [18]. Moreover, dosing regimens for *P. aeruginosa* infection were different depending on MICs used in the simulations (Table 5). It explained that cefepime dosing regimens were associated with local MIC values in each setting.

The pharmacokinetic changes of hydrophilic drugs in critically ill patients such as increased volume of distribution due to fluid accumulation, decreased protein binding and metabolism can cause lower drug concentrations especially when conventional dosing regimens were used [5]. The cefepime volume of distribution gathered from critically ill patients and used in this study was approximately 30 L (0.5 ± 0.23 L/kg). The value was larger than that reported in normal population (4–20 L) [2–4]. As volume of distribution is taken into account in a mathematical equation of drug clearance as $CL = k \times V_d$, it affects drug clearance and the probability of target attainment

Table 3 PTAs of all recommended cefepime dosing regimens for Gram-negative infections in two CRRT modalities with different effluent rates and various MICs

Cefepime dosing regimen	Pre-dilution CVVH					CVVHD				
	Effluent rates (mL/kg/h)	PTA (%)				Effluent rates (mL/kg/h)	PTA (%)			
		MIC (mg/L)					MIC (mg/L)			
		1	2	4	8		1	2	4	8
250 mg Q8H	10	98.62	53.10	0.22	0.00	10	98.64	49.90	0.04	0.00
	15	98.50	43.78	0.02	0.00	15	98.46	40.86	0.00	0.00
	20	98.02	36.10	0.00	0.00	20	97.68	29.3	0.00	0.00
	25	98.12	27.06	0.00	0.00	25	96.52	16.58	0.00	0.00
	35	96.42	13.72	0.00	0.00	35	91.62	3.52	0.00	0.00
750 mg LD then 500 mg Q12H	10	100	95.24	20.88	0.00	10	99.98	94.42	17.96	0.00
	15	100	91.44	11.00	0.00	15	99.98	89.06	8.12	0.00
	20	99.96	86.86	5.12	0.00	20	99.88	80.80	1.54	0.00
	25	99.80	81.28	1.64	0.00	25	99.52	71.46	0.14	0.00
	35	99.38	66.48	0.10	0.00	35	98.72	42.06	0.00	0.00
1 g LD then 500 mg Q12H	10	100	98.42	38.36	0.00	10	100	98.02	33.30	0.00
	15	99.96	96.88	25.34	0.00	15	99.98	95.60	18.52	0.00
	20	99.96	94.00	14.22	0.00	20	99.86	90.26	7.24	0.00
	25	99.90	90.24	6.86	0.00	25	99.84	83.04	1.96	0.00
	35	99.74	80.30	1.00	0.00	35	99.08	58.44	0.04	0.00
750 mg Q12H	10	100	99.30	51.16	0.06	10	100	99.18	47.34	0.00
	15	100	98.70	38.72	0.00	15	100	98.36	33.6	0.00
	20	100	97.98	29.42	0.00	20	100	96.66	20.50	0.00
	25	99.98	96.78	18.30	0.00	25	99.94	93.58	8.90	0.00
	35	99.86	91.54	6.72	0.00	35	99.76	80.52	0.98	0.00
1 g Q12H	10	100	99.96	83.58	6.30	10	100	100	82.72	5.52
	15	100	99.92	76.62	2.42	15	100	99.86	72.94	1.12
	20	100	99.82	68.78	0.62	20	100	99.52	61.14	0.06
	25	100	99.52	61.18	0.10	25	100	99.00	47.26	0.00
	35	99.98	98.78	42.26	0.00	35	99.94	96.74	19.50	0.00
750 mg Q8H	10	100	99.98	92.48	19.38	10	100	99.98	92.08	16.34
	15	100	99.98	90.78	12.92	15	100	100	87.92	8.86
	20	100	99.94	86.92	6.56	20	100	99.96	83.70	3.14
	25	100	99.98	83.92	0.26	25	100	99.96	77.50	0.56

Table 3 PTAs of all recommended cefepime dosing regimens for Gram-negative infections in two CRRT modalities with different effluent rates and various MICs *(Continued)*

Cefepime dosing regimen	Pre-dilution CVVH					CVVHD				
	Effluent rates (mL/kg/h)	PTA (%) MIC (mg/L)				Effluent rates (mL/kg/h)	PTA (%) MIC (mg/L)			
		1	2	4	8		1	2	4	8
	35	100	99.98	73.96	0.52	35	100	99.88	54.20	0.00
1 g LD then 750 mg Q8H	10	100	100	96.12	28.10	10	100	100	95.98	26.90
	15	100	100	94.92	18.86	15	100	100	94.26	14.62
	20	100	100	93.08	11.82	20	100	99.98	91.14	7.50
	25	100	100	90.62	7.00	25	100	100	84.68	1.98
	35	100	99.98	82.84	1.30	35	100	99.92	66.64	0.02
1 g Q8H	10	100	100	98.58	54.02	10	100	100	98.60	51.60
	15	100	100	98.20	45.68	15	100	100	98.14	40.96
	20	100	100	97.96	35.56	20	100	100	97.54	29.68
	25	100	100	97.96	29.46	25	100	100	96.50	18.22
	35	100	100	96.56	13.88	35	100	100	91.62	3.58
1.75 g then 1.5 g Q 8 H	10	100	100	100	94.38	10	100	100	100	94.28
	15	100	100	100	92.44	15	100	100	99.98	91.72
	20	100	100	100	90.04	20	100	100	99.98	88.04
	25	100	100	99.96	87.46	25	100	100	99.92	79.64
	35	100	100	99.96	78.62	35	100	100	99.98	61.84
2 g LD then 1.5 g Q8H	10	100	100	100	96.04	10	100	100	100	95.3
	15	100	100	100	95.24	15	100	100	100	94.36
	20	100	100	99.98	93.26	20	100	100	99.98	90.66
	25	100	100	100	90.50	25	100	100	99.98	84.60
	35	100	100	100	82.96	35	100	100	99.96	66.70
1.75 g Q8H	10	100	100	100	96.94	10	100	100	100	96.22
	15	100	100	100	96.34	15	100	100	100	95.70
	20	100	100	100	95.42	20	100	100	100	94.64
	25	100	100	100	94.58	25	100	100	100	92.00
	35	100	100	100	89.48	35	100	100	99.98	77.76
2 g LD then 1.75 g Q8H	10	100	100	100	97.80	10	100	100	100	97.44
	15	100	100	100	97.36	15	100	100	99.98	96.60
	20	100	100	100	96.70	20	100	100	100	95.46

Table 3 PTAs of all recommended cefepime dosing regimens for Gram-negative infections in two CRRT modalities with different effluent rates and various MICs *(Continued)*

Cefepime dosing regimen	Pre-dilution CVVH					CVVHD				
	Effluent rates (mL/kg/h)	PTA (%) MIC (mg/L)				Effluent rates (mL/kg/h)	PTA (%) MIC (mg/L)			
		1	2	4	8		1	2	4	8
	25	100	100	99.98	95.90	25	100	100	100	93.20
	35	100	100	100	92.52	35	100	100	99.98	82.22
2 g Q8H	10	100	100	100	98.60	10	100	100	100	98.36
	15	100	100	100	98.32	15	100	100	100	98.18
	20	100	100	100	98.44	20	100	100	100	97.54
	25	100	100	100	98.00	25	100	100	100	97.02
	35	100	100	100	96.66	35	100	100	100	91.24

PTA probability of target attainment, *CVVH* continuous venovenous hemofiltration, *CVVHD* continuous venovenous hemodialysis, *LD* loading dose

Table 4 The probability of developing neurotoxicity from selected cefepime dosing regimens

Cefepime dosing regimens	Pre-dilution CVVH		CVVHD	
	Effluent rate (mL/kg/h)	48-h trough probability ≥ 70 mg/L (%)	Effluent rate (mL/kg/h)	48-h trough probability ≥ 70 mg/L (%)
1 g Q8H	10	0.18	10	0.04
	15	0.00	15	0.00
	20	0.00	20	0.00
	25	0.00	25	0.00
	35	0.00	35	0.00
1.75 g LD then 1.5 g Q8H	10	26.28	10	22.30
	15	11.54	15	7.02
	20	4.46	20	1.44
	25	1.26	25	0.08
	35	0.14	35	0.00
2 g LD then 1.5 g Q8H	10	26.04	10	21.7
	15	13.36	15	7.40
	20	5.12	20	0.98
	25	1.50	25	0.06
	35	0.08	35	0.00
1.75 g Q8H	10	45.44	10	41.30
	15	29.14	15	22.24
	20	16.84	20	7.82
	25	7.96	25	1.94
	35	1.22	35	0.04
2 g LD then 1.75 g Q8H	10	45.12	10	42.10
	15	32.46	15	22.30
	20	17.16	20	7.78
	25	8.04	25	1.76
	35	1.38	35	0.04
2 g Q8H	10	61.04	10	58.10
	15	47.86	15	40.52
	20	33.48	20	20.84
	25	20.90	25	8.98
	35	6.52	35	0.26

CVVH continuous venovenous hemofiltration, *CVVHD* continuous venovenous hemodialysis, *LD* loading dose

when volume of distribution increases. Given that AKI patients may have well-preserved non-renal drug clearance [32], an average non-renal clearance gathered from previously published studies (24.33 ± 11.25 mL/min) was similar to the values reported from healthy volunteers and patients with renal insufficiency in a range of 10–30 mL/min [3, 4, 33]. Additionally, hypoalbuminemia occurred in ICU patients was reported in a range of 40–50% [34] and could increase free drug concentrations that would be removed by CRRT, the liver, and the kidney. Given these reasons described earlier, the loading dose concept is very crucial to attain the PTA target in these situations.

An effluent rate contributes to extracorporeal clearance defined by the described equation. Higher effluent rate requires a higher dose to compete the PTA target in the population. When CRRT setting was prescribed with an effluent rate of 35 mL/kg/h, cefepime doses would be 2 g LD followed by 1.75–2 g every 8 h for *P. aeruginosa* (MIC of 8 mg/L) to achieve the PTA target. Undoubtedly, if the lower effluent rates of 10–15 mL/kg/h were utilized, the lower cefepime loading dose of 1.75 g was suggested with same maintenance doses as compared with using KDIGO-recommended effluent rates of 20–25 mL/kg/h (Table 5).

Table 5 Recommendations of cefepime dosing regimens for treating *P. aeruginosa* infections with various MICs in critically ill patients receiving CRRT

Actual MIC (mg/L)	Target MIC* (mg/L)	Effluent rates (mL/kg/h)	CVVH (pre-hemofilter dilution)	CVVHD
1	4	10–15	250 mg Q8H	250 mg Q8H
		20–25	250 mg Q8H	250 mg Q8H
		35	250 mg Q8H	250 mg Q8H
2	8	10–15	750 mg LD then 500 mg Q12H	1 g LD then 500 mg Q12H
		20–25	1 g LD then 500 mg Q12H	750 mg Q12H
		35	750 mg Q12H	1 g Q12H
4	16	10–15	750 mg Q8H	1 g LD then 750 mg Q8H
		20–25	1 g LD then 750 mg Q8H	1 g Q8H
		35	1 g Q8H	1 g Q8H
8	32	10–15	1.75 g LD then 1.5 g Q8H	1.75 g LD then 1.5 g Q8H
		20–25	2 g LD then 1.5 g Q8H	1.75 g Q8H
		35	2 g LD then 1.75 g Q8H	2 g Q8H

CVVH continuous venovenous hemofiltration, *CVVHD* continuous venovenous hemodialysis, *LD* loading dose
*Pharmacodynamic target defined as at least 70% of the cumulative percentage of a 48-h period with four times MIC (70% $fT_{>4MIC}$)

Some drugs can be removed by membrane interaction known as the adsorption phenomenon. Although the clinical significance has not been evaluated, CRRT hemofilter types do not significantly affect extracorporeal drug clearance and selection of drug dosing regimen due to early saturation of this phenomenon [20].

Owing to the assumption of MCS that generates only adult patients using pharmacokinetic parameters from previously published studies and ICU patient's body weights, those recommendations of cefepime should be applied for only patients who match our assumption such as anuric patients, same effluent flow rates. Another limitation of our study is the MIC breakpoint from

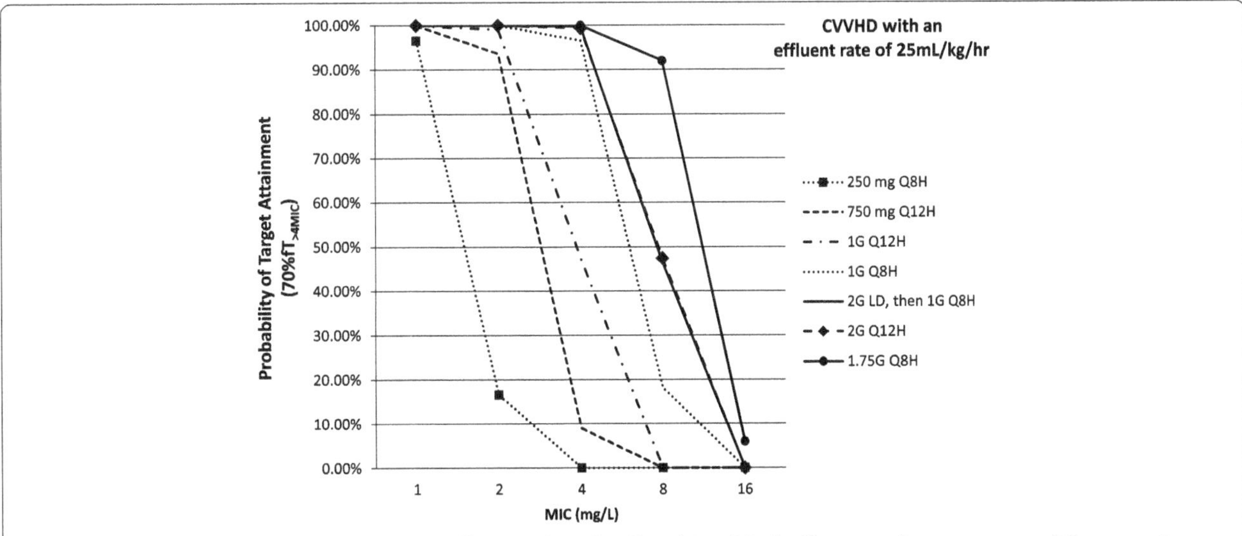

Fig. 1 PTA results of cefepime dosing regimens at different MICs in CVVHD and 25 mL/kg/h effluent rate for management of Gram-negative infections caused by *P. aeruginosa* (> 70% $fT_{>4MIC}$; MIC of 8 mg/L) in virtual patients for the first 48 h

the Clinical Laboratory Standards Institute [31] used in the models. This value of 8 mg/L in the study implies a worst situation of when a susceptible *P. aeruginosa* for cefepime is reported. The dosing recommendations therefore would be adjusted for the settings that have lower reported MICs as shown in Table 5 and Fig. 1. In addition, Su and colleagues conducted a hospital-based retrospective study in 90 hospitalized patients. The results showed that the survival rate of patients with a positive blood culture for susceptible *P. aeruginosa* receiving cefepime as the primary therapy was significantly lower in a group with a higher MIC (> 4 mg/L) compared with that in the lower MIC group (< 4 mg/L) (72.6% vs 23.5%, $p < 0.0001$) [35]. Consequently, we suggested to dose cefepime based on MIC values of each setting (Table 5). An alternative therapy might be considered when a patient who has *P. aeruginosa* infection with a cefepime MIC of > 4 mg/L was identified.

Clinical validation of these results is warranted. Reconsidering using these regimens from clinically available resources in critically ill patients would be suggested, and close monitoring of efficacy when prescribing the conventional dosing regimen is very important.

Conclusion

The MCS technique can be a valuable tool for evaluating drug dosing in critically ill patients receiving CRRT when limited pharmacokinetic data is a major concern. These results revealed that the optimal doses for critically ill patient receiving CRRT were higher than recommended doses form clinical available resources for treating *P. aeruginosa*. The dosing regimen of 2 g LD was followed by 1500–1750 mg every 8 h for critically ill patients receiving CRRT with KDIGO-recommended effluent rates. If the higher effluent rate is prescribed, drug doses should be increased. The MIC values of each setting were an important factor to design cefepime dosing regimens. Clinical study is absolutely needed to validate our recommendations.

Abbreviations

AKI: Acute kidney injury; CL: Clearance; CL_{HD}: Transmembrane clearance; CL_{HF}: Transmembrane clearance; CL_{NR} : Non-renal clearance; CLSI: Clinical Laboratory Standards Institute; CRRT: Continuous renal replacement therapy; CVVH: Continuous venovenous hemofiltration; CVVHD: Continuous venovenous hemodialysis; $fT_{>4MIC}$: The cumulative percentage of a 48-h period with four times MIC; g: Gram; h: Hour; ISN: International Society of Nephrology; k: Elimination rate constant; KDIGO: Kidney Disease: Improving Global Outcomes; kg: Kilogram; L: Liter; LD: Loading dose; MCS: Monte Carlo simulations; mg: Milligram; MIC: Minimum inhibitory concentration; mL: Milliliter; *N*: Number; PTA: Probability of target attainment; q: Every; Q_{blood}: Blood flow rate; Q_d: Dialysate flow rate; Q_{plasma}: Plasma flow rate; $Q_{replacement}$: Replacement fluid flow rate; Q_{uf}: Ultrafiltrate flow rate; r^2: Population-specific correlation; SA: Saturation coefficient; SC: Sieving coefficient; SD: Standard deviation; SEA-AKI: Southeast Asia entitled The Epidemiology and Prognostic Factors for Mortality in Intensive Care Unit Patients with Acute Kidney Injury in Southeast Asia; V_d: Volume of distribution

Acknowledgements

We would like to thank Associate Professor Dr. Wibul Wongpoowarak for the helpful comments of our simulations in the study and Associate Professor Dr. Chalermsri Pummangura for all great advice and support. We also would like to thank Assistant Professor Dr. Dhakrit Rungkitwattanakul for proof reading the article.

Funding

This study was supported by a grant from the Siam University. The funding source had no role in the study design, the collection, analysis and interpretation of data, the writing of the article, and the decision to submit it for publication.

Authors' contributions

WC contributed to the conception and design, acquisition of data, analysis and interpretation of data, and drafting and revising the manuscript. TC and AB analyzed and interpreted the data regarding simulations and probability of target attainment. NS was involved in data collection and drafting and revising the manuscript. SP interpreted the data regarding simulations and probability of target attainment and was also involved in drafting and revising the manuscript. All authors read and approved the final manuscript.

Competing interests

The authors declare that they have no competing interests.

Author details

[1]Faculty of Pharmacy, Siam University, 38 Petkasem Road, Bangwa, Pasicharoen, Bangkok 10160, Thailand. [2]Division of Nephrology, Department of Medicine, Faculty of Medicine, Chulalongkorn University, and King Chulalongkorn Memorial Hospital, Bangkok, Thailand. [3]Department of Clinical Pharmacy, Faculty of Pharmaceutical Sciences, Prince of Songkla University, Songkhla, Thailand. [4]School of Pharmaceutical Sciences, University of Phayao, Phayao, Thailand.

References

1. Kidney Disease: Improving global outcomes (KDIGO) acute kidney injury work group. KDIGO clinical practice guideline for acute kidney injury. Kidney Inter Suppl 2012; 2: 1–138.
2. Maxipime® [package insert]. Lake Forest, IL: Hospira, Inc; 2012.
3. Nye KJ, Shi YG, Andrews JM, Wise R. Pharmacokinetics and tissue penetration of cefepime. J Antimicrob Chemother. 1989;24:23–8.
4. Barbhaiya RH, Knupp CA, Forgue ST, Matzke GR, Guay DRP, Pittman KA. Pharmacokinetics of cefepime in subjects with renal insufficiency. Clin Pharmacol Ther. 1990;48:268–76.
5. Shaw AR, Chaijamorn W, Mueller BA. We underdose antibiotics in patients on CRRT. Semin Dial. 2016;29(4):278–80.
6. Kollef MF, Sherman G, Ward S, Fraser VJ, et al. Inadequate antimicrobial treatment of infections: a risk factor for hospital mortality among critically ill patients. Chest. 1999;115:462–74.
7. Lewis SJ, Mueller BA. Antibiotic dosing in patients with kidney injury; "enough but not too much". J Intensive Care Med. 2016;31:164–76.
8. Isla A, Gascon AR, Maynar J, Arzuaga A, Toral D, Pedraz JL. Cefepime and continuous renal replacement therapy (CRRT): in vitro permeability of two

CRRT membranes and pharmacokinetics in four critically ill patients. Clin Ther. 2005;27(5):599–608.
9. Malone RS, Fish DN, Abraham E, Teitelbaum I. Pharmacokinetics of cefepime during continuous renal replacement therapy in critically ill patients. Antimicrob Agents Chemother. 2001;45(11):3148–55.
10. Li AM, Gomersall CD, Choi G, Tian Q, Joynt GM, Lipman J, et al. A systematic review of antibiotic dosing regimens for septic patients receiving continuous renal replacement therapy: do current studies supply sufficient data? J Antimicrob Chemother. 2009;64:929–37.
11. Barbey F, Bugnon D, Wauters JP. Severe neurotoxicity of cefepime in uremic patients (letter). Ann Intern Med. 2001;135:1011.
12. Chatellier D, Jourdain M, Mangalaboyi J, Ader F, Chopin C, Derambure P, et al. Cefepime-induced neurotoxicity: an underestimated complication of antibiotherapy in patients with acute renal failure. Intensive Care Med. 2002; 28:214–7.
13. Lam S, Gomolin IH. Cefepime neurotoxicity: case report, pharmacokinetic considerations, and literature review. Pharmacotherapy. 2006;26:1169–74.
14. Durand-Maugard C, Lemaire-Hurtel AS, Gras-Champel V, Hary L, Maizel J, Prud'homme-Bernardy A, et al. Blood and CSF monitoring of cefepime-induced neurotoxicity: nine case reports. J Antimicrob Chemother. 2012; 67(5):1297–9.
15. Wong KM, Chan WK, Chan YH, Li CS. Cefepime-related neurotoxicity in a haemodialysis patient. Nephrol Dial Transplant. 1999;14:2265–6.
16. Allaouchiche B, Breilh D, Jaumain H, Gaillard B, Renard S, Saux MC. Pharmacokinetics of cefepime during continuous venovenous hemodiafiltration. Antimicrob Agents Chemother. 1997;41(11):2424–7.
17. Beumier M, Casu GS, Hites M, Seyler L, Cotton F, Vincent JL, et al. Beta-lactam antibiotic concentrations during continuous renal replacement therapy. Crit Care. 2014;18(3):R105.
18. Seyler L, Cotton F, Taccone FS, De Backer D, Macours P, Vincent JL, et al. Recommended beta-lactam regimens are inadequate in septic patients treated with continuous renal replacement therapy. Crit Care. 2011;15(3):R137.
19. Carlier M, Taccone FS, Beumier M, Seyler L, Cotton F, Jacobs F, et al. Population pharmacokinetics and dosing simulations of cefepime in septic shock patients receving continuous renal replacement therapy. Int J Antimicrob Agents. 2015;46:413–9.
20. Schetz M. Drug dosing in continuous renal replacement therapy: general rules. Curr Opin Crit Care. 2007;13(6):645–51.
21. International Society of Nephrology (ISN). Clinical research: the epidemiology and prognostic factors for mortality in intensive care unit patients with acute kidney injury in South East Asia. Available from https://www.theisn.org/component/k2/item/2645-clinical-research-the-epidemiology-and-prognostic-factors-for-mortality-in-intensive-care-unit-patients-with-acute-kidney-injury-in-south-east-asia. Accessed 2 Feb 2018.
22. Legrand M, Darmon M, Joannidis M, Payen D. Management of renal replacement therapy in ICU patients: an international survey. Intensive Care Med. 2013;39:101–8.
23. Aronoff GR, Bennett WM, Berns JS, Brier ME, Kasbekar N, Mueller BA, et al. Drug prescribing in renal failure: dosing guidelines for adults and children. 5th ed. Philadephia: American College of Physicians; 2007.
24. Trotman RL, Williamson JC, Shoemaker DM, Salzer WL. Antibiotic dosing in critically ill adult patients receiving continuous renal replacement therapy. Clin Infect Dis. 2005;41(8):1159–66.
25. Heintz BH, Matzke GR, Dager WE. Antimicrobial dosing concepts and recommendations for critically ill adult patients receiving continuous renal replacement therapy or intermittent hemodialysis. Pharmacotherapy. 2009; 29(5):562–77.
26. Lewis SJ, Chaijamorn W, Shaw AR, Mueller BA. In silico trials using Monte Carlo simulation to evaluate ciprofloxacin and levofloxacin dosing in critically ill patients receiving prolonged intermittent renal replacement therapy. Ren Replace Ther. 2016;2:45.
27. Lewis SJ, Kays MB, Mueller BA. Use of Monte Carlo simulations to determine optimal Carbapenem dosing in critically ill patients receiving prolonged intermittent renal replacement therapy. J Clin Pharmacol. 2016;56(10):1277–87.
28. Mouton JW, Dudley MN, Cars O, Derendorf H, Drusano GL. Standardization of pharmacokinetic/pharmacodynamics (PK/PD) terminology for anti-infective drugs: an update. J Antimicrob Chemother. 2005;55:601–7.
29. Tam VH, McKinnon PS, Akins RL, Rybak MJ, Drusano GL. Pharmacodynamics of cefepime in patients with gram-negative infections. J Antimicrob Chemother. 2002;50:425–8.
30. Drusano GL. Antimicrobial pharmacodynamics: critical interactions of 'bug and grug'. Nat Rev Microbiol. 2004;2:289–300.
31. Clinical Laboratory Standards Institute. Performance Standards for Antimicrobial Susceptibility Testing, ed 26. CLSI supplement M100S. Wayne: CLSI; 2016.
32. Lewis SJ, Mueller BA. Antibiotic dosing in critically ill patients receiving CRRT: underdosing is overprevalent. Semin Dial. 2014;27(5):441–5.
33. Barbhaiya RH, Knupp CA, Tenney J, Martin RR, Weidler DJ, Pittman KA. Safety, tolerance, and pharmacokinetics of cefepime administered intramuscularly to healthy subjects. J Clin Pharmacol. 1990;30:900–10.
34. Finfer S, Bellomo R, McEvoy S, Lo SK, Myburgh J, Neal B, et al. Effect of baseline serum albumin concentration on outcome of resuscitation with albumin or saline in patients in intensive care units: analysis of data from the saline versus albumin fluid evaluation (SAFE) study. BMJ. 2006;333:1044.
35. Su TY, Ye JJ, Yang CC, Huang CT, Chia JH, Lee MH. Influence of borderline cefepime MIC on the outcome of cefepime-susceptible Pseudomonas aeruginosa bacteremia treated with a maximal cefepime dose: a hospital-based retrospective study. Ann Clin Microbiol Antimicrob. 2017;16(1):52.

22

Accuracy of the first interpretation of early brain CT images for predicting the prognosis of post-cardiac arrest syndrome patients at the emergency department

Mitsuaki Nishikimi[1*], Takayuki Ogura[2], Kota Matsui[3], Kunihiko Takahashi[3], Kenji Fukaya[1], Keibun Liu[2], Hideo Morita[4], Mitsunobu Nakamura[2], Shigeyuki Matsui[3] and Naoyuki Matsuda[1]

Abstract

Background: Early brain CT is one of the most useful tools for estimating the prognosis in patients with post-cardiac arrest syndrome (PCAS) at the emergency department (ED). The aim of this study was to evaluate the prognosis-prediction accuracy of the emergency physicians' interpretation of the findings on early brain CT in PCAS patients treated by targeted temperature management (TTM).

Methods: This was a double-center, retrospective, observational study. Eligible subjects were cardiac arrest patients admitted to the intensive care unit (ICU) for TTM between April 2011 and March 2017. We performed the McNemar test to compare the predictive accuracies of the interpretation by emergency physicians and radiologists and calculated the kappa statistic for determining the concordance rate between the interpretations by these two groups.

Results: Of the 122 eligible patients, 106 met the inclusion criteria for this study. The predictive accuracies (sensitivity, specificity) of the interpretations by the emergency physicians and radiologists were (0.34, 1.00) and (0.41, 0.93), respectively, with no significant difference in either the sensitivity or specificity as assessed by the McNemar test. The kappa statistic calculated to determine the concordance between the two interpretations was 0.66 (0.48–0.83), which showed a good conformity.

Conclusions: The emergency physicians' interpretation of the early brain CT findings in PCAS patients treated by TTM was as reliable as that of radiologists, in terms of prediction of the prognosis.

Keywords: Cardiac arrest, Post-cardiac arrest syndrome, Neurological prognosis, Brain CT scan, Targeted temperature management

Background

One of the most important clinical considerations in patients with post-cardiac arrest syndrome (PCAS) is to estimate the neurological prognosis [1, 2]. A definitive estimation of the prognosis of PCAS patients undergoing targeted temperature management (TTM) should be performed 72 h after the return to normal body temperature according to the guideline [3]. But a few previous studies have reported the usefulness of early estimation of the prognosis in PCAS patients at the time of the arrival at the emergency department (ED) [4–6].

Early brain CT is one of the most useful tools for estimating the prognosis of PCAS patients at the ED [7]. Although a few small studies have shown that signs of loss of gray-white matter differentiation and brain swelling on brain CT are reliable signs of a poor prognosis, the interpreters in these studies were imaging specialists, or radiologists, and not emergency physicians [8–11]. Considering that it is impossible for radiologists to evaluate the CT scans in real time at the ED in many countries [12, 13], there is no doubt about the importance of accurate interpretation by

* Correspondence: m0528332626@yahoo.co.jp
[1]Department of Emergency and Critical Care, Nagoya University Graduate School of Medicine, Tsurumai-cho 64, Syowa-ku, Nagoya, Aichi 466-8560, Japan
Full list of author information is available at the end of the article

emergency physicians. But no study has been conducted to determine the accuracy of interpretation of early brain CT images by emergency physicians for estimating the prognosis in PCAS patients. Thus, the aim of this study was to evaluate the accuracy of interpretation of early brain CT by emergency physicians in comparison with that by expert radiologists in PCAS patients treated by TTM.

Methods

Study design

A double-center, retrospective, observational study was performed. We retrospectively reviewed the clinical management charts of the patients with cardiac arrest admitted to the Nagoya University Hospital or Japan Red Cross Maebashi Hospital between April 2011 and March 2017. All eligible patients were more than 20 years old and had lived independently prior to the development of the cardiac arrest. Subjects were included in this study if they had undergone a brain CT at the ED after return of spontaneous circulation (ROSC) following cardiac resuscitation, and these CT images had been interpreted by both the emergency physicians at the ED and radiologists. Note that a brain CT examination is routinely performed for PCAS patients before the initiation of TTM in these two hospitals. After the admission, TTM was undertaken in all the patients at the intensive care unit (ICU) by cold infusion and a surface cooling device with computerized automatic temperature control.

Dataset

Data were collected retrospectively by reviewing the electronic medical charts of the patients, including the clinical histories, cardiac rhythms, physical examination findings, blood examination results, brain CT image findings, and clinical courses after admission.

To compare the interpretations of the CT images by the emergency physicians and radiologists, we conducted a retrospective review of the records of the findings of the emergency physicians and reports of the radiologists. We only reviewed those findings that had been entered by the emergency physicians before the radiologists' reports became available, so as to exclude the possibility of the latter influencing the interpretation by the emergency physicians. When phrases such as "signs of loss of gray-white matter differentiation or brain swelling was seen" were found in the records, we judged that the interpreter had recognized the signs of the hypoxic encephalopathy. At the two participant hospitals, emergency physicians at the ED must interpret the findings on early brain CT while having no access to the reports by radiologists, because the radiologists provide their reports only after (within 2 days) the emergency physicians' interpretation. The emergency physicians in this study were defined as specialists and fellows working on a regular basis at our ED, and all of them had the experience of working at the ED as residents for at least 2 years.

The calculation of the gray matter attenuation to white matter attenuation ratio

One blinded critical care fellow calculated the gray matter attenuation to white matter attenuation ratio (GWR) by retrospectively reviewing the CT images of all subjects. It was measured using the method described in Torbey et al.'s report [14]. The GWR was compared with the predictive accuracy of the interpretation by the emergency physicians in order to validate the latter with objective indices. The intensities of circular areas of interest (about 10 mm2) were measured for both the gray and white matter on three axial slices (5-mm slice thickness) at a basal ganglia level, a centrum semiovale level, and a high convexity level. Then, the GWR was calculated as shown below:

GWR basal ganglia = [PU + CN]/[CC + PIC]

GWR cortex = [MC1 + MC2]/[MWM1 + MWM2]

GWR = [GWR basal ganglia + GWR cortex]/2

where PU indicates putamen, CN caudal nucleus, CC corpus callosum, PIC posterior limb of internal capsule, MC1 medial cortex at centrum semiovale, MC2 medial cortex at high convexity level, MWM1 medial white matter at centrum semiovale, and MWM2 medial white matter at high convexity level. Each value was the average of the right and left hemisphere values.

Protocol for targeted temperature management

TTM was undertaken in the eligible patients according to the protocol in place at each of the hospitals. TTM was considered as being indicated for cardiac arrest patients who were in a coma (GCS ≤ 8) after ROSC without remarkable hemodynamic instability or a "Do-Not-Attempt to Resuscitate" directive. The temperature was maintained at the target level of 34–36 °C by infusion of cold fluids in combination with surface cooling with an ice pack and/or a cold blanket or using a surface cooling device with computerized automatic temperature control (Arctic Sun 2000 TTM; Bard Medical Louisville, CO). After the targeted temperature had been maintained for 24 h, rewarming to 36 °C was performed at the rate of 0.2 °C/4 h at Nagoya University Hospital or 1.0 °C/24 h at Japan Red Cross Maebashi Hospital. Propofol, midazolam, dexmedetomidine, fentanyl, and rocuronium were used for sedation, analgesia, and muscle relaxation, according to individual clinician preferences.

Neurological outcome

The Cerebral Performance Categories (CPC) at 30 days was used to estimate the neurological outcome as follows: CPC 1, full recovery; CPC 2, moderate disability; CPC 3, severe disability; CPC 4, coma or vegetative state; and CPC 5, death [15]. CPC 1 and CPC 2 were considered as representing a good outcome, and CPC 3, CPC 4, and CPC 5 were considered as representing a poor outcome.

Statistical analysis

For outcome, we derived the sensitivity and specificity of the interpretations by the emergency physicians and radiologists. We performed McNemar's test to compare the sensitivity and specificity of the two interpretations. Next, in order to investigate the concordance rate between the two interpretations, we calculated the kappa statistic and its 95% confidence interval. All the statistical analyses were conducted using R software version 3.3.1 [16].

Results

During the study period, 122 PCAS patients were admitted to the ICU at either of the participant institutions for TTM, of whom 119 had undergone early brain CT prior to the initiation of the TTM. Of these 119 patients, 13 were excluded because of the lack of availability of the records of CT image interpretation by the emergency physicians and/or radiologists, and the remaining 106 were included in this study (Fig. 1).

The baseline characteristics of the subjects are summarized in Table 1. TTM at 34–36 °C was undertaken for all the patients at the ICU by infusion of cold fluids and use of a surface cooling device with computerized automatic temperature control. Most of the subjects were male (82.1%), with a median age of 64.0 (52.0–71.0) years and median hospital stay of 29.0 (19.0–54.0) days. Forty-five subjects (42.5%) showed good outcomes, while 61 subjects (57.5%) showed poor outcomes.

The accuracies (sensitivity, specificity) of the emergency physicians' and radiologists' interpretation were (0.34, 1.00) and (0.41, 0.93), respectively. To evaluate these accuracies objectively, we calculated the GWRs and also examined the accuracy of the prediction using the GWR cutoff values of 1.16 and 1.13 (Table 2). The exact McNemar test showed no significant differences in either the sensitivity or the specificity between the two interpretations (sensitivity: p value = 0.34, specificity: p value = 0.25). Also, good conformity was confirmed between the two interpretations, with a calculated kappa statistic of 0.66 (95% CI 0.48–0.83, Table 3).

Discussion

Because of the shortage of radiologists in many countries, it is often not possible for radiologists to evaluate CT scans in real time at the ED [12, 13]. In such cases, emergency physicians have to interpret the images and manage the patients accordingly before the radiologists' report becomes available. While several studies have compared the predictive accuracy of the interpretation by emergency physicians with that by the radiologists [17, 18], there was no study about the predictive accuracy of the interpretation of early brain CT by emergency physicians in PCAS patients who underwent TTM. Our study is the first study to examine the predictive accuracy of the interpretation by emergency physicians.

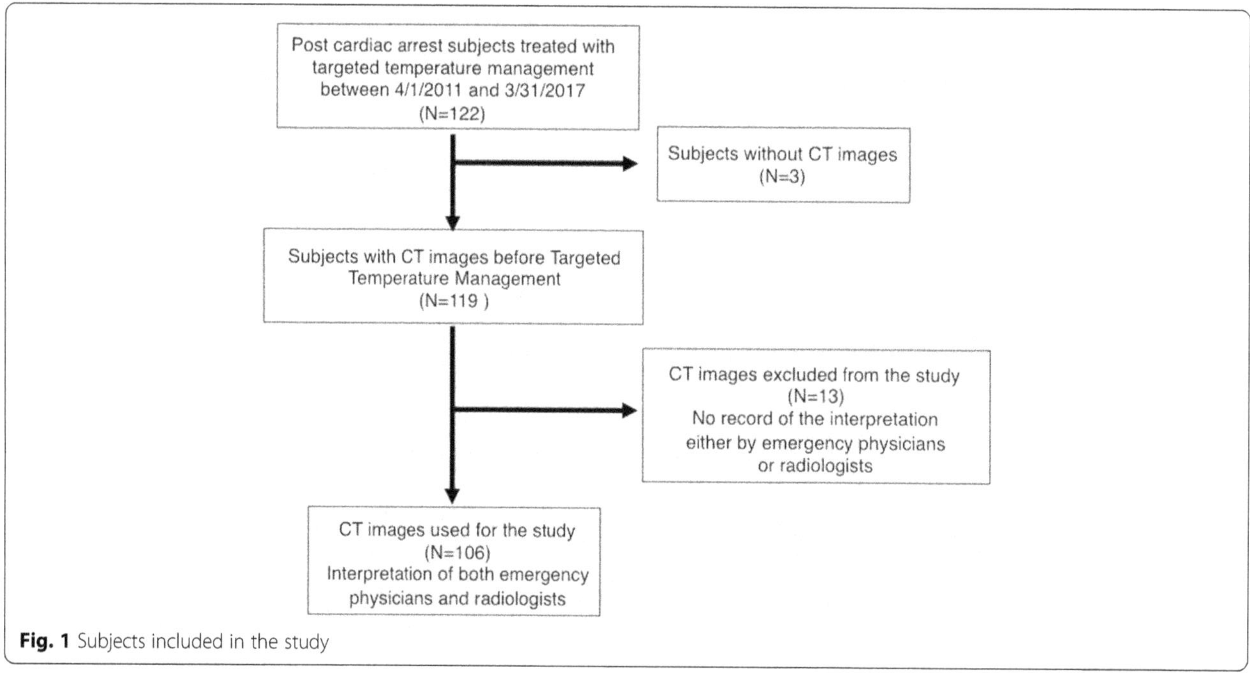

Fig. 1 Subjects included in the study

Table 1 Baseline characteristics of the subjects

Variable	Nagoya $n = 48$	Maebashi $n = 58$	Total $n = 106$
Demographics			
Age, years	64.0 (52.0–70.8)	64.0 (52.0–71.0)	64.0 (52.0–71.0)
Sex, male, *n* (%)	41 (85.4)	46 (79.3)	87 (82.1)
Length of stay in hospital, days	28.0 (19.0–51.0)	32.5 (19.3–57.8)	29.0 (19.0–54.0)
Condition of cardiac arrest			
Witness, *n* (%)	39 (81.3)	49 (84.5)	88 (83.0)
Bystander, *n* (%)	29 (60.4)	32 (55.2)	61 (57.5)
Initial rhythm, shockable, *n* (%)	27 (56.3)	39 (67.2)	66 (62.3)
Duration of resuscitation effort, min	18.0 (12.5–28.5)	18.0 (8.0–28.0)	18.0 (10.0–28.8)
Presumed cardiac etiology, *n* (%)	29 (60.4)	38 (65.5)	67 (63.2)
GCS, $M \geq 2$, *n* (%)[a]	29 (61.7)	38 (66.7)	67 (64.4)
pH[b]	7.07 ± 0.03	7.14 ± 0.03	7.11 ± 0.02
Time to initiation of targeted temperature management, hours	2.5 (1.5–3.0)	2.5 (2.0–3.0)	2.5 (1.5–3.0)
Time to targeted setting temperature, hours	4.5 (3.4–6.0)	5.0 (3.0–9.0)	5.0 (3.0–7.0)
Outcome			
Good (CPC ≤ 2), *n* (%)	21 (43.8)	24 (41.4)	45 (42.5)
Poor (CPC ≥ 3), *n* (%)	27 (56.2)	34 (58.6)	61 (57.5)

Data are presented as the median and interquartile ranges (25–75% percentile) or as absolute frequencies with percentages. Data are presented as mean ± standard error, as the median and interquartile ranges (25–75% percentile) or as absolute frequencies with percentages

Nagoya Nagoya University Hospital, *Maebashi* Japan Red Cross Maebashi Hospital, *GCS* Glasgow Coma Scale

[a]$n = 2$

[b]$n = 2$

We investigated the predictive ability of the GWR using two cutoff values, as well as the predictive accuracies of the interpretations by emergency physicians and radiologists. GWR is one of the most reliable objective indices of hypoxic encephalopathy, and several studies (with small sample sizes) have reported the usefulness of calculation of the GWR for predicting the prognosis in PCAS patients using different cutoff points (1.10 to 1. 20) [19–22]. In our study, we confirmed that the accuracy of poor prognosis prediction based on a GWR of < 1.13 was good, consistent with previous reports, while that based on a GWR of < 1.16 was inadequate. A study with a large sample size would be needed for detecting the best cutoff points.

In this study, the specificity of the emergency physicians' interpretation for a poor prognosis sign was 1.00, which means that the likelihood of good recovery of the PCAS patients was extremely low if the emergency physicians interpreted the findings on early brain CT as being predictive of a poor prognosis. Previous study showed that a hypoxic encephalopathy sign on their brain CT was a reliable sign for a poor prognosis [9, 10], but few studies took into account whether the patients included in the study had undergone/not undergone TTM. Our study showed that, even if the PCAS patients underwent TTM, the predictive accuracy of the interpretation for poor prognosis was still high. From the viewpoint of cost-effectiveness, in patients in whom the emergency room physicians interpret the early brain CT findings in PCAS patients as being predictive of a poor prognosis, TTM may fail to be of benefit, although further studies are needed.

There were some limitations of this study. First, it was a retrospective study that involved a review of the electronic charts of the patients. The interpretations from their CT could have been biased by other information

Table 2 Predictive accuracies of emergency physicians' interpretation, radiologists' interpretation, and the cutoff value of GWR < 1.16 and 1.13

	Interpreters		GWR < 1.16	GWR < 1.13
	By emergency physicians	By radiologists		
Sensitivity	0.34 (0.23–0.48)	0.41 (0.29–0.54)	0.54 (0.41–0.67)	0.28 (0.17–0.41)
Specificity	1.00 (0.92–1.00)	0.93 (0.82–0.99)	0.64 (0.49–0.78)	0.98 (0.88–1.00)

Data are presented as mean and 95% confidence interval

GWR gray matter attenuation to white matter attenuation ratio

Table 3 The conformity between these two interpretations

		Radiologists		
		Poor	Good	Total
Emergency physicians	Poor	17.0% (18/106)	2.8% (3/106)	21
	Good	9.4% (10/106)	70.8% (75/106)	85
	Total	28	78	106

Kappa statistics: 0.66 (95% CI 0.48–0.83). Data are presented as absolute frequencies with percentages
95% CI 95% confidence interval

that could have influenced the prognosis, such as the clinical histories and physical examination findings of the patients. Second, the study was performed at only two participant hospitals, and further multicenter studies would be needed. It would be a great interest to conduct a prospective multicenter study to evaluate the accuracy of interpretation of early brain CT, obtained before the initiation of TTM, so as to optimize the management in patients with PCAS.

Conclusions

The emergency physicians' interpretation of the early brain CT findings in PCAS patients treated by TTM was as reliable as that of radiologists, in terms of prediction of the prognosis.

Abbreviations

95% CI: 95% confidence interval; CPC: Cerebral Performance Categories; ED: Emergency department; GWR: Gray matter attenuation to white matter attenuation ratio; ICU: Intensive care unit; PCAS: Post-cardiac arrest syndrome; ROSC: Return of spontaneous circulation; TTM: Targeted temperature management

Acknowledgements

This work was supported by the Clinical Research Program at Nagoya University. We thank the residents, fellows, paramedic staff, and the secretary Teruko Mizutani in our ICU and emergency department for the data collection and treatment support.

Authors' contributions

MNi, TO, KM, MNa, and SM designed the study. MNi, KM, KT, and SM performed the analyses. MNi, KL, and HM collected the data. MNi, TO, KM, KF, SM, and NM drafted the manuscript. All authors critically reviewed the manuscript. All authors read and approved the final version of this manuscript.

Competing interests

The authors declare that they have no competing interests.

Author details

[1]Department of Emergency and Critical Care, Nagoya University Graduate School of Medicine, Tsurumai-cho 64, Syowa-ku, Nagoya, Aichi 466-8560, Japan. [2]Advanced Medical Emergency Department and Critical Care Center, Japan Red Cross Maebashi Hospital, Maebashi, Japan. [3]Department of Biostatistics, Nagoya University Graduate School of Medicine, Nagoya, Japan. [4]Department of Diagnostic Radiology, Japan Red Cross Maebashi Hospital, Maebashi, Japan.

References

1. Grossestreuer AV, Abella BS, Leary M, Perman SM, Fuchs BD, Kolansky DM, et al. Time to awakening and neurologic outcome in therapeutic hypothermia-treated cardiac arrest patients. Resuscitation. 2013;84(12):1741–6.
2. Young GB. Clinical practice. Neurologic prognosis after cardiac arrest. N Engl J Med 2009;361(6):605–611.
3. Soar J, Callaway CW, Aibiki M, Bottiger BW, Brooks SC, Deakin CD, et al. Part 4: advanced life support: 2015 international consensus on cardiopulmonary resuscitation and emergency cardiovascular care science with treatment recommendations. Resuscitation. 2015;95:e71–120.
4. Oddo M, Rossetti AO. Early multimodal outcome prediction after cardiac arrest in patients treated with hypothermia. Crit Care Med. 2014;42(6):1340–7.
5. Hayakawa K, Tasaki O, Hamasaki T, Sakai T, Shiozaki T, Nakagawa Y, et al. Prognostic indicators and outcome prediction model for patients with return of spontaneous circulation from cardiopulmonary arrest: the Utstein Osaka Project. Resuscitation. 2011;82(7):874–80.
6. Nishikimi M, Matsuda N, Matsui K, Takahashi K, Ejima T, Liu K, et al. A novel scoring system for predicting the neurologic prognosis prior to the initiation of induced hypothermia in cases of post-cardiac arrest syndrome: the CAST score. Scand J Trauma Resusc Emerg Med. 2017;25(1):49.
7. Gutierrez LG, Rovira A, Portela LA, Leite Cda C, Lucato LT. CT and MR in non-neonatal hypoxic-ischemic encephalopathy: radiological findings with pathophysiological correlations. Neuroradiology. 2010;52(11):949–76.
8. Yamamura H, Kaga S, Kaneda K, Yamamoto T, Mizobata Y. Head computed tomographic measurement as an early predictor of outcome in hypoxic-ischemic brain damage patients treated with hypothermia therapy. Scand J Trauma Resusc Emerg Med. 2013;21:37.
9. Inamasu J, Nakatsukasa M, Hayashi T, Kato Y, Hirose Y. Early CT signs of hypoxia in patients with subarachnoid hemorrhage presenting with cardiac arrest: early CT signs in SAH patients presenting with CA. Acta Neurochir Suppl. 2013;118:181–4.
10. Fugate JE, Wijdicks EF, Mandrekar J, Claassen DO, Manno EM, White RD, et al. Predictors of neurologic outcome in hypothermia after cardiac arrest. Ann Neurol. 2010;68(6):907–14.
11. Inamasu J, Miyatake S, Nakatsukasa M, Koh H, Yagami T. Loss of gray-white matter discrimination as an early CT sign of brain ischemia/hypoxia in victims of asphyxial cardiac arrest. Emerg Radiol. 2011;18(4):295–8.
12. Hunter TB, Krupinski EA, Hunt KR, Erly WK. Emergency department coverage by academic departments of radiology. Acad Radiol. 2000;7(3):165–70.
13. Torreggiani WC, Nicolaou S, Lyburn ID, Harris AC, Buckley AR. Emergency radiology in Canada: a national survey. Can Assoc Radiol J. 2002;53(3):160–7.
14. Torbey MT, Selim M, Knorr J, Bigelow C, Recht L. Quantitative analysis of the loss of distinction between gray and white matter in comatose patients after cardiac arrest. Stroke. 2000;31(9):2163–7.
15. Ajam K, Gold LS, Beck SS, Damon S, Phelps R, Rea TD. Reliability of the Cerebral Performance Category to classify neurological status among survivors of ventricular fibrillation arrest: a cohort study. Scand J Trauma Resusc Emerg Med. 2011;19:38.
16. Team RDC. R: a language and environment for statistical computing. 2011.
17. Idil H, Kirimli G, Korol G, Unluer EE. Are emergency physicians competent to interpret the cranial CT of patients younger than the age of 2 years with mild head trauma? Am J Emerg Med. 2015;33(9):1175–7.
18. Kartal ZA, Kozaci N, Cekic B, Beydilli I, Akcimen M, Guven DS, et al. CT interpretations in multiply injured patients: comparison of emergency physicians and on-call radiologists. Am J Emerg Med. 2016;34(12):2331–5.
19. Metter RB, Rittenberger JC, Guyette FX, Callaway CW. Association between a quantitative CT scan measure of brain edema and outcome after cardiac arrest. Resuscitation. 2011;82(9):1180–5.

20. Takahashi N, Satou C, Higuchi T, Shiotani M, Maeda H, Hirose Y. Quantitative analysis of brain edema and swelling on early postmortem computed tomography: comparison with antemortem computed tomography. Jpn J Radiol. 2010;28(5):349–54.
21. Scheel M, Storm C, Gentsch A, Nee J, Luckenbach F, Ploner CJ, et al. The prognostic value of gray-white-matter ratio in cardiac arrest patients treated with hypothermia. Scand J Trauma Resusc Emerg Med. 2013;21:23.
22. Cristia C, Ho ML, Levy S, Andersen LW, Perman SM, Giberson T, et al. The association between a quantitative computed tomography (CT) measurement of cerebral edema and outcomes in post-cardiac arrest—a validation study. Resuscitation. 2014;85(10):1348–53.

23

Epidemiology, clinical characteristics, resistance, and treatment of infections by *Candida auris*

Andrea Cortegiani[1*], Giovanni Misseri[1], Teresa Fasciana[2], Anna Giammanco[2], Antonino Giarratano[1] and Anuradha Chowdhary[3]

Abstract

Candida spp. infections are a major cause of morbidity and mortality in critically ill patients. *Candida auris* is an emerging multi-drug-resistant fungus that is rapidly spreading worldwide. Since the first reports in 2009, many isolates across five continents have been identified as agents of hospital-associated infections. Independent and simultaneous outbreaks of *C. auris* are becoming a major concern for healthcare and scientific community. Moreover, laboratory misidentification and multi-drug-resistant profiles, rarely observed for other non-albicans *Candida* species, result in difficult eradication and frequent therapeutic failures of *C. auris* infections. The aim of this review was to provide an updated and comprehensive report of the global spread of *C. auris*, focusing on clinical and microbiological characteristics, mechanisms of virulence and antifungal resistance, and efficacy of available control, preventive, and therapeutic strategies.

Keywords: *C. auris*, *Candida*, Candidemia, Invasive fungal infection, Antimicrobial resistance, Antifungal resistance

Introduction

Candida spp. infections are a major cause of morbidity and mortality in critically ill patients [1–3]. Yeasts of genus *Candida* are associated with a wide range of different clinical manifestations, including bloodstream infections (BSIs), intra-abdominal candidiasis, deep-seated candidiasis, and superficial infections [1, 4, 5]. Infections caused by *Candida* spp. have progressively increased over the last decades, and this phenomenon is mainly associated with the increasing rate of invasive procedures, the extensive use of broad-spectrum antimicrobials, and the more frequent immunocompromised status of critically ill patients [6–8]. Although *Candida albicans* still remains the main agent of hospital-acquired fungal infection, several species of non-albicans *Candida* namely *C. tropicalis*, *C. glabrata*, *C. parapsilosis*, and *C. krusei* account for increasing incidence of invasive infections with high rates of therapeutic failure, mainly related to echinocandins and azoles resistance [9–11]. Current increase in antifungal drug resistance is not only linked to the acquired mechanism following administration of antifungal agents but intrinsic resistance to several classes of antimicrobials among different non-*albicans* species has also been recorded [12].

C. auris is an emerging multi-drug-resistant fungus that is rapidly spreading worldwide. Since the first reports in 2009, many isolates have been identified across five continents as agents of hospital-associated infections [11, 13, 14]. Reported cases are characterized by high overall mortality [15, 16] and high rate of antifungal resistance [17]. Of note, most reported infections involved critically ill patients [15, 18]. Moreover, difficulty in microbiological identification [19, 20], high virulence [21–23], multi-drug resistance profile [24, 25], and rapid global spread with several reported outbreaks ([11, 26, 27]; (https://www.cdc.gov/fungal/diseases/candidiasis/tracking-c-auris.html); [28]) lead the healthcare and scientific communities to consider *C. auris* as one of the most serious emerging pathogen that critical care physicians should be aware of.

* Correspondence: andrea.cortegiani@unipa.it
[1]Department of Surgical, Oncological and Oral Science (Di.Chir.On.S.). Section of Anesthesia, Analgesia, Intensive Care and Emergency. Policlinico Paolo Giaccone. University of Palermo, Italy, University of Palermo, Via del vespro 129, 90127 Palermo, Italy
Full list of author information is available at the end of the article

The aim of this review is to provide an updated report of the global spread of *C. auris* focusing on clinical and microbiological characteristics, mechanisms of virulence and antifungal resistance, and efficacy of available control, preventive, and therapeutic strategies.

Main text

Systematic review

For the purpose of this review, we performed a systematic review of the literature using "Candida" AND "auris" as keywords. We searched the PubMed, Scopus, and Web of Science. We excluded articles in languages other than English. Two authors (A. C. and G. M.) independently performed the search. Differences in selections were solved by consensus, with the help of the third author (T. F.). We included peer-review articles and meeting abstracts, concerning epidemiology, clinical manifestations and risk factors, virulence, genotypic characteristics, and therapeutic management. Concerning clinical cases, we included all cases of isolation of *C. auris* in humans reported in literature. Cases were defined as patients in whom *C. auris* was isolated, and this definition includes both superficial and deep-seated infections. We also checked references of relevant articles to find potential articles not retrieved by the databases search. After excluding not relevant articles and duplicates, we included 131 relevant articles published from 2009 to 30 May 2018. Articles retrieved were further categorized as shown in the flow diagram, following PRISMA guidelines (Additional file 1).

Microbiological characteristics of *C. auris*

On Sabouraud's agar, *C. auris* produces smooth and white cream-colored colonies, which are germ tube test negative. On CHROMagar *Candida* medium, *C. auris* produces colonies that may appear pale to dark pink, or rarely beige. The yeast *C. auris* is able to grow at 42 °C, and this characteristic helps differentiate *C. auris* from *C. haemulonii*, which does not grow at these temperatures [19]. The microscopic morphology of *C. auris* cells appears to be oval without pseudohyphae formation. However, *C. auris* might exhibit multiple morphological phenotypes under different cultures conditions, including round-to-ovoid, elongated, and pseudohyphal-like forms. For instance, high concentrations of sodium chloride induce the formation of a pseudohyphal-like form [29]. Cycloheximide 0.1% and 0.01% inhibits its growth [30]. The phenotypic, chemotaxonomic, and phylogenetic characteristics (Fig. 1) have therefore clearly suggested that it was a new species affiliated to the genus *Candida* (anamorphic) and therefore to the class of *Ascomycetes* even if the perfect form is not known (teleomorphic). Whole genome phylogeny of *C. auris*, *C. haemulonii*, *C. duobushaemulonii*, and *C. pseudohaemulonii* showed that they represent a single clade, confirming the close relationship of these species [31]. Due to the close genetic relatedness with *C. haemulonii* complex, *C. auris* is often commonly misidentified as *C. haemulonii* in routine diagnostic laboratories using biochemical methods. In fact, commercially available biochemical-based tests, including API AUX 20C, VITEK-2 YST, BD Phoenix, and MicroScan, misidentify *C. auris* as a wide range of *Candida* species and other genera. Misidentifications yielding *C. famata*, *C. sake*, *Rhodotorula glutinis*, *Rhodotorula mucilaginosa*, *Saccharomyces*, *C. catenulate*, *C. lusitaniae*, *C. guilliermondii*, and *C. parapsilosis* have been reported [19, 20, 26]. Recently, BioMerieux has updated the database [32, 33] and inclusion of *C. auris* spectra in the VITEK-2 system yields to its correct identification. Matrix-assisted laser desorption/ionization time-of-flight (MALDI-TOF) mass spectrometry can reliably differentiate *C. auris* from other *Candida* species, provided *C. auris* spectrum is included in the reference database and by selecting appropriate extraction method [34, 35]. The development of specific PCR assays for *C. auris* and for *C. auris*-related species using cultured colonies seems promising for its rapid and accurate identification, particularly in outbreak settings [36, 37]. Molecular identification of *C. auris* can be performed by sequencing various genetic loci (including *D1/D2*, *RPB1*, *RPB2*, and internal transcribed spacer *ITS1*, *ITS2*), but it is not routinely used [38, 39].

Epidemiology trends and world outbreaks

The real prevalence and the epidemiology of *C. auris* still remain uncertain. One of the causes may be the underestimation of its isolation due to the limited accuracy of available conventional diagnostic tools [40]. With the purpose to investigate whether *C. auris* emerged in recent times or had been misidentified in the past, an extensive investigation was conducted within the pool of uncommon *Candida* spp. included in the SENTRY global fungal collection (15,271 isolates of *Candida* spp. from four continents) [41]. This study identified a single *C. auris* isolate from Pakistan dating back to 2008, which had not been previously recognized [41]. In 2011, Lee et al. reported the first three cases of bloodstream fungemia caused by *C. auris* highlighting antifungal resistance and the ability to cause invasive infections [42]. One of these cases was incidentally recognized by molecular identification of a microbiological sample obtained in 1996 as invasive fungal infection isolate. To our knowledge, there are no other unidentified *C. auris* strains prior to 1996.

The first "named" description of *C. auris* as a new emergent pathogen has been reported in 2009 by Satoh et al. [13]. The authors reported a single isolate from the discharge of the external ear canal of a 70-year-old

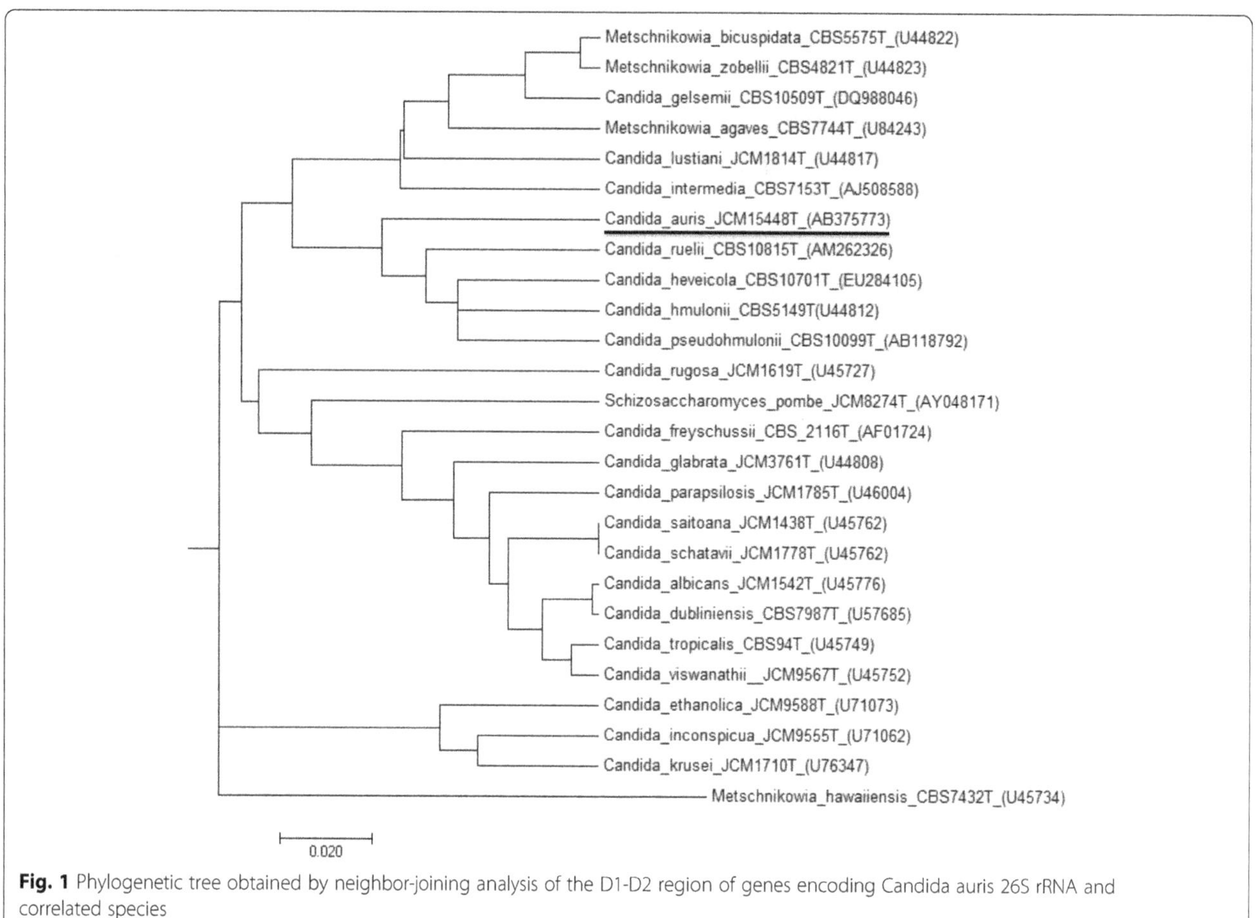

Fig. 1 Phylogenetic tree obtained by neighbor-joining analysis of the D1-D2 region of genes encoding Candida auris 26S rRNA and correlated species

inpatient at Tokyo Metropolitan Geriatric Hospital (Tokyo, Japan). Phenotypic, chemotaxonomic, and phylogenetic analyses indicated an affiliation to *Candida* genus, with a close relation to other unusual species [13] such as *C. haemulonii* and *C. pseudohaemulonii*. Later, in South Korea [14], 15 patients affected by chronic otitis media were identified to be infected by unusual and clonally related yeast isolates of *C. auris* confirmed by genomic sequencing [43]. Since the first isolation, *C. auris* infections have been reported from many countries, including India [15, 24, 38, 44], Pakistan [41], South Korea [42], Malaysia [45], South Africa [46], Oman [47, 48], Kenya [49], Kuwait [50], Israel [51], United Arab Emirates [52], Saudi Arabia [53], China [54], Colombia [55–57], Venezuela [58], the United States (US) ((https://www.cdc.gov/fungal/diseases/candidiasis/tracking-c-auris.html); [59–61]), Russia [62], Canada [63], Panama [64, 65], the United Kingdom (UK) [66], and continental Europe [28, 67–70]. Figure 2 shows *C. auris* reported isolations in chronological order. Figure 3 shows the worldwide distribution.

Europe's burden of *C. auris* outbreaks appears to be increasing, although the epidemiological profile is not completely defined [28]. Recently, the ECDC published a survey on reported cases of *C. auris* and laboratory capacity in Europe, with the purpose to implement surveillance and to control its further spread [28]. Six hundred and twenty cases of *C. auris* were reported in a period from 2013 to 2017, with two countries experiencing four hospital outbreaks. Sporadic cases have been identified since 2013 from different patients throughout England. The first outbreak of *C. auris* in Europe occurred in a London cardio-thoracic center between April 2015 and July 2016; 50 cases were identified, with ability for rapid colonization and transmissibility within the healthcare setting, leading to a serious and prolonged outbreak [66]. The first *C. auris* invasive infection in continental Europe occurred in Spain, where four patients admitted to the surgical intensive care unit of Valencia La Fe University and Polytechnic Hospital (Valencia, Spain) between April and June 2016 were diagnosed with deep-seated infection caused by this "super-fungus" [67]. Despite efforts in limiting diffusion of this pathogen, new colonization cases have continued to appear until now, with a tendency to acquire an endemic pattern. During the study period from April 2016 to January 2017, 140 patients were colonized by *C. auris* and 41 patients underwent candidemia episodes, with 5 patients

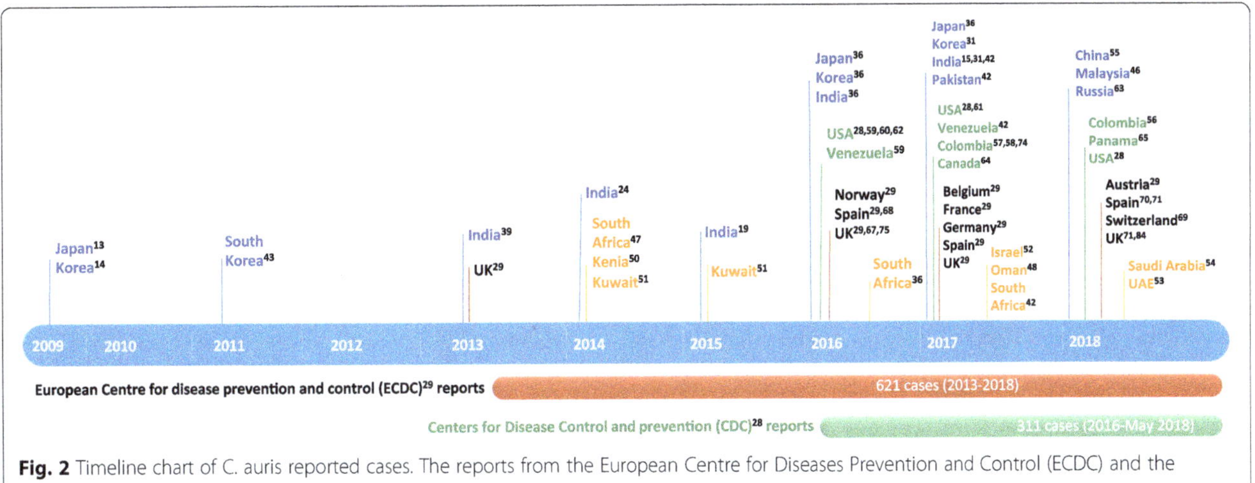

Fig. 2 Timeline chart of C. auris reported cases. The reports from the European Centre for Diseases Prevention and Control (ECDC) and the Centers for Disease Control and Prevention are ongoing

developing septic metastatic complications. This is the largest ongoing European clonal outbreak [69], involving a different strain from those previously reported, as demonstrated by genotype analysis.

Chowdhary et al. in 2013 were the first to report an outbreak of *C. auris* infection in India, identifying 12 patients with positive microbiological clinical samples collected between 2009 and 2012 [38]. Since then, there has been a progressive increase in the number of clinical cases reported. The high prevalence of invasive infections due to *C. auris* has become a great concern in India, as inter- and intra-hospital spreading of this multi-resistant pathogen has been demonstrated [15]. Public Indian institutions are characterized by higher prevalence of *C. auris* isolation than private hospitals, possibly connected to overcrowding and compromised infection control measures [15], with *C. auris* prevalence ranging from 5 to 30% of all candidemia cases in certain institutions [15, 24, 38, 44]. Recently, *C. auris* was found to be the second most prevalent species causing candidemia in a tertiary care trauma center in Delhi, India, warranting more effective infection control practices to prevent its spread [43]. Moreover, outbreaks of candidemia in Pakistan could be related to the interregional spread of the pathogen, as demonstrated by genomic sequencing of Indian and Pakistani isolates [41].

In US, the Center of Disease Control and Prevention (CDC) issued a clinical alert in June 2016 informing

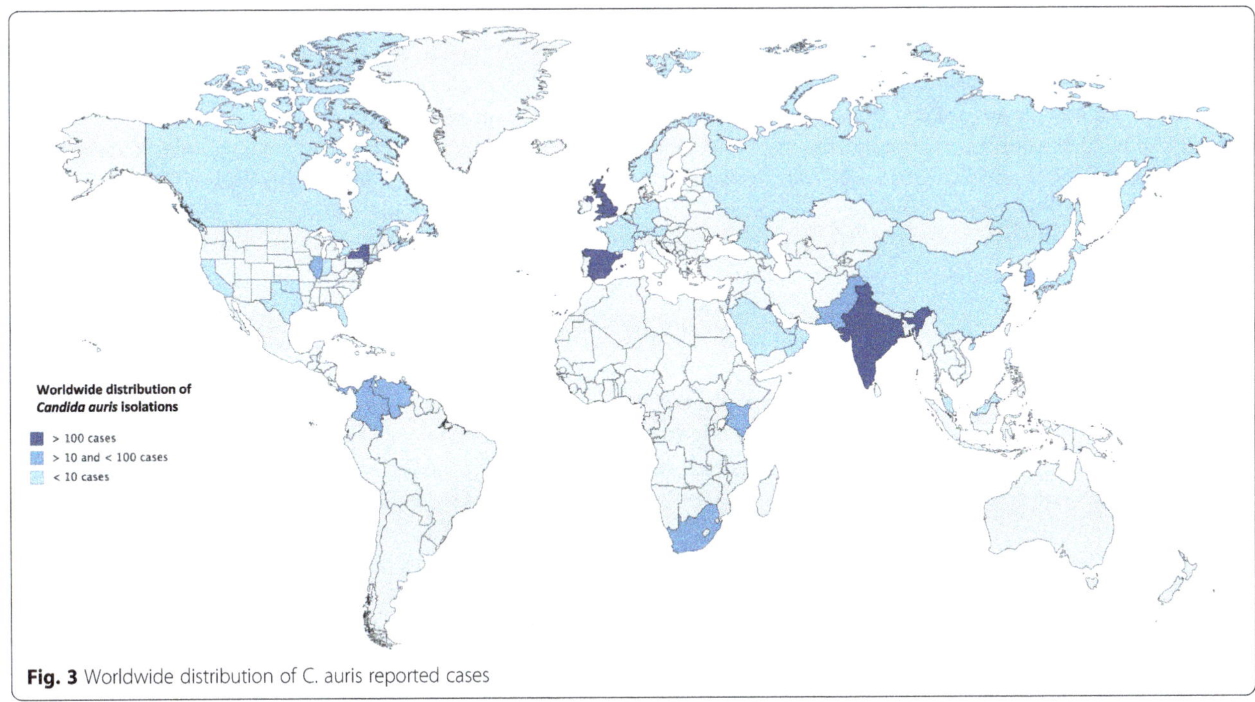

Fig. 3 Worldwide distribution of C. auris reported cases

clinicians, laboratories, infection control practitioners, and public health authorities about *C. auris*. It requested that all cases be adequately reported to authorities and to the CDC [71, 72]. This report describes the first seven US cases of *C. auris* infection occurring during May 2013 and August 2016. Six of seven cases were identified through retrospective review of microbiology records from reporting hospitals and reference laboratories [60]. As of May 2018, CDC recorded 311 confirmed and 29 probable cases of *C. auris* infection. Most *C. auris* isolates in the US have been detected in the New York City area and New Jersey (https://www.cdc.gov/fungal/diseases/candidiasis/tracking-c-auris.html). Available epidemiological information suggests that most strains of *C. auris* isolated in the United States were introduced from abroad. Isolates from Illinois and New York were of the same clade as those from South America and South Asia respectively [61]. However, it is not possible to exclude that most of these cases were acquired in the US following local transmission in healthcare settings [60].

Although imported cases have been demonstrated as in US healthcare outbreaks, one of the major questions regarding *C. auris* spread is whether it emerged independently in different countries or if a single outbreak spread from an original source [40]. Using WGS (whole genome sequencing) and SNP (single-nucleotide polymorphism) analysis together with epidemiological observation [25, 41], it was possible to demonstrate an independent and simultaneous emergence of different *C. auris* clonal populations on different geographical areas. Specifically, it was possible to identify the emergence of four different clades (East and South Asian, African, South American) in as many different regions. Transmission within the healthcare setting is suggested by the clonal relatedness of isolates in different institutions [24, 38, 40, 67].

Different reports have been published from South America. The first outbreak was reported in Venezuela between March 2012 and July 2013 [58]. All the isolates were initially identified as *C. haemulonii*. However, isolation of *C. auris* was later confirmed by genome sequencing. The Venezuelan outbreak resulted in *C. auris* being the sixth most common cause of candidemia in the involved institution. In Colombia, sporadic cases have been reported since 2012 [55–57]. Interestingly, an outbreak was reported in a pediatric intensive care unit in 2016, where five cases of invasive infections were identified. Shortly after, nine cases have been isolated in Panama, where patterns of resistance detected by both microdilution method were similar to those observed among *C. auris* isolates in Colombia [65].

In Africa, the first identification of sporadic cases and outbreaks were in South Africa and Kenya. The first four South African cases were isolated in 2012–2013 [46]. Other 10 isolates have been detected, demonstrating a close relation but phylogenetically distinct from Pakistan, India, and Venezuela [41]. Instead, according to other studies, isolates from South Africa had sequence similarity with those from UK [73]. *C. auris* has been considered as the most common pathogen responsible for candidemias in a reference hospital in Kenya, accounting for 45 (38%) episodes over a nearly 3-year period [49].

Only a single report of *C. auris* candidaemia has been published to date in Israel [17]. Collected strains were phylogenetically different from those from East Asia, Africa, and the Middle East, indicating an independent emergence of the pathogen. Infections have been reported in different Gulf States, including Kuwait [50], Oman [47, 48], and United Arab Emirates [52]. Recently, the first three cases in Saudi Arabia have been reported [53].

Clinical characteristics, risk factors, and outcome

In most cases, clinical presentation is non-specific and it is often difficult to differentiate between other types of systemic infections. Most of the reported cases in the last 5 years were isolated from blood and other deep-seated sites of infection (including invasive devices and catheters tips) [16]. Different clinical conditions including bloodstream infections, urinary tract infection, otitis, surgical wound infections, skin abscesses (related to insertion of the catheter), myocarditis, meningitis, bone infections, and wound infections have been related to *C. auris* [15, 18]. However, isolations from non-sterile body sites such as lungs, urinary tract, skin and soft tissue, and genital apparatus may more likely represent colonization rather than infections [18, 74]. As for other *Candida* spp., the presence of signs and symptoms of infections of the site where *C. auris* has been isolated from can help to differentiate between simple colonization and infection [4]. It is important to identify *C. auris* even from a non-sterile body site because colonization poses the risk of transmission, which requires implementation of infection control precautions [71, 72].

To investigate risk factors associated to *C. auris* infections, Rudramurthy et al. conducted a subgroup analysis and comparison of the clinical manifestations of *C. auris* and non-auris cases in 27 Indian ICUs [15]. In accordance with previous studies, risk factors were not different from those associated with invasive infection due to other *Candida* spp. [22], including prior or continuous exposure to broad-spectrum antibiotics and antifungal agents, diabetes mellitus, abdominal and vascular surgery, presence of central venous catheters, urinary catheterization, post-operative drain placement, chronic kidney disease, chemotherapy, blood transfusions, hemodialysis, total parenteral nutrition, immunosuppressive state [75] and neutropenia [45], and length of ICU stay [15, 18, 76]. The incidence of *C. auris* is significantly higher in patients with primary or acquired altered immune response, secondary to therapeutic management of hematologic malignancies, bone marrow transplantation, and other condition requiring immunosuppressive agents [60]. Interestingly, Azar et al. reported the first case of donor-derived transmission of *C. auris* in a lung transplant patient [75], highlighting several implications on microbiological surveillance before transplants.

The crude in-hospital mortality rate for *C. auris* candidemia is estimated to range from 30 to 72% [16, 26, 41, 44, 69]. Available data suggest that the vast majority of infections affects adults, with a propensity for critically ill patients in intensive care unit (ICU) settings. Pediatric patients have only been reported in Asia and South America [77]. A better outcome was seen in this population [42, 58, 77].

Infection prevention and control

The progressive increase of outbreaks and sporadic cases of *C. auris* infection emphasize the need for adequate prevention measures. According to reports of recent outbreaks, colonization is difficult to eradicate and it tends to persist for months [66, 69]. Prevention of outbreaks has to be based on the early recognition of sporadical cases, identification of reservoirs and prompt notification. Guidance has been released by international organizations such as Public Health England (PHE-UK) [78], the CDC [79], the ECDC [70], and the Center for Opportunistic Tropical and Hospital Infections (COTHI-South Africa) [80], with recommendations regarding the isolation of patients, contact precautions, and cleaning of equipment and environments in contact with affected patients. Prevention and infection control policies are empirical and mainly based on indications formulated for containment strategies for other multi-drug-resistant pathogens. Table 1 summarizes recommendations by the CDC and the ECDC for prevention and control of *C. auris* transmission.

Although the exact mode of transmission has to be identified, early evidence suggests that *C. auris* spread is mainly related to exposure to contaminated facilities and transmission from healthcare personnel. Persistent outbreaks have been associated with hand transmission and contamination of surfaces [61, 66, 81, 82]. However, the

Table 1 Key points for *C. auris* prevention and control by the European Centre for Diseases Prevention and Control (ECDC) and Centers for Disease Control and Prevention (CDC)

ECDC	CDC
Correct identification (MALDI-TOF; DNA sequencing of the D1/D2 domain); Clinicians and microbiologists alertness; Notification and retrospective case-finding	Correct identification (MALDI-TOF; molecular methods) Confirmed isolates of *C. auris* should be reported to local and state public health officials and to CDC
Good standard infection control measures (including environmental cleaning, reprocessing of medical devices and patient isolation) and prompt notification	Infection control measures: • Placing the patient with *C. auris* in a single-patient room and using contact precautions • Emphasizing adherence to hand hygiene • Cleaning and disinfecting the patient care environment (daily and terminal cleaning) with recommended products • Screening contacts of newly identified case patients to identify *C. auris* colonization
Early identification of carriers by using active surveillance cultures (sites considered for sampling include nose/throat, axilla, groin, rectum, insertion sites of venous catheters; clinical samples such as urine, feces, wound drain fluid, and respiratory specimens)	Screening should be performed to identify colonization among potentially epidemiologically linked patients, including: • Current roommates • Roommates at the current or other facilities in the prior month (even if they have been discharged from the facility) Screening for *C. auris* should be done using a composite swab of the patient's axilla and groin (sites of consistent colonization). Patients have also been found to be colonized with *C. auris* in nose, external ear canals, oropharynx, urine, wounds, and rectum.
Establish the source of the outbreak (epidemiological investigation, cross-sectional patient screening and environmental sampling); prevention of inter-hospital and cross-border transmission Enhanced control measures to contain outbreaks (such as contact precautions, single room isolation or patient cohorting, and dedicated nursing staff for colonized or infected patients)	All laboratories, especially laboratories serving healthcare facilities where cases of *C. auris* have been detected, should: • Review past microbiology records to identify cases of confirmed or suspected *C. auris* • Conduct prospective surveillance to identify *C. auris* cases in the future • Consider screening close contacts of patients with *C. auris* for presence of colonization
Education and practice audits (for healthcare workers and contacts)	Education of all healthcare personnel, including staff working with environmental cleaning services about *C. auris* and need for appropriate precautions; Monitor adherence to infection control practices
Antifungal stewardship	Antibiotic and antifungal stewardship

role of healthcare workers still remains difficult to determine. A recent study sampled patients and their contacts, healthcare workers, and environment in four hospitals in Colombia that had previously reported *C. auris* outbreaks, and found *C. auris* on different objects and facilities, such as bedrails, a bed hand-controller, a mobile phone, and floors. Interestingly, positive samples were collected from surfaces with infrequent patient contact but frequent healthcare workers contact (i.e., chairs, bed trays, and medical equipment), and from surfaces with little to no patient contact and infrequent healthcare workers contact (i.e., closet cabinets, door handles, alcohol gel dispensers) [83]. Thus, once *C. auris* is introduced in the hospital setting, environmental contamination evolves well beyond the patient bedside, resulting in recurrent cases of new colonizations.

C. auris is able to survive on a wide range of dry and moist surfaces, including plastic where the pathogen may reside for up to 14 days [84]. *C. auris* seems to be resistant to quaternary compounds disinfectants and cationic surface-active products. Disinfectants with sporicidal activity and hydrogen peroxide-based products are indicated to clean surfaces and healthcare facilities, resulting in highest reduction of *C. auris* colony-forming unit (CFU) [81, 85, 86]. Chlorine-based detergents, ultraviolet light, and hydrogen peroxide vapor demonstrated their efficacy in environmental decontamination procedures after patient discharge [61, 66, 87]. However, persistence of *C. auris* within the hospital environment despite disinfection procedures also suggests an involvement of the interaction between the pathogen and surfaces and the length of exposure to disinfectants [88].

In order to curb transmission, authorities recommend adherence to central and peripheral catheter care bundles, urinary catheter care bundle, and care of tracheostomy sites [78, 79]. If feasible, removal of central catheters or other invasive devices may resolve persistent candidemia and improve clinical outcome [58, 67]. Patients colonized or with proven or suspected *C. auris* infection should be kept in isolation under strict contact precautions until microbiological screening and diagnostic results are available [66]. Incoming patients from institutions where proven *C. auris* isolation has been determined should be screened [78]. Suggested screening sites are groin and axilla, urine, nose and throat, perineal and rectal swab or stool sample. Other high-risk sites may be of consideration, including wounds, cannula entry sites, endotracheal secretions, and drain fluids [70].

C. auris virulence factors

C. auris possesses virulence factors, such as germination, adherence, formation of biofilms, and production of phospholipases and proteinases [30]. Table 2 summarizes

Table 2 *C. auris* virulence and resistance factors

Virulence genes encoding for: Hemolysin, secreted aspartyl proteinases, secreted lipases, phosphatases, mannosyl transferases, phospholipase, integrins, adhesins, Zn(II) 2 cys 6 transcription factor (strain-specif degree of activity)
Resistance genes: Azoles resistance Transport proteins and efflux pumps (ATP-binding cassette *ABC*; major facilitator superfamilies *MFS*; upregulation of *CDR1*, *CDR2*, *MDR1*) *ERG 11* mutations (substitutions *Y132F*, *K143R*, and *F126T*) and *ERG 11* upregulation Echinocandin resistance *FKS1/2* (encoding echinocandin drug target 1,3-beta-glucan synthase)
Adherence to surfaces and plastic materials (e.g., catheters)
Biofilm formation
Cellular morphology (aggregating and non-aggregating forms)
Rudimentary pseudohyphae formation

C. auris virulence and resistance factors. Although compared to *C. albicans*, *C. auris* forms significantly reduced biofilms, nevertheless, it has the capacity to form adherent biofilm communities on a range of clinically important substrates. Larkin et al. studied 16 different *C. auris* isolates obtained from patients in Japan, India, South Korea, and Germany and characterized their morphology and virulence factors [30]. *C. auris* produces phospholipase and proteinase in a strain-dependent manner and exhibited a significantly reduced ability to adhere to catheter material as compared to that of *C. albicans*. Further, *C. auris* biofilms were mainly composed of yeast cells adhering to catheter material. In contrast, *C. albicans* showed a highly heterogeneous architecture of biofilms with yeast cells and hyphae embedded within the extracellular matrix [30]. Sherry et al. described the ability of *C. auris* to form antifungal-resistant biofilms, against all three main classes of antifungals [87]. These biofilms were shown to be resistant to chlorhexidine and hydrogen peroxide, displaying a less susceptible phenotype than *C. albicans* and *C. glabrata* [87, 89]. More recently, Kean et al. using a molecular approach investigated the genes that are important in causing the *C. auris* cells to be resistant within the biofilm [89]. Transcriptomic analysis of temporally developing *C. auris* biofilms was shown to exhibit phase- and antifungal class-dependent resistance profiles. Differential expression analysis demonstrated that 791 and 464 genes were upregulated in biofilm formation and planktonic cells, respectively, with a minimum twofold change. Notably, in the intermediate and mature stages of biofilm development, a number of genes encoding efflux pumps were upregulated, including ATP-binding cassette (*ABC*) and major facilitator superfamily (*MFS*) transporter suggesting efflux-mediated resistance in *C. auris* [89]. Previously, Ben-Ami et al. also reported significantly greater ABC-type efflux activity, as evidenced by Rhodamine 6G transport, among *C. auris* than *C. glabrata* isolates suggesting efflux-mediated intrinsic resistance of *C. auris* to azoles [17]. Virulence of *C. auris* and *C. haemulonii* has been recently compared with *C. glabrata* and *C. albicans* in an immunocompetent murine model of invasive infection. In this study, authors reported that virulence in *C. auris* appears to be similar to *C. albicans* and *C. glabrata*, suggesting that common gene sequences could play a pivotal role [23]. The whole genome data of the emerging multidrug resistant species and other related *Candida* revealed that *C. auris* shares some notable expansions of gene family described as related to virulence (including transporters and secreted lipases) in *C. albicans* and related pathogens [31]. The pathogenicity of *C. auris* compared to that of other common pathogenic yeast species in the invertebrate *Galleria mellonella* infection demonstrated strain-specific differences in the behavior of *C. auris* in *G. mellonella*, with the aggregate-forming isolates exhibiting significantly less pathogenicity than their non-aggregating counterparts. Importantly, the non-aggregating isolates exhibited pathogenicity comparable to that of *C. albicans* [29]. Finally, the ability of salt tolerance and cell clumping into large and difficult to disperse aggregates of *C. auris* can contribute to its resistance in the hospital environments. Despite the ability to possess the virulence factors, it is observed that the capacity of *C. auris* to express those is much weaker than that of other *Candida* spp., suggesting that this emerging species is not as virulent as the latter species [30, 87].

C. auris profile of antifungal resistance and their mechanisms

The ability of *C. auris* to develop resistance to multiple commonly used antifungal agents may be responsible for its high rates of mortality [76]. Antifungal susceptibility data published so far points out that some *C. auris* strains exhibit elevated minimum inhibitory concentration (MIC) for three major classes of antifungal drugs, i.e. azoles, polyenes, and echinocandins [41]. Table 3 shows *C. auris* MICs and tentative MICs breakpoint for the most common antifungal drugs.

C. auris is frequently resistant to fluconazole although isolates with low MICs against fluconazole (2–8 mg/L) have also been recorded in India and Colombia [57, 83, 90, 91]. Recently, reports have also documented high MICs to amphotericin B, voriconazole, and caspofungin. Antifungal susceptibility testing of 350 isolates of *C. auris* in 10 hospitals in India over an 8-year period showed that 90% of strains were resistant to fluconazole (MIC 32 to ≥ 64 mg/L), 2% to echinocandins (MIC ≥ 8 mg/L), 8% to amphotericin B (MIC ≥ 2 mg/L) and 2.3% to voriconazole (MIC 16 mg/L) [90]. In a recent report of *C. auris* candidemia in a tertiary care trauma center in Delhi, India, 45% of *C. auris* isolates exhibited low MICs of fluconazole [91]. Antifungal susceptibility testing of clinical blood isolates and isolates recovered from environmental and body swabs from hospitals in Colombia revealed that all isolates had low MICs to voriconazole, itraconazole, isavuconazole, and echinocandins [83]. The variable rates of azole resistance in different geographic regions suggest localized evolvement of resistance. Although, data underlying the molecular mechanisms related to resistance to common antifungal drug classes in *C. auris* is scarce, the following update is based on a few recent studies:

a) *Azole*

The resistance is mediated by point mutations in the lanosterol 14 α-demethylase (*ERG11*) gene. Substitutions *Y132F*, *K143R*, and *F126L* in the gene were detected. Moreover, *ERG11* gene expression can be increased five- to sevenfold in the presence of fluconazole [90]. This gene, in some strains, can be present in an increased copy number, suggesting that increased copy number may be a mechanism of drug resistance in *C. auris* [91].

Table 3 Minimum inhibitory concentration (MIC) range and tentative MIC breakpoints of *C. auris* for most common antifungal drugs. Data retrieved by Centers of Disease Control and Prevention (CDC) website—https://www.cdc.gov/fungal/candida-auris/recommendations.html

Drugs	MIC range (mcg/ml)	Tentative MIC breakpoints (mcg/ml)
Triazoles		
Fluconazole	0.12 to > 64	≥ 32
Voriconazole (and other 2° generation azoles)	0.032–16	N/A
Polyenes		
Amphotericine B	0.06–8	≥ 2
Echinocandins		
Anidulafungin	0.015–16	≥ 4
Caspofungin	0.03–16	≥ 2
Micafungin	0.015–8	≥ 4

Mutations in *ERG11* gene associated with the development of fluconazole resistance in *C. albicans* have been detected in a global collection of 54 *C. auris* isolates including amino-acid substitutions specific with geographic clades: *F126T* with South Africa, *Y132F* with Venezuela, and *Y132F* or *K143F* with India and Pakistan [41]. The *ERG11* sequences of Indian *C. auris* showed amino acid substitutions at position *Y132* and *K143* for strains that were resistant to fluconazole, whereas genotypes without substitution at these positions were observed in isolates with low MICs of fluconazole (MIC 1–2 mg/L) [90]. These results suggest that these substitutions would give a phenotype of fluconazole resistance. Specific *ERG11* substitutions in *C. albicans*, including *F126T*, *Y132F*, and *K143R*, are directly associated with resistance and have been shown to exhibit reduced susceptibilities to azoles upon heterologous expression in *S. cerevisiae* [92, 93].

Other mechanisms of azole resistance have been described in *C. albicans*, including upregulation of *ERG11* and upregulation of drug efflux pumps (e.g., *CDR1*, *CDR2*, *MDR1*) due to gain of function mutations in transcription factors (e.g., *TAC1*, *MRR1*) that induce their expression [94]. The orthologs of transporters from the ATP-binding cassette (*ABC*) and major facilitator superfamily (*MFS*) classes of efflux proteins have been reported in *C. auris*. Further, the overexpression of *CDR* genes members of the *ABC* family and *MDR1* member of the *MFS* transporters has been recorded in *C. auris* isolates. Also, a single copy of the multidrug efflux pump *MDR1* and 5–6 copy numbers of multidrug transporters such *CDR1*, *SNQ2*, and related genes have been identified in *C. auris* using WG sequence data [31], while the *TAC1* transcription factor that regulates expression of *CDR1* and *CDR2* is present in two copies in *C. auris* [31].

b) *Echinocandins*

Main mechanisms of echinocandins resistance are mutations in the *FKS1* gene encoding echinocandin drug target 1,3-beta-glucan synthase. *FKS1* gene analysis using *C. auris*-specific *FKS* primers in 38 Indian *C. auris* isolates showed that four *C. auris* isolates exhibited pan-echinocandin resistance (MICs > 8 mg/L). All four resistant isolates had *S639F* amino acid substitution equivalent to the mutation at position *S645* of the hot-spot 1 of *FKS1*, which is associated with resistance to echinocandins in *C. albicans* [90]. In contrast, in the remaining 34 *C. auris* isolates, wild-type phenotype was observed and the isolates exhibited low echinocandin MICs. Also, a single *C. auris* isolate resistant to both echinocandins and 5-flucytosine obtained from London Cardiothoracic outbreak was investigated for mutation analysis in the later study using *WGS* displayed *SNP*, causing a serine to tyrosine substitution (*S652Y*) in the *FKS1* gene [95]. A recent study highlighted the challenges with the antifungal susceptibility testing of *C. auris* with caspofungin, as *FKS1* wildtype isolates exhibited an Eagle effect (also known as the paradoxical growth effect). Resistance caused by *FKS1 S639F* in *C. auris* was further confirmed in vivo in the mouse model of invasive candidiasis [96]. All isolates were susceptible at a human therapeutic dose of caspofungin, except for those exhibiting the *S639F* aminoacid substitution. This result suggests that isolates demonstrating echinocandin resistance are characterized by mutations in *FKS1* and that routine caspofungin antifungal susceptibility testing by broth microdilution method for *C. auris* isolates should be cautiously applied or even avoided [96]. However, micafungin is the most potent echinocandin in MIC testing and susceptibility testing with micafungin or FKS1 sequence analysis would be better indicators for detection of echinocandin resistance in *C. auris* [96].

c) Amphotericin B

The underlying mechanism of amphotericin B resistance has not been investigated so far in *C. auris*. A recent study by Escandon et al. aimed to describe the overall molecular epidemiology and resistances among Colombian *C. auris* isolates. The authors found that despite *WSG* revealed that isolates are genetically related throughout the country, higher resistance rates to amphotericin B were identified in northern regions if compared to central Colombia. Moreover, resistance to amphotericin B has been found to be significantly associated to four newly identified non-synonymous mutations [83]. Furthermore, reported data on susceptibility tests demonstrated that commercial systems (Vitek AST-YS07) could also detect false elevated MICs of amphotericin B. Thus, a cautious approach is recommended for laboratories to perform antifungal susceptibility testing for this yeast [19].

Therapy: general concepts and new insights

Echinocandins are the first-line therapy for *C. auris* infection, given resistance to azoles and amphotericine B. As resistance to echinocandins has also been described, patients should undergo close follow-up and microbiological culture-based reassessment to detect therapeutic failure and eventual development of resistances. In cases of unresponsiveness to echinocandins, liposomial amphotericin B (as single or combination therapy with an echinocandin) should be prescribed [60, 61, 67, 75] and consultation with an infectious diseases expert is recommended. Furthermore, MICs of azoles, such as itraconazole, posaconazole, and isavuconazole, are low and these drugs show good in vitro activity, possibly explained by the absence of previous exposure of yeast isolates to these agents, or because of the different structure of the azole-target-protein [41].

Drug associations have already been used with success [60, 67]. Synergistic interactions may have a possible role, as demonstrated for micafungin and voriconazole association [23]. Considering the high prevalence and continuous spread of multi-drug resistant isolates of *C. auris*, there is the need to expand the classes of available antifungals. *SCY-078* showed growth inhibition and anti-biofilm activity against *C. auris* isolates, with activity against echinocandin-resistant strains. Moreover, this drug is not affected by common mutations in protein targets and is orally bioavailable [97]. Recently, Basso et al. described the antifungal properties of θ-defensins, 18-aminoacid macrocyclic peptides with potential applications for therapeutic treatment of systemic MDR infections, representing a template for the future development of new antifungals generation [98]. APX001 is a broad-spectrum antifungal agent for the treatment of invasive fungal infections, including species resistant to other antifungal drug classes, inhibiting an enzyme (*Gwt1*) part of the glycosylphosphatidylinositol (GPI) biosynthesis pathway [99]. Results of a study in a murine model of neutropenic disseminated candidiasis conducted by Zhao et al. may have potential relevance for clinical dose selection and breakpoints identification [100]. CD101 is a novel echinocandin with a prolonged half-life and an improved safety profile, allowing once weekly intravenous administration because of its enhanced pharmacokinetic properties [101]. In a recent study, Berkow et al. demonstrated an encouraging in vitro activity against most *C. auris* isolates, including strains resistant to other echinocandins [101].

Conclusions

Scientific community and clinicians are facing increasing incidence of antifungal resistance. Non-*albicans Candida* spp. infections are progressively emerging in hospitals and ICUs' settings. *C. auris* with high mortality rates, multi-drug resistance, environmental resilience, and horizontal transmission has become an issue in clinical practice. *C. auris* MDR strains may continue to emerge independently and simultaneously throughout the world in next few years. High level of knowledge and alertness by physicians and healthcare workers, especially in critical care settings, would help to control the spread and improve diagnostic and therapeutic strategies.

Abbreviations

ABC: ATP-binding cassette; AmB: Amphotericin B; BSI: Bloodstream infection; CDC: Center of Disease Control and Prevention; CFU: Colony-forming unit; COTHI-South Africa: Center for Opportunistic Tropical and Hospital Infections; ECDC: European Centre for Disease Prevention and Control; GPI: Glycosylphosphatidylinositol; ICU: Intensive care unit; MALDI-TOF: Matrix-assisted laser desorption/ionization time-of-flight; MDR: Multidrug resistant; MIC: Minimum inhibitory concentration; MRSA: Methicillin-resistant *Staphylococcus aureus*; PHE-UK: Public Health England; UK: United Kingdom; US: United States

Acknowledgements

None.

Funding

None.

Authors' contributions

AC, GM, TF, A Giammanco, A Giarratano, and A Chowdhary conceived the content and wrote the manuscript. All authors read and approved the final version of the manuscript.

Competing interests

The authors declare that they have no competing interests.

Author details

[1]Department of Surgical, Oncological and Oral Science (Di.Chir.On.S.). Section of Anesthesia, Analgesia, Intensive Care and Emergency. Policlinico Paolo Giaccone. University of Palermo, Italy, University of Palermo, Via del vespro 129, 90127 Palermo, Italy. [2]Department of Sciences for Health Promotion and Mother and Child Care, University of Palermo, Palermo, Italy. [3]Department of Medical Mycology, Vallabhbhai Patel Chest Institute, University of Delhi, Delhi, India.

References

1. Kullberg BJ, Arendrup MC. Invasive candidiasis. N Engl J Med. 2015;373: 1445–56.
2. Cortegiani A, Russotto V, Maggiore A, Attanasio M, Naro AR, Raineri SM, et al. Antifungal agents for preventing fungal infections in non-neutropenic critically ill patients. Cochrane Database Syst Rev. 2016;1:CD004920.
3. Cortegiani A, Russotto V, Giarratano A. Associations of antifungal treatments with prevention of fungal infection in critically ill patients without neutropenia. JAMA. 2017;317:311–2.
4. Pappas PG, Kauffman CA, Andes DR, Clancy CJ, Marr KA, Ostrosky-Zeichner L, et al. Clinical practice guideline for the management of candidiasis: 2016 update by the Infectious Diseases Society of America. Clin Infect Dis. 2016; 62:e1–50.
5. Cortegiani A, Russotto V, Raineri SM, Gregoretti C, De Rosa FG, Giarratano A. Untargeted antifungal treatment strategies for invasive candidiasis in non-neutropenic critically ill patients: current evidence and insights. Curr Fung Infect Rep. 2017;11:84–91.
6. Kett DH, Azoulay E, Echeverria PM, Vincent J-L. Candida bloodstream infections in intensive care units: analysis of the extended prevalence of infection in intensive care unit study. Crit Care Med. 2011;39:665–70.
7. Calandra T, Roberts JA, Antonelli M, Bassetti M, Vincent J-L. Diagnosis and management of invasive candidiasis in the ICU: an updated approach to an old enemy. Crit Care. 2016;20:125.
8. Bassetti M, Righi E, Ansaldi F, Merelli M, Scarparo C, Antonelli M, et al. A multicenter multinational study of abdominal candidiasis: epidemiology, outcomes and predictors of mortality. Intensive Care Med. 2015;41:1601–10.

9. Cortegiani A, Misseri G, Chowdhary A. What's new on emerging resistant Candida species. Intensive Care Med. 2018 Online First doi: https://doi.org/10.1007/s00134-018-5363-x.
10. Lepak AJ, Zhao M, Berkow EL, Lockhart SR, Andes DR. Pharmacodynamic optimization for treatment of invasive Candida auris infection. Antimicrob Agents Chemother. 2017;61:e00791–17.
11. Chowdhary A, Sharma C, Meis JF. Candida auris: a rapidly emerging cause of hospital-acquired multidrug-resistant fungal infections globally. PLoS Pathog. 2017;13:e1006290.
12. Alexander BD, Johnson MD, Pfeiffer CD, Jimenez-Ortigosa C, Catania J, Booker R, et al. Increasing echinocandin resistance in Candida glabrata: clinical failure correlates with presence of FKS mutations and elevated minimum inhibitory concentrations. Clin Infect Dis. 2013;56:1724–32.
13. Satoh K, Makimura K, Hasumi Y, Nishiyama Y, Uchida K, Yamaguchi H. Candida auris sp. nov., a novel ascomycetous yeast isolated from the external ear canal of an inpatient in a Japanese hospital. Microbiol Immunol. 2009;53:41–4.
14. Kim M-N, Shin JH, Sung H, Lee K, Kim E-C, Ryoo N, et al. Candida haemulonii and closely related species at 5 university hospitals in Korea: identification, antifungal susceptibility, and clinical features. Clin Infect Dis. 2009;48:e57–61.
15. Rudramurthy SM, Chakrabarti A, Paul RA, Sood P, Kaur H, Capoor MR, et al. Candida auris candidaemia in Indian ICUs: analysis of risk factors. J Antimicrob Chemother. 2017;72:1794–801.
16. Osei SJ. Candida auris: a systematic review and meta-analysis of current updates on an emerging multidrug-resistant pathogen. MicrobiologyOpen. 2018. https://doi.org/10.1002/mbo3.578.
17. Ben-Ami R, Berman J, Novikov A, Bash E, Shachor-Meyouhas Y, Zakin S, et al. Multidrug-resistant Candida haemulonii and C. auris, Tel Aviv, Israel. Emerg Infect Dis. 2017;23:195–203.
18. Chowdhary A, Voss A, Meis JF. Multidrug-resistant Candida auris: "new kid on the block" in hospital-associated infections? J Hosp Infect. 2016; 94:209–12.
19. Kathuria S, Singh PK, Sharma C, Prakash A, Masih A, Kumar A, et al. Multidrug-resistant Candida auris misidentified as Candida haemulonii: characterization by matrix-assisted laser desorption ionization-time of flight mass spectrometry and DNA sequencing and its antifungal susceptibility profile variability by Vitek 2, CLSI broth microdilution, and Etest method. J Clin Microbiol. 2015;53:1823–30.
20. Kim T-H, Kweon OJ, Kim HR, Lee M-K. Identification of uncommon Candida species using commercial identification systems. J Microbiol Biotechnol. 2016;26:2206–13.
21. Finn T, Novikov A, Zakin S, Bash E, Berman J, Ben-Ami R. Candida haemulonii and Candida auris: emerging multidrug-resistant species with distinct virulence and epidemiological characteristics. Open Forum Infect Dis. 2016;3:124.
22. Sarma S, Upadhyay S. Current perspective on emergence, diagnosis and drug resistance in Candida auris. Infect Drug Resist. 2017;10:155–65.
23. Fakhim H, Vaezi A, Dannaoui E, Chowdhary A, Nasiry D, Faeli L, et al. Comparative virulence of Candida auris with Candida haemulonii, Candida glabrata and Candida albicans in a murine model. Mycoses. 2018;61:377–82.
24. Chowdhary A, Anil Kumar V, Sharma C, Prakash A, Agarwal K, Babu R, et al. Multidrug-resistant endemic clonal strain of Candida auris in India. Eur J Clin Microbiol Infect Dis. 2014;33:919–26.
25. Sharma C, Kumar N, Pandey R, Meis JF, Chowdhary A. Whole genome sequencing of emerging multidrug resistant Candida auris isolates in India demonstrates low genetic variation. New Microbes New Infect. 2016;13:77–82.
26. Jeffery-Smith A, Taori SK, Schelenz S, Jeffery K, Johnson EM, Borman A, et al. Candida auris: a review of the literature. Clin Microbiol Rev. 2018; 31:e00029–17.
27. Bougnoux M-E, Brun S, Zahar J-R. Healthcare-associated fungal outbreaks: new and uncommon species, new molecular tools for investigation and prevention. Antimicrob Resist Infect Control. 2018;7:45.
28. Kohlenberg A, Struelens MJ, Monnet DL, Plachouras D. Candida auris: epidemiological situation, laboratory capacity and preparedness in European Union and European Economic Area countries, 2013 to 2017. Euro Surveill. 2018;23:18–00136.
29. Borman AM, Szekely A, Johnson EM. Comparative pathogenicity of United Kingdom isolates of the emerging pathogen Candida auris and other key pathogenic Candida species. mSphere. 2016;1:e00189–16.
30. Larkin E, Hager C, Chandra J, Mukherjee PK, Retuerto M, Salem I, et al. The emerging pathogen Candida auris: growth phenotype, virulence factors, activity of antifungals, and effect of SCY-078, a novel glucan synthesis inhibitor, on growth morphology and biofilm formation. Antimicrob Agents Chemother. 2017;61:e02396–16.
31. Munoz JF, Gade L, Chow NA, Loparev VN, Juieng P, Farrer RA, et al. Genomic basis of multidrug-resistance, mating, and virulence in Candida auris and related emerging species. bioRxiv. 2018:299917. https://doi.org/10.1101/299917.
32. Girard V, Mailler S, Chetry M, Vidal C, Durand G, van Belkum A, et al. Identification and typing of the emerging pathogen Candida auris by matrix-assisted laser desorption ionisation time of flight mass spectrometry. Mycoses. 2016;59:535–8.
33. Mizusawa M, Miller H, Green R, Lee R, Durante M, Perkins R, et al. Can multidrug-resistant Candida auris be reliably identified in clinical microbiology laboratories? J Clin Microbiol. 2017;55:638–40.
34. Wattal C, Oberoi JK, Goel N, Raveendran R, Khanna S. Matrix-assisted laser desorption ionization time of flight mass spectrometry (MALDI-TOF MS) for rapid identification of micro-organisms in the routine clinical microbiology laboratory. Eur J Clin Microbiol Infect Dis. 2017;36:807–12.
35. Prakash A, Sharma C, Singh A, Kumar Singh P, Kumar A, Hagen F, et al. Evidence of genotypic diversity among Candida auris isolates by multilocus sequence typing, matrix-assisted laser desorption ionization time-of-flight mass spectrometry and amplified fragment length polymorphism. Clin Microbiol Infect. 2016;22:277.e1–9.
36. Kordalewska M, Zhao Y, Lockhart SR, Chowdhary A, Berrio I, Perlin DS. Rapid and accurate molecular identification of the emerging multidrug-resistant pathogen Candida auris. J Clin Microbiol. 2017;55:2445–52.
37. Leach L, Zhu Y, Chaturvedi S. Development and validation of a real-time PCR assay for rapid detection of Candida auris from surveillance samples. J Clin Microbiol. 2018;56:e01223–17.
38. Chowdhary A, Sharma C, Duggal S, Agarwal K, Prakash A, Singh PK, et al. New clonal strain of Candida auris, Delhi, India. Emerg Infect Dis. 2013;19: 1670–3.
39. Chatterjee S, Alampalli SV, Nageshan RK, Chettiar ST, Joshi S, Tatu US. Draft genome of a commonly misdiagnosed multidrug resistant pathogen Candida auris. BMC Genomics. 2015;16:686.
40. Lockhart SR, Berkow EL, Chow N, Welsh RM. Candida auris for the clinical microbiology laboratory: not your grandfather's Candida species. Clin Microbiol Newsl. 2017;39:99–103.
41. Lockhart SR, Etienne KA, Vallabhaneni S, Farooqi J, Chowdhary A, Govender NP, et al. Simultaneous emergence of multidrug-resistant Candida auris on 3 continents confirmed by whole-genome sequencing and epidemiological analyses. Clin Infect Dis. 2017;64:134–40.
42. Lee WG, Shin JH, Uh Y, Kang MG, Kim SH, Park KH, et al. First three reported cases of nosocomial fungemia caused by Candida auris. J Clin Microbiol. 2011;49:3139–42.
43. Oh BJ, Shin JH, Kim M-N, Sung H, Lee K, Joo MY, et al. Biofilm formation and genotyping of Candida haemulonii, Candida pseudohaemulonii, and a proposed new species (Candida auris) isolates from Korea. Med Mycol. 2011; 49:98–102.
44. Chakrabarti A, Sood P, Rudramurthy SM, Chen S, Kaur H, Capoor M, et al. Incidence, characteristics and outcome of ICU-acquired candidemia in India. Intensive Care Med. 2015;41:285–95.
45. Mohd Tap R, Lim TC, Kamarudin NA, Ginsapu SJ, Abd Razak MF, Ahmad N, et al. A fatal case of Candida auris and Candida tropicalis Candidemia in neutropenic patient. Mycopathologia. 2018;183:559–64.
46. Magobo RE, Corcoran C, Seetharam S, Govender N, Naicker S. Candida auris: an emerging, azole-resistant pathogen causing candidemia in South Africa. Int J Infect Dis. 2014;21:215. https://doi.org/10.1016/j.ijid.2014.03.869.
47. Mohsin J, Hagen F, Al-Balushi ZAM, de Hoog GS, Chowdhary A, Meis JF, et al. The first cases of Candida auris candidaemia in Oman. Mycoses. 2017;60: 569–75.
48. Al-Siyabi T, Busaidi Al I, Balkhair A, Al-Muharrmi Z, Al-Salti M, Al'Adawi B. First report of Candida auris in Oman: clinical and microbiological description of five candidemia cases. J Inf Secur. 2017;75:373–6.
49. Okinda N, Kagotho E, Castanheira M, Njuguna A, Omuse G, Makau P. P0065 Candidemia at a referral hospital in sub-Saharan Africa: emergence of Candida auris as a major pathogen. 2014. 24th ECCMID.
50. Emara M, Ahmad S, Khan Z, Joseph L, Al-Obaid I, Purohit P, et al. Candida auris candidemia in Kuwait, 2014. Emerg Infect Dis. 2015;21:1091–2.

51. Belkin A, Gazit Z, Keller N, Ben-Ami R, Wieder-Finesod A, Novikov A, et al. Candida auris infection leading to nosocomial transmission, Israel, 2017. Emerg Infect Dis. 2018;24:801.
52. Alatoom A, Sartawi M, Lawlor K, AbdelWareth L, Thomsen J, Nusair A, et al. Persistent candidemia despite appropriate fungal therapy: first case of Candida auris from the United Arab Emirates. Int J Infect Dis. 2018;70:36–7.
53. Abdalhamid B, Almaghrabi R, Althawadi S, Omrani A. First report of Candida auris infections from Saudi Arabia. J Infect Public Health. 2018;11:598–9.
54. Wang X, Bing J, Zheng Q, Zhang F, Liu J, Yue H, et al. The first isolate of Candida auris in China: clinical and biological aspects. Emerg Microbes Infect. 2018;7:93.
55. Parra-Giraldo CM, Valderrama SL, Cortes-Fraile G, Garzon JR, Ariza BE, Morio F, et al. First report of sporadic cases of Candida auris in Colombia. Int J Infect Dis. 2018;69:63–7.
56. Morales-Lopez SE, Parra-Giraldo CM, Ceballos-Garzon A, Martinez HP, Rodriguez GJ, Alvarez-Moreno CA, et al. Invasive infections with multidrug-resistant yeast Candida auris, Colombia. Emerg Infect Dis. 2017;23:162–4.
57. Escandón P. Notes from the field: surveillance for Candida auris—Colombia, September 2016–May 2017. MMWR Morb Mortal Wkly Rep. 2018;67:459–60.
58. Calvo B, Melo ASA, Perozo-Mena A, Hernandez M, Francisco EC, Hagen F, et al. First report of Candida auris in America: clinical and microbiological aspects of 18 episodes of candidemia. J Inf Secur. 2016;73:369–74.
59. McCarthy M. Hospital transmitted Candida auris infections confirmed in the US. BMJ. 2016;355:i5978.
60. Vallabhaneni S, Kallen A, Tsay S, Chow N, Welsh R, Kerins J, et al. Investigation of the first seven reported cases of Candida auris, a globally emerging invasive, multidrug-resistant fungus-United States, May 2013-August 2016. Am J Transplant. 2017;17:296–9.
61. Tsay S, Welsh RM, Adams EH, Chow NA, Gade L, Berkow EL, et al. Notes from the field: ongoing transmission of Candida auris in health care facilities - United States, June 2016-May 2017. MMWR Morb Mortal Wkly Rep. 2017; 66:514–5.
62. Vasilyeva N, Kruglov A, Pchelin I, Riabinin I, Raush E, Chilina G, et al. P0311 the first Russian case of candidaemia due to Candida auris. 2018. 28th ECCMID.
63. Schwartz IS, Hammond GW. First reported case of multidrug-resistant Candida auris in Canada. Can Commun Dis Rep. 2017;43:150.
64. Ramos R, Caceres DH, Perez M, Garcia N, Castillo W, Santiago E, et al. Emerging multidrug-resistant Candida duobushaemulonii infections in Panama hospitals: importance of laboratory surveillance and accurate identification. J Clin Microbiol. 2018;56:e00371–18.
65. Arauz AB, Caceres DH, Santiago E, Armstrong P, Arosemena S, Ramos C, et al. Isolation of Candida auris from 9 patients in Central America: importance of accurate diagnosis and susceptibility testing. Mycoses. 2018;61:44–7.
66. Schelenz S, Hagen F, Rhodes JL, Abdolrasouli A, Chowdhary A, Hall A, et al. First hospital outbreak of the globally emerging Candida auris in a European hospital. Antimicrob Resist Infect Control. 2016;5:35.
67. Ruiz Gaitan AC, Moret A, Lopez Hontangas JL, Molina JM, Aleixandre Lopez AI, Cabezas AH, et al. Nosocomial fungemia by Candida auris: first four reported cases in continental Europe. Rev Iberoam Micol. 2017;34:23–7.
68. Riat A, Neofytos D, Coste A, Harbarth S, Bizzini A, Grandbastien B, et al. First case of Candida auris in Switzerland: discussion about preventive strategies. Swiss Med Wkly. 2018;148:w14622.
69. Ruiz-Gaitan A, Moret AM, Tasias-Pitarch M, Aleixandre-Lopez AI, Martinez-Morel H, Calabuig E, et al. An outbreak due to Candida auris with prolonged colonisation and candidaemia in a tertiary care European hospital. Mycoses. 2018;61:498–505.
70. https://ecdc.europa.eu/en/publications-data/rapid-risk-assessment-candida-auris-healthcare-settings-europe. Accessed 22 July 2018.
71. https://www.cdc.gov/fungal/diseases/candidiasis/c-auris-alert-09-17.html. Accessed 22 July 2018.
72. https://www.cdc.gov/fungal/diseases/candidiasis/candida-auris-alert.html. Accessed 22 July 2018.
73. Borman AM, Szekely A, Johnson EM. Isolates of the emerging pathogen Candida auris present in the UK have several geographic origins. Med Mycol. 2017;55:563–7.
74. Kumar D, Banerjee T, Pratap CB, Tilak R. Itraconazole-resistant Candida auris with phospholipase, proteinase and hemolysin activity from a case of vulvovaginitis. J Infect Dev Ctries. 2015;9:435–7.
75. Azar MM, Turbett SE, Fishman JA, Pierce VM. Donor-derived transmission of Candida auris during lung transplantation. Clin Infect Dis. 2017;65:1040–2.
76. Navalkele BD, Revankar S, Chandrasekar P. Candida auris: a worrisome, globally emerging pathogen. Expert Rev Anti-Infect Ther. 2017;15:819–27.
77. Warris A. Candida auris, what do paediatricians need to know? Arch Dis Child. 2018. https://doi.org/10.1136/ archdischild-2017-313960.
78. https://www.gov.uk/government/publications/candida-auris-laboratory-investigation-management-and-infection-prevention-and-control. Accessed 16 July 2018.
79. https://www.cdc.gov/fungal/candida-auris/recommendations.html. Accessed 22 July 2018.
80. http://www.nicd.ac.za/index.php/interim-guidance-for-the-management-of-candida-auris-infections-in-south-african-hospitals/. Accessed 22 July 2018.
81. Biswal M, Rudramurthy SM, Jain N, Shamanth AS, Sharma D, Jain K, et al. Controlling a possible outbreak of Candida auris infection: lessons learnt from multiple interventions. J Hosp Infect. 2017;97:363–70.
82. Eyre D, Sheppard A, Madder H, Moir I, Moroney R, Quan TP, et al. O0172 Epidemiology and successful control of a Candida auris outbreak in a UK intensive care unit driven by multi-use patient monitoring equipment. 2018. 28th ECCMID.
83. Escandón P, Chow NA, Caceres DH, Gade L, Berkow EL, Armstrong P, et al. Molecular epidemiology of Candida auris in Colombia reveals a highly-related, country-wide colonization with regional patterns in amphotericin B resistance. Clin Infect Dis. 2018. https://doi.org/10.1093/cid/ciy411.
84. Welsh RM, Bentz ML, Shams A, Houston H, Lyons A, Rose LJ, et al. Survival, persistence, and isolation of the emerging multidrug-resistant pathogenic yeast Candida auris on a plastic health care surface. J Clin Microbiol. 2017; 55:2996–3005.
85. Cadnum JL, Shaikh AA, Piedrahita CT, Sankar T, Jencson AL, Larkin EL, et al. Effectiveness of disinfectants against Candida auris and other Candida species. Infect Control Hosp Epidemiol. 2017;38:1240–3.
86. Ku TSN, Walraven CJ, Lee SA. Candida auris: disinfectants and implications for infection control. Front Microbiol. 2018;9:726.
87. Sherry L, Ramage G, Kean R, Borman A, Johnson EM, Richardson MD, et al. Biofilm-forming capability of highly virulent, multidrug-resistant Candida auris. Emerg Infect Dis. 2017;23:328–31.
88. Kean R, Sherry L, Townsend E, McKloud E, Short B, Akinbobola A, et al. Surface disinfection challenges for Candida auris: an in-vitro study. J Hosp Infect. 2018;98:433–6.
89. Kean R, McKloud E, Townsend EM, Sherry L, Delaney C, Jones BL, et al. The comparative efficacy of antiseptics against Candida auris biofilms. Int J Antimicrob Agents. 2018. https://doi.org/10.1016/j.ijantimicag.2018.05.007.
90. Chowdhary A, Prakash A, Sharma C, Kordalewska M, Kumar A, Sarma S, et al. A multicentre study of antifungal susceptibility patterns among 350 Candida auris isolates (2009-17) in India: role of the ERG11 and FKS1 genes in azole and echinocandin resistance. J Antimicrob Chemother. 2018;73:891–9.
91. Mathur P, Hasan F, Singh PK, Malhotra R, Walia K, Chowdhary A. Five-year profile of candidemia at an Indian trauma center: high rates of Candida auris blood stream infections. Mycoses. 2018. https://doi.org/10.1111/myc.12790.
92. Morio F, Loge C, Besse B, Hennequin C, Le Pape P. Screening for amino acid substitutions in the Candida albicans Erg11 protein of azole-susceptible and azole-resistant clinical isolates: new substitutions and a review of the literature. Diagn Microbiol Infect Dis. 2010;66:373–84.
93. Xiang M-J, Liu J-Y, Ni P-H, Wang S, Shi C, Wei B, et al. Erg11 mutations associated with azole resistance in clinical isolates of Candida albicans. FEMS Yeast Res. 2013;13:386–93.
94. Cowen LE, Sanglard D, Howard SJ, Rogers PD, Perlin DS. Mechanisms of antifungal drug resistance. Cold Spring Harb Perspect Med. 2014;5:a019752.
95. Rhodes J, Abdolrasouli A, Farrer RA, Cuomo CA, Aanensen DM, Armstrong-James D, et al. Genomic epidemiology of the UK outbreak of the emerging human fungal pathogen Candida auris. Emerg Microbes Infect. 2018;7:43.
96. Kordalewska M, Lee A, Park S, Berrio I, Chowdhary A, Zhao Y, et al. Understanding echinocandin resistance in the emerging pathogen Candida auris. Antimicrob Agents Chemother. 2018;62:e00238–18.
97. Berkow EL, Angulo D, Lockhart SR. In vitro activity of a novel glucan synthase inhibitor, SCY-078, against clinical isolates of Candida auris. Antimicrob Agents Chemother. 2017;61:e00435–17.
98. Basso V, Garcia A, Tran DQ, Schaal JB, Tran P, Ngole D, et al. Fungicidal potency and mechanisms of theta-Defensins against multidrug-resistant Candida species. Antimicrob Agents Chemother. 2018;62:e00111–8.
99. Hager CL, Larkin EL, Long L, Zohra Abidi F, Shaw KJ, Ghannoum MA. In vitro and in vivo evaluation of the antifungal activity of APX001A/APX001 against Candida auris. Antimicrob Agents Chemother. 2018;62:e02319–7.

100. Zhao M, Lepak AJ, VanScoy B, Bader JC, Marchillo K, Vanhecker J, et al. In vivo pharmacokinetics and pharmacodynamics of APX001 against Candida in a neutropenic disseminated candidiasis mouse model. Antimicrob Agents Chemother. 2018;62:e02542–17.
101. Berkow EL, Lockhart SR. Activity of CD101, a long-acting echinocandin, against clinical isolates of Candida auris. Diagn Microbiol Infect Dis. 2018;90:196–7.

24

Transient hyperlactatemia during intravenous administration of glycerol

Shinshu Katayama*, Ken Tonai, Yuya Goto, Kansuke Koyama, Toshitaka Koinuma, Jun Shima, Masahiko Wada and Shin Nunomiya

Abstract

Background: Intravenous glycerol treatment, usually administered in the form of a 5% fructose solution, can be used to reduce intracranial pressure. The administered fructose theoretically influences blood lactate levels, although little is known regarding whether intravenous glycerol treatment causes transient hyperlactatemia. This study aimed to evaluate blood lactate levels in patients who received intravenous glycerol or mannitol.

Methods: This single-center prospective observational study was performed at a 14-bed general intensive care unit between August 2016 and January 2018. Patients were excluded if they were < 20 years old or had pre-existing hyperlactatemia (blood lactate > 2.0 mmol/L). The included patients received intravenous glycerol or mannitol to reduce intracranial pressure and provided blood samples for lactate testing before and after the drug infusion (before the infusion and after 15 min, 30 min, 45 min, 60 min, 90 min, 120 min, and 150 min).

Results: Among the 33 included patients, 13 patients received 200 mL of glycerol over 30 min, 13 patients received 200 mL of glycerol over 60 min, and 7 patients received 300 mL of mannitol over 60 min. Both groups of patients who received glycerol had significantly higher lactate levels than the mannitol group (2.8 mmol/L vs. 2.2 mmol/L vs. 1.6 mmol/L, $P < 0.0001$), with the magnitude of the increase in lactate levels corresponding to the glycerol infusion time. There were no significant inter-group differences in cardiac index, stroke volume, or stroke volume variation. In the group that received the 30-min glycerol infusion, blood lactate levels did not return to the normal range until after 120 min.

Conclusions: Intravenous administration of glycerol leads to higher blood lactate levels that persist for up to 120 min. Although hyperlactatemia is an essential indicator of sepsis and/or impaired tissue perfusion, physicians should be aware of this phenomenon when assessing the blood lactate levels.

Keywords: Glycerol, Hyperlactatemia, Intensive care unit, Mannitol

Background

Lactate is a sensitive indicator of tissue perfusion and metabolism that helps quantify the balance between aerobic and anaerobic metabolism [1–3]. In addition, lactate is correlated with intravascular volume and sepsis status and is associated with circulatory shock severity [4–6]. In this context, lactate levels of > 2.0 mmol/L are included in the Sepsis-3 criteria for septic shock [7], and lactate level measurements are widely recognized as important in the critical care setting. In clinical practice, it is recommended that attempts be made to increase cardiac output using fluid resuscitation or inotropes, which is called lactate-guided resuscitation [8–11].

Intravenous glycerol treatment can be used to reduce intracranial pressure and is usually administered in the form of a 5% fructose solution with concentrated glycerin. Despite low-quality evidence of the efficacy [12, 13], glycerol is widely used in Japan for patients with acute stroke

* Correspondence: shinsyu_k@jichi.ac.jp
Division of Intensive Care, Department of Anesthesiology and Intensive Care Medicine, Jichi Medical University School of Medicine, 3311-1, Yakushiji, Shimotsuke, Tochigi 329-0498, Japan

or brain trauma, without significant side effects [14]. Although children with some congenital metabolic diseases experience hyperlactatemia (i.e., congenital glycerin metabolic disorders), little is known about intravenous glycerol-induced hyperlactatemia [15]. However, fructose can theoretically influence lactate metabolism [16, 17], and lactate levels might change during the administration of glycerol, which could lead to a misdiagnosis or overestimation of disease severity. Therefore, the present study evaluated the blood lactate levels in patients who received intravenous glycerol or mannitol and whether the rate of the intravenous glycerol infusion influenced blood lactate concentrations.

Methods

This single-center, prospective, observational study was performed at a 14-bed general intensive care unit in a university hospital (Tochigi, Japan). The study protocol was approved by the institutional ethics committee of Jichi Medical University Hospital (16-120). Written informed consent was obtained from the participants or their nearest relatives.

Participants

This study included patients who were admitted to the intensive care unit and received intracranial pressure-reducing therapy using intravenous glycerol or mannitol between August 2016 and January 2018. Patients were excluded if they were < 20 years old, had an end-stage renal failure and were receiving chronic dialysis, had hepatic dysfunction, or had abnormal lactate levels (> 2.0 mmol/L) before starting the intracranial pressure-reducing therapy.

Administration of glycerol or mannitol

The intravenous glycerol (GLYCEREB®; Terumo, Japan) was administered at a volume of 200 mL over 30 min or 60 min. The intravenous mannitol (20% MANNITOL INJECTION®; Yoshindo, Japan) was administered at a volume of 300 mL over 60 min. The selection of the drug and infusion rate was made by the attending physician.

Lactate measurement

Blood samples were obtained for lactate measurements at eight time points (before the infusion and after 15 min, 30 min, 45 min, 60 min, 90 min, 120 min, and 150 min) and were immediately transferred to the laboratory for testing. The blood gas analyses, which included lactate measurements, were performed using an ABL800 FLEX device (Radiometer Medical ApS, Denmark) or a RAPIDLAB1265 device (Siemens Healthcare Diagnostics Inc., Tarrytown, NY, USA).

Data collection

The following information was collected for all patients: age, sex, body weight, body height, present disease, Acute Physiology and Chronic Health Evaluation II (APACHE II) score [18], and Sequential Organ Failure Assessment (SOFA) score [19]. We also recorded data regarding the requirement for mechanical ventilation and the 28-day survival status. A FloTrac device (version 1.5, Edwards LifeSciences, Irvine, USA) was used to measure cardiac index (CI), stroke volume index (SVI), and stroke volume variation (SVV).

Statistical analysis

Variables were compared among these groups using Pearson's chi-square test, the Kruskal-Wallis test, or the Steel-Dwass test as appropriate. All analyses were performed using JMP software (version 13; SAS Institute Inc., Cary, NC, USA). Data were presented as median and interquartile range or as number and percentage. Differences were considered statistically significant at P values of < 0.05.

Results

Enrollment and baseline characteristics

During the study period, 37 patients were enrolled and 4 patients were excluded based on the pre-existing high lactate levels (> 2.0 mmol/L). The characteristics of the 33 included patients are summarized in Table 1. Thirteen patients received 200 mL of glycerol over 30 min, 13 patients received 200 mL of glycerol over 60 min, and 7 patients received 300 mL of mannitol over 60 min. Although the groups' APACHE II and SOFA scores were not significantly different, the group that received a 30-min glycerol infusion had a significantly lower 28-day survival rate compared to the other two groups (69.2% vs. 100% vs. 100%; $P = 0.03$). Table 2 shows the laboratory findings from before the start of the infusions, with no evidence of significant inter-group differences. There were no significant differences in parameters of hepatic function between the groups.

Comparing the groups that received glycerol or mannitol

Both groups of patients who received glycerol had significantly higher lactate levels than the mannitol group (2.8 mmol/L vs. 2.2 mmol/L vs. 1.6 mmol/L, respectively; $P < 0.0001$), with the magnitude of the increase in lactate levels corresponding to the glycerol infusion time. Compared to the mannitol group, the 30-min glycerol group had significantly higher lactate levels at all measured time points between 15 and 120 min, and all of these patients had high lactate levels (> 2.0 mmol/L) during the infusions. The 60-min glycerol group had significantly higher lactate levels at the 45-min and 60-min measurements, relative to the mannitol group, and 9 patients (69.2%) in the 60-min glycerol group

Table 1 Patient characteristics

	Glycerol 200 mL/30 min $n = 13$	Glycerol 200 mL/60 min $n = 13$	Mannitol 300 mL/60 min $n = 7$	*P* value
Age, years	57 (47–66)	46 (38–69)	58 (45–62)	0.592
Male, sex	6 (46.1%)	5 (38.5%)	4 (57.2%)	0.724
Height, cm	161 (154–166)	155 (154–164)	170 (155–170)	0.229
Body weight, kg	60 (51–65)	60 (55–69)	62 (54–67)	0.731
Body mass index, kg/m^2	23.9 (19.4–25.7)	25.0 (21.2–26.9)	21.7 (21.1–27.9)	0.573
Diseases, %				0.426
Brain tumor	7.7%	23.1%	0.0%	
Intracranial hemorrhage	15.4%	23.1%	14.3%	
Sub-arachnoid hemorrhage	23.1%	7.7%	42.9%	
Cerebral infarction	38.5%	38.5%	28.6%	
Traumatic brain injury	0.0%	7.7%	14.3%	
Other	15.4%	0.0%	0.0%	
IHD	7.7%	0.0%	0.0%	0.452
CHF	0.0%	15.4%	0.0%	0.194
Atrial fibrillation	15.4%	15.4%	0.0%	0.542
Diabetes mellitus	15.4%	23.1%	14.3%	0.840
Hypertension	30.8%	23.1%	42.9%	0.655
APACHE II	19 (13–22)	16 (13–28)	18 (11–22)	0.858
28-day survival, %	69.2%	100.0%	100.0%	0.030

APACHE II Acute Physiology and Chronic Health Evaluation II score, *CHF* chronic heart failure, *IHD* ischemic heart disease

had high lactate levels during the infusions. None of the patients in the mannitol group had high lactate levels during the infusions (100% vs. 69.2% vs. 0.0%, respectively; $P < 0.0001$) (Fig. 1). None of the patients exhibited signs of intravenous hemolysis.

Hemodynamics and blood gas analyses

During the glycerol or mannitol treatment, no significant inter-group differences were observed in terms of CI, SVI, SVV, pH, or HCO_3^- levels (Figs. 2 and 3).

Table 2 Laboratory findings immediately before the administration of intracranial pressure-reducing agents

	Glycerol 200 mL/30 min	Glycerol 200 mL/60 min	Mannitol 300 mL/60 min	*P* value
WBC, 10^9/L	12.5 (10.2–14.7)	10.1 (9.1–12.2)	1.4 (8.1–13.4)	0.228
Hb, g/dL	9.5 (8.6–11.3)	8.2 (7.8–10.4)	9.4 (8.9–10.0)	0.256
CRP, mg/dL	8.1 (3.8–14.5)	5.7 (0.7–9.5)	5.1 (2.7–9.5)	0.271
Alb, g/dL	2.3 (2.1–2.7)	2.6 (2.3–3.2)	3.0 (2.5–3.4)	0.143
BUN, mg/dL	10 (9–13)	12 (8–19)	14 (10–16)	0.502
Creatinine, mg/dL	0.67 (0.49–0.87)	0.51 (0.43–1.11)	0.61 (0.50–0.97)	0.790
T-Bil, mg/dL	0.75 (0.47–1.08)	0.95 (0.56–1.68)	1.01 (0.67–1.24)	0.420
AST, U/L	28 (18–48)	26 (21–37)	29 (23–83)	0.634
ALT, U/L	18 (13–37)	19 (14–43)	20 (15–57)	0.699
LDH, U/L	249 (182–328)	231 (166–269)	216 (182–246)	0.530
P, mg/dL	2.6 (2.0–2.8)	2.8 (1.9–3.3)	2.7 (2.2–3.1)	0.828
ChE, U/L	205 (155–234)	139 (115–185)	195 (79–232)	0.211
SOFA	3 (2–5)	6 (3–7)	3 (3–4)	0.182
Mechanical ventilation	46.1%	76.9%	71.4%	0.235

Alb albumin, *ALT* alanine aminotransaminase, *AST* aspartate transaminase, *BUN* blood urea nitrogen, *ChE* choline esterase, *CRP* C-reactive protein, *Hb* hemoglobin, *LDH* lactate dehydrogenase, *P* phosphate, *SOFA* Sequential Organ Failure Assessment, *T-bil* total bilirubin, *WBC* white blood cells

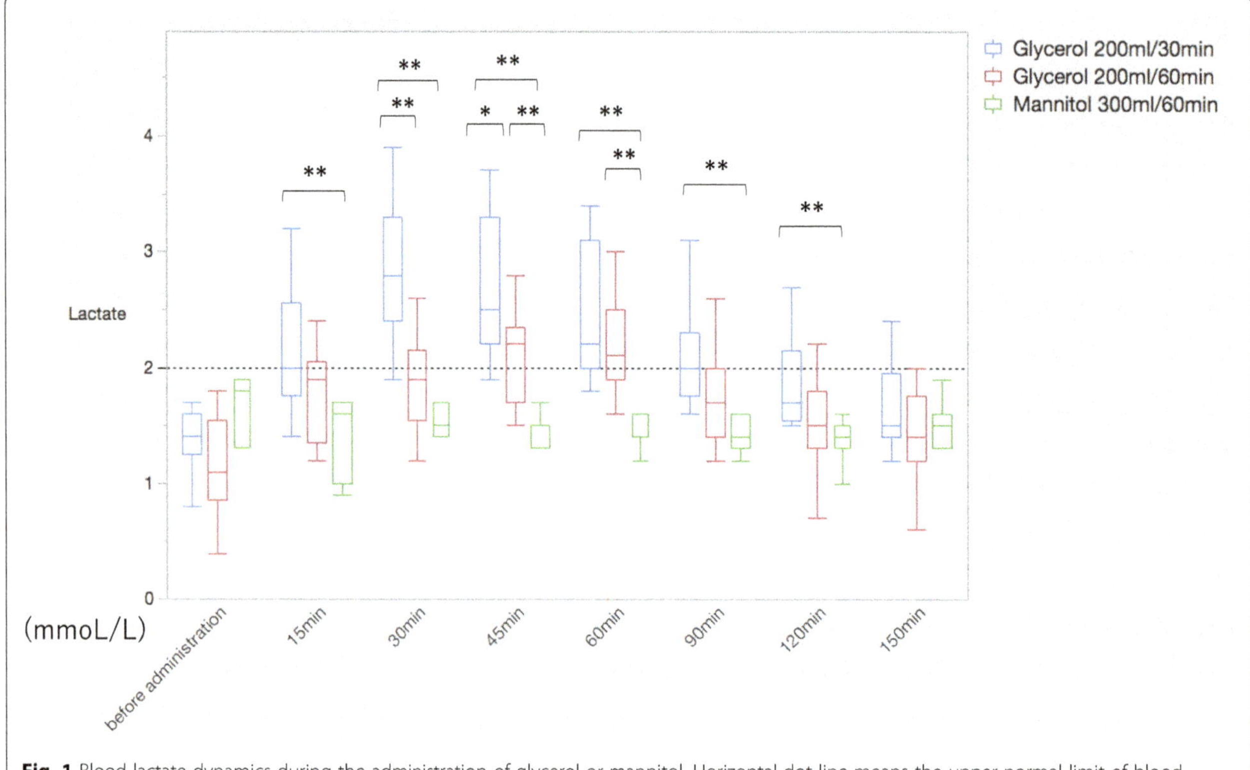

Fig. 1 Blood lactate dynamics during the administration of glycerol or mannitol. Horizontal dot line means the upper normal limit of blood lactate level. *$P < 0.05$, **$P < 0.01$

Discussion

The present study revealed that intravenous glycerol treatment increased the lactate levels in all patients, and 84.6% of these patients developed lactate levels of > 2.0 mmol/L. This study also revealed that lactate levels differed significantly according to the duration of glycerol infusion. However, intravenous mannitol treatment did not influence the lactate levels, and there were no inter-group differences in cardiac output and stroke volume parameters. Therefore, the effects of osmotic diuresis seem unrelated to the increased lactate levels.

Hyperlactatemia during glycerol administration is caused by the fructose that is added to the glycerol solution. Intravenously administered fructose is metabolized by the liver and converted by fructokinase into fructose-1-phosphate, which then enters the glycolytic or gluconeogenesis cycle before being metabolized into lactate, glucose, or glycogen. Fructokinase activity remains unchanged in a state of insulin deficiency, and fructose is quickly metabolized, which causes pyruvate accumulation. This occurs even in the presence of reduced glucose tolerance because fructose metabolism does not involve glucokinase or phosphofructokinase, which has decreased the activities in an insulin-deficient state. Furthermore, metabolism of fructose into pyruvate in the liver is rapid enough to cause significant accumulation of un-metabolized pyruvate by the tricarboxylic acid cycle, which causes hyperlactatemia. Approximately 30% of the administered fructose is converted into glucose [17], with the intravenous fructose stimulating splanchnic lactate release both at rest [16] and during exercise [20], as well as glucose-stimulated extrasplanchnic lactate production [21]. Moreover, the lactate concentration increases that are induced by fructose are positively correlated with muscle glycogen resynthesis [22], which accelerates nucleic acid turnover and uric acid production, and then causes hyperlactatemia [23].

The fructose infusion rate should not exceed 0.3 g/kg/h [24], and the recommended glycerol infusion rate should not exceed 300 mL over 30 min for a 60-kg patient, as rapid glycerol administration increases the risk of intravascular hemolysis [25]. It has been shown that administering 0.5 g/kg glycerol for 90 min is superior to 30 min for reducing intracranial pressure [26]. Although the present study did not measure haptoglobin to quantify hemolysis, we did not detect any apparent signs of intravascular hemolysis among the included patients. However, we found that the increase in lactate levels was larger at higher infusion rates. Thus, physicians should be aware of this phenomenon and ideally wait for at least 120 min when assessing the illness severity in patients who received glycerol. Conversely, the glycerol infusion rate should be moderated and lactate levels tested frequently in patients with pre-existing hyperlactatemia.

Hyperlactatemia can occur under several physiological conditions, although it is often correlated with oxygen

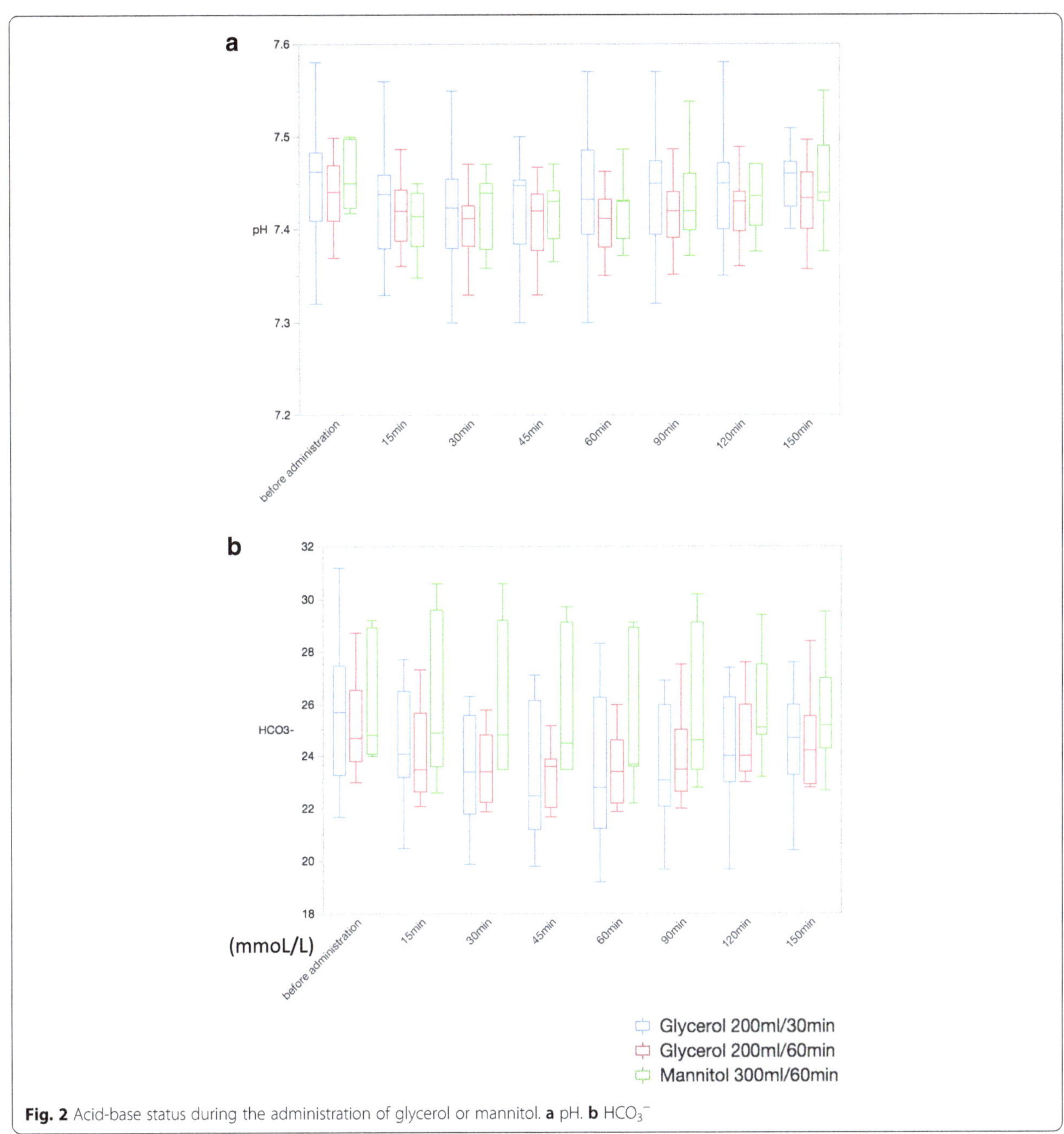

Fig. 2 Acid-base status during the administration of glycerol or mannitol. **a** pH. **b** HCO_3^-

delivery, cardiac function, intravascular volume, and hemoglobin levels. For example, hemodynamically unstable patients are likely to present with increased lactate levels. In this context, agents that reduce intracranial pressure (e.g., glycerol or mannitol) induce strong osmotic diuresis that can cause reduced stroke volume and intravascular volume that lead to elevated lactate levels. However, the present study did not detect significant relationships between the various hemodynamic parameters and hyperlactatemia, and none of the patients developed active bleeding or desaturation during the administration of glycerol or mannitol. Therefore, it appears unlikely that hyperlactatemia caused by intravenous glycerol administration is related to impaired hemodynamics or oxygen delivery.

The present study has several limitations. First, this was a small single-center observational study; nevertheless, we were still able to detect a significant relationship between intravenous glycerol treatment and elevated blood lactate levels. Second, we did not evaluate whether the patients had congenital metabolic disorders, although these conditions are very rare. Finally, we did not evaluate

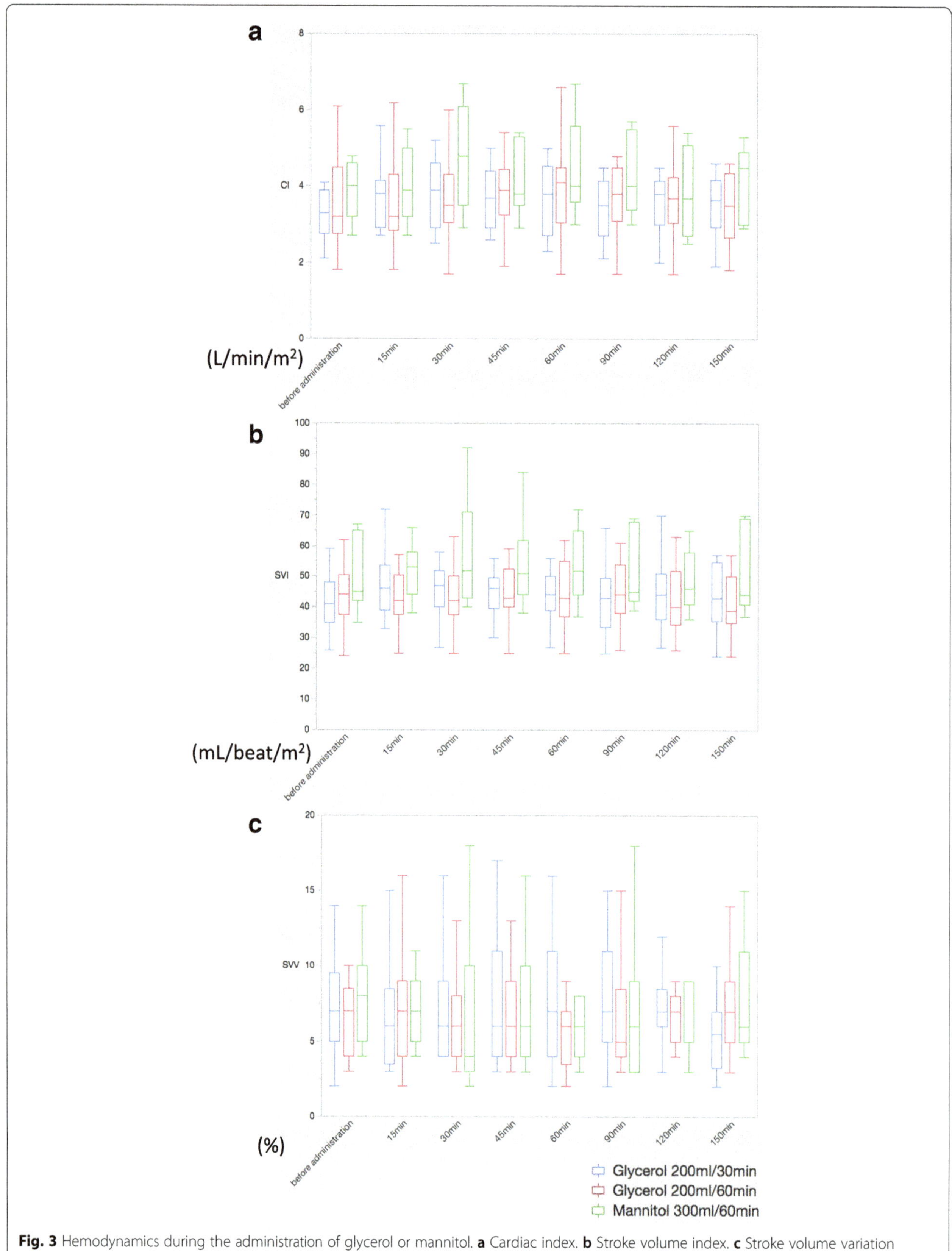

Fig. 3 Hemodynamics during the administration of glycerol or mannitol. **a** Cardiac index. **b** Stroke volume index. **c** Stroke volume variation

any increases in lactate levels among patients with pre-existing hyperlactatemia (who were excluded from the study). Although the effects of glycerol on lactate levels disappeared after at least 120 min had passed in patients with normal baseline lactate levels, it is plausible that in patients with hyperlactatemia, the effects of glycerol may be prolonged past 120 min due to the impaired lactate metabolism, thus warranting a longer observation period than used in this study. Therefore, further studies are needed to evaluate blood lactate levels during glycerol administration in patients with pre-existing hyperlactatemia.

Conclusions

Intravenous administration of glycerol induced an increase in blood lactate levels that persisted for up to 120 min. Although hyperlactatemia is an essential indicator of sepsis and/or impaired tissue perfusion, this phenomenon should be considered when assessing the blood lactate levels.

Abbreviations

APACHE II: Acute Physiology and Chronic Health Evaluation II; CI: Cardiac index; SOFA: Sequential Organ Failure Assessment; SVI: Stroke volume index; SVV: Stroke volume variation

Acknowledgements

We acknowledge the assistance of the intensive care nursing staff at Jichi Medical University Hospital, Tochigi, Japan.

Funding

The study was supported by research funding from Jichi Medical University.

Authors' contributions

SK collected and interpreted the data and wrote the first draft. SN contributed to the protocol's design and revised the manuscript. KT, YG, KK, TK, JS, and MW collected the data and revised the manuscript. All authors are accountable for all aspects of the work and have approved the final manuscript.

Competing interests

The authors declare that they have no competing interests.

References

1. Levy B. Lactate and shock state: the metabolic view. Curr Opin Crit Care. 2006;12:315–21.
2. Hernandez G, Bruhn A, Castro R, Regueira T. The holistic view on perfusion monitoring in septic shock. Curr Opin Crit Care. 2012;18:280–6.
3. Garcia-Alvarez M, Marik P, Bellomo R. Sepsis-associated hyperlactatemia. Crit Care. 2014;18:503.
4. Aduen J, Bernstein WK, Khastgir T, Miller J, Kerzner R, Bhatiani A, et al. The use and clinical importance of a substrate-specific electrode for rapid determination of blood lactate concentrations. JAMA. 1994;272:1678–85.
5. Weil MH, Afifi AA. Experimental and clinical studies on lactate and pyruvate as indicators of the severity of acute circulatory failure (shock). Circulation. 1970;41:989–1001.
6. Bakker J, Coffernils M, Leon M, Gris P, Vincent JL. Blood lactate levels are superior to oxygen-derived variables in predicting outcome in human septic shock. Chest. 1991;99:956–62.
7. Singer M, Deutschman CS, Seymour CW, Shankar-Hari M, Annane D, Bauer M, et al. The Third International Consensus Definitions for Sepsis and Septic Shock (Sepsis-3). JAMA. 2016;315:801–10.
8. Jansen TC, van Bommel J, Schoonderbeek FJ, Sleeswijk Visser SJ, van der Klooster JM, Lima AP, et al. Early lactate-guided therapy in intensive care unit patients: a multicenter, open-label, randomized controlled trial. Am J Respir Crit Care Med. 2010;182:752–61.
9. Ryoo SM, Lee J, Lee YS, Lee JH, Lim KS, Huh JW, et al. Lactate level versus lactate clearance for predicting mortality in patients with septic shock defined by Sepsis-3. Crit Care Med. 2018;46:e489–95.
10. De Backer D, Creteur J, Dubois MJ, Sakr Y, Koch M, Verdant C, et al. The effects of dobutamine on microcirculatory alterations in patients with septic shock are independent of its systemic effects. Crit Care Med. 2006;34:403–8.
11. Rhodes A, Evans LE, Alhazzani W, Levy MM, Antonelli M, Ferrer R, et al. Surviving Sepsis Campaign: International Guidelines for Management of Sepsis and Septic Shock: 2016. Intensive Care Med. 2017;43:304–77.
12. Fawer R, Justafre JC, Berger JP, Schelling JL. Intravenous glycerol in cerebral infarction: a controlled 4-month trial. Stroke. 1978;9:484–6.
13. Bayer AJ, Pathy MS, Newcombe R. Double-blind randomised trial of intravenous glycerol in acute stroke. Lancet. 1987;1:405–8.
14. Tsubokawa T, Katayama Y, Ishii S. Fructose-added glycerol (Glyceol) for therapy of elevated intracranial pressure: analysis of the side effects of long-term administration in a multi-institutional trial. Neurol Res. 1989;11: 249–52.
15. Katayama S, Nunomiya S, Wada M, Misawa K, Tanaka S, Koyama K, et al. Hyperlactatemia caused by intra-venous administration of glycerol: a case study. Indian J Crit Care Med. 2012;16:241–4.
16. Bjorkman O, Gunnarsson R, Hagstrom E, Felig P, Wahren J. Splanchnic and renal exchange of infused fructose in insulin-deficient type 1 diabetic patients and healthy controls. J Clin Invest. 1989;83:52–9.
17. Atwell ME, Waterhouse C. Glucose production from fructose. Diabetes. 1971; 20:193–9.
18. Knaus WA, Draper EA, Wagner DP, Zimmerman JE. APACHE II: a severity of disease classification system. Crit Care Med. 1985;13:818–29.
19. Vincent JL, Moreno R, Takala J, Willatts S, De Mendonca A, Bruining H, et al. The SOFA (sepsis-related organ failure assessment) score to describe organ dysfunction/failure. On behalf of the working group on sepsis-related problems of the European Society of Intensive Care Medicine. Intensive Care Med. 1996;22:707–10.
20. Ahlborg G, Bjorkman O. Splanchnic and muscle fructose metabolism during and after exercise. J Appl Physiol. 1990;69:1244–51.
21. Youn JH, Bergman RN. Conversion of oral glucose to lactate in dogs. Primary site and relative contribution to blood lactate. Diabetes. 1991;40: 738–47.
22. Rosset R, Lecoultre V, Egli L, Cros J, Dokumaci AS, Zwygart K, et al. Postexercise repletion of muscle energy stores with fructose or glucose in mixed meals. Am J Clin Nutr. 2017;105:609–17.
23. Fox IH, Kelley WN. Studies on the mechanism of fructose-induced hyperuricemia in man. Metabolism. 1972;21:713–21.
24. Wang YM, van Eys J. Nutritional significance of fructose and sugar alcohols. Annu Rev Nutr. 1981;1:437–75.
25. Yu YL, Kumana CR, Lauder IJ, Cheung YK, Chan FL, Kou M, et al. Treatment of acute cerebral hemorrhage with intravenous glycerol. A double-blind, placebo-controlled, randomized trial. Stroke. 1992;23:967–71.
26. Node Y, Nakazawa S. Clinical study of mannitol and glycerol on raised intracranial pressure and on their rebound phenomenon. Adv Neurol. 1990; 52:359–63.

25

High red blood cell distribution width as a marker of hospital mortality after ICU discharge

Rafael Fernandez[1,2,3*], Silvia Cano[1,2,3], Ignacio Catalan[1,2,3], Olga Rubio[1,2,3], Carles Subira[1,2,3], Jaume Masclans[1,2,3], Gina Rognoni[1,2,3], Lara Ventura[1,2,3], Caroline Macharete[1,2,3], Len Winfield[1,2,3] and Josep Mª. Alcoverro[1,2,3]

Abstract

Background: High red blood cell distribution width (RDW) is associated with worse outcome in diverse scenarios, including in critical illness. The Sabadell score (SS) predicts in-hospital survival after ICU discharge. We aimed to determine RDW's association with survival after ICU discharge and whether RDW can improve the accuracy of the SS.

Design: Retrospective cohort study. Setting: general ICU at a university hospital.

Patients: We included all patients discharged to wards from January 2010 to October 2016.

Methods: We analyzed associations between RDW and variables recorded on admission (age, comorbidities, severity score), during the ICU stay (treatments, complications, length of stay (LOS)), and at ICU discharge (SS). The primary outcome was hospital mortality. Statistical analysis included multivariable logistic regression and receiver operating characteristic curve (ROC) analyses.

Results: We discharged 3366 patients to wards; median ward LOS was 7 [4–13] days; ward mortality was 5.2%. Mean RDW at ICU discharge was 15.4 ± 2.5%. Ward mortality was higher at each quartile of RDW (0.7%, 2.9%, 7.5%, 10.3%; area under ROC 0.81). A logistic regression model with Sabadell score obtained an excellent accuracy for ward mortality (area under ROC 0.863), and the addition of RDW slightly improved accuracy (AUROC 0.890, $p < 0.05$). Recursive partitioning demonstrated higher mortality in patients with high RDW at each SS level (1.6% vs. 0.3% in SS0, 9.7% vs. 1.1% in SS1, 21.9% vs. 9.7% in SS2), but not in SS3.

Conclusion: High RDW is a marker of severity at ICU discharge and improves the accuracy of Sabadell score in predicting ward mortality except in the more extreme SS3.

Keywords: Scoring systems, Mortality prediction, Biomarkers

Introduction

The primary mission of intensive care units (ICU) is to improve the survival of critically ill patients. The first severity scores to predict mortality in patients admitted to the ICU were based on the maximum deviations of physiological variables. These scores have been periodically refined by including new variables or by adjusting the weight of each variable. In the most recent versions, the weight of physiological variables has decreased while the weight of patients' comorbidities and health status has increased [1].

One physiological variable with the potential to improve the accuracy of severity and prognostic scores is red blood cell distribution width (RDW). Simple and inexpensive to obtain, RDW reflects the degree of heterogeneity of erythrocyte volume (anisocytosis); RDW has traditionally been used in the differential diagnosis of anemias. An increased RDW mirrors a profound deregulation of erythrocyte homeostasis involving both impaired erythropoiesis and abnormal red blood cell survival, which may be attributed to a variety of underlying metabolic abnormalities such as shortening of telomere length, oxidative stress, inflammation, poor nutritional status, dyslipidemia, hypertension, erythrocyte

* Correspondence: rfernandezf@althaia.cat
[1]Intensive Care Department, Hospital Sant Joan de Deu – Fundacio Althaia, Dr. Joan Soler 1, 08243 Manresa, Spain
[2]Universitat Internacional de Catalunya, Barcelona, Spain
Full list of author information is available at the end of the article

fragmentation, and alteration of erythropoietin function [2]. Many clinical conditions are associated with RDW above the upper limit, commonly accepted as 14.5%. Some of these conditions are inflammatory, others are hematological, and others are comorbidities (e.g., obesity, aging, smoking) [2]. High RDW has been associated with worse outcome in various conditions, such as community-acquired pneumonia [3, 4], myocardial infarction, cardiac arrest [5], and cerebral infarction [6], and in very different scenarios (e.g., critically ill patients on admission [7–9], during the ICU stay [10, 11], and long-term after hospital discharge [12]). Nevertheless, adding high RDW failed to improve the accuracy of common severity scores [13], suggesting that factors associated with high RDW (e.g., fever, leukocytosis, or cancer) may already be included in severity scores.

Our group investigates outcomes of patients in the ward after ICU discharge; this research led to the Sabadell score in 2006 [14]. A multicenter validation study confirmed that the Sabadell score classifies patients into four groups with very different ward mortality [15]. A trial is underway to elucidate whether intensivist surveillance can improve ward survival in different Sabadell score groups [16]. The real value of studying this population is that ICU surveillance after discharge is a growing wave, but needs to clearly frame those patients with a higher likelihood for complications and mortality. The follow-up of the entire ICU-discharged population is not worthy and unrealistic. Outreach teams need sensitive markers to identify ward patients at risk, and biomarkers like RDW are promising candidates [17, 18].

We aimed to determine the association of RDW with ward survival after ICU discharge and whether RDW can improve the accuracy of the Sabadell score. We hypothesized that adding RDW would improve the accuracy of the Sabadell score for predicting ward mortality after ICU discharge.

Methods

We retrospectively studied all patients registered in our computerized database between January 2010 and October 2016; accordingly, informed consent was waived.

Our 16-bed mixed ICU admits patients with all kinds of medical and surgical conditions except those who have undergone cardiac surgery, neurosurgery, or transplantation and also serves as a coronary unit and stroke unit for a population of 200,000 inhabitants.

We excluded patients who died during the ICU stay and those who were not discharged to the ward, mainly due to transfer to other hospitals or nursing homes or direct discharge to their homes. Patients needing ICU readmission during the index hospitalization were not included twice; their outcomes were attributed to their first ICU admission.

On ICU admission, we recorded age, sex, diagnosis, SAPS3 score, and comorbidities. During the ICU stay, we recorded major ICU procedures (mechanical ventilation, renal replacement therapy, vasoactive drugs, tracheostomy, and blood transfusion) and adverse events (nosocomial pneumonia, acute renal failure, and delirium). At discharge from the ICU (or step-down unit, when applicable), the attending physician classified the patient according to the Sabadell score, a subjective tool explained in detail elsewhere [14]. Briefly, it has four levels of expected prognosis based on the clinician perception taking into account the illness evolution, comorbidities, sequelae, and socio-familiar support: score 0 is for patients with good prognosis, score 1 is for patients with poor prognosis in the medium-to-long term and acceptable ICU readmission, score 2 is for patients with poor prognosis in the short-term and debatable ICU readmission, and score 3 is for patients who are expected to die before discharge from the hospital.

Routine laboratory reports of blood work ordered by attending physicians as clinically required always included RDW. Based on previous references (4, 9, 10), high RDW was defined as greater than 14.5%. For the purpose of the present study, we used the last RDW recorded before discharge to the ward.

Variables are reported as means ± standard deviations, medians [interquartile ranges], or percentages and odds ratios, as appropriate. We used t tests to compare the means of continuous normal variables, Mann-Whitney U tests to compare the medians of continuous non-normal variables, and Fisher's exact test to compare categorical variables; significance was set at $p < 0.5$.

Variables at ICU admission, during ICU stay, and at ICU discharge were compared between patients with and without high RDW values. Variables that were significant in the univariable analyses were included in a multivariable logistic regression analysis with ward mortality as the dependent (outcome) variable. The discrimination of the multivariate model was assessed using the area under the receiver operating characteristic curve (AUROC). Accuracy was considered to be good if the area under the curve was more than 0.75 and excellent if more than 0.85. To evaluate the contribution of high RDW to the prognostic value, we calculated the increase in the AUROC of the logistic model after including high RDW. Areas under the ROC curves (AUC) from logistic models were compared with Stata's "roccomp" command (chi-squared test).

Results

In the 6-year study period, we admitted 4675 patients to our ICU. Of these, 621 (13.3%) died during the ICU stay, 349 (7.5%) were directly discharged home, 329 (7.0%) were transferred to other hospitals or nursing homes, 10

(0.2%) were lost, and 3366 (72.0%) were discharged to the ward. The median length of ward stay was 7 [4–13] days, and 177 (5.3%) patients died in the wards.

Table 1 compares the recorded variables in patients with high RDW versus patients without high RDW. All the variables recorded at ICU admission (age, cancer, hepatic cirrhosis, and SAPS3 mortality risk), during ICU stay (blood transfusion, delirium, vasoactive drugs, mechanical ventilation, and acute renal failure), and at ICU discharge (ICU length of stay and Sabadell score) were worse in patients with high RDW, suggesting a profile of sicker patients.

After ICU discharge, patients with high RDW had longer ward stay (9 [5–16] vs. 6 [4–10.5] days; $p < 0.001$) and higher ward mortality (154 (8.4%) vs. 22 (1.4%); $p < 0.001$), as depicted in Fig. 1. For ward mortality, high RDW showed a sensitivity of 0.87 (0.81–0.92), specificity of 0.471 (0.468–0.474), positive predictive value of 0.084 (0.078–0.088), and negative predictive value 0.986 (0.979–0.991). A closer look at RDW and ward mortality demonstrated a stepwise correlation between RDW and ward mortality (Table 2). Partitioning the total population in quartiles of RDW, ward mortality ranged from 0.7% for RDW < 13.8% to 10.3% for RDW > 16.1%. The SAPS3 score was progressively worse at each quartile, and the standardized mortality ratio was also worse at higher quartiles of RDW (Table 2).

Variables associated with ward mortality in the univariable analysis were age, cancer, SAPS3, delirium, acute renal failure, blood transfusion, vasoactive drugs, mechanical ventilation, ICU length of stay, Sabadell score, and high RDW (Table 3).

Sabadell score for prediction of ward mortality showed an AUROC of 0.863, and the inclusion of high RDW improved the AUROC to 0.890 ($p < 0.05$).

The best multivariable logistic regression model, which included age, SAPS3, and Sabadell score, yielded an AUROC of 0.901, with good calibration (Lemeshow goodness-of-fit = 0.118). Moreover, the addition of RDW slightly improved the accuracy of the model only marginally (AUROC 0.908; $p = 0.047$).

Additionally, when patients were grouped according to Sabadell score, high RDW identified patients with significantly higher ward mortality (Fig. 2). High RDW was

Table 1 Characteristics on admission, during the intensive care unit (ICU) stay, at ICU discharge, and at hospital discharge in patients with normal versus high red cell distribution width

Variable	Normal RDW (≤ 14.5%) $n = 1525$	High RDW (> 14.5%) $n = 1841$	p
At ICU admission			
Age	61.8 ± 17.5	67.7 ± 15.1	< 0.001
Female sex	502 (33%)	742 (40%)	< 0.001
Cancer	86 (5.6%)	298 (16.2%)	< 0.001
Hepatic cirrhosis	14 (0.9%)	106 (5.8%)	< 0.001
SAPS3 mortality risk, %	11 [5.0–21.9]	25 [12.6–44.6]	< 0.001
During ICU stay			
Blood transfusion	45 (2.9%)	347 (18.8%)	< 0.001
Delirium	68 (4.5%)	144 (7.8%)	< 0.001
Vasoactive drugs	209 (14%)	608 (33%)	< 0.001
Mechanical ventilation	239 (16%)	585 (32%)	< 0.001
Acute renal failure	170 (11%)	533 (29%)	< 0.001
At ICU discharge			
ICU length of stay, days	2.3 [1.6–4.0]	3.3 [1.9–5.9]	< 0.001
Sabadell score:			< 0.001
0	1272 (79.8%)	1084 (57.4%)	
1	176 (11.0%)	465 (24.6%)	
2	62 (3.9%)	216 (11.4%)	
3	15 (0.9%)	76 (4.0%)	
Red cell distribution width, %	13.7 ± 0.54	16.9 ± 2.56	< 0.001
At hospital discharge:			
Ward length of stay, d	6 [4–10.5]	9 [5–16]	< 0.001
Ward mortality	21 (1.3%)	155 (8.2%)	< 0.001

RDW red cell distribution width, *SAPS3* Simplified Acute Physiologic Score 3, *ICU* intensive care unit

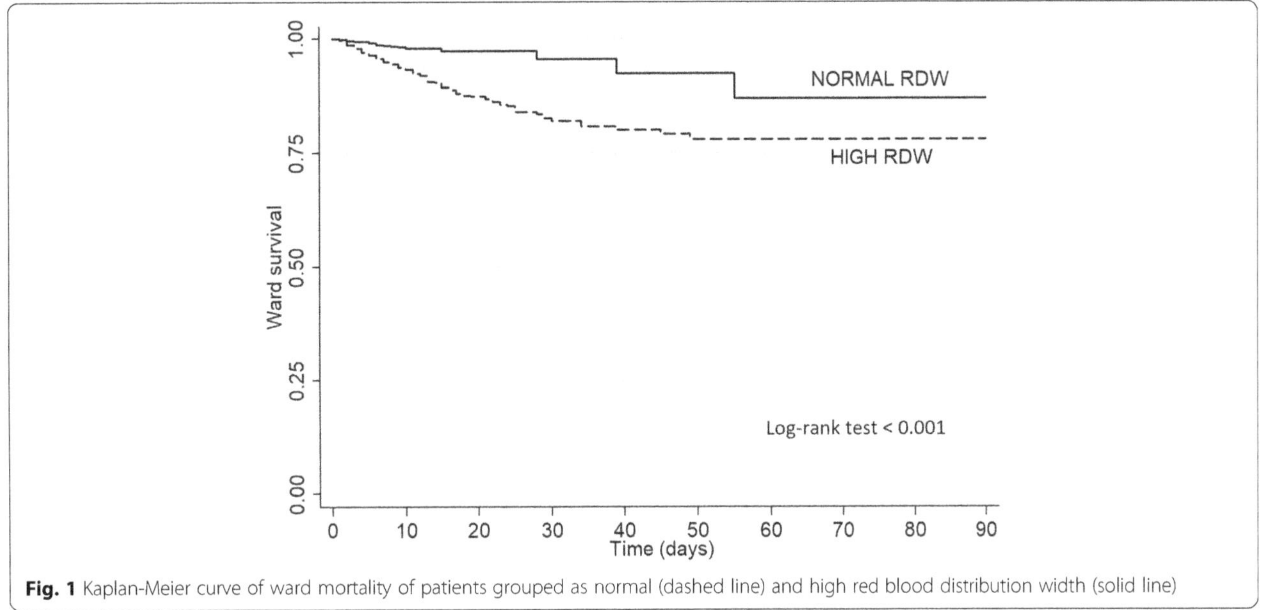

Fig. 1 Kaplan-Meier curve of ward mortality of patients grouped as normal (dashed line) and high red blood distribution width (solid line)

significantly associated with higher ward mortality in patients with Sabadell score 0 (1.6% vs. 0.3%, OR 5.0 [1.6–17.8]), Sabadell score 1 (9.7% vs. 1.1%, OR 9.3 [2.1–53.2]), and Sabadell score 2 (21.9% vs. 9.7%, OR 2.6 [1.0–7.2]), but not in Sabadell score 3.

Discussion

To our knowledge, this is the first study to show that high RDW is a marker of severity in patients discharged from the ICU to the wards. Additionally, high RDW identified patients with higher ward mortality at each level of prognosis depicted by the Sabadell score, except the most extreme SS3.

Our results in a wide sample of critically ill patients are in line with previous reports demonstrating high RDW as a marker of severity. Sadaka et al. [7] retrospectively studied 279 patients with septic shock and demonstrated that each quintile of RDW increase was associated with higher ICU mortality. Meynaar et al. [8] retrospectively studied 2915 patients in a mixed ICU and found that high RDW on admission was associated with hospital mortality; in multivariate analysis, RDW remained an independent risk factor for mortality after correction for APACHE II score, age, admission type, and mechanical ventilation (odds ratio 1.04 for each femtoliter of RDW). Bazick et al. [9] retrospectively studied a wide population of ICU patients and found that each quintile of RDW increase was associated with increased mortality and with an increased risk of acquiring a bloodstream infection. Zhang et al. [11] retrospectively studied 1539 ICU patients and found that high RDW on admission was associated with mortality, but its predictive performance was suboptimal (AUROC 0.62). Last year, Otero et al. [19] studied 500 critically ill surgical patients; 47% had high RDW on admission, and high RDW was associated with a twofold increase in mortality. In our study, ward mortality increased with RDW at ICU discharge. Beyond what would be expected considering the association between high RDW and severity of illness as defined by the SAPS3 score, the standardized mortality ratio was worse at higher RDW levels (Table 2).

The dynamic nature of RDW precludes firmly establishing the best time for RDW determination. Kim et al. [10] prospectively studied 329 septic patients and found that an increase in RDW >0.2% from baseline during

Table 2 Ward mortality, severity score on admission, and standardized mortality ratio for patients classified by quartiles of red cell distribution width at ICU discharge

Quartile	Red cell distribution width	Ward mortality	SAPS3 predicted risk of death	Standardized mortality ratio
1	< 13.8%	6 (0.7%)	14%	0.13
2	13.9–14.8%	25 (2.9%)	21%	0.32
3	14.9–16.3%	59 (7.5%)	28%	0.50
4	> 16.1%	86 (10.3%)	34%	0.77

SAPS3 Simplified Acute Physiologic Score 3, *ICU* intensive care unit

Table 3 Variables associated with ward mortality

Variable	Univariable OR	AUC	*p*	Multivariable OR	*p*
Age, years	1.07 [1.06–1.09]	0.73	< 0.001	1.03 [1.02–1.05]	< 0.001
Cancer	2.1 [1.4–3.1]	0.55	< 0.001		
SAPS3	1.04 [1.03–1.05]	0.78	< 0.001	1.012 [1.004–1.021]	< 0.005
Delirium	2.5 [1.6–3.9]	0.54	< 0.001		
Acute renal failure	2.7 [2.0–3.7]	0.60	< 0.001		
Blood transfusion	1.9 [1.3–2.8]	0.54	< 0.005		
Vasoactive drugs	2.2 [1.6–3.1]	0.59	< 0.001		
Mechanical ventilation	1.9 [1.3–2.5]	0.56	< 0.001		
ICU length of stay, days	1.03 [1.02–1.04]	0.62	< 0.001		
Sabadell score	5.1 [4.3–6.0]	0.86	< 0.001	3.8 [3.1–4.6]	< 0.001
High RDW	6.3 [3.9–9.9]	0.67	< 0.001	2.8 [1.7–4.6]	< 0.001

SAPS3 Simplified Acute Physiologic Score 3, *RDW* red cell distribution width, *ICU* intensive care unit, *OR* odds ratio, *AUC* area under ROC

the first 72 h after hospitalization was significantly associated with higher mortality, even after adjusting for SOFA score and other covariates. Nevertheless, other investigators found no differences attributable to the evolution of RDW during the ICU stay [11]. We analyzed RDW at ICU discharge rather than at ICU admission, with the aim of attaining a better picture of the at-risk population just before discharge to the ward. To our knowledge, no other studies have focused on RDW at ICU discharge, although Purtle et al. [12] concluded that high RDW at hospital discharge is a robust predictor of subsequent all-cause patient mortality in critical care patients that survive hospitalization.

Another issue is whether high RDW can improve current mortality prediction models. In specific subgroups, some investigators [7, 20] found that adding high RDW resulted in statistically significant improvements in the predictive performance of severity scores, but that these increases were of little practical usefulness. In septic patients, Sadaka et al. [7] found that adding high RDW increased the AUROC from 0.69 to 0.77 in APACHE II. In patients treated with continuous renal replacement, Oh et al. [21] found that adding high RDW to SOFA increased the AUROC from 0.69 to 0.75. However, other investigators found that adding high RDW brought about only marginal improvement in APACHE II [8] and APACHE III [13]. In our study, adding high RDW improved the predictive performance of SAPS3 risk of death only marginally (AUC 0.778 vs. 0.798, data not shown).

Ward survival after ICU discharge remains an unresolved issue. In some scenarios, it appears to be a quality indicator, with higher mortality suggesting suboptimal treatment in the ward or premature ICU discharge. Nevertheless, some patients who survive the ICU stay have severe derangements that preclude significant recovery, and ward physicians and outreach teams would benefit from better classification of patients at ICU discharge [17, 18, 22]. A decade ago, Fernandez et al. [14, 15] devised a subjective score that classifies patients at

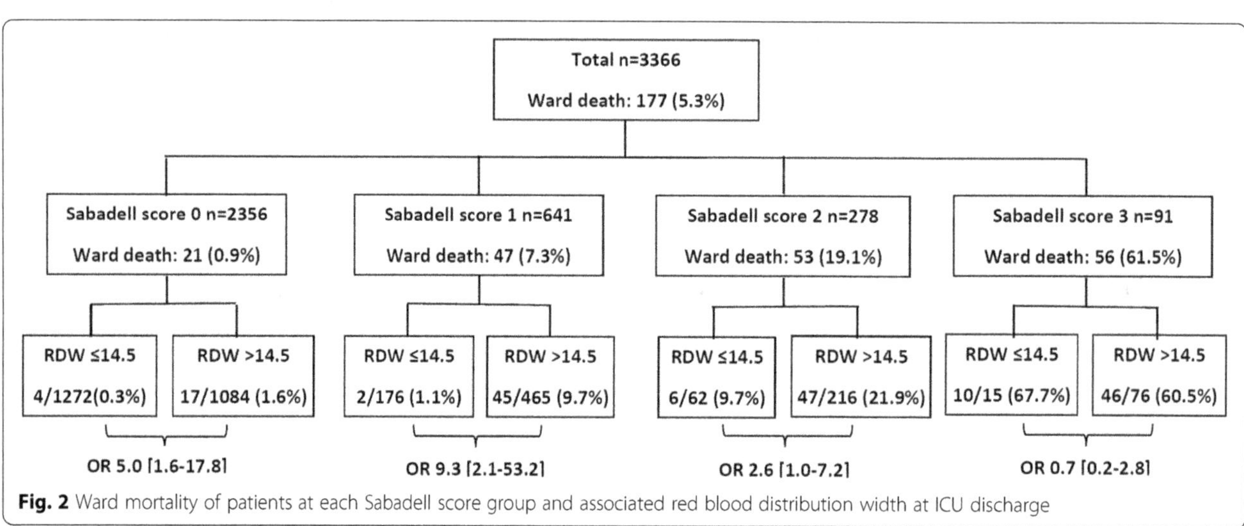

Fig. 2 Ward mortality of patients at each Sabadell score group and associated red blood distribution width at ICU discharge

ICU discharge into four groups with very different mortality in the ward, the Sabadell score. In the present study, adding high RDW to the Sabadell score improved the prediction of outcome in patients discharged to the ward. In each Sabadell score group except the worst (patients with null expected survival in the ward), patients with high RDW had substantially higher mortality than those with normal RDW.

Whether or not outreach teams should target patients with high RDW will depend on further investigations about the feasibility of treating the underlying conditions responsible for high RDW (inflammation, underperfusion states, or occult cancer).

Limitations of the study

Our analysis of outcome at hospital discharge did not include patients transferred from the ward to other community hospitals or nursing homes. Nevertheless, in our public system, these transfers account for a minority of patients.

The lack of impact of high RDW in the more extreme SS3 patients may be related either to a small sample size or to the fact that mortality in this specific condition in mostly related to other variables (severe brain damage, refractory heart failure, and decisions to withhold/withdraw life support treatments).

We conclude that high RDW is a marker of severity in patients discharged from the ICU and improves the accuracy of the Sabadell score in predicting ward mortality except in the more extreme SS3. Whether outreach teams should target high patients with RDW remains to be determined.

Abbreviations

APACHE: Acute physiologic and chronic health evaluation; AUROC: Area under the ROC curve; ICU: Intensive care unit; LOS: Length of stay; OR: Odds ratio; RDW: Red blood cell distribution width; ROC: Receiver-operator characteristic; SAPS3: Severity Acute Physiologic Score; SOFA: Sequential organ failure assessment; SS: Sabadell score

Acknowledgements

None.

Funding

None.

Authors' contributions

RF was responsible for the conception of the study. SC, IC, OR, CS, JM, GR, LV, CM, and JMA were responsible for the acquisition of data. RF and LW were responsible for the analysis of data. RF was responsible for the interpretation of data and for drafting the manuscript. RF, SC, IC, OR, CS, JM, GR, LV, CM, and JMA were responsible for revising the manuscript critically for important intellectual content, final approval of the version to be published, and agreement to be accountable for all aspects of the work. All authors read and approved the final manuscript.

Competing interests

The authors declare that they have no competing interests.

Author details

[1]Intensive Care Department, Hospital Sant Joan de Deu – Fundacio Althaia, Dr. Joan Soler 1, 08243 Manresa, Spain. [2]Universitat Internacional de Catalunya, Barcelona, Spain. [3]CIBERES, Madrid, Spain.

References

1. Metnitz PG, Moreno RP, Almeida E, et al. SAPS 3--from evaluation of the patient to evaluation of the intensive care unit. Part 1: objectives, methods and cohort description. Intensive Care Med. 2005;31:1336–44.
2. Salvagno GL, Sanchis-Gomar F, Picanza A, et al. Red blood cell distribution width: a simple parameter with multiple clinical applications. Crit Rev Clin Lab Sci. 2015;52:86–105.
3. Lee SM, Lee JH, Kim K, et al. The clinical significance of changes in red blood cell distribution width in patients with community-acquired pneumonia. Clin Exp Emerg Med. 2016;3:139–47.
4. Ku NS, Kim HW, Oh HJ, et al. Red blood cell distribution width is an independent predictor of mortality in patients with gram-negative bacteremia. Shock. 2012;38:123–7.
5. Kim J, Kim K, Lee JH, et al. Red blood cell distribution width as an independent predictor of all-cause mortality in out of hospital cardiac arrest. Resuscitation. 2012;83:1248–52.
6. Kim J, Kim YD, Song TJ, et al. Red blood cell distribution width is associated with poor clinical outcome in acute cerebral infarction. Thromb Haemost. 2012;108:349–56.
7. Sadaka F, O'Brien J, Prakash S. Red cell distribution width and outcome in patients with septic shock. J Intensive Care Med. 2013;28:307–13.
8. Meynaar IA, Knook AH, Coolen S, et al. Red cell distribution width as predictor for mortality in critically ill patients. Neth J Med. 2013;71:488–93.
9. Bazick HS, Chang D, Mahadevappa K, et al. Red cell distribution width and all-cause mortality in critically ill patients. Crit Care Med. 2011;39:1913–21.
10. Kim CH, Park JT, Kim EJ, et al. An increase in red blood cell distribution width from baseline predicts mortality in patients with severe sepsis or septic shock. Crit Care. 2013;17:R282.
11. Zhang Z, Xu X, Ni H, et al. Red cell distribution width is associated with hospital mortality in unselected critically ill patients. J Thorac Dis. 2013;5: 730–6.
12. Purtle SW, Moromizato T, McKane CK, et al. The association of red cell distribution width at hospital discharge and out-of-hospital mortality following critical illness. Crit Care Med. 2014;42:918–29.
13. Loveday S, Sinclair L, Badrick T. Does the addition of RDW improve current ICU scoring systems? Clin Biochem. 2015;48:569–74.
14. Fernandez R, Baigorri F, Navarro G, et al. A modified McCabe score for stratification of patients after intensive care unit discharge: the Sabadell score. Crit Care. 2006;10:R179.
15. Fernandez R, Serrano JM, Umaran I, et al. Ward mortality after ICU discharge: a multicenter validation of the Sabadell score. Intensive Care Med. 2010;36: 1196–201.
16. Cano S. To survive after ICU discharge. ClinicalTrials.gov Identifier: NCT02599636. https://clinicaltrials.gov/show/NCT02599636 (Accessed 24 Apr 2017).
17. Ranzani OT, Prada LF, Zampieri FG, et al. Failure to reduce C-reactive protein levels more than 25% in the last 24 hours before intensive care unit discharge predicts higher in-hospital mortality: a cohort study. J Crit Care. 2012;27:525.e9–15.
18. Matsumura Y, Nakada TA, Abe R, et al. Serum procalcitonin level and SOFA score at discharge from the intensive care unit predict post-intensive care unit mortality: a prospective study. PLoS One. 2014;9:e114007.
19. Otero TM, Canales C, Yeh DD, et al. Elevated red cell distribution width at initiation of critical care is associated with mortality in surgical intensive care unit patients. J Crit Care. 2016;34:7–11.
20. Hunziker S, Celi LA, Lee J, et al. Red cell distribution width improves the simplified acute physiology score for risk prediction in unselected critically ill patients. Crit Care. 2012;16:R89.
21. Oh HJ, Park JT, Kim JK, et al. Red blood cell distribution width is an independent predictor of mortality in acute kidney injury patients treated with continuous renal replacement therapy. Nephrol Dial Transplant. 2012; 27:589–94.

26

Studying the effect of abdominal massage on the gastric residual volume in patients hospitalized in intensive care units

Farzad Momenfar[1], Alireza Abdi[1,4*], Nader Salari[4], Ali Soroush[2] and Behzad Hemmatpour[3]

Abstract

Background: The main problem of hospitalized patients in intensive care units is feeding, and if the patient does not receive the daily caloric intake required to his body, he will have malnutrition and problems related to it. Abdominal massage is a method used to improve digestive function in various studies, but few studies have been conducted in intensive care units, and sometimes, contradictory results have been obtained. Therefore, the present study is conducted with the aim of determining the effect of abdominal massage on the gastric residual volume in patients hospitalized in intensive care units.

Methods: This study was conducted as a clinical trial in Ahwaz, in 2017. Samples were 60 patients hospitalized in intensive care units who were randomly divided into case and control groups. The intervention period for the case group was 3 days and twice daily for 20 min. Measuring the gastric residual volume was investigated before the intervention and 1 hour after the second massage each day. Data were entered into the checklist designed by the researcher and were analyzed using SPSS version 24 and descriptive and inferential tests.

Results: The gastric residual volume on the second and third day after the intervention was less than before the intervention (p value< 0.05), the gastric residual volume before intervention with after intervention in the control group during different days, on each of the 3 days after the intervention, was more than before the intervention (p value< 0.05), and the gastric residual volume after the intervention in different days and the mean of different days in the case group was lower than the control group (p value> 0.05).

Conclusion: Results represent the effect of abdominal massage on reducing the gastric residual volume in patients hospitalized in intensive care units. Therefore, it is suggested that this method can be considered as a caring method in the daily care program for these patients.

Keywords: Abdominal massage, Residual volume, Intensive care unit

Background

Food support has a vital role in taking care of patients in intensive care units [1]. This is one of the important goals in taking care of these patients [2]. Feeding with nasogastric (NG) tube is used for patients who are unable to feed through mouth [3], and in this case, after the inserting the NG tube, during the first 24 h, the gastric residual volume (GRV) is measured every 6 h. If the GRV is greater than 250 cc, the nurse should inform the doctor for further investigation and will not receive a meal in that session [4]; even this method is omitted based on the newest guidelines, [5] but it still is implemented in Iran as a routine measure [6]. Feeding method through NG tube tract helps to maintain peristalsis, improves blood supply, and strengthens the immune system [7], and timely and adequate nutritional support plays an important role in improving recovery, reducing physiological stress, and increasing the immunity capacity [8]. Likewise, this approach accelerates wound healing, reduces the

* Correspondence: A_abdi61@yahoo.com
[1]Nursing and Midwifery School, Students Research Committee, Kermanshah University of Medical Sciences, Kermanshah, Iran
[4]Nursing and Midwifery school, Kermanshah university of medical sciences, Kermanshah, Iran
Full list of author information is available at the end of the article

number of hospitalization days, reduces the infection risk, and in cases where the patient is hospitalized due to ulcers or injuries, reduces catabolic responses [9]. In fact, the aim of nutritional support through the NG tube for patients in intensive care units is to reduce or eliminate malnutrition because malnutrition can cause muscle atrophy and loss of body mass [7].

Among the factors that prevent adequate feeding of patients, in this way, we can refer to delay in initializing feeding, reduction in rate of gavage, not gavaging the volume prescribed by the physician, and increasing the frequency of discontinuation of feeding [10]. Nurses working in intensive care units play a key role in implementing nutritional support in patients with decreased levels of consciousness that include: timely initializing the feeding, correct feeding, surveying gastric intolerance, examining the emplacement of NG tube, determining the amount of calories necessary for the patient, and measuring the GRV [1].

Among the most important digestive complications in patients fed by the NG tube method, food intolerance and delayed gastric emptying can be referred [11]. To find out the delay in gastric emptying, usually the best way is to measure GRV bedside the patient [12]. Studies show that 10 to 63% of patients fed with this method have stomach intolerance, which causes only 43–64% of these patients receive their daily needed calories [9]. Food intolerance in these patients is associated with the increased risk of mortality and malnutrition-related complications [13], and lack of needed nutrition intake results in loss of body mass, excessive weight loss [7], progression of infection, bedsore, the increased duration of hospitalization, the increased risk of mortality, and increased costs [14], and ultimately lead to cachexia and sarcopenia in these patients [15].

Various methods have been suggested for preventing and treating food intolerance and increasing the rate of gastric emptying, among which the use of prokinetic drugs such as metoclopramide can be referred. But these drugs have many side effects such as abdominal cramps, allergies, bronchospasm, heart disorders, and disorders in pancreas [9]. For 38.8% of hospitalized patients in intensive care units in Germany, abdominal massage is used for managing complications following immobility and improving food tolerance [9]. In this regard, the research conducted by Kahraman and Ozdemir [16] showed that the GRV on the last day had a significant reduction compared to the first day. But in the study of Tekgündüz et al. [17], the GRV after abdominal massage did not show any difference between the two test and control groups. Other researchers also believed that abdominal massage with stimulated peristaltic movements of digestive system, altered intra-abdominal pressure and induced mechanical and reflexive effects on the intestines, reducing the transit time of nutrition in the intestines and increasing the number of intestinal movements and easier food movement along the gastrointestinal tract can be considered as a palliative treatment to prevent the complications caused by this feeding method [9, 18]. Considering the few studies in intensive care units and existing controversy studies, the present study was conducted with the aim of determining the effect of abdominal massage on the GRV in patients hospitalized in intensive care units.

Methods

This study was conducted as a clinical trial in intensive care units of Fatemeh Zahra Hospital (Ahvaz, Iran) in 2017. The research population was all the patients hospitalized in intensive care units, and samples were 60 patients hospitalized in intensive care units that were first included as convenience and then were divided into two groups by simple random method, case group (abdominal massage recipients) and control group (normal care recipients). In this method, 60 cards having the same appearance were provided, and on 30 of them, the letter A was written that identified the case group "abdominal massage," and on the other 30, B was written to indicate the control group "usual care." Then, another person accidentally took one of these cards, with the code written on it, so that the random allocation of patients to each group was determined.

Sample size was estimated based on the formula of comparing a quantitative feature in two groups, the 95% confidence coefficient (1-α), power 90% (1-β), as well as the mean and standard deviation (SD) of GRV in abdominal massage (105 ± 15.30 cc) and control (142.91 ± 66.7 cc) groups after intervention in Uysal et al. [9]; thus, 28 individuals were calculated to each group, so, considering the probability of attrition, 30 individuals were recruited in each group, following formula.

Inclusion criteria included having NG tube (for check the GRV), Glasgow coma scale less than 7 (because usually these patients need gavage), not having abdominal radiotherapy during last 6 weeks, and not having abdominal surgery (because the massages are forbidden for these patients). The patients who took prokinetic medications (due to interfering with massage effects) or discharged during the study (these patients did not complete the intervention course) were excluded.

To collect the data, the researcher, after obtaining permission from the Deputy of Research and Information Technology of Kermanshah University of Medical Sciences and the hospital of research location, went to the place where samples were hospitalized (intensive care units) and selected those who had the criteria for inclusion in the study, then the individual accompanied with the patient (one of the first-class relatives who was responsible for the patient) was asked to complete a written informed consent after a complete explanation of the study goals and the method of work. Samples were randomly divided into two case and control groups. Every day, the researcher went to the intensive care unit of Fatemeh Zahra Hospital in the morning from 8 am to 12 noon for a period of 3 months and conducted the study. The initial information was collected in a designed checklist, using file information and questioning from the individual accompanying the patient.

Data collection tools

Data were collected using a researcher-designed checklist containing two parts, one including demographic information (age, sex, marital status, education, occupation) and the other for pursuing the record of gastric nutrition status (in relation to the type of nutrition, the amount of food each time, number of feeding times, number of vomiting times, GRV in different times, and medication). The form of pursuing the patient's nutritional status was adjusted and used after a detailed study of the books and scientific publications and using available articles on the subject of the study. The qualitative content validity method was used to investigate the validity of the checklist; thus, the forms were distributed to ten faculty members of nursing and intensive care field, and their opinions were applied.

Intervention

In the present study, massages based on the tensegrity principles were used, and the primary outcome was the change of GRV after abdominal massage. The intervention period for the case group was 3 days. These patients received 20 min of abdominal massage intervention twice a day, and the interval between two massages was 2 h. Each day, before the intervention and 1 hour after the second massage, the GRV was measured and investigated. This type of massage technique consists of five steps. The first stage of massage starts with movements like brushing the skin in the abdominal area (Fig. 1); in the second stage, elastic deformation of the thoracolumbar fascia will be performed in the form of displacement, the dominant hand is placed on the abdominal skin, and the other hand is placed on it, and with an adequate pressure of hand, the skin of under pressure area is squeezed (Fig. 2). In the third stage, the skin of the abdominal skin is elastically deformed by massage, the abdominal skin is picked, and kneaded by the fingers (like kneading dough) (Fig. 3). The fourth stage involves shock movements along the armpit from top to bottom and bottom to the top (Fig. 4), and the last stage contains deformation of the muscles in the intercostal spaces of false ribs (the fingers are placed between the intercostal spaces and pulled on the skin with an appropriate pressure) (Fig. 5); the lubricant gel is used to facilitate the massaging. The patient's position is asleep to the back while undergoing massage. The angle between the bed and the patient's head is 30 to 45 degrees, and the patient's legs are placed on a pillow. This condition helps to relax the abdominal muscles.

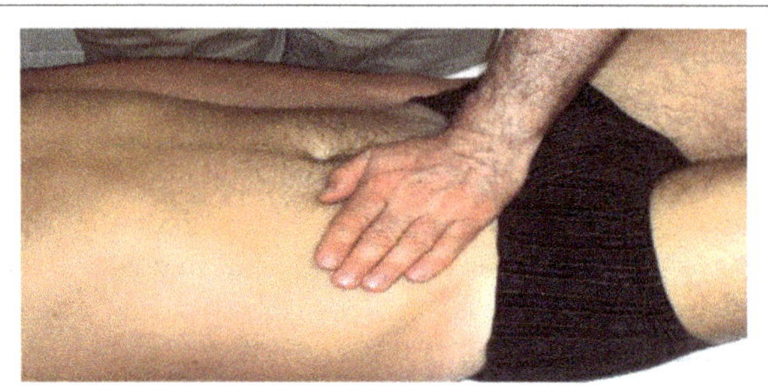
Fig. 1 Stage one, brushing on the abdomen skin

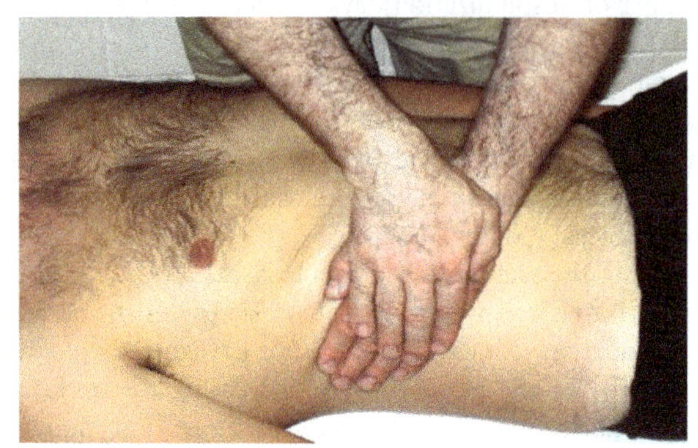
Fig. 2 Stage two, the dominant hand is placed on the abdominal skin and the other hand on it with appropriate presser, the skin drown

Patients hospitalized in intensive care unit were gavaged every 3 h according to the protocol, and the studied patients were fed in the same way. First, using a special 50 ml gavage syringe, 5 cc of air was quickly injected into the stomach, and using a stethoscope, the voice in the stomach was heard, and after confirmation of the insertion of the NG tube, first lavage was performed and the gastric volume residual was measured,

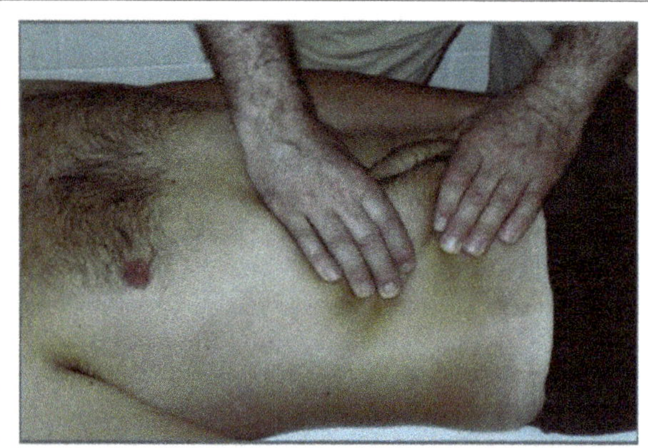
Fig. 3 Stage three, the abdominal skin shape is changed with rubbing

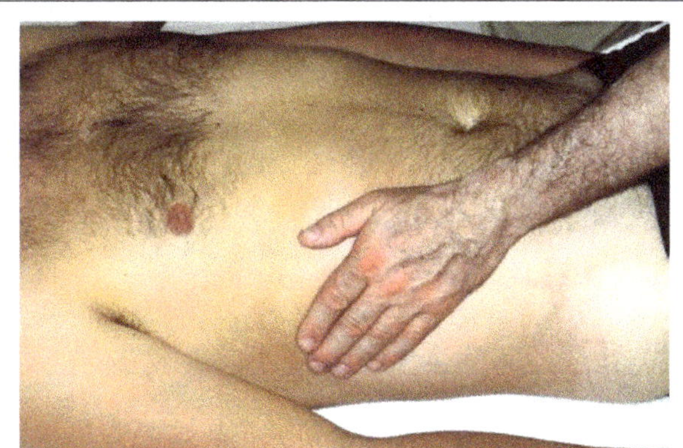

Fig. 4 Stage four, the shake movements in line with armpit from top to down and vice versa

and this amount was returned to the stomach with any amount it has, and a certain amount of food was gavaged into the stomach in such a way that the final volume in each patient should reach 300 cc.

Data collection from intervention group

After confirmation of the NG tube placement in the stomach, the lavage was performed, and the amount of gastric residual was measured and recorded, then this amount of lavaged food was returned to the stomach. In the next stage, abdominal massage was performed at 8 o'clock in the morning for 20 min, and after massage, the gavage was performed, and the gastric volume was increased to 300. After 2 h, the second stage of abdominal massage was performed, and finally, 1 h after the second massage, at 12 o'clock, the GRV was examined.

Data collection from the control group

After confirmation of the insertion of NG tube into the stomach, lavage was performed for each patient at 8 am, and the GRV was measured and recorded, then this amount of lavaged food was returned to the stomach, and eventually, the volume of food in the stomach was increased to 300 cc by gavage, and 3 h later, at 12 o'clock, the GRV was checked and recorded.

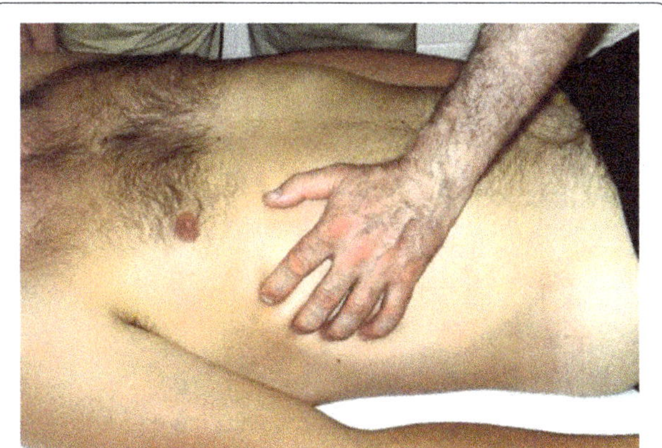

Fig. 5 Stage five, the fingers are placed between intercostal spaces and pulled appropriately

Ethical considerations

This study was registered in Iranian Registry of Clinical Trials, IRCT2017062134641N2. Also, the approval code from Ethics Committee of Kermanshah University of Medical Sciences was obtained, kums.rec.1396.31, and written informed consent was received from the individual accompanying the patient. The necessary assurance was given to the individual accompanying the patient and hospital officials about confidential information of patients and the anonymity right of them.

Data analysis

Data were analyzed by SPSS version 24 and descriptive and inferential tests. Descriptive statistics such as frequency, frequency percentage, mean and median, and standard deviation were used for this purpose. The demographic information of the two groups was investigated based on qualitative variables (sex, marital status, educational level, and occupation) using chi-square test. Wilcoxon test was used to compare the mean of the intended quantitative feature before and after the intervention in each of the two control and test groups (to compare changes within groups). The U Mann-Whitney test was used to compare the mean rank of the quantitative intended feature in the two control and test groups before and after the intervention (in order to compare the variations between the groups). Independent and paired t tests were used to compare the mean of the total GRV in both groups before and after intervention. The significance level of the tests was considered 0.05.

Results

In this study, 76 patients were recruited into the study, and among them, 16 (21%) were excluded because of death (3 patients), transfer to other hospital or ward (3 patients), NG tube extraction (3 patients), cardiopulmonary resuscitation (1 patient), discharge (2 patients), and change in feeding approach (4 patients). Thus, analysis was conducted onto 60 individuals (79%). Among the patients, 60% (36 patients) were male. The mean and standard deviation of age was 59.72 ± 16.02 years. The majority of the subjects in both groups were married (83.3%). Regarding the educational degree, most of the participants had diploma (30%), and the number of illiterate ones was less than the rest (8.3%). Regarding their occupation, most of them were unemployed (30%), and the number of those who were employed was less than the rest (8.3%). The intervention and control groups were similar in terms of demographic variables including gender, marital status, educational level, and employment status, and there was not any significant difference (p value < 0.05), and also, the two groups did not differ in terms of age (Table 1).

Comparing the mean of the total GRV before and after the intervention in both groups, the results showed that the mean of the total GRV before the intervention between the two groups was not statistically significant ($p < 0.05$). However, in comparison of the mean of the total GRV after the intervention in the case group (97.30 cc) was less than the control group (143.46 cc) (p value < 0.05, $t = 3.62$). In addition, the mean of GRV was not changed in case group before and after of intervention, significantly; however, it was increased in the control group ($p < 0.001$) (Table 2).

Comparing the GRV before intervention in the case and control groups in different days, the results showed that the mean gastric volume before intervention in the case and control groups in different days had no significant difference (Table 3), but the mean of the GRV after the intervention in the case and control group was significant in the different days, and it was less in the case group in all 3 days (p value < 0.05) (Table 4).

Discussion

The results of this study showed that tensegrity type of abdominal massage can have an important effect on the reduction of GRV in patients hospitalized in intensive care units who are fed through NG tube, as the total mean of GRV in all days was significantly less than the control group, and also, it was low in all days in the case group. Controlling and reducing the GRV could be an important measure for improving nutritional status and reducing complications in critically ill patients [19], and consequently decreasing the rate of malnutrition [20]. Also, this measure could reduce the rate of vomiting and abdominal distention and improve weight gain and defecation pattern [17]. In this regard, a study by Kahraman and Ozdemir [16] in Turkey, conducted on the effect of abdominal massage on the GRV of patients hospitalized in intensive care unit, showed that the GRV on the last day compared to the first day had a significant reduction, but there was an increase in GRV in the control group. The results of this study are in line with our study. In a randomized control trial study by Dehghan et al. [21] in Iran on 70 patients by the tracheal tube, there were no differences between the two groups in terms of gastric residual volume after abdominal massage intervention. The results are not in line with our study, which may be related to the difference in massage time (15 min). In another similar study conducted by Uysal et al. [9] in İzmir on patients with neurology and neurosurgery, the results showed that in the test group, GRV was increased two times, and in the control group, it was more than eight times. The results of this study showed that the increase in the GRV in the control group was more than that in the case group, and the results were in line with our study. Another study was conducted by

Table 1 Demographic characteristics of two groups based on the variables of sex, marital status, education, job, and age

Variables	Case *N* (%)	Control *N* (%)	Total *N* (%)	Statistical test
Sex				
Male	18 (60)	18 (60)	36 (60)	χ^2=0 $p = 0.604$
Female	12 (40)	12 (40)	24 (40)	
Marital status				
Single	5 (16.7)	5 (16.7)	10 (16.7)	χ^2=0 $p = 0.635$
Married	25 (83.3)	25 (83.3)	50 (83.3)	
Level of education				
Illiterate	3 (10)	2 (6.7)	5 (8.3)	χ^2=1.132 $p = 0.889$
Elementary	8 (26.7)	6 (20)	14 (23.3)	
Diploma	8 (26.7)	10 (33)	18 (30)	
Associate	6 (20)	5 (16.7)	11 (18.3)	
Bachelor	5 (16.7)	7 (23)	12 (20)	
Employment status				
Unemployed	7 (23.3)	11 (36.7)	18 (30)	N/A
Retired	7 (23.3)	5 (16.7)	12 (20)	
Housewife	8 (26.7)	4 (13.3)	12 (20)	
Employee	2 (6.7)	3 (10)	5 (8.3)	
Free job	6 (20)	7 (23.3)	13 (21.7)	
Age (mean and SD)	60.76 ± 17.38	58.66 ± 14.75	59.72 ± 16.02	$t = 0.508$ $p = 0.616$

N/A not applicable

Table 2 Comparison of the total average of GRV before and after intervention in both groups

Groups Time of GRV measurement	Case group Mean (SD) of GRV (cc)	Control group Mean (SD) of GRV (cc)	Statistical test
Before	106.76 (58.56)	108.63 (26.58)	$t = 0.159$ $p = 0.874$
After	97.30 (54.06)	143.46 (39.93)	$t = 3.62$* $p < 0.001$
Statistical test	$t = 0.964$ $p = 0.343$	$t = 4.70$ $p < 0.001$*	

*is significant

Table 3 Comparison of the average of GRV before intervention in the case and control groups in different days

Variables	Groups	Average rating	Statistical test
Average of GRV before intervention in first day	Case	29.03	$p = 0.514$ $Z = -0.562$
	Control	31.97	
Average of GRV before intervention in second day	Case	30.45	$p = 0.982$ $Z = -0.022$
	Control	30.55	
Average of GRV before intervention in third day	Case	29.02	$p = 0.509$ $Z = -0.660$
	Control	31.98	

Table 4 Comparison of the average of GRV after intervention in the case and control groups in different days

Variables	Groups	Average rating	Statistical test
Average of GRV after intervention in first day	Case	21.52	*$p < 0.001$ $Z = -3/994$
	Control	39.48	
Average of GRV after intervention in second day	Case	24.53	*$p = 0.008$ $Z = -2.651$
	Control	36.47	
Average of GRV after intervention in third day	Case	20.25	*$p < 0.001$ $Z = -4.563$
	Control	40.75	

*is significant

Warren [22] in America on the effect of abdominal massage on the GRV in patients connected to the ventilator system. The measurement results of the GRV in the first measurement, compared to the last one in the case group, showed a significant reduction in comparison to the control group, which is in line with the current research. In a study performed by Tekgündüz et al. [17] on premature infants, the results of the Wilcoxon test showed that the GRV in the case group, in the last day compared to the first day, had a significant decrease (*P* value< 0.05), but after comparing the experimental group with the control group in terms of the volume of residual stomach food, the results showed that there was no statistically significant difference. The results of other researches, such as the study by Uysal [23] on patients hospitalized in the neurosurgical department, represented the effect of abdominal massage on the gastric residual volume in patients hospitalized in intensive care units, which is in line with the present study.

Various studies shown that abdominal massage can play an important role in reducing the GRV, and it is through the stimulation mechanism of the peristaltic movements, intra-abdominal pressure changes, mechanical and reflexive effects on the intestines, shortening the food transition time in intestines, increased intestinal movements, and easier food flow through the digestive tract [9, 18]. Also, the effect of abdominal massage may be due to the parasympathetic stimulation that is followed by the stomach and intestine stimulation, and movements of digestive system increases, and this increase in activity leads to easier digestion of food in the stomach and its easier movement in the intestine. In a study on premature infants to show how massage leads to weight gain, the results of the study showed that abdominal massage increases the activity of vagus nerve and stomach movements [24]. In another study by McClurg et al. [25], which was conducted on a patient with multiple sclerosis, the results of the study showed that abdominal massage through the activation of parasympathetic divisions in the autonomic nervous system increased muscle movements in the intestine and increased digestive system secretions and relaxation of the sphincters of digestive tract, by affecting digestive system function, and had an important role in relieving constipation symptoms in these patients. Turan and Ast [26] also showed that abdominal massage by increasing peristalsis movements increases the intestinal movements, has a positive role in reducing constipation following surgery, and also increases the quality of life of postoperative patients.

Patients hospitalized in the intensive care unit connected to the ventilator, and also fed through the NG tube, due to aspiration of food following an increase in the GRV have pneumonia associated with ventilator. Regarding this, a study by Kahraman and Ozdemir [16] was conducted, and the results showed that pneumonia associated with ventilator in the group receiving abdominal massage was five times lower, although this result is not statistically significant compared to the control group, but abdominal massage can reduce the gastric residual volume and food regurgitation to esophagus, reduce the risk of aspirating this food into the lungs, and reduce the risk of pneumonia associated with mechanical ventilation in these patients [16]. Also, in another study by Le Blanc et al. [27] on patients undergoing colectomy with pain and ileus of the intestine, the results showed that the abdominal massage performed by a mechanical device also reduces the pain and also the duration of intestinal paralysis in these patients.

Limitations

In this study, the researcher had a little knowledge about abdominal massage. Therefore, for this limitation, he was trained by a sports medicine specialist to perform abdominal massage. Also, it was not possible to obtain satisfaction of the patient due to their unconsciousness. Therefore, for this limitation, the consent of the individual accompanying the patient was sought, in case of referring to the hospital. In addition, we did not take any other information about some variables such as surgical/medical status, main diagnosis, organ failures, severity scores, elective/emergency admission, and requirement of mechanical ventilation and vasopressors, which may affect GRV in intensive care patients.

Conclusion

The purpose of this study was to evaluate the effect of abdominal massage on the GRV in patients hospitalized in intensive care unit. The results of this study represented the effect of abdominal massage on reducing the gastric residual volume, so this procedure is recommended to be considered as a care method to improve nutrition status in patients hospitalized in these units.

Abbreviations

GRV: Gastric residual volume; SD: Standard deviation

Acknowledgements
This article is the result of a master's degree dissertation on critical care. Hereby, thanks and gratitude will be given to the officials and professors of the Nursing and Midwifery Faculty, the Chancellor of Technology and Information of Kermanshah University of Medical Sciences, and the officials of Fatemeh Zahra Hospital in Ahvaz, as well as the patients and individuals accompanying them helping the researcher in this study.

Funding
The study was funded by Kermanshah University of Medical Sciences.

Authors' contributions
FM, AA, NS, AS, and BH contributed in designing the study. FM collected the data. FM, AA, and NS analyzed the data. FM and AA wrote the final report and article, and all authors read and approved the paper. All authors read and approved the final manuscript.

Competing interests
The authors declare that they have no competing interests.

Author details
[1]Nursing and Midwifery School, Students Research Committee, Kermanshah University of Medical Sciences, Kermanshah, Iran. [2]Department of Sports Medicine and Rehabilitation, Imam Reza Hospital, Kermanshah University of Medical Sciences (KUMS), Kermanshah, Iran. [3]Department of Anesthesiology, Taleghani Hospital, Kermanshah University of Medical Sciences, Kermanshah, Iran. [4]Nursing and Midwifery school, Kermanshah university of medical sciences, Kermanshah, Iran.

References

1. Morphet J, Clarke AB, Bloomer MJ. Intensive care nurses' knowledge of enteral nutrition: a descriptive questionnaire. Intensive Crit Care Nurs. 2016;37:68–74.
2. Gupta B, Agrawal P, Soni KD, Yadav V, Dhakal R, Khurana S, et al. Enteral nutrition practices in the intensive care unit: understanding of nursing practices and perspectives. J Anaesthesiol Clin Pharmacol. 2012;28(1):41.
3. Pancorbo-Hidalgo PL, García-Fernandez FP, Ramírez-Pérez C. Complications associated with enteral nutrition by nasogastric tube in an internal medicine unit. J Clin Nurs. 2001;10(4):482–90.
4. Wilson S, Madisi NY, Bassily-Marcus A, Manasia A, Oropello J, Kohli-Seth R. Enteral nutrition administration in a surgical intensive care unit: achieving goals with better strategies. World J Crit Care Med. 2016;5(3):180–6.
5. McClave SA, Taylor BE, Martindale RG, Warren MM, Johnson DR, Braunschweig C, McCarthy MS, Davanos E, Rice TW, Cresci GA, Gervasio JM. Guidelines for the provision and assessment of nutrition support therapy in the adult critically ill patient: Society of Critical Care Medicine (SCCM) and American Society for Parenteral and Enteral Nutrition (ASPEN). J Parenter Enter Nutr. 2016;40(2):159–211.
6. Rezae J, Kadivarian H, Abdi A, Rezae M, Karimpour K, Rezae S. The effect of body position on gavage residual volume of gastric in intensive care units patients. Iran J Nurs. 2018;30(110):58–67.
7. Ros C, McNeill L, Bennett P. Review: nurses can improve patient nutrition in intensive care. J Clin Nurs. 2009;18(17):2406–15.
8. Elpern EH, Stutz L, Peterson S, Gurka DP, Skipper A. Outcomes associated with enteral tube feedings in a medical intensive care unit. Am J Crit Care. 2004;13(3):221–7.
9. Uysal N, Eser I, Akpinar H. The effect of abdominal massage on gastric residual volume: a randomized controlled trial. Gastroenterol Nurs. 2012; 35(2):117–23.
10. Zhang Z, Li Q, Jiang L, Xie B, Ji X, Lu J, et al. Effectiveness of enteral feeding protocol on clinical outcomes in critically ill patients: a study protocol for before-and-after design. Ann Transl Med. 2016;4(16):308.
11. Montejo J, Minambres E, Bordeje L, Mesejo A, Acosta J, Heras A, et al. Gastric residual volume during enteral nutrition in ICU patients: the REGANE study. Intensive Care Med. 2010;36(8):1386–93.
12. Deane A, Chapman M, Fraser R, Bryant L, Burgstad C, Nguyen Q. Mechanisms underlying feed intolerance in the critically ill: implications for treatment. 2007.
13. Nguyen NQ. Pharmacological therapy of feed intolerance in the critically ills. World J Gastrointest Pharmacol Therapeutics. 2014;5(3):148.
14. Mosquera C, Koutlas NJ, Lee KC, Strickland A, Vohra NA, Zervos EE, et al. Impact of malnutrition on gastrointestinal surgical patients. J Surg Res. 2016; 205(1):95–101.
15. Barker LA, Gout BS, Crowe TC. Hospital malnutrition: prevalence, identification and impact on patients and the healthcare system. Int J Environ Res Public Health. 2011;8(2):514–27.
16. Kahraman BB, Ozdemir L. The impact of abdominal massage administered to intubated and enterally fed patients on the development of ventilator-associated pneumonia: a randomized controlled study. Int J Nurs Stud. 2015;52(2):519–24.
17. Tekgündüz KŞ, Gürol A, Apay SE, Caner İ. Effect of abdomen massage for prevention of feeding intolerance in preterm infants. Ital J Pediatr. 2014;40(1):1.
18. Sinclair M. The use of abdominal massage to treat chronic constipation. J Bodyw Mov Ther. 2011;15(4):436–45.
19. Kozeniecki M, Pitts H, Patel JJ. Barriers and solutions to delivery of intensive care unit nutrition therapy. Nutr Clin Pract. 2018;33(1):8–15.
20. Heydari A, Zeydi AE. Is gastric residual volume monitoring in critically ill patients receiving mechanical ventilation an evidence-based practice? Indian journal of critical care medicine. 2014;18(4):259.
21. Dehghan M, Mehdipoor R, Ahmadinejad M. Does abdominal massage improve gastrointestinal functions of intensive care patients with an endotracheal tube?: a randomized clinical trial. Complement Ther Clin Pract. 2017;30:122–8.
22. Warren M. Abdominal massage may decrease gastric residual volumes and abdominal circumference in critically ill patients. Evid Based Nurs. 2016;19(3):76.
23. Uysal N. The effect of abdominal massage administered by caregivers on gastric complications occurring in patients intermittent enteral feeding–a randomized controlled trial. Eur J Integrative Med. 2017;10:75–81.
24. Lämås K, Lindholm L, Stenlund H, Engström B, Jacobsson C. Effects of abdominal massage in management of constipation—a randomized controlled trial. Int J Nurs Stud. 2009;46(6):759–67.
25. McClurg D, Hagen S, Hawkins S, Lowe-Strong A. Abdominal massage for the alleviation of constipation symptoms in people with multiple sclerosis: a randomized controlled feasibility study. Mult Scler J. 2011;17(2):223–33.
26. Turan N, Ast TA. The effect of abdominal massage on constipation and quality of life. Gastroenterol Nurs. 2016;39(1):48–59.
27. Le Blanc-Louvry I, Costaglioli B, Boulon C, Leroi A-M, Ducrotte P. Does mechanical massage of the abdominal wall after colectomy reduce postoperative pain and shorten the duration of ileus? Results of a randomized study. J Gastrointest Surg. 2002;6(1):43–9.

Permissions

All chapters in this book were first published in JIC, by BioMed Central; hereby published with permission under the Creative Commons Attribution License or equivalent. Every chapter published in this book has been scrutinized by our experts. Their significance has been extensively debated. The topics covered herein carry significant findings which will fuel the growth of the discipline. They may even be implemented as practical applications or may be referred to as a beginning point for another development.

The contributors of this book come from diverse backgrounds, making this book a truly international effort. This book will bring forth new frontiers with its revolutionizing research information and detailed analysis of the nascent developments around the world.

We would like to thank all the contributing authors for lending their expertise to make the book truly unique. They have played a crucial role in the development of this book. Without their invaluable contributions this book wouldn't have been possible. They have made vital efforts to compile up to date information on the varied aspects of this subject to make this book a valuable addition to the collection of many professionals and students.

This book was conceptualized with the vision of imparting up-to-date information and advanced data in this field. To ensure the same, a matchless editorial board was set up. Every individual on the board went through rigorous rounds of assessment to prove their worth. After which they invested a large part of their time researching and compiling the most relevant data for our readers.

The editorial board has been involved in producing this book since its inception. They have spent rigorous hours researching and exploring the diverse topics which have resulted in the successful publishing of this book. They have passed on their knowledge of decades through this book. To expedite this challenging task, the publisher supported the team at every step. A small team of assistant editors was also appointed to further simplify the editing procedure and attain best results for the readers.

Apart from the editorial board, the designing team has also invested a significant amount of their time in understanding the subject and creating the most relevant covers. They scrutinized every image to scout for the most suitable representation of the subject and create an appropriate cover for the book.

The publishing team has been an ardent support to the editorial, designing and production team. Their endless efforts to recruit the best for this project, has resulted in the accomplishment of this book. They are a veteran in the field of academics and their pool of knowledge is as vast as their experience in printing. Their expertise and guidance has proved useful at every step. Their uncompromising quality standards have made this book an exceptional effort. Their encouragement from time to time has been an inspiration for everyone.

The publisher and the editorial board hope that this book will prove to be a valuable piece of knowledge for researchers, students, practitioners and scholars across the globe.

List of Contributors

Toru Kameda
Department of Emergency Medicine, Red Cross Society Azumino Hospital, 5685 Toyoshina, Azumino, Nagano 399-8292, Japan

Nobuyuki Taniguchi
Department of Clinical Laboratory Medicine, Jichi Medical University, 3311-1, Yakushiji, Shimotsuke, Tochigi 329-0498, Japan

Sujay Samanta, Ratender Kumar Singh, Arvind K. Baronia, Banani Poddar, Afzal Azim and Mohan Gurjar
Department of Critical Care Medicine, Sanjay Gandhi Post Graduate Institute of Medical Sciences (SGPGIMS), Raebareli Road, Lucknow, Uttar Pradesh 226014, India

Shigeki Kushimoto, Daisuke Kudo and Yu Kawazoe
Division of Emergency and Critical Care Medicine, Tohoku University Graduate School of Medicine, Seiryo-machi 2-1, Aoba-ku, Sendai, Miyagi 980-8574, Japan
Department of Emergency and Critical Care Medicine, Tohoku University Hospital, Seiryo-machi 1-1, Aoba-ku, Sendai, Miyagi 980-8574, Japan

Alexander F. van der Sluijs, Margreeth B. Vroom and Dave A. Dongelmans
Department of Intensive Care Medicine, Academic Medical Center, Room C3-343, Meibergdreef 9, Amsterdam 1105 AZ, The Netherlands.

Eline R. van Slobbe-Bijlsma
Department of Intensive Care Medicine, Ter Gooi Ziekenhuizen, Hilversum, The Netherlands

Stephen E. Chick and Alexander P. J. Vlaar
INSEAD Healthcare Management Initiative, INSEAD, Fontainebleau, France

Kota Hoshino, Taisuke Kitamura, Yoshihiko Nakamura, Yuhei Irie, Norihiko Matsumoto, Yasumasa Kawano and Hiroyasu Ishikura
Department of Emergency and Critical Care Medicine, Faculty of Medicine, Fukuoka University, 7-45-1 Nanakuma, Jonan-ku, Fukuoka 814-0180, Japan

Shunsuke Taito
Division of Rehabilitation, Department of Clinical Practice and Support, Hiroshima University Hospital, 1-2-3, Kasumi, Minami-ku, Hiroshima 734-8551, Japan

Nobuaki Shime and Kohei Ota
Department of Emergency and Critical Care Medicine, Institute of Biomedical and Health Sciences, Hiroshima University, 1-2-3, Kasumi, Minami-ku, Hiroshima 734-8553, Japan

Hideto Yasuda
Department of Intensive Care Medicine, Kameda Medical Center, 929, Higashi-cho, Kamogawa, Chiba 296-8602, Japan

Michael P. Catalino and Nathan Davis
Department of Neurosurgery, University of North Carolina School of Medicine, 170 Manning Drive, Campus Chapel Hill, NC 27599-7025, USA

Feng-Chang Lin
Department of Biostatistics, Gillings School of Global Public Health, Chapel Hill, NC, USA

Keith Anderson
School of Medicine, University of North Carolina School of Medicine, Chapel Hill, NC, USA

Casey Olm-Shipman and J. Dedrick Jordan
Department of Neurology, University of North Carolina, 170 Manning Drive, Campus Chapel Hill, NC, USA

Lukas Buendgens, Jan Bruensing, Ulf Herbers, Christer Baeck, Christian Trautwein, Alexander Koch and Frank Tacke
Department of Medicine III, RWTH-University Hospital Aachen, Pauwelsstrasse 30, 52074 Aachen, Germany

Eray Yagmur
Medical Care Center, Dr. Stein and Colleagues, 41061 Mönchengladbach, Germany

Shunji Kasaoka
Department of Emergency and General Medicine, Kumamoto University Hospital, 1-1-1 Honjo, Chuo-ku, Kumamoto 860-8556, Japan

Yasumitsu Mizobata
Department of Traumatology and Critical Care Medicine, Graduate School of Medicine, Osaka City University, 1-4-3 Asahimachi, Abeno-ku, Osaka City, Osaka 545-8585, Japan

Ka Leung Mok
Accident and Emergency Department, Ruttonjee Hospital, 266 Queen's Road East, Wanchai, Hong Kong SAR

Kwok M. Ho and Yusrah Harahsheh
Department of Intensive Care Medicine, Royal Perth Hospital, 4th Floor, North Block, Wellington Street, Perth, Western Australia 6000, Australia

Kwok M. Ho
School of Population and Global Health, University of Western Australia, Perth, Western Australia, Australia

Yusrah Harahsheh
School of Medicine and Pharmacology, University of Western Australia, Perth, Western Australia, Australia

Kwok M. Ho
School of Veterinary and Life Sciences, Murdoch University, Perth, Western Australia, Australia

Yuichiro Sakamoto, Hiroyuki Koami and Toru Miike
Department of Emergency and Critical Care Medicine, Faculty of Medicine, Saga University, 5-1-1 Nabeshima, Saga City, Saga 849-8501, Japan

Francis Chun Yue Lee
Acute and Emergency Care Centre, Khoo Teck Puat Hospital, Singapore, Singapore
Yong Loo Lin School of Medicine, National University of Singapore, Singapore, Singapore

Ashitha L. Vijayan, Vanimaya, Shilpa Ravindran, R. Saikant, S. Lakshmi, R. Kartik and Manoj. G
Diagnostic Products Division, Corporate R&D Centre, HLL Lifecare Limited, Akkulam, Sreekariyam (P.O), Trivandrum, Kerala, India

Anton Krige and Martin Bland
Department of Anaesthesia and Critical Care, Royal Blackburn Hospital, Haslingden Road, Blackburn, UK

Thomas Fanshawe
Nuffield Department of Primary Care Health Sciences, University of Oxford, Oxford, UK

Takahiro Nakashima and Yoshio Tahara
Department of Cardiovascular Medicine, National Cerebral and Cardiovascular Center, 5-7-1 Fujishirodai, Suita 565-8565, Japan

Christopher Duplessis, Michael Gregory, Kenneth Frey, Matthew Bell, Luu Truong, Kevin Schully, James Lawler and Danielle Clark
Biological Defense Research Directorate, Naval Medical Research Center, 503 Robert Grant Avenue, Silver Spring, MD 20910, USA

Raymond J. Langley
Department of Pharmacology and Center for Lung Biology, University of South Alabama College of Medicine, Mobile, USA

Stephen F. Kingsmore
Rady Pediatric Genomic and Systems Medicine Institute, Rady Children's Hospital, Encinitas, USA

Christopher W. Woods and Ephraim L. Tsalik
Division of Infectious Diseases and International Health, Department of Medicine, Duke University School of Medicine, Durham, USA
Center for Applied Genomics and Precision Medicine, Department of Medicine, Duke University School of Medicine, Durham, USA

Christopher W. Woods
Section on Infectious Diseases, Durham Veteran's Affairs Medical Center, Durham, USA

Emanuel P. Rivers and Anja K. Jaehne
Department of Emergency Medicine, Henry Ford Hospital, Wayne State University, Detroit, USA

Eugenia B. Quackenbush
Department of Emergency Medicine, University of North Carolina Health Care, Chapel Hill, USA

Ephraim L. Tsalik
Emergency Medicine Service, Durham Veteran's Affairs Medical Center, Durham, USA

Hadrien Winiszewski, François Aptel, François Belon, Nicolas Belin, Claire Chaignat, Cyrille Patry, Cecilia Clermont, Elise David, Jean-Christophe Navellou, Guylaine Labro, Gaël Piton and Gilles Capellier
Medical Intensive Care Unit, Besançon, France

Hadrien Winiszewski
Service de Réanimation Médicale, CHU de Besançon, 25030 Besançon, France

Gilles Capellier
Department of Epidemiology and Preventive Medicine, School of Public Health and
Preventive Medicine, Faculty of Medicine, Nursing and Health Sciences, Clayton, Australia

Gaël Piton and Gilles Capellier
Research Unit EA 3920 and SFR FED 4234, University of Franche Comté, Besançon, France

Takayuki Ogura and Daisuke Kobashi
Department of Emergency Medicine and Critical Care Medicine, Japan RedCross Maebashi Hospital, Asahi-cho 3-21-36, Maebashi, Gunma 371-0014, Japan

Yoshihiko Nakamura
Department of Emergency and Critical Care Medicine, Faculty of Medicine, Fukuoka University, Fukuoka, Japan

Kunihiko Takahashi, Kazuki Nishida and Shigeyuki Matsui
Department of Biostatistics, Nagoya University Graduate School of Medicine, Nagoya, Japan

Weerachai Chaijamorn and Taniya Charoensareerat
Faculty of Pharmacy, Siam University, 38 Petkasem Road, Bangwa, Pasicharoen, Bangkok 10160, Thailand

Nattachai Srisawat
Division of Nephrology, Department of Medicine, Faculty of Medicine, Chulalongkorn University, and King Chulalongkorn Memorial Hospital, Bangkok, Thailand

Sutthiporn Pattharachayakul
Department of Clinical Pharmacy, Faculty of Pharmaceutical Sciences, Prince of Songkla University, Songkhla, Thailand

Apinya Boonpeng
School of Pharmaceutical Sciences, University of Phayao, Phayao, Thailand

Mitsuaki Nishikimi, Kenji Fukaya and Naoyuki Matsuda
Department of Emergency and Critical Care, Nagoya University Graduate School of Medicine, Tsurumai-cho 64, Syowa-ku, Nagoya, Aichi 466-8560, Japan

Takayuki Ogura, Keibun Liu and Mitsunobu Nakamura
Advanced Medical Emergency Department and Critical Care Center, Japan Red Cross Maebashi Hospital, Maebashi, Japan

Kota Matsui, Kunihiko Takahashi and Shigeyuki Matsui
Department of Biostatistics, Nagoya University Graduate School of Medicine, Nagoya, Japan

Hideo Morita
Department of Diagnostic Radiology, Japan Red Cross Maebashi Hospital, Maebashi, Japan

Andrea Cortegiani, Giovanni Misseri and Antonino Giarratano
Department of Surgical, Oncological and Oral Science (Di.Chir.On.S.). Section of Anesthesia, Analgesia, Intensive Care and Emergency. Policlinico Paolo Giaccone. University of Palermo, Italy, University of Palermo, Via del vespro 129, 90127 Palermo, Italy

Teresa Fasciana and Anna Giammanco
Department of Sciences for Health Promotion and Mother and Child Care, University of Palermo, Palermo, Italy

Anuradha Chowdhary
Department of Medical Mycology, Vallabhbhai Patel Chest Institute, University of Delhi,
Delhi, India

Shinshu Katayama, Ken Tonai, Yuya Goto, Kansuke Koyama, Toshitaka Koinuma, Jun Shima, Masahiko Wada and Shin Nunomiya
Division of Intensive Care, Department of Anesthesiology and Intensive Care Medicine, Jichi Medical University School of Medicine, 3311-1, Yakushiji, Shimotsuke, Tochigi 329-0498, Japan

Rafael Fernandez, Silvia Cano, Ignacio Catalan, Olga Rubio, Carles Subira, Jaume Masclans, Gina Rognoni, Lara Ventura, Caroline Macharete, Len Winfield and Josep M[a]. Alcoverro
Intensive Care Department, Hospital Sant Joan de Deu – Fundacio Althaia, Dr. Joan Soler 1, 08243 Manresa, Spain
Universitat Internacional dec Catalunya, Barcelona, Spain
CIBERES, Madrid, Spain

Farzad Momenfar and Alireza Abdi
Nursing and Midwifery School, Students Research Committee, Kermanshah University of Medical Sciences, Kermanshah, Iran

Ali Soroush
Department of Sports Medicine and Rehabilitation, Imam Reza Hospital, Kermanshah University of Medical Sciences (KUMS), Kermanshah, Iran

Behzad Hemmatpour
Department of Anesthesiology, Taleghani Hospital, Kermanshah University of Medical Sciences, Kermanshah, Iran

Alireza Abdi and Nader Salari
Nursing and Midwifery school, Kermanshah university of medical sciences, Kermanshah, Iran

Index

A
A-lines, 117, 119-120, 122
Abdominal Massage, 228-234
Abdominal Ultrasound, 1
Acs, 106, 111, 146-153
Acute Kidney Injury, 2, 7-8, 94, 98, 105, 185-186, 194-195, 227
Acute Myocardial Infarction, 67-68, 70, 81, 95, 153-155
Acute Respiratory Distress Syndrome, 42, 47-48, 62, 65-66, 77, 117, 125, 128-129, 167, 173-174, 182-183
Acute Traumatic Coagulopathy, 19-22, 24, 72-73, 78, 115-116
Antibiotic Therapy, 130, 133-134, 136
Antifungal Resistance, 202-203, 209, 211
Antimicrobial Resistance, 202
Arrhythmia, 46, 67, 140

B
B-lines, 117, 120-122, 125-128
Biomarker, 36, 40, 58-59, 63, 65, 130-136, 153, 156-157, 160-165
Brain Ct Scan, 196

C
C-terminal Proendothelin-1, 58, 60, 64-65
C. Auris, 202-212
Candidemia, 202, 204-206, 208-209, 212-213
Cardiac Arrest, 25, 68-71, 90, 93, 95-96, 146, 148, 151-152, 154-155, 196-197, 199-201, 223, 227
Cardiac Output Monitoring, 137
Cardiovascular Disease, 67, 70
Cardiovascular Intensive Care, 67-71
Cefepime, 185-195
Cell-free Dna, 156-157, 164-166
Chronic Obstructive Pulmonary Disease, 117, 148, 167, 169, 173-174
Continuous Renal Replacement Therapy, 36-37, 185-186, 194-195, 227
Coronary Care Unit, 67-68, 70-71
Critical Care, 1, 6-7, 10, 19, 24, 26-28, 32-34, 40-42, 47, 71-72, 81, 95, 97, 105-106, 117, 137-138, 143, 165, 167, 175, 183, 196-197, 200, 202, 215, 226-227, 234
Critical Illness, 10, 47-48, 58, 61, 64-66, 80, 222, 227, 235, 243
Critically Ill Patients, 2, 8, 15, 17-18, 26-30, 32-33, 41, 43, 47-48, 50, 57-63, 65-66, 69, 78, 95, 97-99, 105, 116, 132, 135, 144-145, 171, 183, 185-188, 202, 211, 222, 225, 227, 232
Ct-proet-1, 58-65
Curtain Sign, 117-119, 121, 123-124, 126, 129

D
Damage Control Resuscitation, 24-25, 72-73, 78-80
Damage Control Surgery, 21, 23, 25, 72, 80, 115
Decompression, 49, 51, 55-57
Diagnostic Marker, 130, 136
Diaphragm Thickening Fraction, 10, 15-17
Diaphragm Ultrasound, 10-11, 17-18
Disseminated Intravascular Coagulation, 19-20, 22, 24-25, 34, 37, 39-41, 78, 115, 175-176, 179, 181, 183
Dosing, 185-195

E
Echocardiography, 65, 68, 81-86, 89, 92, 95-97, 138, 143-144, 147-148
Edwards Vigileo Flotrac Monitoring, 137
Emergency Department, 2, 5, 8, 19, 40, 81, 85, 94-97, 108, 133, 136, 144, 146, 152-153, 196, 200
Exacerbation, 127-129, 167-169, 174, 239
Extracorporeal Co2 Removal, 167, 173-174

F
Fibrinolysis, 20-21, 23-25, 34-40, 73, 75, 77, 79, 90, 108-109, 111, 115-116, 149-150, 152, 154, 164-165
Fluid Responsiveness, 82, 85, 88, 96, 137-138, 141-144

G
Glycerol, 215-221

H
Hemorrhagic Stroke, 49
Hyperlactatemia, 215-216, 218-219, 221

I
I-lines, 117, 120, 126, 128
Icu, 8, 10-14, 16-17, 26-35, 42-65, 69-70, 72-73, 77-78, 93, 95, 98, 100, 105, 130, 132-134, 136, 143-144, 156, 162-164, 167-170, 175-183, 192-193, 195-198, 200, 206-207, 211-212, 222-227, 234
Intensive Care Department, 26-27, 32
Intensivist, 11, 27-29, 32-33, 48, 56, 175-176, 183, 223
Invasive Fungal Infection, 202-203
Ischemic Stroke, 49, 53, 57

L
Lung Ultrasound, 97, 117, 121, 125, 128-129

M
Mannitol, 215-221
Massive Transfusion Protocol, 21, 72, 76, 78-79
Mechanically Ventilated Patients, 18, 42-43, 47-48
Mortality Prediction, 156-157, 161, 163, 222, 226

N

Neurological Prognosis, 196

Nstemi, 146, 149, 152

Nucleosomes, 156-165

P

Passive Leg Raising, 137-138, 144

Pathogen-associated Molecular Patterns, 34, 37

Pci, 68, 70, 146-147, 149-152, 154

Pharmacodynamics, 185, 195, 214

Pharmacokinetics, 185-186, 188, 194-195, 214

Point-of-care Ultrasound, 1, 81, 90, 93, 95-97

Post-cardiac Arrest Syndrome, 69, 196, 200

Procalcitonin, 34, 38, 41, 61, 66, 130-133, 135-136, 156-157, 159, 161, 163-166, 227

R

Rehabilitation, 42-48, 53-54, 168, 234

S

Sepsis Diagnosis, 34, 136

Sepsis Prognostication, 156-157

Sepsis-3, 34-36, 39, 41, 66, 95, 159, 183, 215, 221

Septic Shock, 8, 37, 41, 59, 63, 65-66, 81, 90, 95-96, 130, 132-135, 137, 139-140, 143-145, 156, 159-162, 165-166, 170, 175-176, 179, 183-184, 186, 195, 215, 221, 225, 227

Severe Sepsis, 41, 65-66, 130, 132-136, 144-145, 156, 159-163, 165-166, 183-184, 227

Six Sigma, 26, 33

Stemi, 146-150, 152-154

T

Targeted Temperature, 68-71, 196-197, 199

Total Quality Management, 26, 30, 32

Tracheostomy Timing, 49-51, 57

Trauma-induced Coagulopathy, 19-21, 23-24, 72, 78

V

Vasoplegic Shock, 137

Venous Thromboembolism, 20, 98, 105

Ventilator-associated Pneumonia, 49-50, 53, 56-57

Z

Z-lines, 117, 120, 122